NurseThink® for Students

NCLEX-PN®
Conceptual Review Guide

Clinical-Based for Next Gen Learning

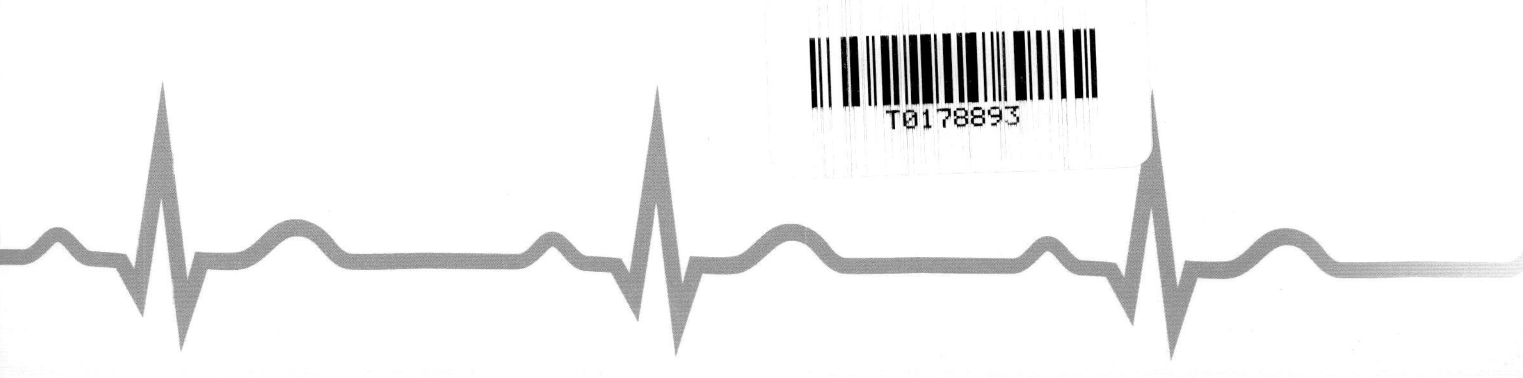

Judith W. Herrman
PhD, RN, CNE, ANEF, FAAN

Stephanie Terry
PhD, RN, CNE

Amy Austin
EdD, MSN, RN

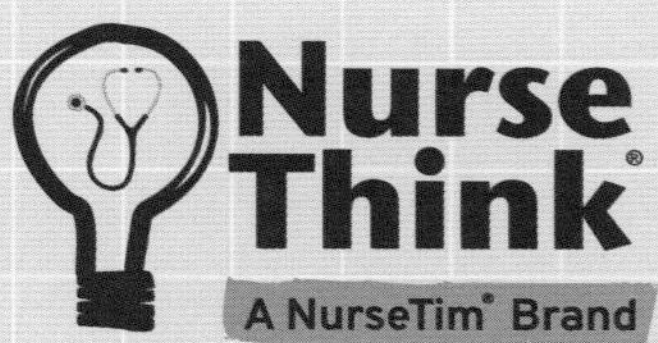

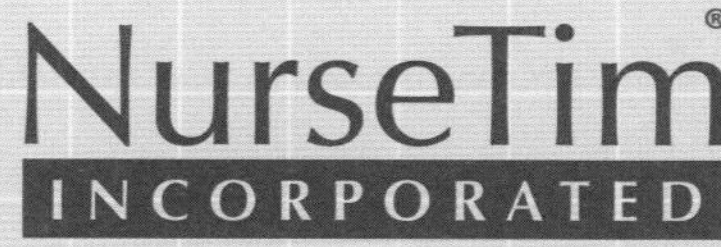

Follow Us On Social Media @NurseThink / NurseThink.com / help@nursethink.com

Executive Editor: Tim Bristol
NurseThink® Manager: Rebecca Synoground
Design Account Director: Cory Dammann
Design, Layout, & Production: Shayla Johnson
Photography: © Shutterstock

Published by NurseTim, Inc., PO Box 505, Victoria, MN 55386

Additional copies of this publication are available at www.NurseThink.com.

ISBN: 978-1-7364762-1-5

eBook ISBN: 978-1-7364762-2-2

Printed in the United States of America

First Edition

Brief Contents

Table of Contents

CH 8: Homeostasis 129

CH 9: Respiration 155

CH 10: Regulation 183

CH 11: Nutrition 213

CH 12: Hormonal 255

CH 13: Movement 287

CH 14: Comfort 337

Table of Contents

SECTION 2
Priority Exemplars

SECTION 3
Closing

NURSETHINK® FOCUSED

Specialties

Children's Health

Mental Health

Women's Health

NURSETHINK® FOCUSED

NCLEX-PN® Client Needs

Priority Exemplars that emphasize different parts of the NCLEX-PN®.

Pharmacological and Parenteral

Reduction of Risk Potential

Physiological Adaptation

About the Authors

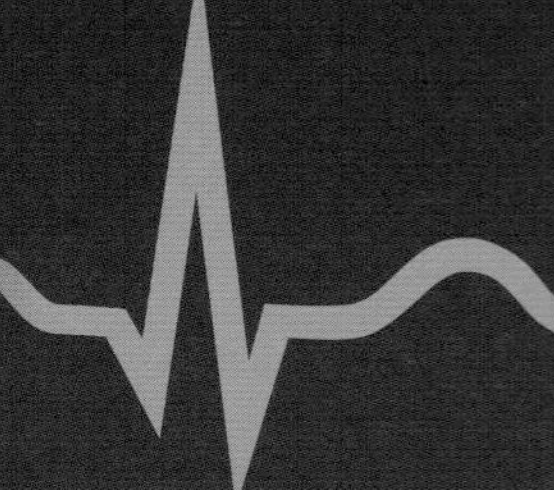

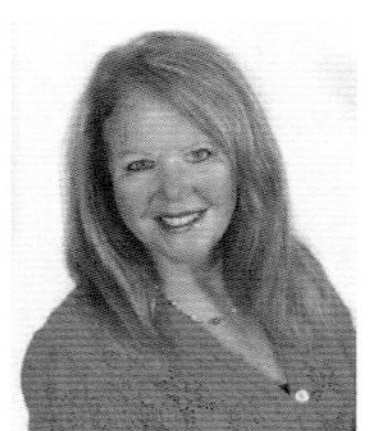

Dr. Judith W. Herrman is a nurse, educator, and researcher with a passion for learning and teaching. Judy's experiences in and love for nursing education provide context for work in creative teaching strategies, curriculum development, evaluation and test development, building positive workplaces, preparing for NCLEX®, and applying the principles of brain science to clinical decision-making. Judy's research interests include healthy decision-making across the lifespan, enhancing sexual health and promoting access to sexual education and healthcare, and advocacy for marginalized populations, especially children with health issues, young parents, and vulnerable youth. Judy has published widely and is excited that the team's hard work on these resources may help students join the great profession of nursing!

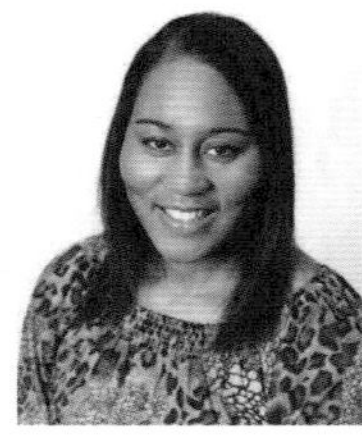

Dr. Stephanie Terry is a nurse educator with over 20 years of nursing and nursing education experience, teaching and serving as an educational leader at the PN, ADN, BSN, and graduate levels of nursing. Her areas of expertise focus on leadership, mentoring nursing faculty, and instructional development, emphasizing clinical judgment, active learning, retention, and student success. Because of her love for mentoring faculty, she has published several articles on this topic. Dr. Terry is passionate about nursing and nursing education and assisting faculty and students around the country in the development of well-trained nurses to provide quality and safe, effective care to clients.

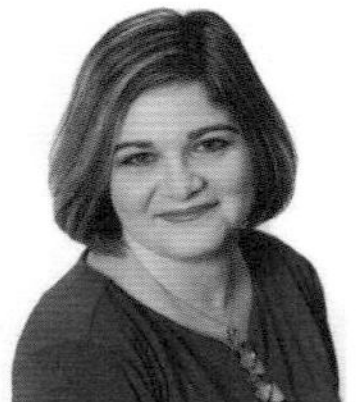

Dr. Amy Austin is a Nurse Educator from Texas, in the greater Houston area. She has worked in nursing education for over a decade with experience at both the Vocational Nursing and Associate Degree level. She has served on numerous college committees, including the accreditation review team, technology task force, and nursing curriculum committee. Dr. Austin specializes in the integration of technology and virtual simulation into nursing programs. She is passionate about bringing technology into the classroom and helping faculty incorporate technology into their curricula.

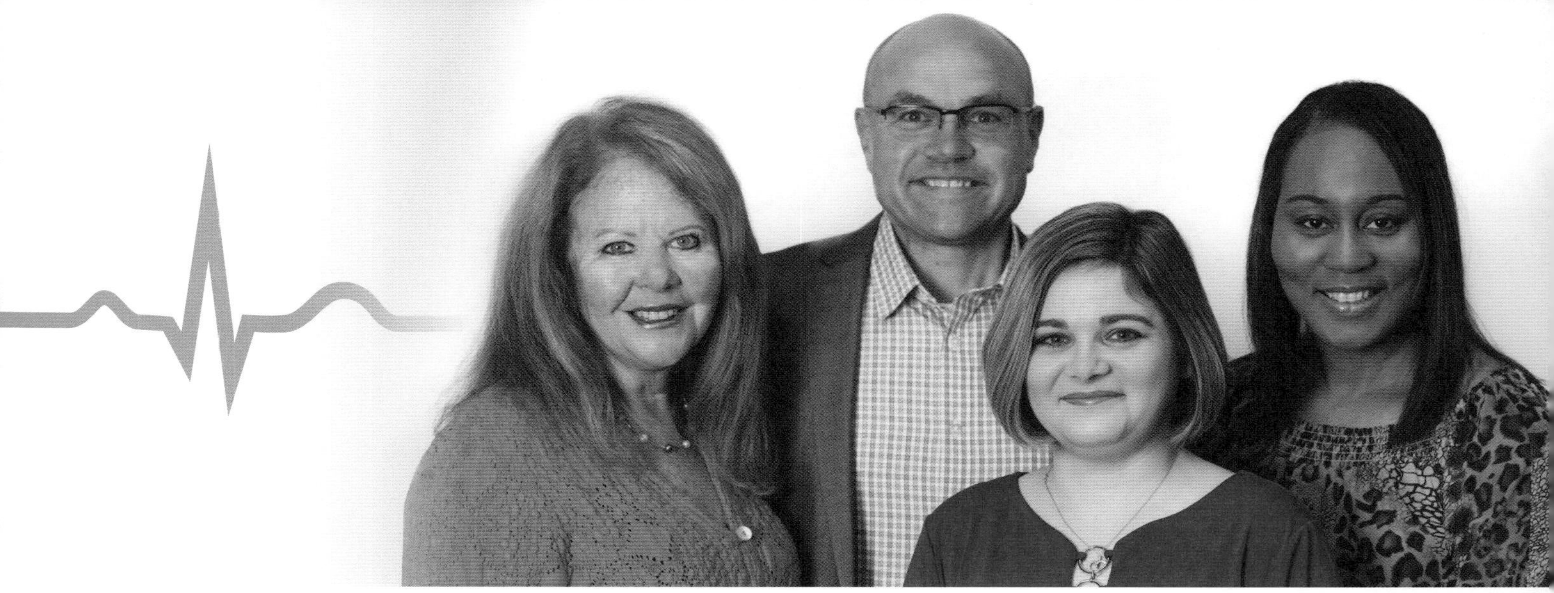

Acknowledgements

I would like to extend my sincere thanks to the entire NurseThink® team, especially Tim, Stephanie, Amy, Anne, and Rebecca, as we embarked upon and completed another great project to add to the NurseThink® tools. I would also like to extend my appreciation to my husband Dan who continues to support me along the way and my amazing family who inspire me to grow and learn. As we watch our eight children develop and navigate the world, the need for educated and thinking nurses becomes apparent and critical for all. I am blessed to be part of this process.

- Judith W. Herrman, PhD, RN, CNE, ANEF, FAAN

I want to thank Judy and Amy for co-authoring this book with me, and Tim Bristol for giving me the opportunity to do so. To the entire NurseTim, Inc., team (too many to name), you are appreciated for your endless contribution to this wonderful product. To all the many contributors and reviewers, thank you for lending your time and expertise in making this happen. And to my family, thank you for your support in all of my endeavors, big or small, and for giving me the room to grow and discover all I can be.

- Stephanie Terry, PhD, RN, CNE

First, I would like to thank John, my husband, for his love and support. I want to thank my two amazing boys; your hugs and smiles are my greatest joy. I would like to think the entire NurseThink team. I could not ask for a better team to work with. It was an honor to work with my co-authors, Judy and Stephanie, and I cannot thank you both enough for all that you did. Thank you to everyone who helped to make this book happen, including the outstanding group of reviewers. We could not have done this without you.

- Amy Austin, EdD, MSN, RN

Letter From the Authors

The profession of nursing is such a rich conundrum, it is both complex but bears its firm foundation on the basics; rooted in science yet truly also practiced as an art; and requiring of deft psychomotor skills yet inherently grounded in thinking and thoughtful practice. Nursing is both difficult and intuitive; focused on the ill yet aiming to prevent illness and trauma; it requires busyness and hard work yet must also be patient and foster peace; and the profession is so rewarding yet sometimes challenging. As you embark on the career of nursing, I hope you embrace all these aspects and that this text offers you a clear path to NCLEX® success. We wish you well!

- Judith W. Herrman, PhD, RN, CNE, ANEF, FAAN

Nursing is about caring, compassion, and providing safe care to your clients. Nursing is a profession that is well respected and life-changing. The day you decided you wanted to be a nurse and made the first step by enrolling in a nursing program, your life was impacted in many ways and now you have the opportunity to impact the lives of others by the nursing care you provide. This book is written to help you on the journey to become safe and resilient nurses. From the Clinical Case Studies to the NextGen Clinical Judgment exercises and quizzes, you will find a rich array of learning activities to help guide you to the fundamental goal of using Clinical Judgment to care for all clients. May you find this book as rewarding as we did writing it.

- Stephanie Terry, PhD, RN, CNE

By pursuing a nursing career, you are joining one of the most trusted professions. As nurses, we have the ability to make positive impacts for our clients, their families, and even the community we serve. Becoming a quality nurse takes hard work and dedication, but you have tools that can help you along the way. We hope that the Go to Clinical cases, Priority Exemplars, and the NurseThink® quizzes help you to develop clinical judgment. Being a nurse is truly an honor and I am so glad you decided to join us.

- Amy Austin, EdD, MSN, RN

Reviewers and Contributors

Emerald Bilbrew, DNP, MSN, BSN, RN, CMSRN
Course Lead, ADN Nursing Instructor
Fayetteville Technical Community College
Fayetteville, NC

Melvina Brandau, PhD, RN
Assistant Professor
Ohio University

Anne Liners Brett, PhD, RN
Consultation Manager
NurseTim, Inc
Germantown, WI

Kristofer Bristol, BSN, RN
Student Success Specialist
NurseTim, Inc.
Minneapolis, MN

Tim Bristol, PhD, RN, CNE, ANEF, FAADN
Faculty Development, Owner
NurseTim, Inc
Victoria, MN

Sheila Chery, RN, BSN
Exam Support Specialist
NurseTim, Inc.
Rock Hill, SC

Kerry DeGroot, RN, MSN
Nursing Instructor
Moraine Park Technical College
West Bend, WI

Debi Erick, MSN, PHN, RN, CNE
Dean of Nursing
Bryant & Stratton College
North Chesterfield, VA

Kimberley Floyd, MSN-Ed, BSN, RN, CCM
Execuive Director of Nursing
Advanced College
South Gate, CA

Colleen M Gordon, MSN/Ed, RN, CNE, CMSRN
Academic Program Coordinator
Fayetteville Technical Community College
Fayetteville, NC

Sandra McCrary-Marshal, RN, MSN
Department Chair, Professor
Austin Community College
Austin, TX

Karin J Sherrill, RN, MSN, CNE, ANEF, FAADN
Faculty Educator, Nursing Education Consultant
Maricopa Community Colleges at Gateway Community College
Phoenix, AZ

Jonette I Talbott, RN,BSN,MSN,FNP-C
Retired, Professor and Director of Practical Nursing
Southside Virginia Community College
Nathalie, VA

Melinda Terry, RN, BSN, MBA-NM
Case Manager
Veterans Health Administration
Emporia, VA

SECTION 1

Introduction

CHAPTER

1

Save Time Studying

Focus on Clinical

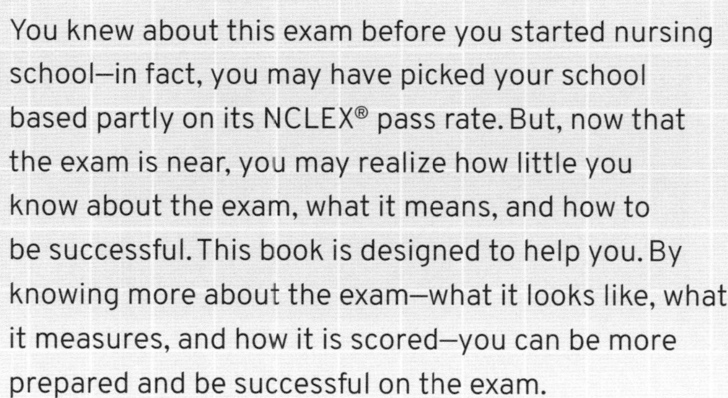

You knew about this exam before you started nursing school—in fact, you may have picked your school based partly on its NCLEX® pass rate. But, now that the exam is near, you may realize how little you know about the exam, what it means, and how to be successful. This book is designed to help you. By knowing more about the exam—what it looks like, what it measures, and how it is scored—you can be more prepared and be successful on the exam.

You've been successful in nursing school and you have used your thinking skills to help you achieve that success! You learned early on that multiple-choice questions in nursing often have four right answers—and you needed to choose the highest priority or the best answer! That is your clinical judgment skills at work! While you were in nursing school you learned NurseThink® and how to process information to perform well on tests AND in the clinical area.

The NCLEX-PN® is all about clinical judgment and that is why NurseThink® is clinically-based. In some states PN stands for Practical Nurse. Other states use the term PN and VN to indicate Licensed Vocational Nurses. These candidates all take the NCLEX-PN® examination. Some of you completed a nursing program based on concepts (perfusion, oxygenation, comfort, homeostasis, etc.). Others learned based on units or medical models. Nonetheless, you learned about concepts in caring for clients clinically.

Experienced nurses, when walking into a client's room, may be aware of the client's medical diagnosis. However, the nurse should provide high-level care based on priority needs of the client. For example, the nurse considers: How is the client oxygenating? What about the client's perfusion? How about the client's pain level? What do the client's vital signs and laboratory data tell us about the client's homeostasis?

Remember, the NCLEX-PN® does not test what you know, it tests how you think.

As you answer questions, consider the concepts in the item—how would a nurse provide care for the client in the question? This book provides **Priority Exemplars** to assist you in building your clinical judgment skills. Simultaneously, this book offers several tools and resources to help you succeed on NCLEX-PN®.

NurseThink® *THIN Thinking*

THIN Thinking is a unique clinical judgment strategy from NurseThink®. *THIN Thinking* allows for processing of the information essential to providing high-level and complex client care. This method promotes higher-order mental processing, rather than memorization. On the exam, candidates often select an answer based on recognition of material rather than analyzing an item for priority client needs. *THIN Thinking* encourages the candidate to read the question and focus on the client.

The candidate will apply the **"THIN"** mnemonic to guide their decision towards the highest priority answer. This strategy is especially valuable when confused by a question or stuck between two answers. To implement *THIN Thinking*, consider this process:

T: TOP THREE

What are the three priority needs, concepts, questions, components, or elements noted in this question? Ask yourself: What is this question addressing? What are the top three needs?" This is where to apply **Prioritization Power**! Consider these prioritization options.

- **Maslow's Hierarchy of Needs:** This is a theory that places basic physiological needs as a higher priority than self-esteem needs. A greater challenge occurs when comparing the priority of safety to physiological needs. For example, if a client is not breathing, that is the priority. But, if the client is not breathing from a car accident and the car is on fire, moving the client to a safe environment should occur before addressing the fact that they are not breathing (making safety a higher priority).
- **ABC's:** This is everyone's favorite. Is there a time when circulation is a higher priority than airway or breathing? Yes, consider a client with diabetic ketoacidosis with a respiratory rate of 28 breaths per minute. Although alarming, this is a good thing as it indicates that they are attempting to compensate for the metabolic acidosis from the ketotic state. In this case, airway and breathing are not a problem, move on to circulation.
- **Actual versus Potential:** In most cases an actual problem will take precedence over a potential problem, unless the actual problem offers low risk, while the potential problem offers a high-risk for safety or injury. For example, an alert client may have an actual problem of vomiting, but the client who is nauseated, in c-spine precautions is a higher priority, since if they begin vomiting there are concerns of airway safety and spinal injuries.
- **Acute versus Chronic:** Acute will be the higher priority. An example would be the client suffering from chronic obstructive pulmonary disease being managed with medication and oxygen. This client is considered chronic until there is evidence of respiratory distress (respiratory rate, ABGs, pulse ox, etc.) at which time the client becomes acute (shows change in their baseline condition).

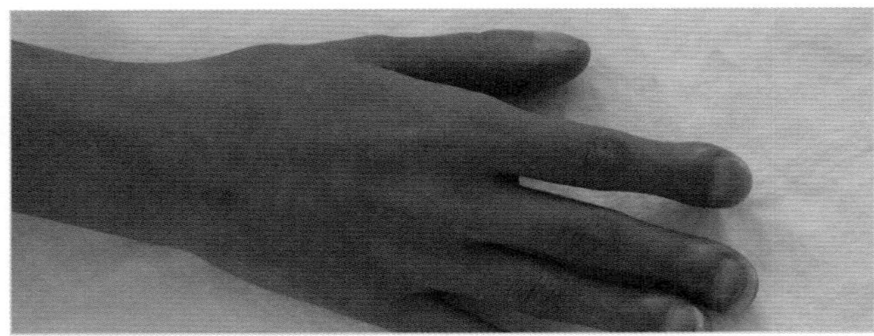

Image 1-1: Is clubbing of the fingers indicative of an acute or chronic health issues? What types of health disorders lead to clubbing? Why does clubbing occur?

- **Least Invasive First:** It is important for the nurse to consider less invasive options before increasing the client risk of injury with an invasive option. For example, standing a male client at the bedside every two hours to use a urinal is a better option than applying protective briefs. Applying protective briefs is a better option than applying a condom catheter. Applying a condom catheter is a better option than placing an indwelling catheter.

- **Safe Practice:** Safety concerns may include evaluation of the risk for falls, prevention of injury when performing a skill, reduction of risk for hospital-acquired infections (HAI), and more.

H: HELP QUICK

What can the nurse do quickly to relieve the problem? What strategies can the nurse use quickly while waiting for another intervention or healthcare professional? What interventions may be implemented quickly? Will it help to elevate the head of the bed? What if oxygen is applied? Will the dizziness be improved if the client sits down? How can the nurse act now to help the client?

I: IDENTIFY RISK TO SAFETY

What are the top safety concerns of the client? The National Council Licensure Examination (NCLEX®) is an exam about safety – many questions are going to address client safety or discuss threats to client safety. Because of this, it is important to consider the highest concerns for safety experienced by the client. Safety concerns may include evaluation of the risk for falls, prevention of injury, reduction of risk for hospital-acquired infections (HAI), and more.

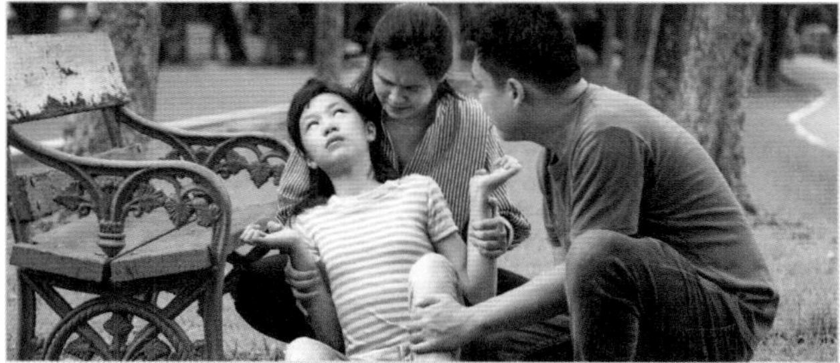

Image 1-2: A client with seizures is at risk for injury. List 5 threats to safety when a client has a seizure. What nursing precautions should be instituted to prevent injury?

N: Clinical Problem Solving Process (Nursing process)

Many questions represent a step of the clinical problem solving process (nursing process). Although it is possible for a test question to refer to any step of the clinical problem solving process, the NCLEX® exam is often focused on nursing action related to the process of data collection or intervention. Reflect on "what action should the nurse take next?" knowing that an action can be data collection or an intervention. When determining a priority action, ask yourself, "Have I collected enough data to safely perform this intervention?" For example, a client with surgical pain rating of 8 out of 10 needs pain medication (intervention). Higher priorities would be to determine when the client last received a pain medication, the type of pain medication prescribed, and if there is a need to consult with the registered nurse.

Prioritization Power

Let's discuss more about **Prioritization Power.** When you looked up your medications for clinical, you tried to learn all twenty side effects or all six indications for a medication. Now that you are preparing for NCLEX-PN®, you want to use **Prioritization Power.** That means you will need to analyze the options and identify the TOP THREE side effects and indications for each medication. In each chapter of this book, you will read the Go To Clinical Case and practice **Prioritization Power.**

In addition, for each *Go To Clinical Case* you will read the details of care for a specific client. Then, you will be asked to identify the TOP THREE: Priority Data Collection or Cues, Priority Labs/Diagnostics, Priority Potential and Actual Complications, Priority Interventions, Priority Medications, Priority Nursing Implications, and Reinforcement of Priority Teaching. In the following pages, you will find the answers to the TOP THREE **represented by NurseThink®** 💡 in the related **Priority Exemplars.** As you progress through the book you will identify concepts, consider key components of nursing care, and develop your clinical judgment skills. This guide will lead you through 20 chapters, over 160 **Priority Exemplar**s requiring nursing care, and more that 500 quiz questions (in book and online). You will be able to check your answers and review extensive rationale for correct/incorrect answers and NurseThink® *THIN Thinking.*

NurseThink® is a tool to develop habits of clinical judgment through prioritization and conceptual processing to meet client needs.

Clinical judgment is the observed outcome of critical thinking and decision making (NCSBN, 2018).

To help you develop your clinical judgment skills, each question is categorized to competencies listed by the Quality and Safety Education for Nurses (QSEN) institute at QSEN.org. These competencies include Patient-Centered Care, Teamwork and Collaboration, Evidence-based Practice, Quality Improvement, Safety, and Informatics. The NCLEX-PN® Client Needs for each question are also identified. They include Coordinated Care, Safety and Infection Control, Health Promotion and Maintenance, Psychosocial Integrity, Basic Care & Comfort, Pharmacological Therapies, Reduction of Risk Potential, and Physiological Adaptation. More discussion of these components of the NCLEX-PN® test plan categories is in Chapter 2 and online at www.NCLEX.org. See Chapter 2 for a brief discussion of Next Generation NCLEX® and the NCSBN® Clinical Judgment Measurement Model.

Alternate Item Formats

To ensure you have the most up-to-date information on the mechanics of the NCLEX-PN®, be sure to visit www.NCLEX.org. In addition to the customary multiple-choice format (e.g. four options with one correct answer), the National Council of State Boards of Nursing (NCSBN) implements other question types using what they call alternate item formats. These questions measure critical thinking and clinical judgment in different ways. They take a little more time and sometimes cause stress for candidates. Therefore, we will explain them briefly. In addition, you can go on the NCLEX® website to learn more about the different formats (more about that in Chapter 2). Alternate format questions include:

> **Chart exhibit questions:** Computer tabs allow you to view client records, including health care provider prescriptions, client flow sheets, diagnostic results, progress notes, and other documents. You will then answer an item about this information.

> **Select all that apply:** These questions, sometimes referred to as multiple response, include a stem and usually five or six options. You will need to pick one or more options as the correct answer. The best strategy is to treat each option as a true/false question. These questions are reported to appear frequently on NCLEX-PN®.

> **Ordered Response / Drag and Drop:** Perhaps the hardest of all question formats—these questions ask you to read an item and put the answer options in order of rank or occurrence. You need to have a good understanding of the steps needed and the correct order! These items may also ask you to prioritize a single client's needs or prioritize the needs of several clients. Again, there is no partial credit.

> **Fill-in-the-blank:** These options are primarily reserved for math calculations (drug dosages, intravenous drip rates, conversions, intake and output). You will be provided the unit of measurement and rounding instructions to type the answer into the provided field.

> **Hot spot:** These questions ask you to use the cursor to identify a place on the screen that answers the question. These can be locations on the body, elements of the environment, components of a medical record, or any other graphic depiction of the question that you are asked to interpret and identify a key spot or location on the picture.

> **Varied multiple choice:** Audio or graphic files may provide information about which candidates must make decisions in related test items.

NurseThink® for Clinical Judgment

We know that NCLEX-PN® tests how you think, not what you know! Therefore, one of the things we know about clinical practice in nursing, and the NCLEX-PN® exam, is that they require us to Think! Think hard from a clinical perspective! The **Priority Exemplars**, **Go To Clinical Cases**, and **NurseThink® Quizzes** will contribute to your NCLEX-PN® preparation! In addition, **Next Gen Clinical Judgment** boxes, and **Clinical Hints** will continue to grow your decision-making skills. Remember, focusing on the **Top-Three** helps you save time studying. We hope you find this book valuable on your road to NCLEX-PN® success!

CHAPTER

2

What is NCLEX-PN® all about?

National Council of State Boards of Nursing

To start out, NCLEX® stands for the National Council Licensure Examination. This exam is written, regulated, and evaluated by the National Council of the State Boards of Nursing (NCSBN). In fact, one of your greatest tools is the NCSBN website (www.nclex.org). You want to be familiar with their website since this organization is responsible for WRITING THE EXAM! There are many resources on this site, including details about the exam, the process of applying, specific policies, and frequently asked questions (FAQs). These FAQs are especially informative! In addition, the website includes important information about exam security and what you will be asked to do and provide as part of your exam experience. For example, there is a strict "No phones" policy such that it is best if you leave it in your car! If not, it will be put in a sealed bag and locked in a locker but you are to have no contact with your phone during the exam. There are also practice tests, alternate item tests, and details about computer adapted testing (CAT). CAT is unique in that it is able to estimate the clinical decision-making and clinical judgment skills of a candidate in as few as 75 questions—candidates will answer between 75 and 145 questions. We'll talk more about that in Chapter 3! Let's discuss the questions first before we address the exam.

Cognitive Level of Exam Questions

There was a time when test-taking "tricks" were shared when teaching about the preparation for standardized exams. These "tricks" were thought to give candidates the advantage when they confronted information they did not know or with which they were not comfortable.

Current testing practices warrant that you must **know** the material and be able to **think critically** about that material in order to pass the exam. Although "tricks" don't work, we will share some strategies in Chapter 4 to help you along!

Before we launch into the exam and the details of how you can be successful, we want to share with you a little more about the NurseThink® approach to critical thinking and answering higher level questions. What are higher level questions? You may have heard through nursing school that, early in your program, you are learning content. You are memorizing, remembering, and comprehending content about the human body, alterations in body systems, and the fundamentals of nursing science. Knowledge level questions ask about these facts and concepts. Building on that, a comprehension level question has you use information you learned to demonstrate how something works or how it is used. For example, a Knowledge/Comprehension level question could be:

Q: A nurse administers a laxative to a client. Which therapeutic effect should the nurse anticipate?

1. The client will breathe easier when walking.
2. The client will urinate without pain.
3. The client will empty his bowels.
4. The client will be able to sleep through the night.

These knowledge and comprehension questions are important. You needed to learn this information so that, as you progress in your education and in your nursing career, you are able to critically think about that information to make important clinical decisions—both in nursing practice and on NCLEX-PN®. So, there was a place for knowledge and comprehension level questions early in your education. In fact, there are some knowledge and comprehension questions in this text.

As you progressed through nursing school the focus changed from learning information to using the Clinical Problem Solving Process to address and treat conditions, essentially asking the question, "What should the nurse do about it?" These questions identified nursing actions, whether data collection or interventions, that were indicated by information given in the test item. These questions are known as application and analysis questions and *these* are the items you will see on NCLEX-PN®. NCSBN tells us that questions will only be at these levels, so we want to make sure you are comfortable with these questions and the thinking involved in answering higher level questions.

First, let's talk about application questions. These questions are more than just about a client or clients—they ask what a nurse should do based on the information or case portrayed in the question:

Q: A nurse notes that a client's abdomen is hard and distended. The client states that he has not had a bowel movement in 5 days. Which intervention should the nurse do next?

1. Administer the prescribed bulk-forming laxative.
2. Calculate the client's total fluid and solid food intake.
3. Encourage the client to ambulate in the hall.
4. Safely administer the prescribed biscodyl suppository.

This question gives you information and you need to establish the highest priority—next thing to do—again, what a nurse should do in this situation. If you remember, back in Chapter 1, we presented the *THIN Thinking* model. This question is a great example of *THIN Thinking*—**Help Quick** is the first thing to do for this client.

Next Gen Clinical Judgment

According the National Council of State Boards of Nursing (NCSBN) clinical judgment is the **doing** part of critical thinking and decision making. As you answer test items, be sure to try and envision what the nurse should be doing. For example, think about:

1. A client falls in the hallway
2. A client vomits 3 times
3. A client pulls out their catheter
4. A client becomes short of breath

What should the nurse do?

The highest level projected on NCLEX-PN® is the Analysis level. These items require reviewing a set of data, analyzing that data, and coming to a conclusion about a nursing action. They tend to include more data than application questions and require high level thinking. These analysis questions may ask you to set priorities between several clients or several competing priorities within one client. Here is an analysis question:

Q: A nurse plans the care of the four clients to which the nurse is assigned. Which client should the nurse care for first?

1. A 75-year-old male who is three days post-op total hip replacement and is receiving intravenous antibiotics to be administered by the registered nurse.
2. A 46-year-old who had abdominal surgery and needs encouragement with the incentive spirometer and has decreased breath sounds and increased work of breathing.
3. A 94-year-old who was admitted four days ago with dehydration and is receiving intravenous hydration.
4. A 68-year-old man who had a rectal prostatectomy yesterday and is ambulating in the hall.

You can see these higher level questions cause you to use **NurseThink**®! Many experts believe that it is not as important for you, as an exam candidate, to differentiate between application and analysis questions. Instead, you need to be able to recognize higher level questions from lower level items. The alternate format items you read about in Chapter 1 may be higher or lower level questions. Although alternate items are often thought of as more difficult, and certainly are more time-consuming than standard items, they are not always at the higher cognitive level. It is important to know about alternate items, to be able to differentiate between knowledge/comprehension and application/analysis ones, and be able to answer these higher level items before you sit down to take the exam.

NCLEX-PN® Client Needs

The NCLEX-PN® exam is computer adapted such that each candidate gets a unique exam experience based on their ability. Items are chosen for the candidate based on level of difficulty of the previous question and the blueprint (see Table 2-1).

Safe and effective care environment	
Coordinated Care	18-24%
Safety and Infection Control	10-16%
Health Promotion and Maintenance	6-12%
Psychosocial Integrity	9-15%
Physiological Integrity	
Basic Care and Comfort	7-13%
Pharmacological Therapies	10-16%
Reduction of Risk Potential	9-15%
Physiological Adaptation	7-13%

Table 2-1: See www.NCLEX.org for more information.

This means that every candidate will answer questions along this blueprint, but each candidate will receive unique questions. Questions are assigned a level of difficulty. If a candidate answers a question correctly, the next question is either the same level of difficulty or a little harder. If the candidate answers it incorrectly, the subsequent question is the same level of difficulty or a little easier.

The blueprint is an excellent example of evidence-based practice! The NCSBN conducts a practice or job analysis and this information, in addition to other analyses, is used to develop the blueprint. For the practice analysis, surveys are sent to newly working practical nurses with a list of tasks. These new practitioners are asked to consider- "What do you do all day?" They rank this list of activities and these rankings inform the components of the blueprint. The exam is reviewed every three years and items undergo rigorous review to ensure accuracy, validity, lack of bias, and readability. In addition, each candidate takes 15 pretest items and the performance on these items by the large pool of candidates informs further revision and validity of the questions. These questions don't count but nor do you know which ones they are in your exam—so do your best on every item! We do know that these pretest questions ensure that each question that counts on the exam is truly valid and that pretest questions are posed to every candidate in the first 75 questions. We usually say, use strategies and knowledge to the best of your ability to answer every question. Even though you don't know which questions "don't count," you may feel some solace in knowing that a truly obscure or difficult question may be a pretest question!

Sometimes the categories of the NCLEX-PN® blueprint seem hard to understand—they may not mesh with how you learned or studied in nursing school. Let's take a question through the process to show you how the Client Needs work. We'll describe a case and consider the types of questions that could be asked under each domain.

Case

A nurse cares for an older adult client who presented to the emergency department with confusion and new-onset incontinence. The client is receiving intravenous antibiotics and intravenous fluids.

If we look at the Client Needs, we can come up with questions that might be seen in each category.

Safe and Effective Care Environment:

- **Coordinated Care:** A question in this section may address the client being unable to articulate his own needs. If the client is confused, unable to speak, or not able to make decisions, the nurse should function as a client advocate. A test item may refer to the nurse's role in contributing to the plan of care and monitoring the care provided by the unlicensed assistive personnel.

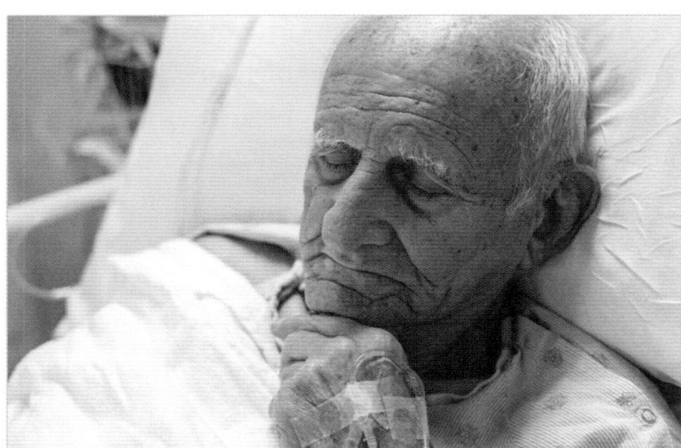

Image 2-1: How should the nurse determine that this client's intravenous access device is patent?

- **Safety and Infection Control:** This client is at risk for injury. Consider the client's confusion and intravenous therapy and how they contribute to this risk. A test item may also address risk for infection. How does his current status increase his risk for infection?

Health Promotion and Maintenance:

An item in this section may address collecting data about the client, considering the client's immunization needs, identifying client's barriers to communication, or providing care that specifically meets the needs of older adults.

Psychosocial Integrity:

Questions in this area may address every client for whom the nurse provides care. Our client would benefit from calm and respectful communication with the nurse. The client's confusion may be lessened by creating a therapeutic environment.

Physiological Integrity:

- **Basic Care and Comfort:** Items related to Basic Care and Comfort may address monitoring this client's intake and output or assisting with activities of daily living. Hygiene, positioning, and safe transfers may be the subjects of test items.
- **Pharmacological Therapies:** Items pertaining to Pharmacological Therapies may address the nurse administering intravenous piggyback (secondary) medications or maintaining safe medication practices by all routes of administration within the scope of practice of a LPN/LVN.
- **Reduction of Risk Potential:** Questions addressing Reduction of Risk Potential may address collecting a urine culture, maintaining the peripheral intravenous (IV) catheter, or identifying client risk and implementing interventions.
- **Physiological Adaptation:** Physiological Adaptation will include items pertaining to the care of a client with a fluid electrolyte imbalance, reinforcing client education about their condition, or recognizing and reporting a change in the client's condition.

You can see how this blueprint or test plan covers the spectrum of nursing care and may apply to any specialty or setting. Clients in NCLEX® questions are from across the well-illness continuum, across the lifespan, and in a variety of clinical settings, including homes, community agencies, hospitals, schools, workplaces, long-term care facilities, and anywhere nurses provide care!

Examples of Topics in Each Client Need

Candidates are encouraged to go to the NCSBN website to review topics under each category and the complete test plan, but they are briefly discussed here for your review.

Safe and Effective Care Environment:

This larger category discusses the role of the practical nurse in providing nursing care in the healthcare delivery setting.

- **Coordinated Care:** This section highlights the aspects of client care related to advocacy, conflict management, priority setting, assigning other healthcare professionals, and working with the healthcare team. Candidates are asked to establish priorities for a single client and also to juggle competing priorities between several clients. The practical nurse collaborates with the healthcare team members to provide client care and works within their scope of practice.
- **Safety and Infection Control:** As indicated in this title, this section discusses injury and infection prevention and the nurse's role in keeping clients safe. One great way to study for this section is to take note of the precautions in the clinical area—these are essentially agency care plans to keep clients safe. Neutropenic, fall, aspiration, suicide, seizure, flight risk, bleeding, and other precautions keep clients safe. These precautions assist nurses to protect clients from health and environmental hazards.

Health Promotion and Maintenance:

This is the wellness aspect of the exam and includes such content as normal labor and delivery, developmental milestones including changes of aging, collection of data on physical status, risk behaviors, screening, and keeping clients healthy across the lifespan. Practical nurses assist clients with prevention and early detection of health problems and questions may address health screening, providing information, or identifying community resources. This client need addresses wellness concepts that may occur with or without concurrent acute or chronic illness.

Psychosocial Integrity:

Therapeutic communication, substance use and abuse, defense mechanisms, dealing with crisis and stress, persistent/chronic mental illness, grief and bereavement, and psychotropic medications are included in this section. Establishing therapeutic relationships and communication questions may be asked in this domain where answers appear in quotation marks and reflect client or nursing statements. Communication questions may be difficult because the response choices may not reflect your usual communication style. Remember that the goal of therapeutic communication is to open up the reciprocal communication pathway and encourage the client to respond. Even if you personally would not say something, you want to follow the accepted styles that reinforce therapeutic communication. Options that foster communication include open-ended questions, and those that reflect empathy, respect, genuine caring, and therapeutic boundaries. Closed-ended questions, that can be answered with a yes or no, do not promote rich discussion.

Clinical Hint

Leading questions should not be used when collecting data from clients. Questions like "You don't smoke cigarettes, do you? rarely yield valid information.

Physiological integrity:

This section, about one-half of the exam, focuses on physiological components of care.

- **Basic care and comfort:** We frequently discuss that, although the quality of today's healthcare is augmented by technology and advances in science, one cannot forget the importance of the basics. Skills you learned in fundamentals, like activities of daily living, hygiene, assistive devices, sleep, body mechanics and moving clients, comfort measures, and nutrition, are also critical components and basics of client care. Basic nutrition and therapeutic/condition-specific dietary recommendations are part of this category. This section also includes alternative/complementary therapies and the nurse's role in ensuring client safety with these treatments.
- **Pharmacological Therapies:** This section, about one-fifth of the exam, is often the most dreaded of all sections! It includes questions about specific medications and classes of drugs, routes of administration, calculations of doses, and priority nursing implications of medications. Medication therapeutic actions and side effects, contraindications, potential interactions, reinforcement of client teaching, and details about administering the medication may be the subjects of these items. Questions may also pertain to the practical nurse's role in administering intravenous piggyback (secondary) medications, monitoring intravenous flow rate, monitoring transfusion of blood products, maintaining pain control devices, and administering injections.
- **Reduction of risk potential:** This section, although perhaps the most abstract of all the blueprint, speaks to the essential role of nursing in monitoring for and preventing complications. Untoward effects from infection, surgery, injury, illness, interventions, immobility, and other conditions may be prevented or reduced in severity if detected and intervened upon early. Here, questions discuss diagnostic procedures, unexpected effects of care, and therapeutic procedures, including psychomotor skills and policies. Practical nurses may also provide interventions to prevent complications, such as the use of sequential compression devices or compression stockings.
- **Physiological adaptation:** This section mirrors what you learned in pathophysiology and about disease processes. Expected signs and symptoms, and therapeutic measures, related to conditions are addressed, along with unexpected responses to treatments, illness management, performing wound care, and fluid and electrolytes.

Integrated concepts

NCLEX-PN® items are also written by attending to what the NCSBN calls the **Integrated Concepts.** These concepts are woven throughout your exam and reflect the beliefs and philosophy of the exam. These provide the foundation for the exam such that each item has some elements addressed as these integrated concepts. The integrated concepts are:

- **The Clinical Problem-Solving Process (Nursing Process)** includes the steps of data collection, planning, implementation, and evaluation. Questions may refer to any step of this process.
- **Caring** is the interaction of the nurse and client in an attitude of mutual respect and trust. It may seem like common sense but choose answers that demonstrate this level of caring!
- **Communication and Documentation** includes both the verbal and non-verbal messages between clients, client's significant others, and members of the healthcare team as well as written/electronic health records.

Next Gen Clinical Judgment

Basic care and comfort includes fundamental skills so critical to safe client care. List 10 basic interventions nurses use to avoid injury or threats to safety for clients and others.

- **Teaching and Learning** is the facilitation of knowledge, skills, and attitudes designed to assist to promote changes in behaviors. The role of the practical nurse is to reinforce the teaching initiated by a registered nurse or other members of the healthcare team. Questions related to reinforcing teaching and learning may have two purposes—to test the candidate's knowledge of the content to be taught and to measure the candidate's ability to adapt material to the level of understanding of the client. It is critical to read the stems of the questions several times, as in all item stems you experience, because the stem itself indicates the type of answer for which you are looking. For example, if a stem states "Which option indicates a need for more teaching?" you are looking for a wrong or incorrect statement or answer. If the stem states: "Which indicates a good understanding of teaching?" you are looking for a correct or valid statement or answer. These questions reinforce the need for careful reading in the NCLEX-PN® exam.
- **Culture and Spirituality** is the interaction of nursing with clients (individuals, families/significant others, groups, and populations) which recognizes and considers client-reported, self-identified unique and individual preferences in client care, within parameters of standards of care and legal implications. The Integrated Concept of Culture and Spirituality was added in 2016. Prior to this, these questions were under Psychosocial Integrity. The NCSBN realized that, in many cases, culture and spirituality may infuse any question and that this elevation to an Integrated Concept reinforced the importance of considering aspects of culture and spirituality in every area of nursing and client care. Cultural awareness, cultural influences on health, spiritual influences on health, and spiritual factors impacting care all infuse the NCLEX-PN® exam. How language and religious and spiritual client needs are met are integral nursing considerations in holistic client care. Culture and spirituality may influence rituals, customs, holidays, dietary practices, manner of dress, relationships with authority, social interactions, gender roles, communication, and decision-making. Critical to this is the need to focus on the client as an individual and respect the client's choices and needs.

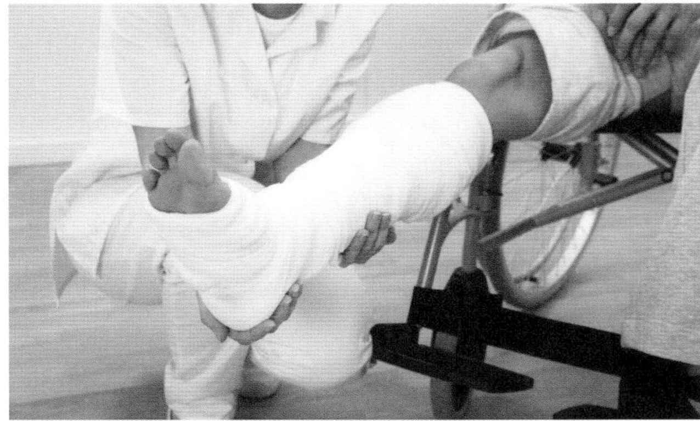

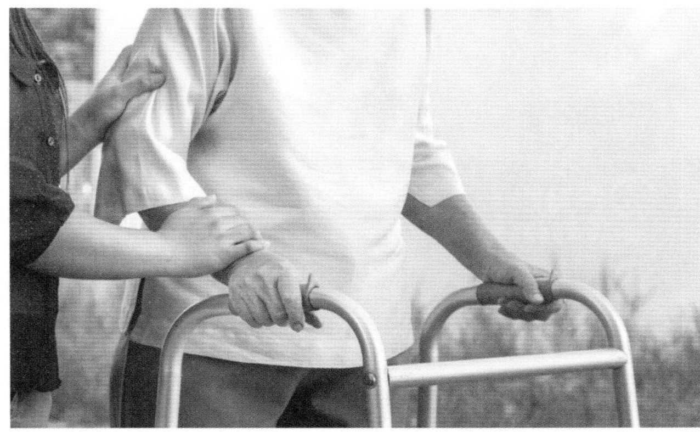

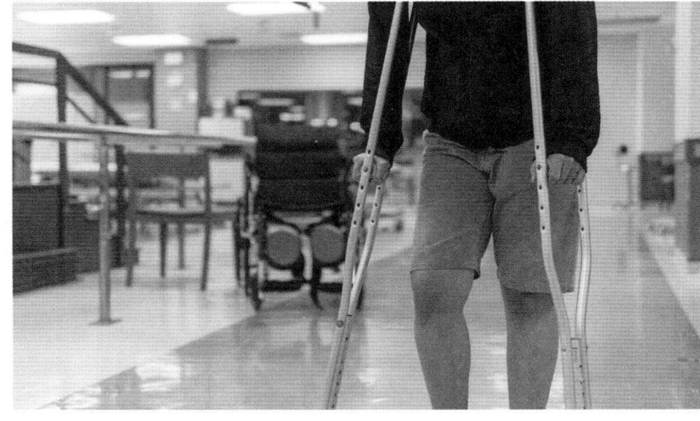

Image 2-2, 2-3, 2-4: The nurse cares for the clients depicted in each of these images. Try to write an NCLEX® style question about each image.

Next Generation NCLEX®

The National Council of State Boards of Nursing (NCSBN) is dedicated to ensuring the health and welfare of the public through the provision of safe nursing care. To best accomplish that goal, the NCSBN launched an initiative to more accurately measure clinical judgment on both the PN and RN exams. These changes are anticipated to occur in 2023, so this may be very relevant to you! When Next Generation NCLEX® is launched, candidates will take the traditional items noted in this chapter and will answer Next Generation items as depicted in the examples on these pages.

The foundation of the Next Generation exam items is the Clinical Judgment Measurement Model. This evidence-based strategy allows the nurse to make high-level decisions as a client's condition changes. Clinical Judgment includes these six items and will measure your ability to apply them to a clinical situation: recognize cues, analyze cues, prioritize hypotheses, generate solutions, take action, and evaluate outcomes. Next Generation exam items will be formatted in case study format with images of client health records. There may be many pages of data to read and review, be sure to analyze all of the material presented! This text blueprints each item to the Clinical Judgment Measurement Model and includes Next Generation Test items.

Here are examples:

After reviewing this information, you will be asked questions that apply clinical judgment. Review the six items (table on page 14) of the Clinical Judgment Measurement Model to determine if you can identify what is happening with this client.

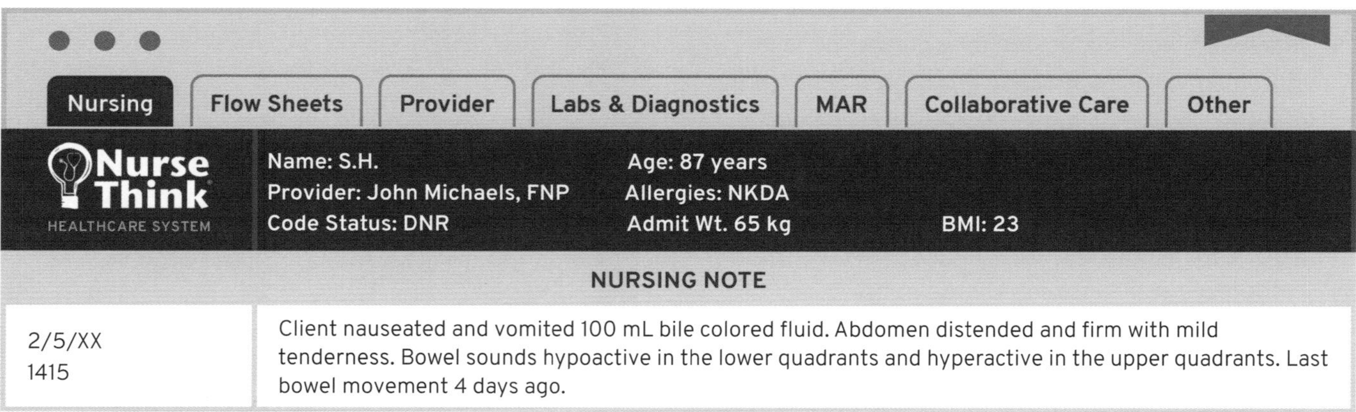

Nursing | Flow Sheets | Provider | Labs & Diagnostics | MAR | Collaborative Care | Other

Nurse Think HEALTHCARE SYSTEM

Name: S.H. | Age: 87 years
Provider: John Michaels, FNP | Allergies: NKDA
Code Status: DNR | Admit Wt. 65 kg | BMI: 23

NURSING NOTE

2/5/XX 1415	Client nauseated and vomited 100 mL bile colored fluid. Abdomen distended and firm with mild tenderness. Bowel sounds hypoactive in the lower quadrants and hyperactive in the upper quadrants. Last bowel movement 4 days ago.

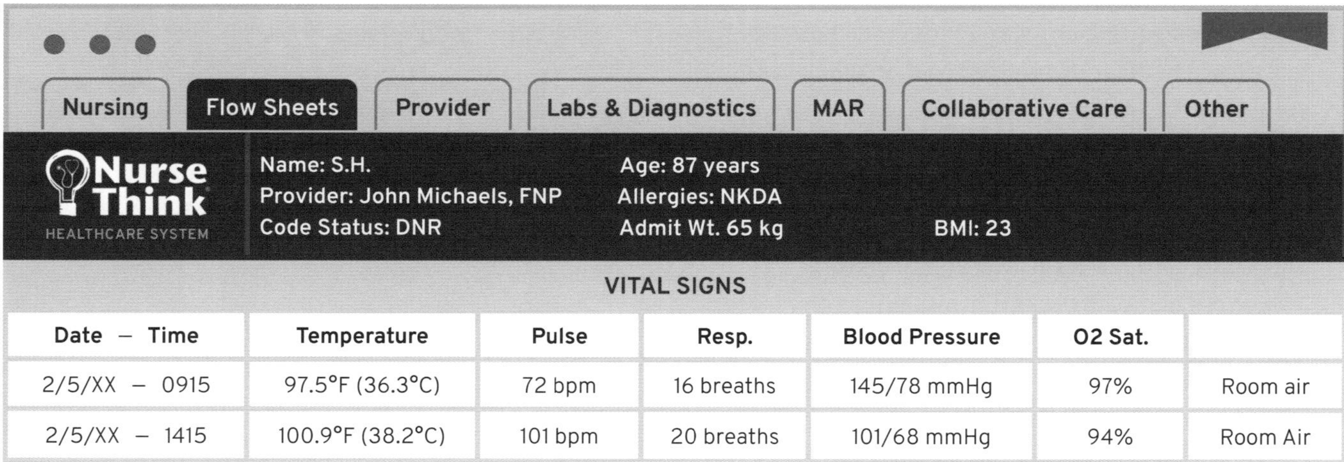

Nursing | Flow Sheets | Provider | Labs & Diagnostics | MAR | Collaborative Care | Other

Nurse Think HEALTHCARE SYSTEM

Name: S.H. | Age: 87 years
Provider: John Michaels, FNP | Allergies: NKDA
Code Status: DNR | Admit Wt. 65 kg | BMI: 23

VITAL SIGNS

Date – Time	Temperature	Pulse	Resp.	Blood Pressure	O2 Sat.	
2/5/XX – 0915	97.5°F (36.3°C)	72 bpm	16 breaths	145/78 mmHg	97%	Room air
2/5/XX – 1415	100.9°F (38.2°C)	101 bpm	20 breaths	101/68 mmHg	94%	Room Air

The style of the Next Generation NCLEX® items are different from traditional exam questions. You should be prepared to answer questions in a variety of formats and styles including extended drag-and-drop, highlight, and close, to name a few. Exposure to a variety of item formats is not as important as reading the information in the client's record and applying the clinical judgment model. It's about applying your THINKING.

Let's try a few items related to S.H.

1. After reviewing the client information in the healthcare records, highlight the areas of the record that are most concerning.

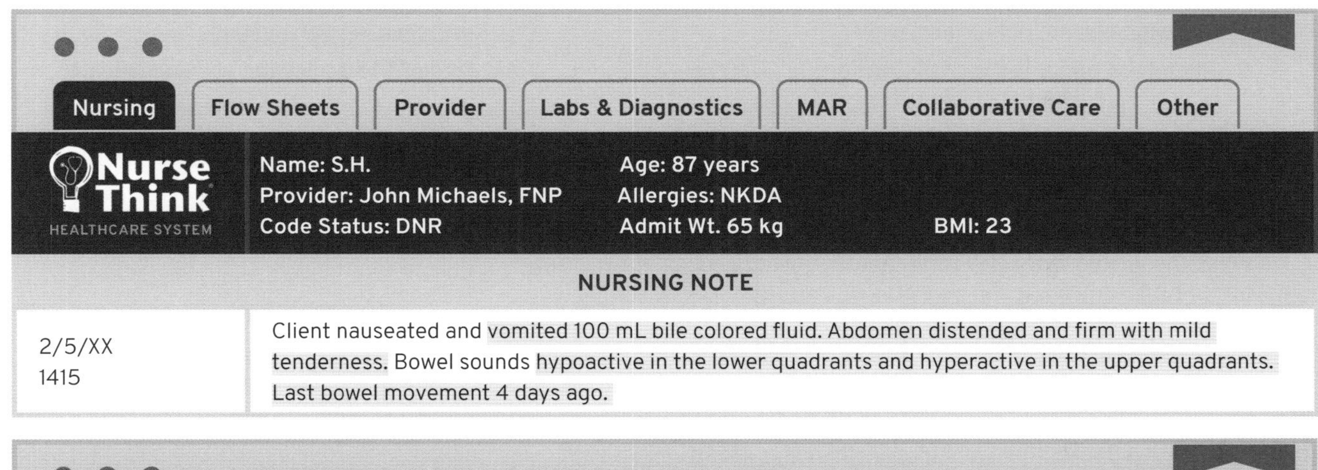

Nursing | Flow Sheets | Provider | Labs & Diagnostics | MAR | Collaborative Care | Other

Nurse Think HEALTHCARE SYSTEM

Name: S.H. | Age: 87 years
Provider: John Michaels, FNP | Allergies: NKDA
Code Status: DNR | Admit Wt. 65 kg | BMI: 23

NURSING NOTE

2/5/XX 1415	Client nauseated and vomited 100 mL bile colored fluid. Abdomen distended and firm with mild tenderness. Bowel sounds hypoactive in the lower quadrants and hyperactive in the upper quadrants. Last bowel movement 4 days ago.

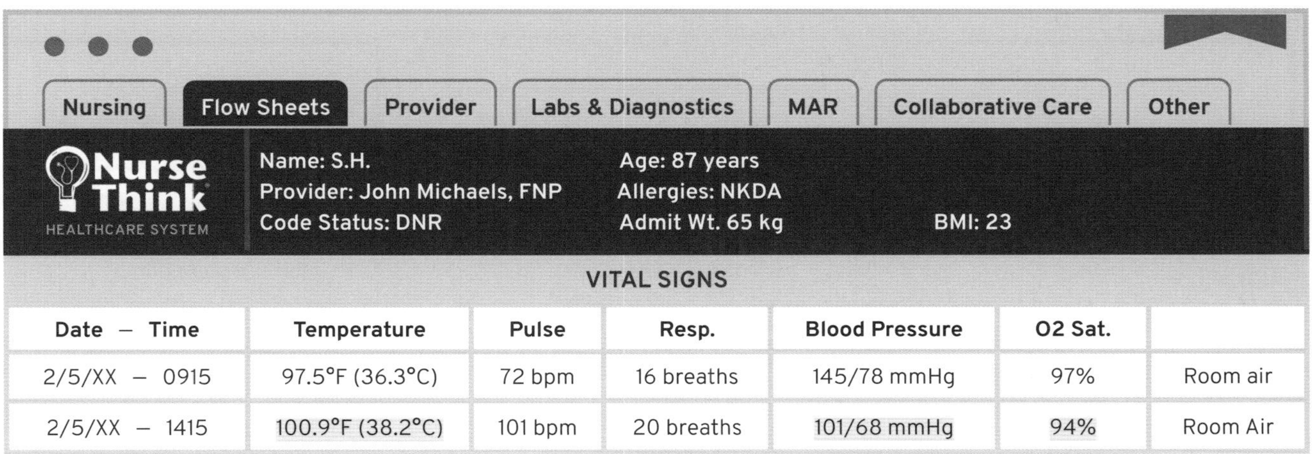

Nursing | Flow Sheets | Provider | Labs & Diagnostics | MAR | Collaborative Care | Other

Nurse Think HEALTHCARE SYSTEM

Name: S.H. | Age: 87 years
Provider: John Michaels, FNP | Allergies: NKDA
Code Status: DNR | Admit Wt. 65 kg | BMI: 23

VITAL SIGNS

Date – Time	Temperature	Pulse	Resp.	Blood Pressure	O2 Sat.	
2/5/XX – 0915	97.5°F (36.3°C)	72 bpm	16 breaths	145/78 mmHg	97%	Room air
2/5/XX – 1415	100.9°F (38.2°C)	101 bpm	20 breaths	101/68 mmHg	94%	Room Air

2. Complete the sentence using the words in the table for each corresponding letter. Select one answer for each letter. Based on the data collected by the nurse, the client is most likely experiencing (A) due to (B).

(A)	(B)
☐ Septicemia	☐ Low fiber diet
☐ Constipation	☐ Infection
☐ Aspiration	☑ Constipation
☑ Bowel Obstruction	☐ Vomiting

3. The health care provider is notified, and prescriptions are received. Review each prescription and determine if it is anticipated or not-anticipated. Select one option for each row.

HCP Prescription	Anticipated	Not-Anticipated
Acetaminophen 2000 mg PO every 6 hours PRN for fever > 101°F (38.3°C)	☐	☑
Flat Plate of the abdomen	☑	☐
Tap water enema until clear	☐	☑
Full liquid diet	☐	☑
Ondansetron 4 mg intravenous, PRN for nausea	☑	☐

4. Which findings indicate that the client's condition has improved? Select 4 items that are correct.

a. Liquid feces is passed.
b. Nausea resolves.
c. Emesis becomes clear and watery.
d. Abdomen becomes less distended.
e. Worsening pain in the right lower quadrant.
f. Blood pressure decreases.
g. Bowel sounds become hypoactive throughout.
h. The client is hungry.
i. The temperature normalizes.
j. Flat plate of the abdomen shows free air.
k. Abdominal tenderness worsens.

5. Identify the data changes, a potential complication, and the medical interventions using the bowtie chart. Select the words from the table below that are most appropriate.

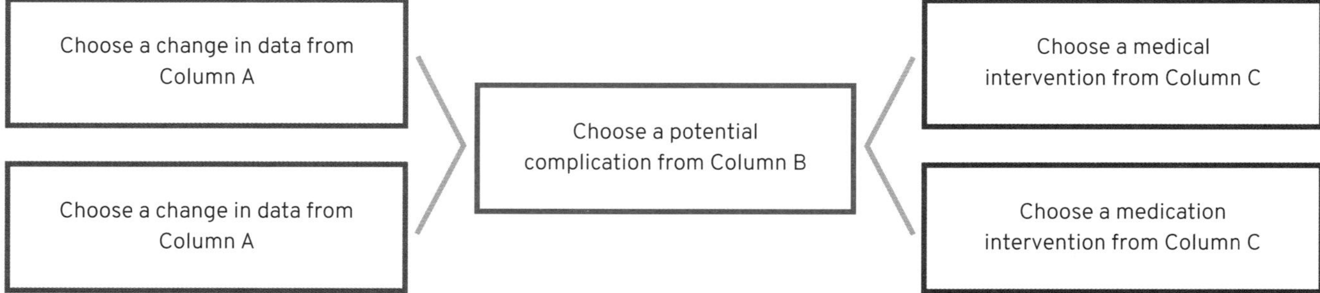

Column A Data Collection Change	Column B Potential Complication	Column C Medical Intervention
Irregular heart rhythm	Atelectasis from hypoventilation	*Surgical preparation
O2 Sat 90%	*Peritonitis from bowel perforation	High-flow oxygen
*Temperature 101.5°F (38.6°C)	Cardiac dysrhythmias from electrolyte imbalance	Continuous cardiac monitoring
Productive cough of clear sputum		*Intravenous antibiotics
*Significant abdominal pain		Small volume nebulizer treatments

Apply the Clinical Judgment Measurement Model	
Recognize Cues: Identify relevant and important information from different sources.	• What information is relevant/irrelevant? • What information is most important? • What is of immediate concern?
Analyze Cues: Organize and link the recognized cues to the client's clinical presentation.	• What client conditions are consistent with the cues? • Are there cues that support or contraindicate a particular condition? • Why is a particular cue or subset of cues of concern? • What other information would help establish the significance of a cue or set of cues?
Prioritize Hypotheses: Evaluate and rank the hypotheses according to priority.	• Which explanations are most/least likely? • Which possible explanations are the most serious?
Generate Solutions: Identify expected outcomes and use hypotheses to define a set of interventions for the expected outcome.	• What are the desirable outcomes? • What interventions can achieve those outcomes? • What should be avoided?
Take Action: Implementing the solution(s) that addresses the highest priorities	• Which intervention or combination of interventions is most appropriate • How should the intervention(s) be accomplished?
Evaluate Outcomes: Compare observed outcomes against expected outcomes.	• What signs point to improving/declining/unchanged status? • Were the interventions effective? • Would other interventions have been more effective?

Table 2-2: (NCSBN® Next Gen NCLEX®)

CHAPTER

3

What can I expect?

The Exam

The NCLEX-PN® exam experience is different for each candidate. Let's talk a little about the exam itself. The exam for each candidate is unique but based on standardized content and is directed toward assessing clinical judgment skills. You will answer between 75 and 145 questions and will have up to 5 hours to complete the exam (please check NCSBN website because there is a possibility this number is changing). This time period includes time for optional breaks. Breaks are offered to each candidate at the two-hour and three and one-half hour point, but it is up to you if you want to take a break or keep on testing! Although this is plenty of time for most people, you may want to limit your review of each question to less than three minutes. Studies tell us that if you think about a question for more than three minutes you risk the potential to "overthink" a question. Make sure you consider the options and answer confidently—moving on to the next question!

As discussed earlier, in Computer Adaptive Testing (CAT), the exam is constructed for each candidate based on items' levels of difficulty and to represent the appropriate percentages of the test plan. If the candidate gets a question correct, the next question is the same or a higher level of difficulty. If the question is answered incorrectly, the next item is the same or an easier difficulty level. Once you have answered the item and press "enter," that item disappears and will not be seen again. You must answer every question, there is no ability to skip or leave a question blank, and there is no penalty for guessing. This means of administration is good news for most people, especially for individuals who often change their answers. Researchers tells us that we often change correct to incorrect options; a good rule to follow is to change your answer with confidence, not with doubt. In other words, if you have a brainstorm that another answer is correct—then change the answer with confidence. On the other hand, if you doubt your thoughts or judgment—leave it! Your first inclination or hunch is often correct. Remember, your educated guess is often correct and, for traditional multiple choice items, you have a 25% chance of getting the question right! The process of elimination is your ally as you take the test, which enables you to increase this percentage even higher! Some candidates use the dry erase board to write down the numbers signifying the answer options (Details about the dry erase board later). These test-takers cross out options as they proceed to think through an item, ultimately yielding a visible reminder of their answer option.

You do not need to have special computer skills for this exam. You should go to the NCSBN (www.nclex.org) website to watch the tutorial video. You will be able to use the drop-down calculator on the computer and the computer has the customary mouse, keyboard, and monitor. There is also a clock/timer on the computer which may be turned on or off based upon your personal preference. The computer will show the number of each question. If you require specific accommodations related to your health, testing skills, or specific abilities/disabilities, you should check the NCSBN website (www.nclex.org) and you are encouraged to contact the testing center well in advance to ensure the best testing situation for you and to allow the center to meet your needs.

You are encouraged to do your best the **first time** you take the exam. We have heard of people taking the exam the first time, without studying, as a way to "try it out" and see how the exam looks and feels. Candidates may do this with the intent of then studying and passing the second time. Not only is this a waste of money and prolongs the time before you can practice as a nurse (and maybe, pay back your school loans!), but there is research that indicates that the passing rate on those taking the second exam is less than **one half** the rate for the first exam. For example, the current PN pass rate is about 83% on the first administration of the exam. Repeat PN examinees have a pass rate of about 36%. It is important that you focus on passing the FIRST TIME you take NCLEX-PN®. Not only is that critical for you and your career, but schools, as you may remember, are evaluated based on their first-time pass rates, among other criteria! On the other hand, if you are not successful the first time, despite your best efforts, we hope this text can continue to build your clinical judgment, competence, knowledge, and skills such that you are successful in subsequent testing experiences!

Application

You are in your last semester of school and are getting ready to graduate and take the NCLEX-PN® exam. The best source of information about your applying for the exam is the NCSBN website (www.nclex.org) and the state/local board of nursing where you plan on living. We will summarize the general principles, although the application process varies slightly.

- The NCSBN website (www.nclex.org) offers the NCLEX-PN® Exam Candidate Bulletin. Make sure you download that first to make sure you get off to the right start!
- You will need to apply for a nursing license with the state in which you are living or plan to be living. If the state you live in or plan to live in is part of the multistate compact, you will be able to work in other compact states, but you must have the license in your state of residence. If you plan to work in a state that is not part of this compact, you will need to get a license for that state. International candidates should check the NCSBN website and their local boards of nursing to ensure compliance with procedures. Although it seems very confusing, check your state board of nursing's website and you will be on your way. Many schools provide this information to students prior to graduation. You will need to pay a fee and complete an application. Each application process is unique and some states/locations require passport-size pictures. Be very careful completing this application and follow the directions completely. You may experience significant delays if the application needs to be returned to you to correct errors.

- You will also need to apply to Pearson Vue or the exam setting (for locations not using Pearson Vue) to take the exam. There is also a fee for this application.
- Once you have graduated, your school provides the information to the state board of nursing indicating that you have graduated and meet the requirements for taking the exam.

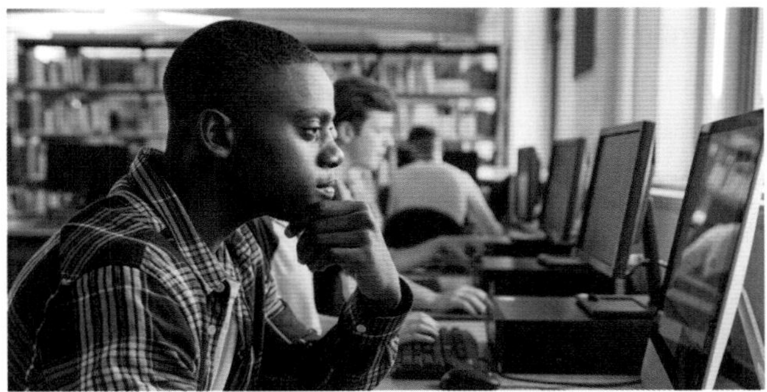

Image 3-1: How comfortable are you with computer-based testing? How does computer-based testing differ from pencil-and-paper testing? How do you need to prepare for the computer testing of NCLEX®?

- Once all records are obtained, you will be sent an authorization to test (ATT). You can call the Pearson Vue or other exam setting (for locations not using Pearson Vue) and enter your ATT. Many sites also provide a mechanism to make an appointment online. You cannot make an appointment without an ATT.

  Things you want to consider when making an appointment:

  - Think about the time of day when you are at your best! Make a morning appointment if you are an early riser... an afternoon appointment if that is when you perform at your peak! You will be asked to make an appointment at least five hours prior to the site's closing time because that is the maximum time allowed for the exam.
  - Consider life events and other scheduling variables—big events, time commitments, your work schedule, and your prospective employer's requests for your start date.
  - Pay attention to the policies related to changing your appointment or if you miss the appointment. If you do not call to cancel your appointment, and don't show up, you will lose your application fees and will need to pay and schedule again.
  - Research studies indicate that candidates who take the exam within 45-90 days after graduation experience the highest success rates. The information is more "fresh in your mind," you are still in the studying/test-taking groove, and there is less of a chance for life and other distractions to divert you from your NCLEX-PN® goals.

Before and the day of the exam

Chapter 4 and Chapter 20 will address how to set study goals, prepare yourself, and get you closer to NCLEX-PN® success. The day before the exam, you may want to do a "trial drive" to make sure you know where you are going and are comfortable with the location, the traffic patterns, and parking options. The night before the exam you want to put your books away and consider means to pamper yourself, clear your mind of distractions, and feel the best about yourself! Many go to a movie, get a massage, spend time with friends or family, read a book, or hunker down in front of the television for some intense relaxation. Make sure you get enough rest—go to bed early and set your alarm, or maybe a few alarms, to ensure that you wake up on time.

The morning of the exam, no matter what time you are scheduled to take the exam, eat a nutritious, light meal. Do not overdo caffeinated or other beverages and make sure you are comfortable but not hungry. There are a few differing thoughts on dressing for the exam. Some recommend the "dress for success" option where you wear professional clothes to gain confidence and positive self-thoughts. Others dictate that comfort is the key such that one small step above pajamas is the best idea! You decide—but make sure you dress in layers to adapt to the climate of the testing center.

Arrive at the testing center thirty minutes early to provide a buffer if you encounter traffic congestion or problems with parking. Bring your ATT and government-issued identification (ID) with you. Make sure this ID matches the name on your application exactly and, if it doesn't match, call the testing center **before you arrive to test** to allay any test day worries! Leave your phone, watch, books, and any other materials out in your car. Anything you bring with you into the testing center will be placed in a locker and you will not be able to access these during testing time. You will not be able to bring any food or water into the setting; if you have medical requirements for a snack or beverage you are encouraged to contact the testing center and you may need to apply for special accommodations. Water is available and may be accessed during breaks. Most centers have you wear a lanyard indicating that you are a testing candidate to curb any access to the lockers during testing and to curtail any conversations. Because centers have very small waiting rooms, and friends or family are not able to wait for you, candidates are encouraged to drive themselves or to be dropped off at the center.

At the testing center you will undergo significant security procedures to confirm your identity and preclude any test compromise. You will be fingerprinted and have palm vein scanning, in addition to being videotaped, photographed, and audio-recorded during the examination. You will receive a dry erase board and marker; should you run out of room on the board you must turn in that board and get a new one rather than erasing your board. You will be placed in a cubicle with a computer with adequate lighting. Because multiple examinees are in the same room, some candidates find the ambient noise disruptive. You may ask for earplugs from the exam proctor. Anytime you wish to contact the proctor, you are encouraged to raise your hand rather than getting out of your seat. Once you have completed the exam, you will receive a message that "Exam ENDED." There is a brief survey after the exam is completed.

Although the test pool available to NCSBN is large, there are a finite number of questions that make up the NCLEX-PN® examinations for a vast number of candidates. For this reason, and to preserve the examination pool for future candidates, each examinee will sign a confidentiality statement. In this document you promise not to discuss specific topics or items on the exam or to provide any information to others that would compromise the integrity of the exam. It is human nature to talk about the experience. It is important, as you begin your professional career, that you adhere to the principles and policies of this confidentiality agreement. In kind, it is critical that you refrain from asking these details of other candidates and ensure that this exam remains a sound mechanism to determine and validate entry-level nursing practice.

Staying calm in the cubicle

We will talk again, in Chapters 4 and 20, about dealing with the stress of life and NCLEX-PN® in the weeks and months prior to the exam. Here we are briefly going to address "calming yourself in the cubicle."

For example, you have just answered #39—it was a really hard question and you start to feel yourself panic. You know your personal, early signs of stress and anxiety. Do you feel a fluttering in your stomach? Perspiration EVERYWHERE? A headache coming on? Are your hands shaking? Do you feel nauseous? Do you feel like you can't think?

These feelings have happened to all of us and we know NCLEX-PN® is stress producing. But this is your chance to demonstrate how much you have learned, how much you know, and how you can use clinical judgment! Rather than letting stress cloud your thoughts and get the best of you, take control in the cubicle and keep on testing.

Instead of seeing stress as a liability in exam taking, think of stress as your friend. That may sound crazy to you, so let us explain. Without any stress, it would be hard for you to take the exam seriously and be primed to do your best! Instead, you may daydream during the exam or be distracted by other competing priorities. Here is where stress helps you out. A moderate level of stress ensures that you are focused and able to fully attend to the task at hand—taking the exam. You filter out distracting thoughts and focus on each question with enthusiasm and peak performance in test-taking. This stress keeps your brain oxygenated and helps you not worry about hunger, fatigue, or other concerns. On the other hand, stress may exceed this moderate level and start to interfere with your ability to think and make connections. Higher levels of stress impair your reasoning and distract you from your focus on the exam. Your physical and emotional symptoms detract from your abilities to rationally think through questions, retrieve memories, and make cogent decisions. Rather than allowing these symptoms to persist, you have to handle them---calm them (and yourself) in the cubicle!

Only you know the EARLY signs of stress you are most likely to manifest and when stress levels start to exceed moderate levels. Take a moment now to write down your symptoms. What do you feel when you first feel stress set in? How do these feelings progress? What goes on in your mind as these symptoms and feelings become apparent during testing? Now that you have that information in mind, consider what you can and should do to address rising stress levels and ensure that you are functioning at your peak level. You may already have a successful means to deal with stress during testing. You were successful in nursing school, so keep it up! If you are not sure you have a favorite method, you aren't confident your method will work with this level of high stakes testing, or you want to try something new, see this list to continue to foster stress reducing techniques. Practice a few before the exam, pick a favorite one, and master the technique prior to the exam. When you FIRST feel stress rising during NCLEX-PN® with the early signs identified previously, call your new stress management strategies into play and then, when you are calm, continue with your testing!

Calming yourself in the cubicle!

- Conjure up and use affirmations, or positive thoughts and messages, and rehearse them prior to the exam. Say to yourself—I am smart! I am qualified! I am competent! I am confident! I am ready! Some candidates "picture themselves as a nurse," wherein they envision the stethoscope around their neck or their name badge with a big LPN/LVN!
- Use muscle relaxation to calm your nerves. For some this is as simple as a neck roll. For others they conduct an ascending, progressive total body muscle contraction and relaxation. Beginning with the toes and ending at the neck, individuals using this strategy contract and relax every muscle in the body as a means to provide respite from the exam and refocus energy to thinking and decision-making.
- For many individuals, prayer or calming chants (silently, of course) may allow for brief interruptions from testing and allow you to reset your testing mindset.
- Researchers tell us that deep breaths enable us to lower our heart rate, focus our mind, and calm negative messages. Consider embracing yoga principles or other breathing techniques that allow for optimal focus and control.

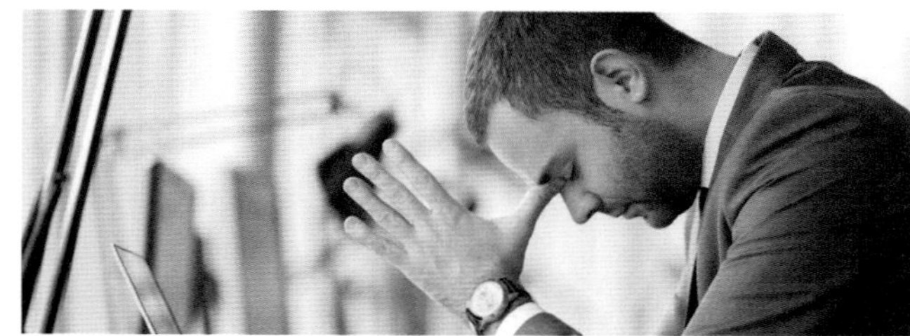

Image 3-2: What methods have you used in the past to "calm yourself in the cubicle?" Were they effective? What other methods might you use to ensure optimal testing performance?

Scoring the exam and passing standards

We believe that gone are the days that you can pass NCLEX-PN® without studying! It is a difficult exam and is more difficult than it used to be. In fact, the NCLEX-PN® exam has been progressively getting more difficult. We don't say this to scare you—but to mobilize you into action to create your own study plan for NCLEX-PN®! One great resource to use to better understand the scoring of the exam is located on the NCSBN website. (https://www.ncsbn.org/356.htm). This brief video explains how items are selected and how performance is scored by comparing exam candidates with individuals working out in a gym—we encourage you to watch it a few times!

When you sit down to NCLEX-PN® you will take between 75 and 145 questions. As discussed, you will be exposed to questions at various levels of difficulty and your computer adaptive test will assess your level of clinical decision making based on your answers to the test questions. Once you "prove" to the computer that you are above the passing standard and have completed at least 75 questions (please check NCSBN website because there is a possibility this number is changing), the test will end. In converse, if a candidate is consistently well below the passing standard the exam will turn off. Many believe that it is a good sign if you are experiencing difficult items—the computer is pushing you to your limit!

The NCSBN describes three scenarios to describe how candidates may pass or fail the exam:

- The 95% confidence interval rule: In this scenario, the computer will end the examination after 75 questions if the candidate is, with 95% confidence, clearly above or below passing standard.
- The maximum length rule: This rule presides when the candidate reaches item 145. If the candidate is above the passing standard at this point, the candidate passes. If the candidate is below the passing standard at this point, the candidate fails.
- The run out of time rule (ROOT): This principle governs the status of the candidate if the candidate uses up the entire 5 hours allowed for the exam. If the candidate completes fewer than 75 items or is below the passing standard for the last 60 items, the candidate will fail. If the candidate was above the passing standard for the last 60 items, the candidate will pass.

Getting my results

Although you will be most eager to get your results after the exam, the testing center will not have any knowledge of your score. Rumors exist about—If you get only 75 questions, you definitely passed—If you get all 145 questions you definitely failed—If you get 145 questions but you knew you passed at question 100, you were a test subject. None of these statements are true and NCSBN has repeatedly refuted the urban legend that some people are randomly selected to take all the questions! Make sure you routinely consult the NCSBN website with questions and be discriminating about believing erroneous rumors about the exam. Instead, here is what we know about getting your results:

- The exam is graded twice before releasing your findings.
- The results are sent to the state or other location board of nursing and mailed to the candidate within one month of the examination.
- Some states provide access to unofficial, quick results services which make results available to candidates within 2 days for an additional fee.
- Some states or locations have a verification of licensure pathway, where candidates, employers, and schools can determine if a practical nurse license has been issued under a specific participant's name—this would indicate that the candidate passed.

Candidates who pass the exam will receive a document with the pass determination and indicate the number of items completed. Those examinees who did not pass will receive a candidate report indicating that they failed and documenting personal strengths and weaknesses. The NCSBN website notes that areas of strength or weakness are not provided to individuals passing the exam to avoid employers, schools of higher learning, or individuals using this information to compare successful NCLEX-PN® candidates or provide a means to discriminate between successful candidates. Candidates that are not successful on NCLEX-PN® are guaranteed, depending upon the state or location, to obtain a retake appointment within 45 to 90 days of receiving a new ATT.

Now that we have a firm foundation of knowledge about the exam, let's proceed to Chapter 4 and discuss how you can prepare for NCLEX-PN®: Study what you don't know and the 20/50 rule, test-taking strategies, terms to know, and an introduction to principles of a healthy lifestyle to ensure your success!

CHAPTER

4

How can I prepare?

Know what you don't know with the 20/50 Rule!

It is important to think about your preparation for NCLEX-PN® as a marathon, not a sprint. Every experience you had in nursing school, in simulation and clinical, and all your preparation, add to your clinical judgment and your abilities on the exam. A colleague of ours was once known to say: "We tend to study what we like and are good at knowing and doing." The converse is also true. We tend to avoid those things we find difficult or less than interesting. Our recommendation is that you identify your weaknesses through test-taking and study those topics with which you struggle or on which you perform poorly.

To do this, now is the time to discover what your areas of weakness are and to address them. As you launch into this text, we recommend the 20/50 Rule. While in nursing school, each day you need to take a 20-item quiz and review the questions you get wrong. In addition, once a week take a 50-item test and pursue those topics that you were less sure of or did not answer correctly. When you are in your intense study phase consider increasing this to 50 items each day with 100 item weekly tests. In Chapter 20, we will discuss more about NCLEX-PN® preparation but this text will continue to help you-so read further!

Whether you are still in nursing school, or are in your intense study phase, another strategy is to use E3—what we call Expand Every Event. This strategy helps you engage in material—as you sit in class write down three words that help you understand every question, client, or case you discuss. Reflect on these terms later and try to determine if you have questions about the topic.

E3 helps you perform "mental aerobics" or engage in material three times. Brain researchers tell us that we need to interact with material three times for us to make a memory about, or essentially learn, content. Reading and preparing before class provides you one opportunity. Hearing information in class provides another opportunity. Engaging in the material using a creative learning strategy, like E3, will further assist you to make memories and learn material. During your study phase, make conscious efforts to actively engage in learning material—write it down, say it out loud, or compose exam questions about the material. This is so much better than memorization—it is about learning material and thinking about it to make sound clinical decisions. In Chapter 20, we are going to talk more about using the "mental aerobics" principles to learn and succeed for NCLEX-PN®.

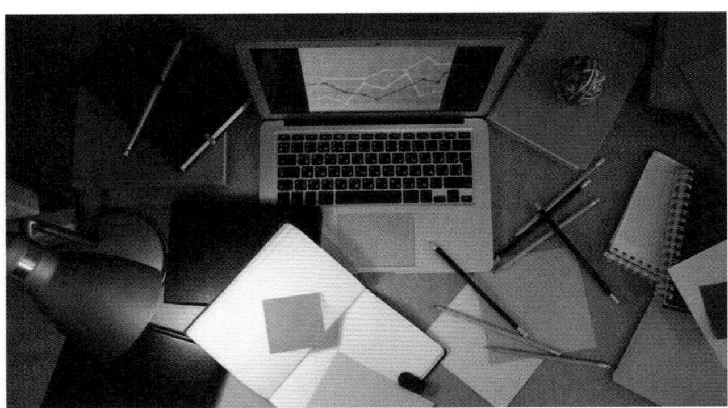

Image 4-1: Many people study in a dedicated spot. What do you need around you to create an effective, quiet, and calm study spot?

Test-taking Strategies

As we discussed, there are no "tricks" to taking NCLEX-PN®—but there are some strategies you can use to identify correct answers.

- We believe your greatest asset for the exam is **careful** and **calm reading**! We often misread questions and the human brain has the capacity to misinterpret questions to get them to be what we want them to be! We have all looked at exams after we completed them and said, "Why did I answer that?" It is often because we misread the question or the answer options. Read questions for critical words and concepts. Words and phrases like changes in level of consciousness, restlessness, increased work of breathing, lethargy, "floppy," a threatened airway, or significant deviations in vital signs may influence how you answer a question! These keywords or concepts may describe a change in client status, so important to recognize on NCLEX-PN®. It is critical to carefully read questions!
- Often candidates do well to visualize the client—and use your intelligent intuition! We often second-guess ourselves and, luckily, on NCLEX-PN® you will not be able to change answers. But often you question your initial, intuitive response. Remember, a good rule of thumb is to "Change your answer with confidence, not with doubt." In this way, you change the answer if you have an ah-hah and come to the right answer, but leave an answer, with your initial response, if you doubt whether the previous or changed answers are correct.

Clinical Hint

When answering a question and visualizing a client, think: How would the client look if interventions were effective? How would the client look if they were not effective?

- Remember the client is always a higher priority than the equipment—when a question tells you that a client's monitor is alarming, it is always critical to collect more data and attend to the client first, then deal with the alarm.
- Sometimes it is hard to understand a question the way it is written—try to rephrase the question in your own words and then try to answer it. In contrast, do not misinterpret the question. It is important to read and verify the meaning of a question when trying to answer. The human brain is amazing in its ability to rewrite a question to the way you "want" the item to look or the way you have seen the concept posed in the past. Make sure you accurately read the question several times. Picture in your mind what the answer might be. Then look at the options and see if it is there. Make sure you don't "read into" a question.

- If the question asks for the "First Nursing Action" it is often about collecting more data. We know that data collection is the first step of the clinical problem solving process and more information is often needed before one can intervene. When you look at a question, do you need more information? Could additional data lead to a more appropriate intervention?
- When questions ask for the "Essential Nursing Action," think safety. We will repeat the **safety message** several times in this text—NCLEX-PN® is an exam of safety! Keeping clients, other healthcare professionals, and ourselves safe is critical on the exam.
- You will be given a piece of paper and pencil or a dry erase board and marker. Use these to help you use your test-taking strategies—whether it is the process of elimination, completing calculations, making notes to yourself or writing down formulas or memorized information for later use.
- Be careful about passing client responsibilities quickly on to other healthcare professionals. It is very rare that a nurse stands at a client's side and does nothing, only to call the health care provider. Nor do nurses initiate a social work consult without communicating with the client. We will collect data, intervene, reassure, communicate with clients and then make the emergency call or referral. NCLEX-PN® is a test of nursing practice and, as such, will ask what the nurse would do!
- Questions about assigning staff may be difficult. As a testing strategy, one thing to remember is to assign away the simplest task to the unlicensed assistive personnel. The practical nurse may assign to an unlicensed assistive personnel or another LPN/LVN within their scope of practice and as dictated by the state in which they practice.
- If numbers are included in a question, take them seriously—interpret them and choose the correct nursing action. Are the numbers telling you the client is stable or unstable? Are the vital signs normal? How do they relate to the client's age? This may be critical information! A client's age may influence an answer based on developmental level, susceptibility to medication or illness, vulnerability, or treatment. For example, urinary tract infections and dehydration are far more grave if they occur in infants or older adults.
- Consider the time frame in every question! Is the client young or old? Did the surgery happen one hour ago or last year? What is the time frame since surgery, injury, admission, diagnosis, or other event? All of these variables may critically inform the decision-making in a test item!
- The NCLEX-PN® exam takes place in "NCLEX® WORLD." In this world, you have enough time, supplies, money, and help to accomplish tasks according to the highest of standards and in exact adherence to policies. That is not to say that, in real nursing practice, these standards are not important—but they are adapted to the capacities and capabilities of the real world. Do not answer questions on the exam based on the limitations that you may have witnessed in practice. Instead, keep to the high level of care you learned about and consider what is SAFEST for the client!
- Questions will not include proper names and will include the level of detail needed to answer the question. If the question cites an age, ethnicity, race, or gender, that information is important to answer the question.
- Questions are all "stand-alone." Except for those questions that are part of the Next Gen of NCLEX-PN®, which are explained in Chapters 2 and 20, all questions are unrelated. Do not be tempted to answer a question based on a previous question's answer. All questions are chosen randomly and are based on your personal performance.
- Questions on medications may be perceived as difficult. One strategy to consider is that side effects of medications are often accentuated expected therapeutic effects. For example, if a medication is prescribed to bring blood pressure down for clients with hypertension, then side effects include hypotension and orthostatic hypotension.

- Make sure you focus on normal values **and** critical values of laboratory studies. Although it is tempting to memorize lab studies norms, remember to focus on when lab values may yield critical signs and symptoms. For example, although a value of 126 mg/dL for blood glucose is not within the normal range, it is not a critical value that warrants emergency care. Consider when lab abnormalities may cause critical changes in status or require nursing care. They are more important to address than lab values that are marginally abnormal.
- Nurses are devoted to supporting clients with the utmost respect and encouraging as much self-care as possible. Although it may seem like common sense, pick an answer that supports respect and self-care for the clients. In this sense, the least invasive measures are often correct. There are times we implement a "least invasive" intervention while preparing for subsequent actions. Remember the *THIN Thinking* Help Quick option. In addition, nurses provide client-centered/family-centered care, this is important to remember as you answer questions!

Terms to know

There are certain words that are used on NCLEX-PN® to communicate to those taking the exam. They include:

- RN: Registered Nurse is the term for licensed registered nurses who may work with or supervise LPN/LVNs. LPN/LVNs are required to report changes in client status to RNs and to assist RNs in carrying out the plan of care.
- UAP: Unlicensed assistive personnel, or UAPs, is the term for any health care provider who does not have a license, including nurse's aides, assistants, or other titles.
- HCP: Health care providers include all professionals with prescriptive privileges, including physicians, nurse anesthetists, physician assistants, nurse practitioners, and nurse midwives.
- Prescriptions is the term used for any "orders" coming from those professionals noted above. In addition to medications, prescriptions may be for diagnostic and lab studies, activity restrictions, diets, procedures, and treatments.
- Rather than saying "complains of" the exam will use another term, thought to be with less judgmental than this phrase such as "presents with" or "states has these symptoms."
- The word "client" will refer to the subject of the question and may refer to the individual, family, group, or population.
- Medications will only be listed by their generic names, not their trade names. No proprietary names will be used.
- Nursing diagnoses are not tested on the NCLEX®. Client needs, and related concepts, are the focus of nursing care.

Healthy lifestyle for healthy testing

Although it is hard to focus on yourself or your own health while going through nursing school and preparing for the exam, we just want to briefly mention how important it is to stay healthy and engage in healthy habits. A healthy body and mind will best be able to think and make connections during the exam. Researchers identified the components of success, calling it "NCLEX-PN® Boot Camp". In this model, candidates focus on personal health (physical, emotional, and spiritual), practice questions, and treat exam preparation like a job—full time and full effort! So, what can you do to prepare?"

- Questions, questions, and more questions! Researchers tell us that you need to complete 2000-3000 questions to be prepared for the NCLEX-PN® exam. There was a time when 5000 questions were recommended, but the evidence now points to the more conservative number. Hooray for science!
- Consider your time and balance your time with work, questions, rest, exercise, and play
- Researchers tell us that you need to take the exam within 45-90 days from graduation and you need to devote designated time to study for the exam—we'll talk more about this in Chapter 20.

Researchers also affirm that having a healthy lifestyle and health-promoting habits contribute to NCLEX-PN® Success. Here are some hints to get you started and to launch into the content sections of this book:

- Remember—you have been successful! You succeeded in nursing school—you have made it this far and you are eligible to take the exam. Now you just need to learn what you don't know and focus study efforts on that material!
- Consider a standard place for studying—set yourself up—with or without music, with or without beverages and snacks, with or without interruptions of your phone and people in your world. Have this book available with plenty of sharpened pencils, your nursing textbooks, and a computer to search for information.
- Try to consider your diet and sleep habits. Studies tell us that a high protein, moderate carbohydrate diet fosters thinking and clear decision-making. A balanced diet with adequate fiber and water is optimal. Researchers indicate that the memories we make and the concepts we learn during the day are processed and organized during our sleep cycles. Adequate sleep is required to lay down memories for retrieval later. Consider your sleep and diet habits as you establish a study plan.
- Make sure you take time to play and have fun—spend time with your family and with yourself in activities that are fun and allow you to relax—and recharge—then go back to studying! Make smart decisions about alcohol, caffeine, and nicotine during this time—you want your mind to be sharp and at its best!
- Remember your affirmations!
    - You are smart! You are ready! You will be a Licensed Practical/Vocational Nurse
- Let's dive into the content sections of the book. Each chapter discusses a set of concepts or a system. **Within each chapter there are:**
    - The **Go To Clinical Cases**—read these and use **Prioritization Power** to complete the NurseThink® Time. These include: the **Top Three** Priority Data Collection or Cues, Priority Labs/Diagnostics, Priority Potential and Actual Complications, Priority Interventions, Priority Medications, Priority Nursing Implications, and Reinforcement of Priority Teaching.
- You can check your answers by looking at the related **Priority Exemplars**—the **Top Three** will designated by a 💡.
- Review the other **Priority Exemplars**. Consider the material you know and don't know. Try to come up with potential exam questions related to that material. Use **Priority Exemplars** as references as you work through the chapters.
- In addition, **Next Gen Clinical Judgment** Boxes and **Clinical Hints** will continue to enhance your decision-making skills.
- At the end of most chapters are **NurseThink® Quizzes.** Take the Quizzes, check your answers, and, for the ones that are incorrect, take a minute to determine what you don't know. This is where you can go back to the **Priority Exemplars** or your other resources to continue to grow your mastered content. Remember to use the E-3 strategy.
- Use the online quizzing and testing resources to continue to hone your skills, identify what you don't know, and direct your studies and ongoing NCLEX® preparation!

So, let's get started!

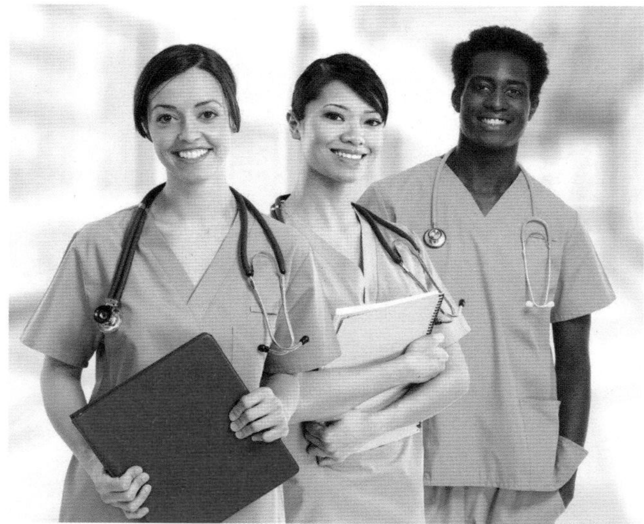

Image 4-2: Talk with your colleagues about how they plan to study. Are they studying alone or with others? Are they taking a review course? How might their thoughts and experiences influence your study plan?

SECTION 2

Priority Exemplars

CHAPTER

5

Sexuality

Reproduction / Sexuality

This chapter addresses pregnancy, labor, and delivery along with conditions that impair or interfere with sexuality and reproduction. Sexuality is a basic human trait and need. Reproduction is a routine process in which nurses support pregnancy, labor, and delivery.

Nurses play a significant role in reinforcing teaching and supporting clients during the reproductive cycle and in conditions that interfere or impair reproduction or sexual functioning.

Study Hint: (GTPAL)

- Gravida: # of pregnancies
- Para/Parity: # of pregnancies in which the fetus reaches 20 weeks of pregnancy
- Term pregnancy: 38 weeks or greater
- Preterm pregnancy: 20 weeks to 37 weeks
- Abortion/miscarriage: Stillborn
- Living: Living at time of birth

Priority Exemplars:

- Pregnancy
- Postpartum hemorrhage
- Abortion/miscarriage
- Breastfeeding
- Contraception
- Dystocia
- Erectile dysfunction
- Hypertensive disorders of pregnancy
- Newborn care
- Placental abruption
- Placenta previa
- Preterm labor
- Stages of labor
- STI: Chlamydia
- STI: Human papillomavirus
- STI: Syphilis

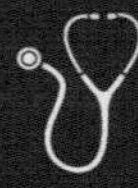

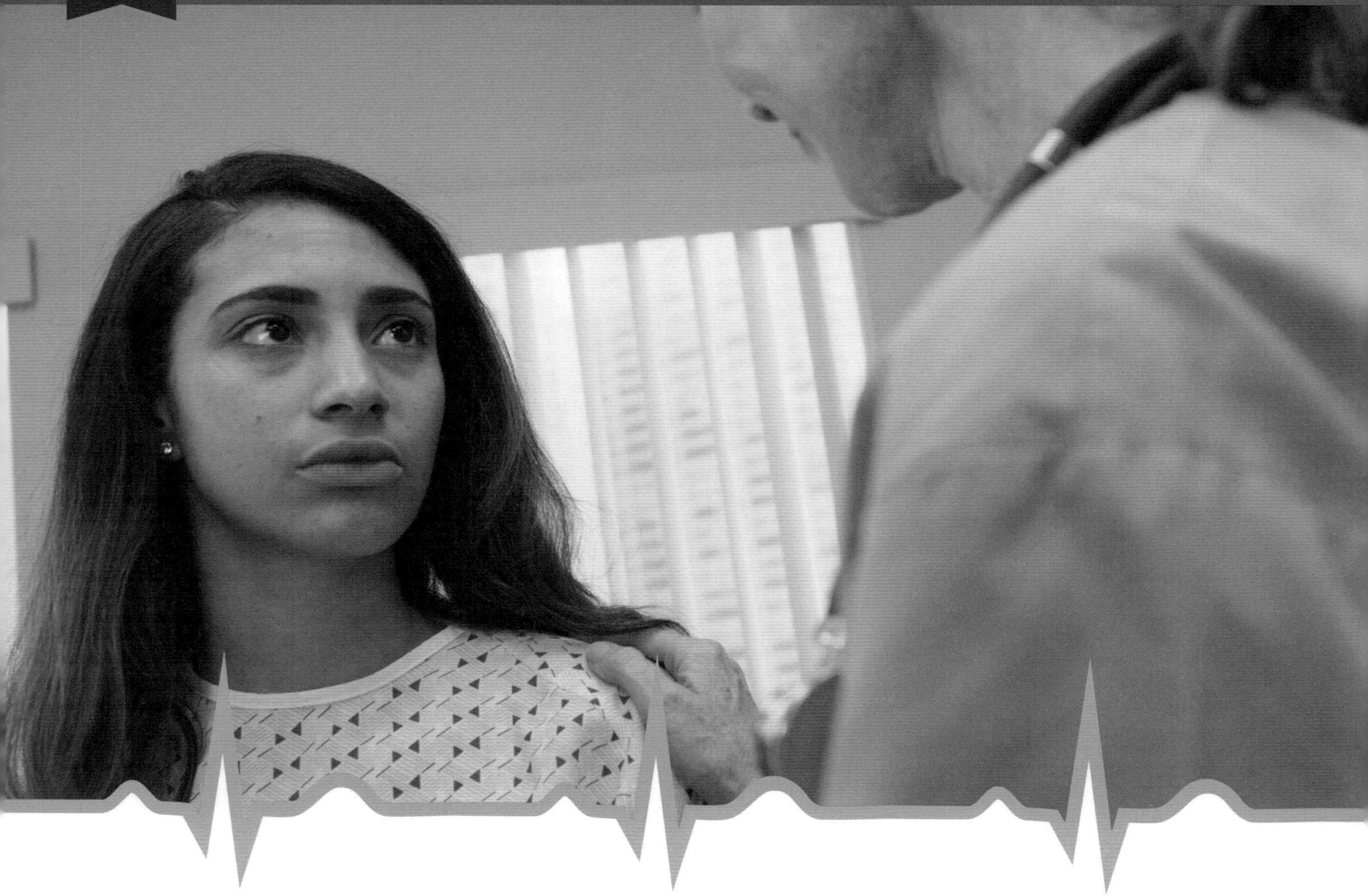

Go To Clinical

Go To Clinical Case 1

S.S. is a 20-year-old college student who is sexually active with her boyfriend of two years. S.S. uses an intrauterine device (IUD) for birth control; however, because she has been away at college, she missed her three-year replacement visit that was scheduled two months prior. S.S. is aware of the risk she is taking missing this appointment and tells her boyfriend, "I'll just get it replaced when we return home for Spring break; in the meantime, we just have to be careful and use condoms."

S.S. is now home visiting her obstetrician with complaints of fatigue, breast tenderness, and a missed menstrual cycle. The nurse cares for S.S. and suspects she may be pregnant.

NurseThink® Time

Using the NurseThink® system, complete the priorities. Check your answers designated by 💡 in the Pregnancy Priority Exemplar.

Clinical Hint

The pregnant woman's body goes through several physiological and psychological changes. These changes are necessary for nourishing and supporting the fetus and preparing the client for childbirth. Nurses must be aware and monitor how these changes will affect the client and their daily living.

NurseThink® Time

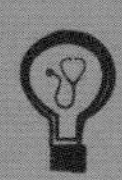

Priority Data Collection or Cues

1.

2.

3.

Priority Laboratory Tests/Diagnostics

1.

2.

3.

Priority Interventions or Actions

1.

2.

3.

Priority Potential & Actual Complications

1.

2.

3.

Priority Nursing Implications

1.

2.

3.

Priority Medications

1.

2.

3.

Reinforcement of Priority Teaching

1.

2.

3.

Pathophysiology/Description

- Described as gestation (approximately 280 days) from fertilization to implantation to birth
- Nagele's rule–subtract 3 months and add seven days to the first day of the last menstrual period–add one year-yields date of delivery

Priority Data Collection or Cues

- Pregnancy outcomes terminology
  - Gravidity–number of pregnancies (nulligravida-no pregnancies, multigravida-two or more pregnancies)
  - Parity–numbers of births (nullipara, primipara, multipara)
  - GTPAL–gravidity, term births, preterm births, abortions/miscarriages, living children
- Signs of pregnancy
  - Presumptive–amenorrhea, nausea/vomiting, breast changes, urinary frequency, quickening, fatigue, change in color of vaginal mucosa
  - Probable–uterine enlargement, Hegar's sign (softening of uterine segment), Goodell's sign (softening of cervix), Chadwick's sign (violet discoloration of the cervix), Ballottement (rebounding of uterus when fetus is unengaged), Braxton Hicks contractions, positive hCG
  - Positive–fetal heart tones, fetal movements, ultrasound confirmation
- Fundal height
  - From 18-30 weeks, fundal height = gestational age
- Maternal physical changes
  - Increase in circulating blood volume, physiological anemia of pregnancy, retention of sodium/water
  - Nausea and vomiting, constipation
  - Urinary frequency
  - Skin changes–linea nigra (dark line down abdomen), melasma (mask of pregnancy), striae gravidarum (stretch marks), vascular spider nevi, palmar erythema pruritis gravidarum
  - Increased lordosis, relaxed muscle tone, posture changes, carpal tunnel syndrome, tingling of hands and feet, diastasis recti abdominis (separation of abdominal muscles), syncope
  - Emotional changes–ambivalence, acceptance, emotional lability, body image changes, preparing emotionally for motherhood
- Collect data on the mother's history
  - Chronic or acute illness/disease and current health status (hypertension, diabetes, cardiac disease, asthma, rubella, other infections: STIs and HIV)
  - Examine family history
  - Examine reproductive history
  - Examine history of or risk for intimate partner violence
  - Look for substance use or abuse/cigarette smoking
  - Look for risk associated with age (< 18 years, > 35 years)
  - Ask about genetic issues
  - Check nutritional history
  - Check use of medications, herbal therapies, and complementary/alternative therapies

Priority Laboratory Tests/Diagnostics

- Pregnancy test for human chorionic gonadotropin (hCG)-appears 8-10 days after conception-via blood, urine, or home urine testing (variations in accuracy of home tests)
- Blood type and Rh factor
- Rubella titer
- Hemoglobin/hematocrit/complete blood count
- Pap smear
- Cultures for STIs (gonorrhea, syphilis, HPV, Chlamydia, trichomoniasis, herpes simplex, HIV)
- Sickle cell screening as indicated
- Tuberculosis screening
- Hepatitis B titer
- Urinalysis and urine culture
- Ultrasounds–gestational age, fetal outlines, amniotic fluid volume, multiple fetuses (abdominal or transvaginal)
- Biophysical profile–monitor fetal breathing movements, fetal movements, fetal tone, amniotic fluid volume, and fetal heart patterns
- Doppler blood flow analysis–blood flow in fetus, umbilical cord, and placenta
- Percutaneous umbilical blood sampling–needle aspiration of blood guided by ultrasound
- Alpha-fetoprotein screening–monitor for spina bifida and Down syndrome
- Lecithin-sphingomyelin (L/S ratio)–maturity of fetus
- DNA testing–monitor for genetic abnormalities
- Chorionic villi sampling–monitor for genetic abnormalities via villi in chorion
- Amniocentesis–aspiration of fluid between 15 and 20 weeks
- Kick counts–fetal movement counting and recording
- Fern test–microscopic slide test to ascertain if vaginal leakage is amniotic fluid
- Nitrazine test–look at pH of vaginal secretions–amniotic fluid is 7.0-7.5; vaginal secretions are 4.5-5.5
- Fetal-Fibronectin–cervical swab, identify risk for preterm labor
- Nonstress test–for fetal well-being, identify changes in heart rate as related to fetal movement
- Contraction stress test–for fetal well-being, monitor changes in heart rate as related contractions or simulated contractions
- Group B streptococcus–vaginal and rectal cultures at 35-37 weeks gestation
- Glucose tolerance test between 24-28 weeks gestation, or as indicated by the health care provider

Priority Interventions or Actions

- Establish health care provider visit schedule–every 4 weeks until 32 weeks, every 2 weeks until 36 weeks, every week until delivery

- Nausea and vomiting—most in first trimester, elevated hCG levels, eat dry crackers, small/frequent meals, drinking liquids apart from meals, if unmanageable-hyperemesis gravidarum-treated with intravenous fluids or total parenteral nutrition (antiemetics with caution)
- Supine hypotension—side sleeping and caution during examination, change positions slowly, ensure safety
- Breast discomfort—wear a supportive bra, wash nipples carefully
- Fatigue/backache—rest periods, regular exercise, yoga, optimal hydration and nutrition
- Heartburn—tailor sitting, upright after meals, small/frequent meals
- Ankle edema—elevate legs, supportive hose, ankle exercises, sleep on side
- Varicose veins—supportive hose, elevate legs, move/exercise often
- Headaches—drink water, change positions slowly, snacks, cool cloth
- Hemorrhoids/constipation—sitz baths, high fiber foods/water, exercise
- Leg cramps—increase calcium intake, regular exercise, dorsiflex foot
- Shortness of breath—rest, sleep with HOB elevated, pace activities
- Pica—eating non-food substances, may result in anemia, nutrition counseling
- Anemia—ensure prenatal vitamins and, if prescribed, iron supplementation, take with vitamin C, nutrition counseling

Priority Potential & Actual Complications

- Hypertensive disorders/gestational hypertension
- Abortion/miscarriage/fetal demise
- Gestational diabetes and DIC
- Infection-TORCH-monitor and manage
  - Toxoplasmosis
  - Other infections: HIV, HBV, STIs, Group B strep, pyelonephritis, UTI, tuberculosis
  - Rubella
  - Cytomegalovirus
  - Herpes simplex
- Ectopic pregnancy is implantation outside of uterus
- Hydatidiform mole is peripheral cells of fertilized ovum proliferate, may be benign or malignant-must be vacuum extracted, pregnancy not recommended for one year
- Incompetent cervix is treated with cervical cerclage

Priority Nursing Implications

- Offer counseling and support to the woman during pregnancy
- Provide sexuality counseling. Pregnancy does not limit intercourse but may require position or activity changes, pregnant women may have decreased desire or body image changes that warrant reinforcement of teaching and discussion
- Pregnancy can offer challenges for women who are obese with complications in pregnancy, delivery, post-delivery
- Observe and intervene related to the emotional tasks of pregnancy including transitioning to motherhood/parenthood/fatherhood, changes in family dynamics, and dealing with body image changes
- Attend to needs of non-pregnant partners/co-mothers
- Observe and intervene with extended family adaptation including siblings, grandparents, etc.
- Counsel mothers that the expected weight gain in pregnancy is 25-35 pounds, increase to 300 kcal/day during pregnancy (may be based on pre-pregnancy BMI)

Priority Medications

- Prenatal vitamins given orally
  - High iron may cause constipation
  - High in folic acid (preconceptual and prenatal recommended to prevent neural tube defects)
  - Taken throughout pregnancy and breastfeeding

Reinforcement of Priority Teaching

- The importance of nutrition and hydration during pregnancy—instruct to avoid high mercury fish (swordfish, tuna), raw or undercooked fish and meat (sushi), cold cuts, soft cheeses, raw eggs, uncooked batter (avoid salmonella, listeria)
- Expected physical and emotional changes of pregnancy, anticipatory guidance for pregnancy, labor, and delivery
- The prevention of urinary tract infections including fluid intake, frequent emptying of bladder, cranberry juice or capsules, Kegel exercises, hygiene
- Ensure attention to dental health including cleaning, examinations, and treatment, gingival health
- Explore birth plan and potential alternatives with client and family including caregivers (physician, midwife, doula) and setting (hospital, birth center, home)
- Exercise as tolerated. Mothers may continue exercises that they were accustomed to until later in pregnancy, now is not the time to start a new exercise regimen; stop exercise if feel shortness of breath, dizzy, numbness, contractions, or vaginal bleeding
- Counsel client on avoidance of alcohol, unprescribed medications, cigarettes, and caffeine

Go To Clinical Answers

Text designated by 💡 are the top answers for the Go To Clinical related to Pregnancy.

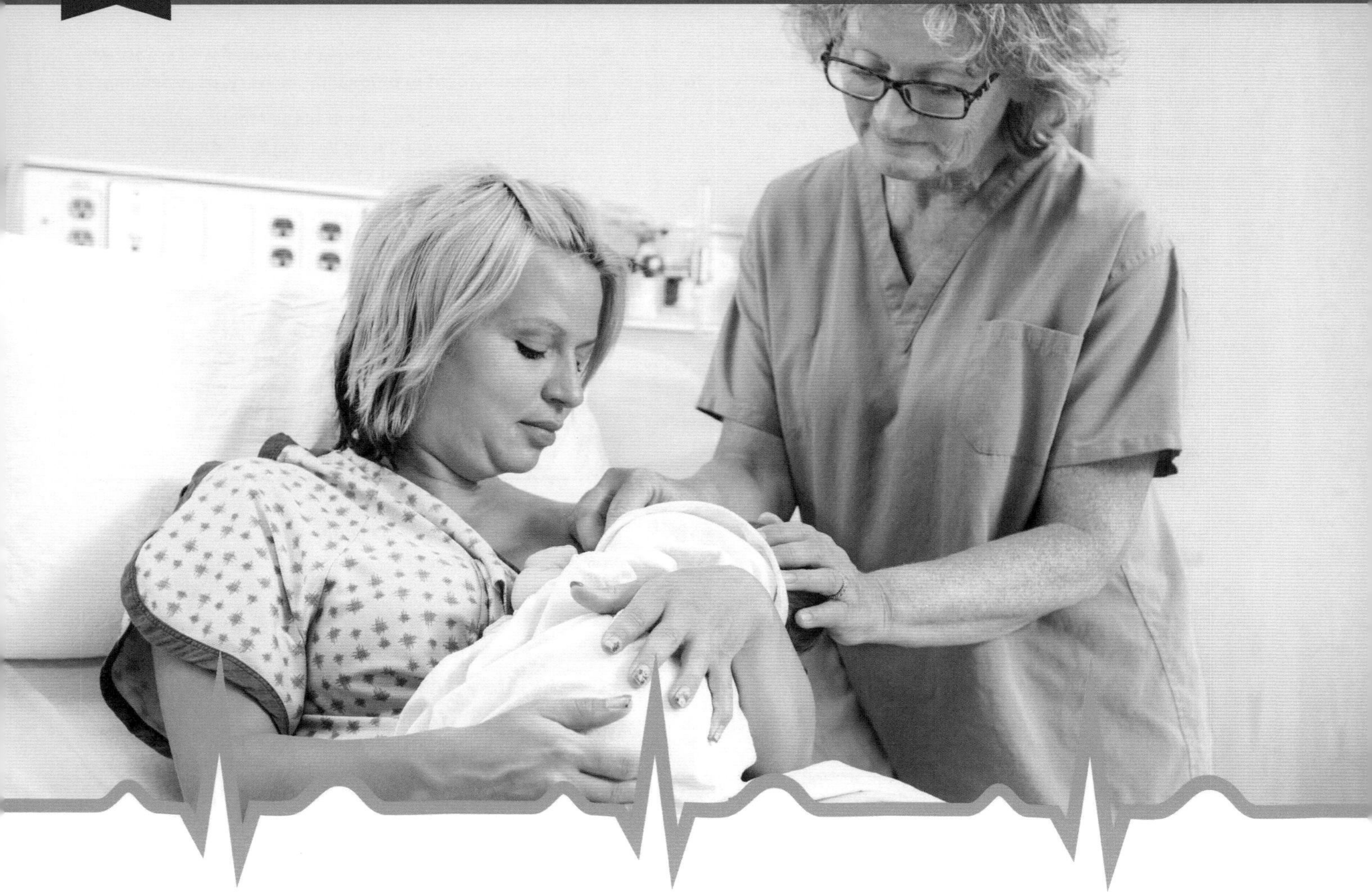

Go To Clinical Case 2

The nurse starting the evening shift cares for Mrs. A., a 26-year-old client, G1 P1, who delivered vaginally an 8lb 2oz (3685 gm) term male infant at 1630. Mrs. A had an uncomplicated pregnancy with forceps delivery. The off-going shift reported that Mrs. A. voided during delivery and has not been up to the restroom. Ibuprofen 600 mg was given p.o. 45 minutes prior for abdominal cramping, and at this time her perineal pad was changed. Heavy lochia rubria noted with small clots. Vital signs taken 20 minutes prior to your arrival revealed pulse 86 beats/minute; blood pressure 120/76 mmHg; respiratory rate 22 breaths/minute; temperature 98.1°F (36.7°C); oxygen saturation on room air 97%.

When the nurse arrives in the room to greet Mrs. A., she is in pain, rating her pain a 7 on a 0-10 pain scale. She states, "I don't feel well." The nurse proceeds to check Mrs. A's abdomen and notes the hospital gown, bed linens, and perineal pad are saturated with blood. The fundus is boggy at 3 cm above the umbilicus. What is the nurse priority nursing actions?

Next Gen Clinical Judgment

Use 10 words to describe how a client would look if they lost a significant amount of blood.

NurseThink® Time

Using the NurseThink® system, complete the priorities. Check your answers designated by in the Postpartum hemorrhage Priority Exemplar.

NurseThink® Time

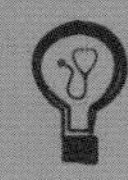

Priority Data Collection or Cues

1.

2.

3.

Priority Laboratory Tests/Diagnostics

1.

2.

3.

Priority Interventions or Actions

1.

2.

3.

Priority Potential & Actual Complications

1.

2.

3.

Priority Nursing Implications

1.

2.

3.

Priority Medications

1.

2.

3.

Reinforcement of Priority Teaching

1.

2.

3.

Postpartum hemorrhage

Pathophysiology/Description

- Leading cause of morbidity and mortality in US and worldwide
- Bleeding of 500 mL or more post-vaginal delivery or 1000 mL or more after a C-section
- May occur as early hemorrhage (first 24 hours) or late hemorrhage (after 24 hours to 6 weeks)
- May be caused by uterine atony, lacerations of the cervix or vagina, retained portions of the placenta, or rupture of hematomas
- Risk factors include history of previous hemorrhage after birth; placental abruption; placenta previa; prolapsed uterus related to multiparity birth, large baby, or polyhydramnios; dystocia or prolonged labor; oxytocin induction or augmentation; administration of magnesium sulfate; operative/invasive delivery; or infections

Priority Data Collection or Cues

- Monitor vital signs. Attend to blood pressure and heart rate
- Monitor perfusion including skin temperature, capillary refill, peripheral pulses, motor/sensory function, and pallor
- Observe for bleeding including source (lacerations, hematomas, or episiotomy), pattern, amount, perineal pad count/weight, watch for and count clots, duration, color (dark red-venous; bright red-arterial/lacerations), and consistency
- Observe for signs of hypotension including restlessness, tachycardia, tachypnea, hypotension, cool/clammy skin, pale or grey skin color
- Monitor for complaints of dizziness, weakness or dyspnea
- Evaluate contractability of uterus (hypotonic/boggy)
- Examine fundal height, firmness, and position
- Monitor bladder for distension

Priority Laboratory Tests/Diagnostics

- CBC—Hemoglobin or hematocrit levels
- Ultrasound of uterus for retained placenta
- Blood type and screen
- Coagulation studies/platelet counts

Priority Interventions or Actions

- Ensure safety precautions and reinforce bedrest
- If lack of uterine tone, gently massage fundus, encourage client to empty her bladder if condition warrants. Health care provider may do bimanual compression, put baby to breast
- Insert a urinary catheter to check renal perfusion and output and empty bladder
- Administer oxygen-non-rebreather 8-10 L/min, monitor pulse ox
- Assist in accessing two intravenous sites and provide fluids, bolus, or transfuse as prescribed (PRBCs preferred)
- Prepare for surgery as indicated-surgical or bedside repair
- If indicated, critical care monitoring and hemodynamic monitoring

Priority Potential & Actual Complications

- Hypovolemic shock/hemorrhagic shock
- Acidosis
- Uterine inversion
- Disseminated intravascular coagulation
- May be fatal

Priority Nursing Implications

- Provide support to client and family with care of critically ill client
- Ensure maternal contact with infant as able
- Consider interventions to address interruption in infant/maternal bonding

Priority Medications

- Oxytocin given intravenous
  - To decrease bleeding
  - 10-40 units/1000 mL lactated ringers or normal saline solution
  - Increases tone of uterus to decrease bleeding
- Prostaglandins
  - To decrease bleeding
  - Misoprostol-per rectum, sublingual, or oral
  - 15-methyl prostaglandin F2 alpha
    - Intramuscular injection
    - Contraindicated with asthma and hypertension
  - Prostaglandin E2–oral or per rectum
- Methylergonovine
  - Intramuscular uterine stimulant
  - Contraindicated with hypertension

Reinforcement of Priority Teaching

- Increased importance of rest in mother after blood loss-superimposed on care of infant/assistance with baby care
- High iron diet to include green, leafy vegetables, meats, and supplements as prescribed
- With lacerations and while on iron prevent constipation, encourage fluids and high fiber diet
- May have difficulty with delays in breastfeeding, refer to lactation counselor

Go To Clinical Answers

Text designated by ● are the top answers for the Go To Clinical related to Postpartum hemorrhage.

Abortion/miscarriage

Pathophysiology/Description

- Spontaneous loss of products of conception prior to period of viability, defined as before 20 weeks gestation (also called miscarriage)
- About 10-20% of pregnancies end in miscarriage, 80% before 12 weeks
- Spontaneous abortions in the first 12 weeks are thought to be related to chromosomal abnormalities, endocrine/thyroid deficiencies, varicella exposure/contraction, genetic factors, type 1 diabetes, systemic conditions (lupus)
- Spontaneous abortions 12-20 weeks (second-trimester loss) are more common in mothers <18 or >40 years or with poor outcomes from previous pregnancies, or related to diet, obesity, alcohol/caffeine consumption
- Differentiated as:
    - Induced—therapeutic or elective ending of pregnancy
    - Spontaneous—occurring by natural causes
    - Threatened—spotting or cramping without cervical changes
    - Inevitable—spotting or cramping and cervix begins to dilate and efface
    - Incomplete—loss of some products of conception, some (usually the placenta) is retained
    - Complete—loss of all products of conception
    - Missed—products of conception retained in the uterus after fetal demise
    - Recurrent/habitual—3 or more pregnancy losses at < 20 weeks gestation in successive pregnancies
    - Septic—spontaneous abortion with infected products of conception

Priority Data Collection or Cues

- Monitor vital signs—focusing on heart rate and blood pressure/related to blood loss
- Observe for bleeding—history, amount, pad count, clots, tissue
- Monitor pain—cramping, lower abdominal pain
- Monitor woman's emotional state, support systems, coping abilities, screen for depression

Priority Laboratory Tests/Diagnostics

- Pregnancy test—hCG—human chorionic gonadotropin to confirm pregnancy/maintained pregnancy along with progesterone levels
- Complete blood count—monitor hemoglobin and hematocrit following blood loss and look for infection
- Ultrasound (abdominal or transvaginal) of uterus to detect contents
- Genetic evaluation of clients with recurrent miscarriages

Priority Interventions or Actions

- Maintain bedrest
- Monitor for bleeding including patterns, amount, pad count, clot count, weigh pads as per agency policy
- Monitor cramps
- Observe for hemorrhage
- If inpatient, save tissue and clots for health care provider observation and to allow mother the option of viewing remains
- Ensure intravenous access, administer prescribed fluids and blood products
- Prepare for dilation and curettage/suction curettage if suspected to be an incomplete abortion
- Administer Rho (D) immune globulin if client is Rh-negative
- Prophylactic cerclage of the cervix may be done if cause is cervical insufficiency

Priority Potential & Actual Complications

- Incomplete abortions without procedure include infection, sepsis
- Emotional and relational implications include depression and anxiety

Priority Nursing Implications

- Clients often report that at less than six weeks pregnancy, the miscarriage may feel like a period. From 6-12 weeks clients report some discomfort along with more substantial blood loss. Greater than 12 weeks, clients usually report severe pain/cramping along with substantial blood loss
- Monitor for risk factors and assist with potential identification of future prevention efforts
- Provide emotional support and assist with potential guilt, depression and anger felt by the client

Priority Medications

- Misoprostol given orally, sublingual, vaginal
    - To medically ensure complete miscarriage if incomplete
    - Side effects include nausea, vomiting, diarrhea
- Oxytocin given intravenous
    - Administered post-curettage to prevent hemorrhage

Reinforcement of Priority Teaching

- Rest after miscarriage
- Avoid tampons, sexual intercourse, or douching for two weeks
- Ensure follow-up with health care provider for birth control, timing of subsequent pregnancies, and importance of prenatal care
- Refer for potential underlying health issues
- Ensure emotional needs of client and family are addressed to refer support groups and/or counseling

Breastfeeding

Pathophysiology/Description

- Benefits of breastfeeding including physical and psychological health advantages for mother and baby, convenience, along with economic and environmental advantages
- Preferred method of nutrition, in accordance with the wishes and abilities of the mother, for the first six months of life

Priority Data Collection or Cues

- Check mother's level of knowledge about breastfeeding
- Check mother's comfort level with breastfeeding and support from others, including partner and family
- While observing breastfeeding, observe the ability of the infant to latch on to the nipple on both breasts, the sucking and swallowing sequence, the optimal position for the mother to hold the infant during feeding, the condition of the nipple and surrounding tissue after feeding, and the mother's expressed comfort and satisfaction with each feeding
- Monitor infant weight gain
- Monitor infant color for physiological jaundice

Priority Interventions or Actions

- Put the baby to breast as soon as stable, preferably in the delivery room
- Provide hygiene care and instruct mothers on breast hygiene
- Provide support and coaching during each of the early feedings, referral to a lactation counselor for every breastfeeding mother is encouraged
- Encourage feeding on each side for 15-20 minutes and to begin each feeding on the side last nursed upon. Mothers often develop creative ways to remember this, including double breast pads on the last used side, hair elastics on the wrist of the side last used, etc
- Encourage use of breast pads to deal with leaking between feedings
- Reinforce education and support for minor and major issues with breastfeeding
- Recommend to mothers methods to encourage latching on: Brush lower lip with nipple, stimulate the lips to open the mouth wide, release suction by placing a clean finger into the infant's mouth or pull down on the infant's chin
- Seek out health care provider's views on vitamin D supplementation for exclusively breastfed infants
- Ensure iron supplementation for exclusively breastfed infants as iron stores are depleted around 4 months

Priority Potential & Actual Complications

- To treat breast engorgement between feedings, use ice packs or chilled cabbage leaves, manually express milk. Immediately before feedings, use warm soaks or a warm shower to encourage let-down during the early days of feeding
- For cracked nipples, leave nipples open to air between feedings, rub nipples with dry washcloth to toughen nipples, ensure that the infant latches onto entire areola of breast and not just nipple, ensure that the mother rotates breast and limits time on each side, and use lanolin cream as needed
- For inverted or flattened nipples, use breast shields

Priority Nursing Implications

- Encourage breastfeeding moms to wear supportive bras (without underwires) after delivery and throughout breastfeeding, even when sleeping
- Notify moms about the potential for uterine cramping during early breastfeedings
- Encourage mothers to observe foods which the infant may not tolerate in breastmilk including strawberries, caffeine, brussels sprouts, chocolate, cauliflower, onions, garlic, etc.
- Encourage mothers to avoid over-the-counter, other medications, and alcohol unless approved by health care provider

Reinforcement of Priority Teaching

- Discuss nutrition and hydration—breastfeeding women should increase intake of water/fluids, continue prenatal vitamins, and consume about 300-500 more calories/day
- Value of handwashing to prevent infection transmission
- Encourage mothers to burp the infant after each breast
- Role of the partner/co-parent/parent to change diapers, burp, console, and cuddle with infant before and after feedings
- Inform client/parents that infants who breastfeed often have loose, frequent, yellow, seedy stools
- Assist client, infant, and family to develop a feeding schedule
- Provide mother with information and reinforcement of teaching on breastmilk pumping and storage, many insurance companies provide breast pumps
- Reinforce feeding readiness cues and means to deal with a fussy or sleepy baby or nursing multiple infants
- Explain to the mother symptoms of and means to prevent plugged milk ducts and mastitis
- Provide access to breastfeeding support groups in the community

Pathophysiology/Description

- Many contraceptive methods are available to clients who choose to prevent or delay childbearing. Cultural, religious, and personal preferences will influence method choice
- Methods are largely described as barrier methods (may be used by women and men) and hormonal methods (largely used by women)
- Contraceptive methods vary in effectiveness, cost, reversibility, effort needed, and use of hormones
- Contraceptive methods require varying levels of capacity for adherence to a schedule, association with sexual activity, participation of sexual partners, ability for discretion, and comfort with body
- Male and female condoms, along with the use of barrier dental dams, are able to prevent exposure to sexually transmitted infections
- Cost may be a factor for some clients
- Hormonal contraceptives may be indicated to treat menstrual irregularities

Priority Data Collection or Cues

- Monitor blood pressure (hormonal methods are contraindicated/used cautiously with hypertension)
- Monitor client's weight (some methods contraindicated with obesity)
- Check desire to prevent pregnancy, level of motivation, and knowledge level
- Examine health status and presence of pre-existing conditions, including thromboembolic disease, history of estrogen feeding cancers, hypertension, cardiac disease, and pregnancy, that contraindicate some hormonal contraceptives
- Determine woman's lifestyle, habits, and risk behaviors, including tobacco smoking and multiple sexual partners
- Consider client's current medications (antibiotics may decrease the effectiveness of oral contraceptives, hormonal methods may interact with anticoagulants)

Priority Laboratory Tests/Diagnostics

- Screen for sexually transmitted infections based on age, symptoms, risk factors, and sexual history

Priority Interventions or Actions

- Many health care providers now prescribe oral and injectable contraception without a vaginal examination, but clients are encouraged to have routine screenings, including clinical breast examinations, based on age, health history, and risk factors
- Nursing interventions with contraception focus on reinforcing teaching about self-administration, side effects, adverse reactions, and when to consult health care providers

Priority Potential & Actual Complications

- Clients with a latex allergy may react to latex condoms
- Complications differ based on method (intrauterine devices complications may include ectopic pregnancy, uterine perforation) and implanted contraceptive rods may migrate
- Complications differ based on client health history (oral contraceptives may increase blood glucose levels in clients with type 1 diabetes)
- Non-barrier methods increase the risk for sexually transmitted infections

Priority Nursing Implications

- Nurses need to ensure that contraceptive methods match the client's needs and that the client is able to safely adhere to the method or medication regimen
- Assist client to develop methods for reminders (phone alarm for daily pills, calendar for injection every 3 months, etc.)
- Need to ensure client's knowledge of, comfort level with, and ability to access a birth control method
- Ensure that the method's effectiveness coincides with client's desire to prevent pregnancy and sexually transmitted infections
- Encourage clients using hormonal methods to wear condoms with all sexual activity
- Observe each client for potential birth control sabotage, reproductive coercion, or intimate partner violence

Reinforcement of Priority Teaching

- Ensure that clients are aware that they need to use back up contraception during initial period of starting contraception
- Explain to clients what to do if a pill or injection is missed (depends upon method) and to use backup method of contraception until birth control levels are re-established
- Conduct self-breast exams monthly
- Make sure clients are aware of need to have blood pressure assessed and for follow-up
- Instruct client on method-specific recommendations related to cessation of method if they desire to become pregnant (for example, the client is recommended to be off of oral contraceptives for one to two months prior to attempting to become pregnant)

Next Gen Clinical Judgment

A client presents to the clinic indecisive on whether to use an oral contraceptive or an intrauterine device (IUD) to prevent pregnancy. What priority measures can the nurse take in helping the client decide the best option?

Dystocia

Pathophysiology/Description

- Dysfunctional, long, difficult, or abnormal labor
- Lack of progress of dilation, descent, and/or expulsion
    - 8-11% of labors, it is most common indication for C-section
- Related to alterations in function or parts of the birth process

1. Powers-ineffective contractions, pushing, or bearing down
    - Maternal fatigue or dehydration
    - Epidural or early analgesia
    - Overstimulation of uterus, uterine dysfunction, hypotonic (short, irregular, weak) or hypertonic (painful, frequent, and uncoordinated) uterine contractions
2. Passage-pelvis/soft tissue obstruction
    - Cephalopelvic disproportion
    - Fetopelvic dystocia
3. Passenger
    - Size, presentation
    - Multiparity
4. Position
    - Maternal body position during labor
    - Restriction of normal activity
5. Psychological
    - Negative past experiences and fear inhibit progress in labor
    - Childbirth preparation and support may allow childbirth to progress more quickly

- Risk factors include obesity, short stature, previous dystocia, malpresentation, malposition, advanced maternal age, infertility

Priority Data Collection or Cues

- Monitor vital signs for maternal tachycardia, monitor maternal temperature
- Monitor fetal heart tones for fetal tachycardia and response to contractions and progress of labor
- Assist in examining for cervical effacement and dilation
- Monitor contraction patterns
- Determine Bishop score which is maternal readiness for labor/induction, (dilation of cervix, effacement of cervix, consistency of cervix, position of cervix, and station of presenting part—each of 5 parameters are scored 0-3, 6 or more is readiness for labor induction)
- Monitor fetal position and presentation
- Assist in checking intactness of amniotic membranes
- Monitor for risk for dystocia throughout labor
- Monitor maternal pain level and effectiveness of management strategies

Priority Laboratory Tests/Diagnostics

- Ultrasound
- Nonstress tests to ensure fetal well-being

Priority Interventions or Actions

- Encourage maternal rest between contractions to ensure energy to deal with labor, provide comfort measures, back rubs, position changes, and encourage ambulation and frequent voiding
- Assist mother in learning breathing and relaxation strategies
- Pain relief may allow client to deal with contractions and allow labor to progress
- Administer prophylactic antibiotics as prescribed
- Administer fluids as prescribed, monitor intake and output
- Monitor color of amniotic fluid
- Monitor for prolapse of cord after membranes break or are ruptured
- Internal or external version to turn a fetus in breech or shoulder presentation
- Cervical ripening
    - Chemical agents
    - Physical and mechanical methods-balloon catheter, hydroscopic dilators, amniotic membrane sweeping
    - Other methods-intercourse, nipple stimulation, walking
- Amniotomy—rupture of membranes
- Episiotomy—incision of posterior vagina/perineum
- Forceps assisted birth or vacuum assisted birth
- Cesarean birth with spinal, epidural, or general anesthesia

Priority Potential & Actual Complications

- Maternal dehydration and infection
- Fetal hypoxia, injury, asphyxia, or demise
- Post-vaginal delivery complications: infection, hemorrhage
- C-section complications include anesthesia reactions, hemorrhage, bowel/bladder injury, aspiration pneumonia, drug reaction, air embolism, amniotic embolism, urinary tract infections, wound hematoma/infection, dehiscence, bowel dysfunction, venous thrombosis. For the neonate, tachypnea, asphyxia, injuries, prematurity
- Complications associated with procedures (forceps, etc.)

Priority Nursing Implications

- Continually monitor mother's comfort, fetal heart tones, and mother's vital signs in response to procedures
- For mothers who are Rh-negative, prepare to administer Rho (D) immune globulin

Reinforcement of Priority Teaching

- Assist client and family/partners to review and debrief birth process, although it may not have replicated the birth plan
- Ensure that client gets the rest needed to heal and provide mothering, feeding, and affection to infant

Erectile dysfunction (ED)

Pathophysiology/Description

- Inability to attain and/or sustain an erection to engage in satisfying sexual activity
- More than 10 million men affected, 50% of men 40-70 years have some level of ED
- Lack of blood flow (vascular impairment) associated with ED
- May be from primary or secondary causations including recreational drug use, alcohol use, smoking, illnesses, or medications (antihypertensives, antilipemics, sedatives, others)
- Causes may also include vascular (hypertension, peripheral vascular disease), endocrine (diabetes, obesity, reduced testosterone level), genitourinary (prostatitis, renal failure, history of a radical prostatectomy), neurological (Parkinson's, stroke, trauma/spinal cord injury, tumors), psychological (depression, stress, fear/anxiety)
- May occur at any age, more prevalent as men age

Priority Data Collection or Cues

- Ask client about ability to attain and sustain an erection
- Ask about frequency and onset and may be episodic, may be gradual onset (illness/medications), or may occur suddenly (fear, anxiety, or emotionally related)
- Ask about emotional impact of ED on intimate relationships
- Assist in collecting data on medical, sexual, and psychosocial aspects of the client; screening may include erectile function, orgasmic function, sexual desire, intercourse satisfaction, and overall satisfaction with sexual experiences
- Examine genitalia for lesions, masses, changes in structure

Priority Laboratory Tests/Diagnostics

- Medical history profile to include serum glucose, lipid profile, complete blood count
- Hormone levels (testosterone, prolactin, luteinizing hormone, thyroid hormone)
- Prostate specific antigen levels
- Non-invasive testing include nocturnal penile tumescence/ rigidity testing, penile blood flow/angiography, and ultrasound

Priority Interventions or Actions

- Address causative factors that are modifiable-change medications, manage illnesses, counseling
- Medications are the most common treatment
- Penile implants
- Intraurethral medication pellets
- Intracavernosal self-injection
- Sexual counseling

Priority Potential & Actual Complications

- Sexual dysfunction
- Impaired relationships
- Mental health issues-stress, depression
- Use of erectogenics with nitrates may cause hemodynamically significant hypotension/bradycardia, cardiopulmonary arrest

Priority Nursing Implications

- Ensure that clients have realistic expectations of treatment–if sensation or function were absent, ejaculation or tactile sensation may not be resumed
- Ensure client safety related to hypotension/dizziness with first doses of medication
- Ask all clients with chest pain about use of erectogenic medications

Priority Medications

- Sildenafil/ tadalafil/ vardenafil given orally
  - Relaxes smooth muscle and increases blood flow/ erectogenic
  - Take 30-60 minutes before anticipated intercourse
  - Do not take more than once per day
  - Potentiates hypotension with nitrates–should not be used with nitroglycerin
  - Side effects include headache, flushing, GI upset, and nasal congestion
  - Tadalafil may be safer with clients with cardiac history
  - All erectogenic drugs may cause priapism (sustained erection for 4 hours or more) and require medical attention
  - Alcohol should be avoided–increases hypotension

Reinforcement of Priority Teaching

- Safe administration and use of erectogenic medications
- Refer clients for assistance with sexual communication with partners and counseling for clients and partners

Clinical Hint

Vardenafil, tadalafil, and avanafil are PDE-5 inhibitors used to treat ED and should not be mixed with nitrates such as nitroglycerin.

Hypertensive disorders of pregnancy

Pathophysiology/Description

- Hypertension occurs in 5-10% of all pregnancies
  - Gestational hypertension is defined as increased blood pressure without proteinuria after 20 weeks gestation; BP >140/90 mmHg, 2 readings 4 hours apart, generally resolves within 12 weeks postpartum
  - Preeclampsia (pregnancy-induced hypertension—PIH) is hypertension after 20 weeks gestation, may or may not include proteinuria. Clients may have no previous history of hypertension and may occur postpartum. May include thrombocytopenia, liver dysfunction, renal insufficiency, pulmonary edema, and cerebral or visual changes
  - Eclampsia is seizures and/or coma not due to other causes
  - Chronic hypertension is when hypertension exists before pregnancy
  - Superimposed preeclampsia is chronic hypertension with preeclampsia
- Pathophysiology includes changes in placental perfusion, vasospasm, decreased liver and kidney perfusion, cerebral edema, central nervous system irritability
- Major cause of morbidity and mortality by uteroplacental insufficiency and preterm birth
- Risk factors include primipara, < 19 or > 40 years, preeclampsia in previous pregnancy, African American descent, multifetal gestation, maternal infection, pre-exsisting chronic hypertension, renal disorders, diabetes mellitus, obesity, connective tissue disorders/systemic lupus erythematosus, chronic hypertension increases risk of eclampsia, pregnancy onset of snoring

Priority Data Collection or Cues

- Monitor blood pressure, compare to baseline values. BP 30 mmHg over systolic or diastolic baseline are diagnostic for preeclampsia
- Ask about symptoms: Headache, epigastric pain, visual changes (scotoma, photophobia, double vision), dizziness

Priority Laboratory Tests/Diagnostics

- 24-hour urine collection for protein most accurate data collection. Value > 300 mg in 24 hours contributes to diagnosis
- Urine dipstick of +1 protein also noted (may be less reliable)
- Platelets < 100,000/mm^3
- Liver enzymes may be twice normal value
- Serum creatinine > 1.1 mg/dL or doubling of the normal serum creatinine, prolonged creatinine clearance

Priority Interventions or Actions

- Prevention for high-risk clients includes low dose aspirin therapy
- All clients: Monitor blood pressure and for seizures
- Maintain a restful and calming environment
- Preeclampsia
  - Monitor fetal and maternal health status—fetal monitoring
  - Look for growth restriction
  - <37 weeks and a BP <160/110—mother and fetus are monitored and mother kept on bed rest
  - > 37 weeks—vaginal induction/cervical ripening
- Chronic hypertension/gestational hypertension
  - Administer medications to decrease blood pressure (Methyldopa—safest with breastfeeding)
- Eclampsia
  - Observe for warning symptoms-headache, blurred vision, epigastric/right upper quadrant pain, changes in level of consciousness
  - Seizures or convulsions
    - Stay with client/call for help
    - Monitor fetal heart tones/heart rate patterns as able
    - Raise and pad side rails
    - Maintain a patent airway-turn and position, prevent aspiration
    - Monitor pulse oximetry, oxygen by mask as able/needed
    - Monitor blood pressure
    - Monitor and document seizure (tonic/clonic) and other signs
    - Maintain intravenous access with a large-bore needle
    - Administer magnesium sulfate
    - Prepare for delivery as indicated
  - After seizure
    - Look for hypotension, halted respirations, twitching, amnesia, post-ictal sleep, and potential for falls after sleep
    - Monitor for stability
    - Monitor fetal heart tones/uterine activity/cervical status
    - Prepare for delivery as indicated

Clinical Hint

HELLP syndrome can be a serious complication of gestational hypertension. HELLP: hemolysis resulting in anemia and jaundice; elevated liver enzymes; and low platelets. HELLP is diagnosed through laboratory tests.

Priority Potential & Actual Complications

- Severe hypertension
- Eclampsia
- Pulmonary edema
- Fetal demise/decline
- Placental abruption
- Disseminated intravascular coagulation (DIC)
- Stroke

Priority Nursing Implications

- Assist the client in dealing with the stress of pregnancy and high-risk status, may feel guilt over lifestyle issues, negative outcomes, or fear related to outcomes
- Create a non-stimulating/low-stress environment—lower lights, maintain quiet, keep away from high activity on the unit or at home
- Observe for risk of seizures. Maintain seizure precautions including suction and oxygen at bedside, padded side rails, call button available
- Have emergency medication and emergency birth pack available

Priority Medications

- Betamethasone
  - Steroid to mature fetal lungs in the event of an emergency or early delivery
  - Given IM every 24 hours times two
  - Works 24 hours after first dose for 7 days
- Nifedipine–given orally
  - Calcium channel blocker/antihypertensive
  - To decrease blood pressure
  - Avoid with magnesium sulfate
  - May cause a headache, flushing of skin, may slow or interfere with labor
  - Must be delivered slowly
- Methyldopa–given orally
  - Antihypertensive
  - To decrease blood pressure
  - Watch for CNS sedation
  - May cause drug-induced fever
  - Monitor fetal heart rate
- Magnesium sulfate
  - Magnesium supplement/prevent seizures
  - Intravenous piggyback via intravenous pump
  - IM avoided due to pain or give with anesthetic
  - Monitor serum magnesium levels (toxic level will be greater than 4 mEq/L)
  - Watch for magnesium toxicity/serum hypermagnesemia. Signs include absence of patellar deep tendon reflexes, decreased level of consciousness, low urine output, bradypnea, and cardiac dysrhythmias
  - Antidote for hypermagnesemia is calcium gluconate
  - May be given for 24-48 hours postpartum

Reinforcement of Priority Teaching

- Home management for hypertension (BP > 150/100) as long as no protein in urine, normal platelets, normal liver enzymes
- BP and urine monitoring
- When to call the health care provider; symptoms to report, and routine appointments
- Tracking of fetal activity by monitoring daily fetal movement count-kick counts
  - Maintain partial bed rest, means to avoid venous thrombosis, and types of gentle exercise
  - Diversional activities, maintaining calm, and stress management
  - Encourage side-lying position
  - Diet should be regular with increased water and fiber, decreased caffeine, decreased sodium, and no tobacco or alcohol
- Blood pressure management and lifestyle patterns that may contribute to preeclampsia, chronic/gestational/ superimposed hypertension, and eclampsia

Next Gen Clinical Judgment

Compare and contrast treatment options for the client with gestational hypertension, chronic hypertension, preeclampsia, and eclampsia.

Clinical Hint

Women who develop preeclampsia during pregnancy can be at increased risk of developing cardiovascular disease later in life; therefore, nurses must stress the importance of regular healthcare visits.

Pathophysiology/Description

- Newborn/neonatal period is initial birth to one month of age
- Care of the newborn includes data collection and assisting with adaptation to extrauterine environment

Priority Data Collection or Cues

- Observe for spontaneous respirations and describe cry (lusty, high-pitched, weak)
- Check, Apgar score, which is a 10 point scale, each of 5 criteria given a 0, 1, or 2—at 1 and 5 minutes (10 minutes if score indicates)
    - Heart rate
    - Respiratory rate and effort
    - Muscle tone
    - Reflex irritability
    - Skin color
- Observe general appearance including respiratory effort and for signs of distress, overt anomalies or trauma, level of alertness
- Monitor vital signs(axillary temperature), body weight, length, and head circumference
- Assist with Ballard scale for gestational data collection based on neuromuscular maturity (posture, range of motion, recoil, limberness) and physical maturity (breast, genitalia, palmar wrinkling, lanugo, ear mobility, eye opening)
- Observe for periods of reactivity at birth to 30 minutes and 2 to 8 hours after birth (between a period of decreased responsiveness/sleep)
- Assist with physical data collection
    - Examine head—sutures, fontanels, molding, masses (caput succedaneum, cephalohematoma), subgaleal hemorrhage
    - Eyes—symmetry, pupils, tracking
    - Ears—symmetry, height compared to eyes
    - Mouth—intactness of soft and hard palates, tongue (connection), ability to suck/gag/swallow
    - Neck—range of motion, midline, torticollis (contraction of one side)
    - Chest—respiratory effort, adaptation to extrauterine environment, patency of nares (newborns breathe mostly through the nose), coughing and sneezing to clear airway, symmetry of thorax/barrel chest, nipples, clavicles for fractures; infant heart sounds
    - Skin—vernix caseosa (cheese-like substance), lanugo (downy hair), milia (small pustules), peeling skin, skin turgor, color (central cyanosis, acrocyanosis, plethoric [deep red color]), lesions, bruising, petechiae, birthmarks, Mongolian spots, nevus vasculosus [strawberry mark], nevus flammeus [port-wine stain], telangiectatic nevi [stork bites], forceps or vacuum marks, Harlequin sign (transient unilateral erythema of newborn, usually benign)
- Check for jaundice/bilirubin (normal < 5.2 mg/dL)
    - Physiological in 60% of newborns
    - Pathological appears within the first 24 hours and requires treatment, if untreated can lead to kernicterus/acute encephalopathy
    - Breastfeeding 2-5 days, related to low milk supply, encourage frequent feeding
    - Breastmilk 5-10 days
    - Measured by transcutaneous bilirubinometers/serum levels
    - Treatment with phototherapy beds or lights (values at which treatment is initiated vary)
- Abdomen—examine umbilical cord (3 vessels—2 arteries, one vein), bleeding, cord site for infection, umbilical hernia, symmetry, bowel sounds, distention
- Genital/Anus—observe patency of anus, labia (pseudomenstruation, smegma), penis/scrotum: placement of meatus (hypospadius, epispadius), for hernia, descent of testes, for void of urine in first 24 hours (uric acid crystals may produce a rust colored urine), for meconium (black/green jelly-like pasty stool)
- Spine—examine tone (hypotonicity/hypertonicity), hair tufts or dimples, neonates should have some head control, movement of all extremities
- Hips—for developmental dysplasia of the hip (no clicks when abducting hips)
- Monitor for hypoglycemia—jitteriness, tremors—treat/prevent with early feeding
- Reflexes
    - Sucking/rooting
    - Swallowing
    - Tonic neck/fencing
    - Palmar/plantar grasp
    - Moro
    - Startle
    - Pull-to-sit response
    - Babinski
    - Stepping/walking
    - Crawling

Priority Laboratory Tests/Diagnostics

- Audiometry screening
- CBC-hemoglobin/hematocrit
- Serum glucose level
- Serum bilirubin/correlate with transcutaneous bilirubinometer
- Arterial blood gases (if warranted)
- Universal newborn screening
    - Varies based on region and state law
    - Many include screening for sickle cell anemia, phenylketonuria, galactosemia, severe combined immunodeficiency—heel sticks
    - Critical congenital heart disease screen-via pulse oximetry
- Culture if infections are suspected

Priority Interventions or Actions

- Results of Apgar if 8-10 (no intervention, supportive care), 4-7 (stimulate the infant, backrub, provide oxygen), 0-3 (full resuscitation)
- Suction mouth and then nares with bulb syringe
- Dry, stimulate, and wrap infant, place cap on head (need to maintain/support thermoregulation—avoid cold stress due to lack of brown fat—infants generate heat via non-shivering thermogenesis)
- Avoid hyperthermia because of neonates' immature sweat gland function
- Initiate skin-to-skin contact or breastfeeding as soon as feasible, if not feasible, place infant in a radiant warmer
- Encourage parental bonding
- Follow agency policy for identification-wrist/ankle bands, foot and hand printing, matching ID bands

Priority Potential & Actual Complications

- Respiratory distress syndrome
- Meconium aspiration syndrome
- Bronchopulmonary dysplasia
- Intraventricular hemorrhage
- Retinopathy of prematurity
- Necrotizing enterocolitis
- Hyperbilirubinemia
- Erythroblastosis fetalis
- Fetal alcohol spectrum disorders
- Addiction/neonatal abstinence syndrome
- Vertical transmission of HIV
- Hypoglycemia
- Transient tachypnea of the newborn

Priority Nursing Implications

- In cases of infant or maternal change in condition, nurses provide support to partners, support persons, and mothers
- Ensure infant safety and identity, protection from abduction
- Gestational age including observe for preterm (before 37 weeks), small for gestational age, large for gestational age
- Support early attachment, skin-to-skin (use overbed warmer as needed) contact, and feeding (breast or bottle)
- Support parents' choice related to circumcision

Next Gen Clinical Judgment

Identify the 4 methods in which newborns experience heat loss and explain how the nurse can prevent heat loss for each of these methods.

Priority Medications

- Phytonadione
  - Vitamin K injection IM vastus lateralis injected in the delivery room
  - Sterile gut of the newborn-bacteria does not produce coagulants
- Hepatitis B vaccine
  - Given IM prior to newborn discharge
  - If mother is Hep B antigen positive, administer hepatitis B immune globulin within 12 hours of birth along with immunization. Provide injections in separate thighs
  - Document on immunization record, obtain parental consent
- Erythromycin
  - Eye prophylaxis
  - Prevent ophthalmia neonatorum-gonorrhea/chlamydia (not as effective treating chlamydia—treated with oral erythromycin)
  - Allow bonding before ointments
  - Required by law

Reinforcement of Priority Teaching

- Reinforce teaching parents about cord care. Check agency protocol for cleaning, antibiotics for infection
- How to manage circumcision or care of uncircumcised penis
- Talk with parents about preferred method of feeding either formula or breastfeeding
- Explain to parents infant care including bathing, dressing, nail care, diaper changes, consoling infant, bonding, infant stimulation
- Discuss maternal and infant return to health care providers
- Explain to parents about infant behaviors including consolability, cuddliness, irritability, crying, use of non-nutritive sucking (pacifiers), and cues
- Infant safety including car seats, safe sleep ("back-to-sleep," in own bed, without stuffed animals or pads, "tummy time" to prevent plagiocephaly (abnormal head shape), holding and carrying, cardiopulmonary resuscitation and management of airway obstruction
- Bathe infant in warm water (test with elbow), dress infant appropriate for weather, and to avoid actions that cause hyper/hypothermia

Clinical Hint

It is rare for a newborn to have an Apgar score of 10 because most newborns have acrocyanosis in which their feet and hands are blue due to peripheral vasoconstriction.

Placental abruption

Pathophysiology/Description

- Detachment of all or part of the placenta from the uterus after implantation
- Occurs between 20 weeks gestation and birth
- High level of morbidity and mortality
- Accounts for 1/3 of antepartum bleeding
- Risk factors include maternal hypertension (chronic or pregnancy-related), multiparity, cocaine use (vascular constriction), abdominal trauma/motor vehicle accident/ domestic violence, cigarette smoking, history of abruptio or premature rupture of membranes with previous pregnancies

Priority Data Collection or Cues

- Ask about risk factors
- Categorized on grade:
  - Grade 1 (10-20% abruption)—minimal bleeding, dark red blood, without tenderness, upper uterine placement
  - Grade 2 (20-50% abruption)—absent to moderate bleeding, dark red blood, increased uterine tone/rigidity without relaxation, pain, mild shock, potential DIC, may impact fetal heart tones
  - Grade 3 (>50% abruption)—absent to moderate bleeding, dark red blood, sudden, significant shock, board-like abdomen, agonizing pain, impacts fetal heart tones, may lead to fetal demise
- Monitor maternal vital signs and fetal heart tones
- Examine fundal height

Priority Laboratory Tests/Diagnostics

- Abdominal and transvaginal ultrasound
- Coagulation studies
- Fetal nonstress test—monitor heart rate patterns in response to fetal movement, uterine contractions, or stimulation
- Biophysical profile—real-time ultrasound assessing amniotic fluid volume, fetal movements, fetal heart tones, fetal breathing movements, and fetal muscle tone
- Type and cross match as needed prior to transfusion
- Kleihauer-Betke test—to detect fetal blood in maternal circulation

Priority Interventions or Actions

- From 20-34 weeks gestation, if there are normal fetal heart tones
  - Client is hospitalized and large-bore intravenous access and a urinary catheter placed to check urine output. Oxygen applied as needed. If there is mild bleeding bedrest is recommended. With no bleeding, bedrest with bathroom privileges is indicated
- > 34 weeks gestation
  - Client is hospitalized and managed as above
  - Betamethasone is administered to mature the fetal lungs
- Large volume bleeding–do all of the above plus
  - Mom and fetus may be in jeopardy
  - Position Trendelenburg to decrease pressure on placenta or lateral if client hypovolemic
  - Birth-vaginal preferred, C-sections are not done with coagulopathy
- All cases: External fetal monitoring, monitor for bleeding, monitor coagulation studies

Priority Potential & Actual Complications

- Fetal loss/demise
- Shock
- Couvelair uterus-decreased contractility
- Disseminated intravascular coagulation (DIC)
- Transplacental hemorrhage
- Renal failure
- Rh sensitization
- Intrauterine growth retardation
- Preterm birth

Priority Nursing Implications

- Nurse provides support and care in the event of fetal demise
- Provide emotional support to deal with stress of critically ill mother and/or fetus
- Provide pain management and replacement fluids

Priority Medications

- Betamethasone–given intramuscular or intravenous
  - Enhance fetal lung maturity
  - Steroid

Reinforcement of Priority Teaching

- Educate family as status of mother and fetus changes
- Provide support of client and infant if preterm
- Support family with an ill neonate and premature infant—neonatal intensive care unit and routines

Next Gen Clinical Judgment

Compare and contrast the difference in treatment regimens for placental abruption and placental previa.

Placenta previa

Pathophysiology/Description

- Placenta is implanted lower than optimal in the uterus—completely or partially/marginally covers the cervix
- Bleeding occurs with dilatation and effacement of the cervix
- Occurs in second and third trimester
- Risk factors include history of C-section, suction curettage, and previous placenta previa; advanced maternal age, multiparity, smoking, and living in a high altitude

Priority Data Collection or Cues

- Ask about risk factors
- Monitor vaginal bleeding—bright red with placenta previa
- Monitor pain—bleeding with placenta previa is usually painless
- Examine abdomen—soft, relaxed and non-tender, fundal height may be greater than expected, often with breech/transverse/oblique lies
- Monitor fetal heart tones—usually normal unless major deterioration
- Monitor urine output

Priority Laboratory Tests/Diagnostics

- Transabdominal ultrasound (check for placental placement—if low then transvaginal)
- Transvaginal ultrasound—done with select cases, avoid uterine stimulation
- Blood studies—hemoglobin/hematocrit, platelets, coagulation studies, type and screen/crossmatch
- Kleihauer-Betke test to detect fetal blood in maternal circulation

Priority Interventions or Actions

- Closely monitor vital signs and monitor for a rapid hemorrhage
- Large bore intravenous access-prepare for fluids and blood products
- Position side-lying, bed rest
- Refrain from unneeded vaginal exams
- < 34 weeks-betamethasone to mature fetal lungs
- Without bleeding and < 36 weeks without labor, implement expectant management including limited activity, pelvic rest, check for bleeding, nonstress test, biophysical profile-twice/week—if no bleeding for 48 hours/stable-may discharge to home with restrictions
- > 36 weeks and no major bleeding—active management including birth. If previa is within 2 cm of cervix, a C-section is indicated; > 2cm away, a vaginal birth is recommended

Priority Potential & Actual Complications

- Hemorrhage (bleeding may also occur postpartum)
- Abnormal placental attachment
- Hysterectomy
- C-section (with concurrent potential side effects)
- Fetal death secondary to preterm birth
- Fetal abnormalities/intrauterine growth retardation

Priority Nursing Implications

- Emotional support for potential stress associated with high-risk pregnancy
- Observe for degree of bleeding by estimating milliliters of blood loss of spots or stains

Priority Medications

- Magnesium sulfate–given intravenous
    - Have available for tocolysis (relax uterus)
    - To prevent preterm delivery
    - Monitor serum magnesium levels (4-7 mEq/L)
    - Look for magnesium toxicity/serum hypermagnesemia. Signs include absence of patellar deep tendon reflexes, decreased level of consciousness, low urine output, bradypnea, and cardiac dysrhythmias
    - Antidote for hypermagnesemia is calcium gluconate
- Betamethasone–given intramuscular or intravenous
    - Steroids administered to mature fetal lungs
    - Given if risk of delivery prior to 34 weeks
- Ferrous sulfate–given orally
    - Increase iron stores in the event of bleeding
    - May cause constipation and gastric upset

Reinforcement of Priority Teaching

- If discharged, home care includes activities restrictions and client must have access to a phone, must be within 20 minutes of the hospital, must have access to transportation, and must have friends/family to assist in care. Clients are told to proceed to the hospital in the event of any vaginal bleeding
- Ensure that mothers understand precautions of pelvic rest-no exams, no sexual intercourse, limited transvaginal ultrasounds
- Counsel client about ways to keep busy and diversional activities—activity restrictions may be very boring and raise anxiety levels

Preterm labor

Pathophysiology/Description

- Labor that occurs after the 20th week but before the 37th week
- Risk factors include history of ongoing or chronic medical conditions, substance use, lack of prenatal care, infection, social and environmental factors, previous preterm labor or other obstetrical complications, multiparity and overdistention of the uterus, anemia, age younger than 18 or over 40 years

Priority Data Collection or Cues

- Consider risk factors for preterm labor
- Check gestational age of infant
- Monitor uterine contractions (painful or painless)
- Monitor for abdominal cramping, low back pain, pelvic pain or heavy feeling, discharge (color, consistency, odor, presence of blood)
- Observe for intactness of membranes
- Observe for presence of fetal fibronectin in vaginal canal
- Assist in examining shape and dilation of cervix

Priority Laboratory Tests/Diagnostics

- Urine culture and sensitivity
- Monitor blood glucose levels
- Monitor complete blood count including WBC
- Ultrasound for fetal position and cervical shape
- Fetal fibronectin (via vaginal swab) associated with placental inflammation/collect specimen before lubricant

Priority Interventions or Actions

- Focus on ceasing contractions
- Treat infections with antibiotics
- Hydrate via oral and intravenous routes
- Maintain bed rest in lateral position
- Provide for continuous fetal monitoring
- Provide steroids to mature fetal lungs
- Provide antibiotics if septic abortion

Priority Potential & Actual Complications

- Issues associated with infant prematurity
- Precipitous delivery
- Postpartum hemorrhage
- Fetal demise

Priority Nursing Implications

- Support the mother during the stress associated with preterm labor
- Carefully assist in fetal monitoring and infant responses to or impact of preterm labor

Priority Medications

- Magnesium sulfate–given intravenous
  - Relaxes smooth muscles and halts preterm labor, prevents preterm birth
  - Look for respiratory depression and depressed deep tendon reflexes
  - Monitor magnesium levels
  - Should be administered via infusion pump
  - Have calcium gluconate available-antidote
  - Monitor urine output throughout infusion
- Nifedipine–given orally
  - Relaxes smooth muscles, including the uterus
  - Watch for maternal hypotension, dizziness, headache, facial flushing, fatigue, nausea, nervousness, tachycardia
  - Do not use with magnesium sulfate
- Betamethasone–given intramuscular or intravenous
  - Increases production of surfactant to accelerate fetal lung maturity
  - Watch for hyperglycemia and maternal immunosuppression
  - Administer deep intramuscular injection
- 17 alpha hydroxyprogesterone caproate
  - Intramuscular injections to prevent preterm labor
- Terbutaline
  - SQ injection
  - Relaxes smooth muscle
  - Duration of not more than 24 hours
  - Contraindicated with cardiac disease, hypertension, hyperthyroid, or hemorrhage
- Antibiotics may be indicated with septic abortions

Reinforcement of Priority Teaching

- Provide support and information about course of labor and birth
- Provide support for infants who are in a NICU due to prematurity
- Encourage maternal and family bonding, breastfeeding, and infant care to support a thriving newborn
- If labor is stopped, provide client with guidelines on bedrest, pelvic rest (no sexual intercourse/vaginal exams/douching), tocolytics, hydration, emptying bladder frequently, and parameters for calling/returning to health care provider
- Notify health care provider of heavy, bright red vaginal bleeding, elevated temperature, or foul-smelling vaginal drainage

Stages of labor

Pathophysiology/Description

- Process of moving fetus, placenta, and membranes out of the uterus and through the birth canal
- Onset of labor
  - Increased estrogen and decreasing progesterone, increased uterine pressure and distention
  - Mechanisms not completely understood
  - Beginning of contractions, effacement/dilation, and descent
- Mechanisms of labor
  - Powers-contractions, pushing, or bearing down
  - Passage
  - Passenger
    - Attitude-flexion, extension
    - Lie-longitudinal or transverse
    - Presentation-cephalic/vertex, breech, shoulder, brow
    - Position-presenting part as compared to maternal pelvis
    - Station-0 at ischial spine (engagement), negative (above), positive (below)
  - Position-mother's position/activity
  - Psychological-fear, anxiety, etc.

Priority Data Collection or Cues

- Data collection of preceding labor
  - Ask about lightening (dropping of infant into the true pelvis) client will feel less pressure on rib cage, and more pressure on bladder
  - May experience low backache or Braxton Hicks contractions
  - Increase in vaginal mucus ("bloody show")
  - Weight loss
  - Increase of energy ("nesting")
  - Rupture of membranes (TACO—Time, amount, color, odor)
  - Diarrhea
  - Differentiate true and false/prodromal labor
- Data collection of first stage of labor
  - Onset of labor to full dilation and effacement
  - Longest stage—usually occurs before mother seeks healthcare
  - Latent phase (0-3 cm cervical dilation)
  - Active phase (4-10 cm cervical dilation)
    - Usually indicates entry to the clinical agency
    - Seek out client history-prenatal data, screening data collection, vital signs, general review of systems, abdominal palpation, vaginal examination, support systems/birth coaches, preparedness for labor
    - Rapid dilation of the cervix; increased rate of descent of the presenting area of the fetus
  - Pain during contractions/relief between/low back pain with posterior position
- Data collection of second stage
  - Full dilation to birth
  - Latent-passive fetal descent and rotation to anterior position
    - Processes include: Engagement, descent, flexion, internal rotation, extension, restitution, external rotation, and expulsion
  - Active-pushing and bearing down; strong urge to push and provide pressure on stretch receptors in the pelvic floor
    - Assist mother into position/observe position of comfort
    - Observe for crowning
    - Assist with delivery and monitor status of mother and fetus/infant
  - Most intense pain level-abdominal and pelvic
  - Observe for shaking extremities, vomiting, restlessness, increase in bloody show
- Data collection of third stage
  - After birth of the fetus to the delivery of the placenta
  - Placenta separates and is delivered 3-4 contractions after birth of infant
  - Pain in perineal area and uterus
- Data collection of fourth stage
  - After delivery of placenta to 2 hours after birth
  - Provide skin-to-skin time with infant (Kangaroo care) bonding/breastfeeding
  - Physical recovery from delivery
  - Provide supplies for episiotomy/repairs as needed
  - Provide newborn care and data collection
  - Monitor for bleeding/hemorrhage and risk factors for postpartum bleeding
  - Monitor lochia (red, pink-brown, yellow-white)/involution of the uterus
- Data collection throughout the labor process
  - Fetal adaptation
    - Fetal heart rate
    - Fetal circulation (pressure on umbilical cord, impact of contractions)
    - Fetal respiration (preparing for and adapting to extrauterine environment)
  - Maternal adaptation
    - Circulatory (increases in cardiac output, supine hypotension, flushing, hemorrhoid protrusion, hot or cold feet)
    - Respiratory (tachypnea, increased oxygen consumption, potential for hyperventilation)
    - Renal (difficulty voiding, proteinuria)
    - Tearing around the vaginal opening
    - Muscle cramping
    - Diarrhea
    - Nausea/vomiting
    - Low blood glucose levels
  - Monitor maternal comfort and the many factors that impact pain perception-anxiety, culture, previous experiences, and support

- Assist in fetal monitoring
  - For low-risk women
  - Every 15-30 minutes in first stage of labor
  - Every 5-15 minutes in second stage of labor
  - Continuous monitoring encouraged for high-risk deliveries
  - Electronic fetal monitoring may be external or internal/ fetal scalp monitoring
  - Baseline heart rate/responses to labor-tachycardia/ bradycardia
  - Variability—absent, minimal, moderate, or marked (absent or minimal may indicate fetal distress, anomalies, or sleep state-[limited to 30 minutes at a time])
  - Accelerations—periodic or episodic, indicate fetal well-being
  - Decelerations
    - Early—in response to uterine contractions
    - Late—does not begin until after contraction started, does not return to baseline until after contraction, may indicate uteroplacental insufficiency-ominous sign with absent/minimal variability. May occur with tachysystole caused by oxytocin
    - Variable—any time in contraction cycle—cord compression; sometimes benign; repetitive may indicate fetal hypoxia
    - Prolonged—fetal hypoxia
- Observe amniotic fluid after rupture of membranes
- Observe vaginal fluids for abnormal bleeding or meconium (could indicate fetal distress)

Priority Laboratory Tests/Diagnostics

- Ultrasound to examine fetal head size to determine feasibility of vaginal delivery
- X-ray of maternal pelvis
- Urinalysis to check hydration, infection
- Complete blood count/Rh testing
- Rapid screen HIV test (unless mother opts-out)
- Group B streptococcus rapid test (if status not known)

Priority Interventions or Actions

- Provide non-pharmacologic pain management
  - Cutaneous stimulation—counterpressure, massage, heat or cold, water therapy, acupressure, acupuncture, intradermal water block
  - Sensory stimulation—music, imagery, aromatherapy, breathing techniques
  - Cognitive strategies—childbirth education, hypnosis, biofeedback
- Provide pharmacologic pain management
  - Sedatives–given intravenous
    - Diazepam–relieve anxiety (may hamper thermoregulation in infant)
  - Metoclopramide–relieve nausea and potentiate analgesics. Given intramuscular or intravenous
  - Analgesia–given intramuscular or intravenous
    - Opioid agonists/agonist-antagonists
    - Patient-controlled analgesia (PCA)
    - May have intense impacts on neonate-respirations, FHR, contractions
    - Administered after labor is well established
    - Should not be administered if delivery expected in 1-4 hours
  - Anesthesia
    - Nerve blocks-epidural, spinal, pudendal
    - Nitrous oxide/general anesthesia
  - C-sections
    - Spinal/epidural blocks
    - General anesthesia
- Provide supplemental oxygen as indicated
- Provide intravenous fluids as prescribed/observe for overhydration
- Provide antibiotics if client is positive for Group B streptococcus
- Encourage voiding every two hours
- Assist in care with nonreassuring heart patterns
  - Identify cause
  - Discontinue oxytocin
  - Change mother's position
  - Increase/apply oxygen
  - Provide intravenous fluids
  - Ensure continuous fetal monitoring
  - Prepare for C-section as indicated

Priority Potential & Actual Complications

- Respiratory depression of mother and fetus secondary to opioids
- Postpartum hemorrhage
- Infection
- Non-progression of labor
- Precipitous delivery
- Fetal hypoxia/asphyxia

Priority Nursing Implications

- Maintain safety precautions with any medication and during active labor
- Support, within agency protocol, women's activity, showering, use of birthing ball, walking, and use of non-pharmacological pain relief
- Maintain mother's hygiene
- Watch for contraction patterns—too rapid contractions, or those without rests in between, may be less effective in dilating cervix
- Although controversial, sources indicate allowing laboring mothers to choose oral food and fluid intake to ensure adequate energy for labor

Priority Medications

- Meperidine–given intravenous
  - Less respiratory depression than morphine
  - Rapid onset when administered intravenous
  - Causes neonatal depression-must be given prior to 1-4 hours from delivery
  - May be used after C-section
  - Have naloxone available
- Fentanyl–given intravenous
  - Fewer neonatal and maternal side effects and less respiratory depression
  - Short half-life, quick action and more frequent dosing
- Nalbuphine–given intramuscular, intravenous, and subcutaneous
  - Opioid agonist-antagonist
  - Less respiratory side effects for mother and fetus, causes sedation
  - Not with those addicted to opioids—stimulates withdrawal in mother and fetus
  - High ceiling medication (higher doses do not increase effect)
- Naloxone–given intramuscular or intravenous
  - Opioid antagonist
  - Administer if birth proceeds rapidly to address impact of narcotics
  - Pain will return with reversal of opioid
  - May delay breastfeeding
- Oxytocin–given intravenous
  - Encourage contraction/tone of uterus
  - 10-40 units/1000 lactated ringers or normal saline solution

Reinforcement of Priority Teaching

- Baby care including feeding, bathing, diaper care, care of umbilicus, circumcision (if done), assessing for jaundice, and follow-up to pediatrician
- Postpartum use of copper intrauterine devices, progestin implants, and progestin-only birth control pills are optimal for first contraception when breastfeeding. Many sources recommend avoiding estrogen methods for 3-6 weeks postpartum in nursing mothers to ensure breast milk supply
- Provide mother with instructions on self-care including avoiding constipation, hygiene, sitz baths, resuming sexual activity, contraception, follow-up, nutrition, pain relief, and hydration
- Monitor and refer for postpartum "blues"
- Assist with transition to parenting for co-mother, father/co-parent, grandparents, and siblings

Next Gen Clinical Judgment

The PN is assisting the RN in caring for a client G3 P2 in active labor who has requested to receive an epidural for pain control during labor. The PN anticipates which adverse side effects once the epidural is placed? What equipment and medications should be readily available for the client?

Clinical Hint

All new parents should be observed for postpartum depression, stress, and difficulties with adjustment. Although parenting is often a joyous time, the lack of sleep, strain, and changes in family dynamics are often overwhelming.

Stages of Birth in Vaginal Delivery

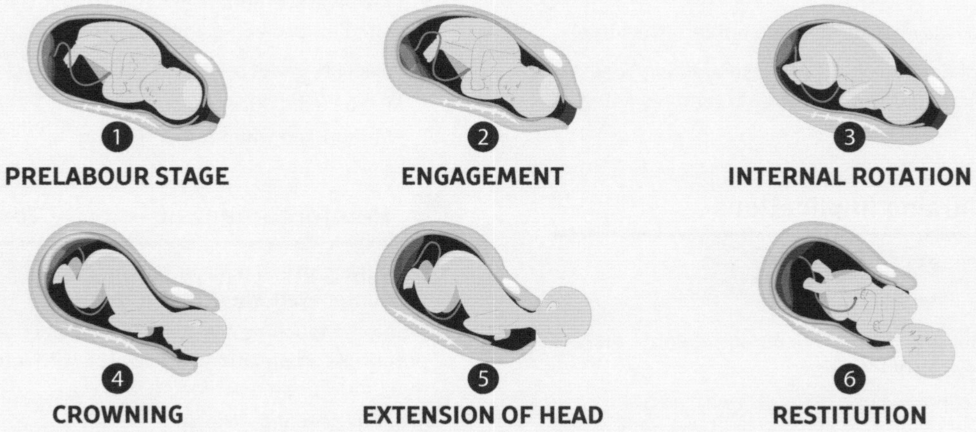

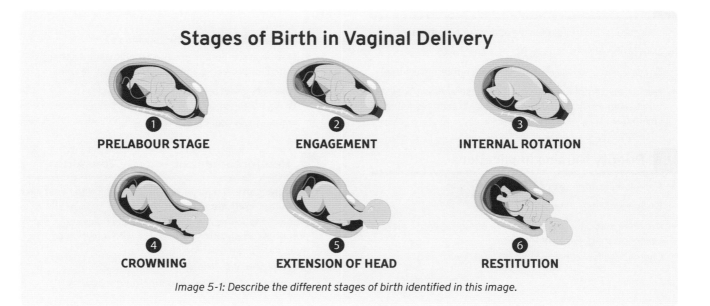

Image 5-1: Describe the different stages of birth identified in this image.

STI: Chlamydia

Pathophysiology/Description

- Bacterial infection caused by *Chlamydia trachomatis*
- Most commonly reported STI in American women, 2 ½ times the rate for men
- Difficult to diagnose, symptoms nonspecific
- Highest rates among sexually active women 15-24 years, peaks at 18-20
- Highest risk among women with multiple sexual partners, nonuse of barrier methods, lower socioeconomic status (less treatment-seeking behaviors)
- Neonatal infection occurs in 25-60% of vaginal births in infected mothers, may also occur with C-sections

Priority Data Collection or Cues

- May have "silent symptoms"
- Ask about risk factors and obtain a culture from women with 2 or more risk factors; screen all women 20-25 years or women with multiple sexual partners
- Screen at first prenatal visit and repeat in late third trimester if women previously tested positive, has a new sexual partner, has multiple sexual partners, had a previous pregnancy complicated with chlamydia, or is < 25 years of age
- May be asymptomatic but ask about potential symptoms including spotting, post-coital bleeding, pelvic pain, mucoid or purulent cervical drainage, or dysuria
- Neonatal chlamydial conjunctivitis includes redness and edema of eyes, untreated may lead to chronic conjunctivitis, scarring, and micro-granulations
- Neonatal chlamydial pneumonia at 4-11 weeks of age, symptoms include progressive rhinorrhea, tachypnea, and coughing

Priority Laboratory Tests/Diagnostics

- Laboratory culture (expensive and more sensitive)
- DNA probe (less expensive but less sensitive)
- Enzyme immunoassay (less expensive but less sensitive)
- Nucleic acid amplification tests (expensive, sensitive) via urine samples—first void and mid-stream samples detect chlamydia

Priority Nursing Implications

- Provide education to clients at risk
- Screen high-risk clients
- Provide emotional support and encourage client to make all sexual partners aware of infection
- Clients may feel ashamed of a diagnosis with an STI

Priority Potential & Actual Complications

- Acute salpingitis
- Pelvic inflammatory disease
- Pelvic abscess
- Increased risk of ectopic pregnancy
- Increase incidence of tubal factor infertility
- Cervical ulcerations which increase susceptibility to HIV
- Neonatal chlamydia conjunctivitis (ophthalmia neonatorum) or pneumonia
- May be associated with premature labor, premature rupture of membranes, stillbirth, and pregnancy loss
- May be related to postpartum endometritis

Priority Medications

- Neonatal ocular prophylaxis
    - Silver nitrate solution or antibiotic ointment
    - May not prevent transmission
    - May not treat infection
- Azithromycin–given orally
    - Single dose for issues with adherence
    - May be more expensive
    - May be used with pregnancy (retest in 3 weeks)
    - May be used with breastfeeding
    - Treatment may be used with clients who are HIV+
- Doxycycline–given orally
    - BID for 7 days
    - Avoid during pregnancy
- Erythromycin
    - Ointment for eyes
    - For prophylaxis—not always effective but is part of routine, preventive newborn care
- Erythromycin
    - Oral
    - For neonatal conjunctivitis/pneumonia
    - May be associated with hypertrophic pyloric stenosis-watch for projectile vomiting, feeding intolerance
- Amoxicillin–given orally
    - May be used during pregnancy
    - May be used when breastfeeding

Reinforcement of Priority Teaching

- Encourage use of male or female condoms with every sexual encounter even when on birth control
- Reinforce teaching client and sexual partners about the potential complications associated with infection and the need for repeated screening
- Treat all sexual partners
- Importance of rescreening during pregnancy

STI: Human papillomavirus (HPV)

Pathophysiology/Description

- Also known as *condylomata acuminata* or genital warts; common viral STI
- Estimate 50% of sexually active women will contract HPV
- Transmitted via sexual contact
- Highest rate in women 20-24 years of age
- HPV has 40 serotypes that are STIs
- May be more common in pregnant women, lesions may enlarge during pregnancy—may affect urination, defecation, mobility and fetal descent

Priority Data Collection or Cues

- Ask client about itching, vaginal discharge, dyspareunia, pruritis, post-coital bleeding, or "bumps" on the labia (or urethra or scrotum in men)
- Look for lesions around posterior part of the vaginal introitus, around the buttocks, vulva, vagina, anus, and cervix (lesions are 2-3 mm in diameter, 10-15 mm in height)—lesions occur singly or in clusters (cauliflower-like mass)
- Cervical lesions—flat topped papules 1-4 cm in diameter
- Lesions are brown to black and are painless but uncomfortable
- Lesions may resolve spontaneously without treatment but warts or cancer may develop later

Priority Laboratory Tests/Diagnostics

- Although viral screening is available, diagnosis is generally done based on history and physical examination
- Papanicolaou (Pap) test to rule out cervical cancer
- HPV-DNA in woman over 30 years
- Histologic evaluation of a biopsy of HPV
- If pregnant, cultures done weekly from 35 weeks until delivery

Priority Interventions or Actions

- No curative therapy exists
- Requires multiple treatments (see medications below)
- Cryotherapy, laser, electrocautery, cytoxic agents or surgical removal of lesions during pregnancy

Priority Potential & Actual Complications

- 2 types of HPV responsible for cervical cancers
- May impede a vaginal delivery and require a C-section
- Neonatal contraction of HPV
- Children may sustain epithelial tumors on the larynx

Priority Nursing Implications

- Because lesions may exist on the labia/vagina and anus, gloves should be changed to avoid cross-contamination
- Lesion care includes bathing with oatmeal solution, blow with cool hair dryer, keep the area clean and dry, cotton underwear/loose-fitting clothing
- Clients need to assume a healthy lifestyle, including rest, diet, and hydration to maximize immune function

Priority Medications

- Imiquimod–given topically
  - Not during pregnancy
  - Immune response modifier
- Trichloroacetic acid (TCA) and bichloroacetic acid (BCA)
  - Applied to warts
  - Use petroleum jelly to protect surrounding skin
  - May be painful upon application
- Podofilox liquid gel
  - Apply to affected area BID x 3 days weekly x 3 to 4 weeks
  - Not for use in pregnancy/breastfeeding

Reinforcement of Priority Teaching

- Transmission and the importance of prevention are critical since there is no cure
- Two doses of HPV vaccine are recommended for children at ages 9-14. Three doses of HPV vaccine over 6 months are recommended for 15 years and older
- HPV vaccination is not recommended for anyone older than age 26 years. For people over the age of 26, the vaccine provides less benefits
- Clients may be taught about barrier methods (male/female condoms) and the benefits of limiting numbers of sexual partners to prevent disease transmission
- Avoid sexual contact until lesions healed

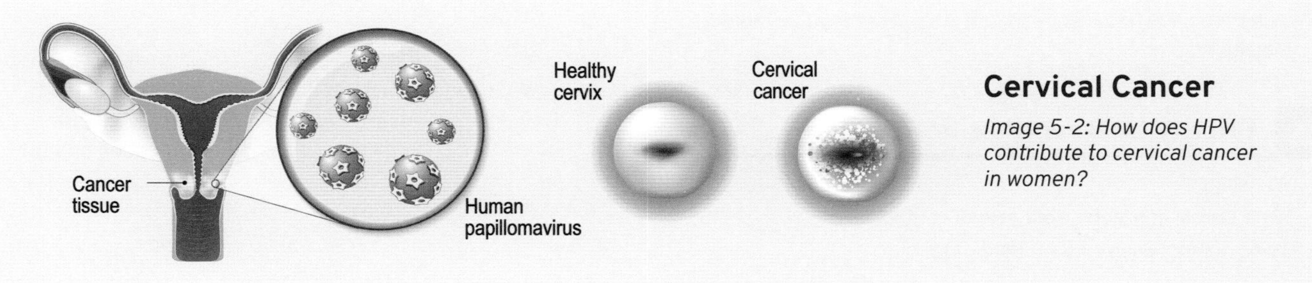

Cervical Cancer

Image 5-2: How does HPV contribute to cervical cancer in women?

STI: Syphilis

Pathophysiology/Description

- Syphilis was one of the earliest STIs identified caused by *Treponema pallidum*
- Known as a chronic infectious disease
- Transmitted via physical contact with subcutaneous lesions that occur during sexual intercourse—kissing, biting, or oral-genital sex (skin, mucous membranes of mouth, anus, and genitals)
- May be transmitted in utero
- Highest risk among women 20-24 years of age

Priority Data Collection or Cues

- Ask about risk factors
- Look for syphilitic lesions—manifestations related to phase of syphilis infections
  - Primary—most infectious
    - Lesion or chancre at point of entry of the spirochete
    - 5-90 days after infection
    - Painless papule becomes a flat, indurated ulcer
  - Secondary—highly infectious
    - 6 weeks to 6 months after infection
    - Maculopapular rash localized on palms, soles, and/or skin and mucous membranes, non-pruritic rash. Mucous patches on mouth, tongue, or cervix
    - Generalized lymphadenopathy
    - Generalized symptoms of fever, headache, and malaise
    - Condylomata lata (wart-like lesions)
  - Tertiary
    - Early latent phase-may be asymptomatic
    - 10-30 years after untreated primary lesion
    - Later-spirochete enters internal organs-neurological (Meningitis, paresis, ataxia, CNS deterioration), cardiovascular (aorta and aortic valve damage), musculoskeletal, and multiorgan system complications
    - Permanent organ damage

Priority Laboratory Tests/Diagnostics

- Microscopic examination of lesion tissue
- Serology during latency and late infection
- VDRL (venereal disease research laboratory test) or rapid plasma reagin

Priority Interventions or Actions

- Penicillin
- Limit sexual contacts/treat sexual contacts
- Symptomatic care for damaged organs

Priority Potential & Actual Complications

- May be fatal
- Systemic implications
- Spontaneous abortion or premature labor if pregnant
- Crosses placenta at 18 weeks-congenital syphilis-physical anomalies, CNS damage, neonatal syphilitic lesions, hearing loss

Priority Nursing Implications

- Screening indicated for all women diagnosed with another STI or HIV
- Provide emotional support for all clients, especially those who are pregnant
- Contact precautions when handling affected infants, most infectious until 24 hours after initiation of antibiotics
- Ensure treatment of all sexual contacts

Priority Medications

- Penicillin–given orally
  - May cause GI upset in high doses
  - May lead to superinfections—encourage eating yogurt or buttermilk
  - High rate of hypersensitivity
  - Encourage fluids to enhance excretion

Reinforcement of Priority Teaching

- The importance of treating in the early stages to avoid permanent damage to organs
- Encourage all partners to be treated
- Ensure pregnant women are tested at first prenatal visit and at 36 weeks gestation if infection is questioned
- Medications and prevention using barrier methods (male or female condoms)

Next Gen Clinical Judgment

1. What health promotion measures are employed to prevent STIs in at risk clients?
2. How does syphilis affect pregnancy?
3. How does infection with syphilis impact a fetus?
4. What education is needed to ensure client comfort and to prevent secondary infections?

NurseThink® Quiz Questions

1. **The nurse assists a new mother in the care of her newborn who was delivered ten hours ago. Which stool sample does the nurse observe when changing the newborn's first diaper?**

   a. 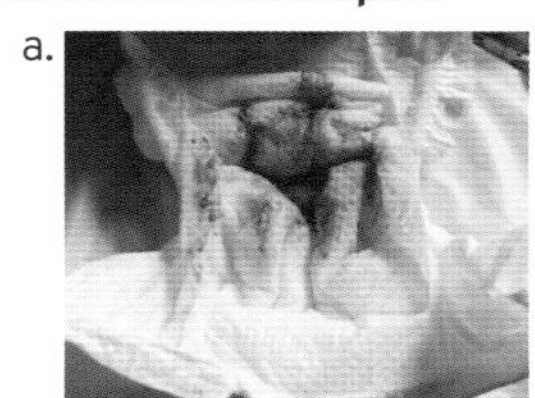
   b. 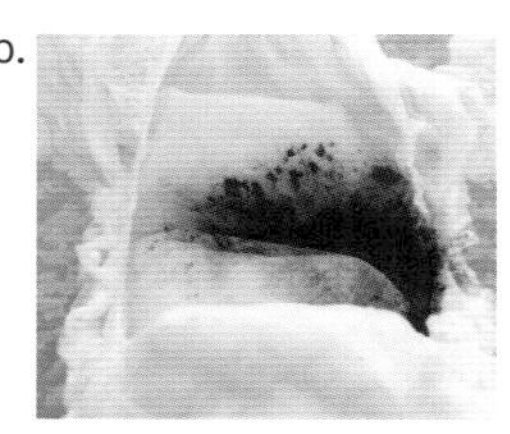
   c. 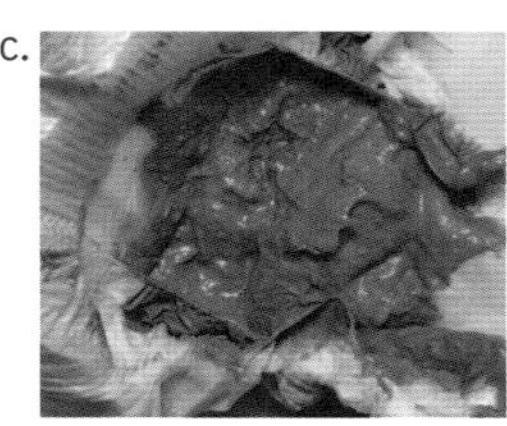
   d. 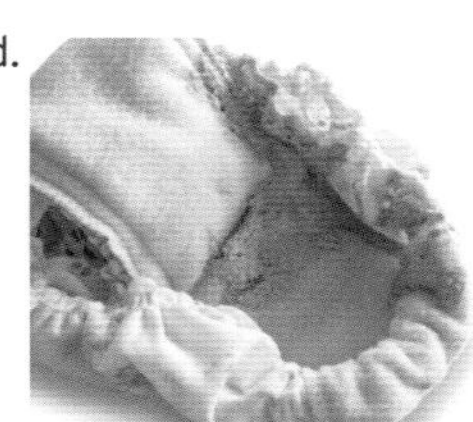

2. **The nurse evaluates a client prescribed combined oral contraceptives for family planning. What finding does the nurse report immediately?**
   a. Blurred vision.
   b. Headaches.
   c. Weight gain.
   d. Heavy menstrual bleeding.

3. **The nurse cares for a client with erectile dysfunction who is newly prescribed tadalafil. What medication does the nurse alert the provider that the client is already taking before the new prescription is filled?**
   a. Intramuscular vitamin B12.
   b. Oral ibuprofen.
   c. Topical nitroglycerin.
   d. Oral metoprolol.

4. **The nurse reviews a client's electronic health record in the early part of her first trimester of pregnancy. What lab values cause the nurse to suspect ectopic pregnancy?**
   a. Low human chorionic gonadotropin.
   b. High thyroid stimulating hormone.
   c. High serum glucose.
   d. Low C-reactive proteins.

5. **The nurse supports a client who just found out she is miscarrying at the fifth week of her pregnancy. What is the most likely cause for early pregnancy miscarriage?**
   a. Diabetes.
   b. Blighted ovum.
   c. Smoking.
   d. Infection.

6. **The nurse cares for a client who is being evaluated for possible preterm labor. What findings are suggestive of preterm labor? *Select all that apply.***
   a. Premature rupture of membranes at 36 weeks.
   b. Positive fetal fibronectin test at 24 weeks.
   c. Regular contractions and progressive dilation at 38 weeks.
   d. Advanced cervical dilation at 20 weeks.
   e. Regular contractions with advanced dilation at 36 weeks.

7. **Place the cardinal movements in order of occurrence as the fetus passes through the birth canal.**
   a. Expulsion.
   b. Extension.
   c. Descent.
   d. Flexion.
   e. External rotation.
   f. Restitution.
   g. Internal rotation.

8. **The nurse monitors the contraction pattern of a client in labor. What pattern does the nurse document as dystocia?**
   a. Regularly spaced strong contractions.
   b. Irregularly spaced weak contractions.
   c. Regularly spaced weak contractions.
   d. Rapid, extremely strong contractions.

9. **Which image illustrates the client experiencing placenta abruption?**

   a. b. 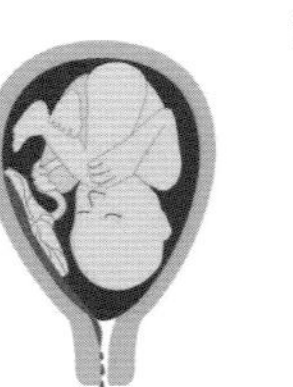
   c. 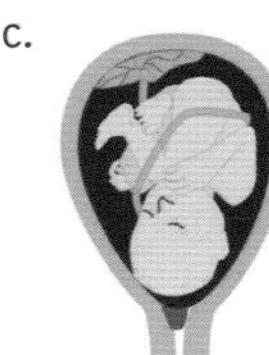

10. **The nurse cares for a client in labor diagnosed with placenta previa. Which degree of previa should the nurse anticipate as the least likely to result in the need for cesarean delivery?**
    a. Total placenta previa.
    b. Partial placenta previa.
    c. Marginal placenta previa.
    d. Low-lying placenta.

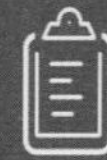

NurseThink® Quiz Questions

11. **The nurse prepares to care for their assigned postpartum clients. Which clients does the nurse consider to be at high risk for postpartum hemorrhage? *Select all that apply.***
    a. Multiple gestation delivery.
    b. Nulliparous.
    c. Prolonged labor.
    d. Induced labor.
    e. Hispanic heritage.

12. **The nurse reinforces breastfeeding education with a new mother. What does the nurse include in the education plan?**
    a. Avoid artificial nipples until breastfeeding is well established.
    b. Breastfeeding should be done five times in 24 hours.
    c. Breast milk should not be given to the infant for the first 24 hours.
    d. Education should only be addressed to the mother.

13. **The nurse cares for a client diagnosed with pelvic inflammatory disease (PID) related to a sexually transmitted infection (STI). What STI does the nurse expect to see in the client's chart as the probable causative factor?**
    a. Syphilis.
    b. Yeast.
    c. Gonorrhea.
    d. Chlamydia.

14. **The nurse evaluates a client for sexually transmitted diseases. Which client below does the nurse document as having human papillomavirus?**

    a. 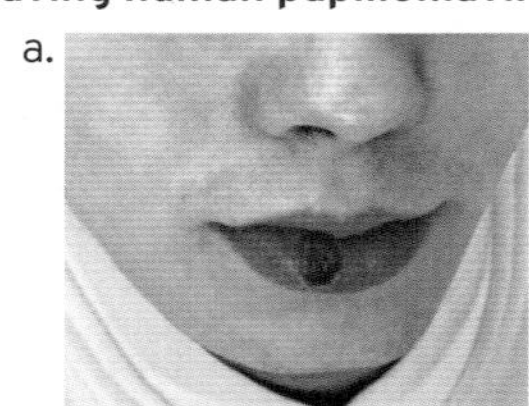
    b. 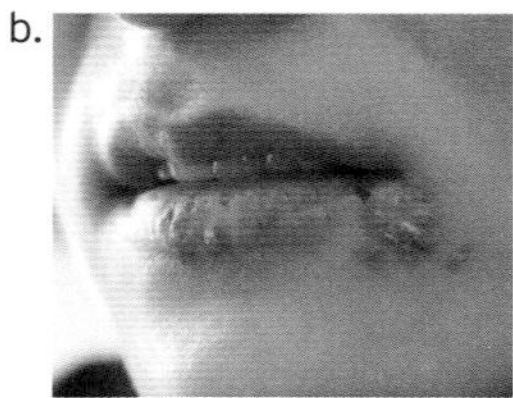
    c. 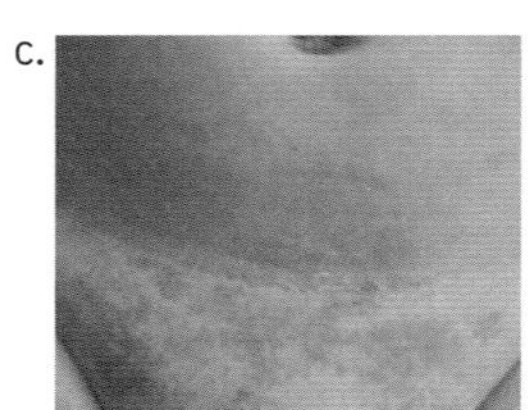
    d. 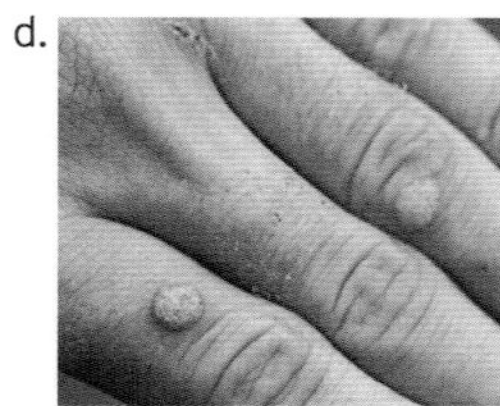

15. **The nurse cares for a client diagnosed with syphilis. What does the nurse expect to be included in the client's treatment plan? *Select all that apply.***
    a. HIV testing.
    b. Follow-up testing in 3 and 6 months.
    c. Recommended abortion due to birth defects.
    d. Sexual activity with condoms only.
    e. Penicillin G injections.

16. **The nurse speaks with a client diagnosed with gestational diabetes about the associated risks. What potential risk is not associated with the client's diagnosis?**
    a. Macrocephaly.
    b. Shoulder dystocia.
    c. Macrosomia.
    d. Cesarean birth.

17. **Which image depicts the most common nonnutritive pica substance related to iron deficiency anemia in pregnant women?**

    a. 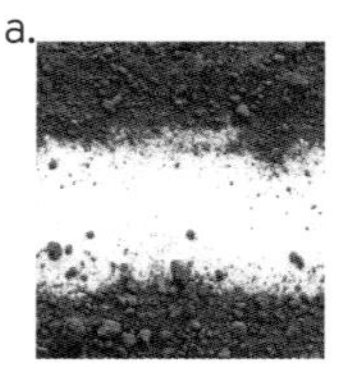
    b. 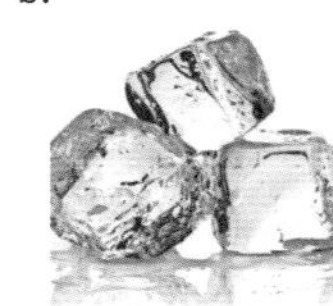
    c. 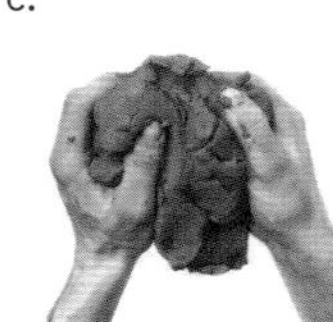

18. **The nurse cares for a pregnant adolescent client. When planning care, what does the nurse consider about adolescent pregnancies that differs from adult pregnancies?**
    a. Young adolescents under 15 need to gain more weight.
    b. Adolescents require less caloric intake daily.
    c. Young adolescents do not require as much calcium as adults.
    d. Folic acid needs are higher for adults than adolescents.

19. **The nurse assists a new mother as she begins to breastfeed her newborn. Rank order the steps to breastfeeding as the nurse walks the mother through the process.**
    a. "Assume a comfortable position with arms supported."
    b. "Lightly brush your baby's mouth with the breast."
    c. "Expose the breast."
    d. "Direct the nipple straight into the baby's mouth."
    e. "Turn the baby's entire body toward you with their mouth adjacent to your nipple."

20. **The nurse cares for a client in the postpartum period and documents this nursing note. What finding does the nurse report immediately to the health care provider?**

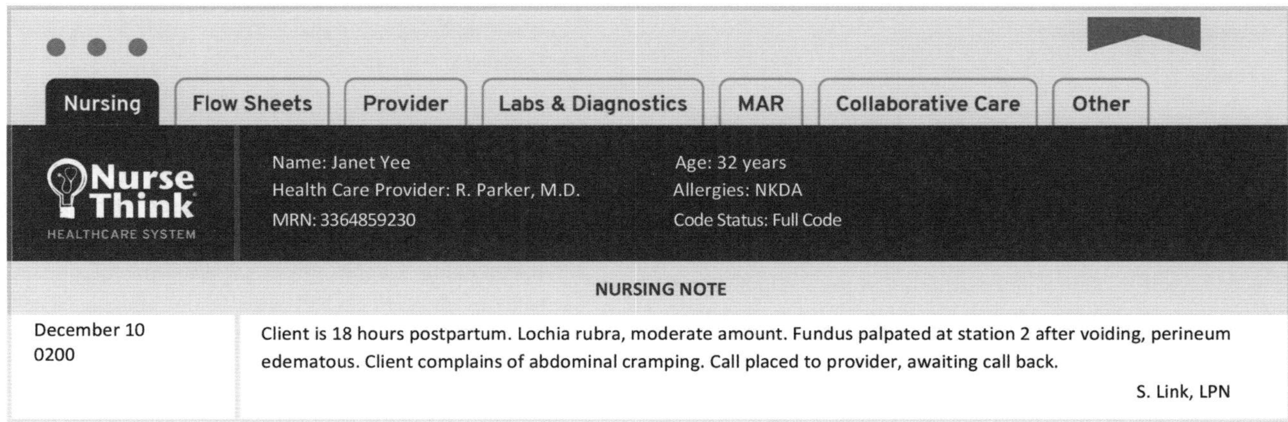

a. Lochia rubra.
b. Abdominal cramping.
c. Fundus at station 2.
d. Perineum edematous.

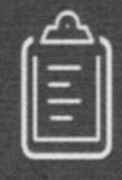

NurseThink® Quiz Answers

1. **The nurse assists a new mother in the care of her newborn who was delivered ten hours ago. Which stool sample does the nurse observe when changing the newborn's first diaper?**

   Answer: b.

   Topic/Concept: Sexuality **Subtopic:** Newborn Care **Bloom's Taxonomy:** Applying **Clinical Problem-Solving Process:** Data Collection **NCLEX-PN®:** Basic Care and Comfort **QSEN:** Evidence-based Practice **CJMM:** Recognize Cues

   Rationale: The first image is what is expected after the second day with a breastfed newborn. The second image is meconium, the expected first stool within 48 hours of birth. The third image is after the second day with a soy formula-fed newborn. The last image is after the second day with a formula-fed newborn.

   THIN Thinking: *Clinical Problem-Solving Process* – Evaluating proper elimination patterns and expectations is imperative in identifying potential congenital abnormalities in the first days of life. If not addressed early on, these could lead to lifelong problems and injury.

2. **The nurse evaluates a client prescribed combined oral contraceptives for family planning. What finding does the nurse report immediately?**
   a. Blurred vision.
   b. Headaches.
   c. Weight gain.
   d. Heavy menstrual bleeding.

   Topic/Concept: Sexuality **Subtopic:** Contraception **Bloom's Taxonomy:** Applying **Clinical Problem-Solving Process:** Evaluation **NCLEX-PN®:** Pharmacological Therapies **QSEN:** Patient-centered Care **CJMM:** Evaluate Outcomes

   Rationale: Although less common, the more serious side effects of combined oral contraceptives can be included in the mnemonic ACHES. Abdominal pain, chest pain, headaches (severe), eye problems (blurred vision), and swelling or aching in the legs and thighs.

   THIN Thinking: *Top Three* – It is very important to identify serious side effects immediately and address them to prevent injury to the client. There are many serious side effects of oral contraceptives; even though not as common in those that do not smoke, they are still a risk that needs to be evaluated.

3. **The nurse cares for a client with erectile dysfunction who is newly prescribed tadalafil. What medication does the nurse alert the provider that the client is already taking before the new prescription is filled?**
   a. Intramuscular vitamin B12.
   b. Oral ibuprofen.
   c. Topical nitroglycerin.
   d. Oral metoprolol.

   Topic/Concept: Sexuality **Subtopic:** Erectile Dysfunction **Bloom's Taxonomy:** Applying **Clinical Problem-Solving Process:** Planning **NCLEX-PN®:** Pharmacological Therapies **QSEN:** Teamwork and Collaboration **CJMM:** Prioritize Hypotheses

   Rationale: Nitroglycerin and tadalafil can react and cause severe hypotension and shock when taken together, so the provider should be alerted to prevent injury. There are not severe side effects between tadalafil and metoprolol, vitamin B12, or ibuprofen.

   THIN Thinking: *Identify Risk to Safety* – Understanding medication side effects can help prevent injury in a client. Drug interactions can be life-threatening in some instances.

4. **The nurse reviews a client's electronic health record in the early part of her first trimester of pregnancy. What lab values cause the nurse to suspect ectopic pregnancy?**
   a. Low human chorionic gonadotropin.
   b. High thyroid stimulating hormone.
   c. High serum glucose.
   d. Low C-reactive proteins.

   Topic/Concept: Sexuality **Subtopic:** Pregnancy **Bloom's Taxonomy:** Analyzing **Clinical Problem-Solving Process:** Data Collection **NCLEX-PN®:** Physiological Adaptation **QSEN:**Evidence-based Practice **CJMM:** Analyze Cues

   Rationale: Low human chorionic gonadotropin levels can indicate ectopic pregnancy and often do not increase as the pregnancy advances. Thyroid hormones indicate thyroid problems, glucose levels can indicate gestational diabetes, and C-reactive proteins can indicate inflammatory illnesses like systemic lupus erythematosus.

   THIN Thinking: *Clinical Problem-Solving Process* – Lab values should be monitored because they can help dictate proper treatment and identify problems that need to be treated.

5. **The nurse supports a client who just found out she is miscarrying at the fifth week of her pregnancy. What is the most likely cause for early pregnancy miscarriage?**
   a. Diabetes.
   b. Blighted ovum.
   c. Smoking.
   d. Infection.

   Topic/Concept: Sexuality **Subtopic:** Miscarriage **Bloom's Taxonomy:** Analyzing **Clinical Problem-Solving Process:** Data Collection **NCLEX-PN®:** Reduction of Risk Potential **QSEN:** Patient-centered Care **CJMM:** Recognize Cues

   Rationale: The most likely cause of early pregnancy miscarriage is blighted ovum. Other causes can include smoking, infection, and uncontrolled diabetes, but these are not as prevalent as a blighted ovum.

THIN Thinking: *Clinical Problem-Solving Process* – Many mothers want to know why they miscarried, feeling like they are somehow at fault. Being able to belay that fear and let them know the most likely cause was out of their control can alleviate some of their guilt and help with the grieving process.

6. **The nurse cares for a client who is being evaluated for possible preterm labor. What findings are suggestive of preterm labor? *Select all that apply.***
   a. Premature rupture of membranes at 36 weeks.
   b. Positive fetal fibronectin test at 24 weeks.
   c. Regular contractions and progressive dilation at 38 weeks.
   d. Advanced cervical dilation at 20 weeks.
   e. Regular contractions with advanced dilation at 36 weeks.

   Topic/Concept: Sexuality **Subtopic:** Preterm Labor **Bloom's Taxonomy:** Applying **Clinical Problem-Solving Process:** Data Collection **NCLEX-PN®:** Reduction of Risk Potential **QSEN:** Evidence-based Practice **CJMM:** Analyze Cues

   Rationale: Preterm labor can occur between 20 and 36 weeks. It can present as premature rupture of membranes, positive fetal fibronectin testing, advanced cervical dilation, and regular and shortening contractions producing dilation. Any signs of labor after 36 weeks is considered full-term labor.

   THIN Thinking: *Identify Risk to Safety* – Evaluation for preterm labor is imperative as efforts to stop premature birth are important in reducing morbidity and mortality in neonates.

7. **Place the cardinal movements in order of occurrence as the fetus passes through the birth canal.**
   a. Expulsion.
   b. Extension.
   c. Descent.
   d. Flexion.
   e. External rotation.
   f. Restitution.
   g. Internal rotation.

   Topic/Concept: Sexuality **Subtopic:** Stages of Labor **Bloom's Taxonomy:** Applying **Clinical Problem-Solving Process:** Data Collection **NCLEX-PN®:** Physiological Adaptation **QSEN:** Evidence-based Practice **CJMM:** Recognize Cues

   Rationale: The cardinal position changes are the needed movements for the expulsion of the fetus from the birth canal and are ordered: descent, flexion, internal rotation, extension, restitution, external rotation, and expulsion. Answer: C, D, G, B, F, E, A

   THIN Thinking: *Clinical Problem-Solving Process* – Understanding the expected outcomes is the best way for the nurse to identify deviation from the normal and address problems as early as possible.

8. **The nurse monitors the contraction pattern of a client in labor. What pattern does the nurse document as dystocia?**
   a. Regularly spaced strong contractions.
   b. Irregularly spaced weak contractions.
   c. Regularly spaced weak contractions.
   d. Rapid, extremely strong contractions.

   Topic/Concept: Sexuality **Subtopic:** Dystocia **Bloom's Taxonomy:** Applying **Clinical Problem-Solving Process:** Planning **NCLEX-PN®:** Physiological Adaptation **QSEN:** Patient-centered Care **CJMM:** Analyze Cues

   Rationale: The first description is a normal pattern. The third description is either earlier in labor or Braxton-Hicks contractions. The last description is hypertonic, in which the contractions are too fast and strong. Dystocia is a uterine contraction pattern in which the contractions are irregular and weak and do not produce efficient dilation patterns.

   THIN Thinking: *Top Three* – Nonprogressive labor can result in the need for cesarean section. This risk will be higher in nulliparous women as dystocia results in emergency cesarean about 50% of the time and only about 5% of the time in multiparous women.

9. **Which image illustrates the client experiencing placenta abruption?**

   Answer: a.

   Topic/Concept: Sexuality **Subtopic:** Placenta abruption **Bloom's Taxonomy:** Analyzing **Clinical Problem-Solving Process:** Implementation **NCLEX-PN®:** Reduction of Risk Potential **QSEN:** Evidence-based Practice **CJMM:** Take Action

   Rationale: The first image is placenta abruption, as evidenced by the clot formation under the separated placenta. The other images are normal presentations.

   THIN Thinking: *Help Quick* – Placenta abruption can happen spontaneously during labor and can be fatal to the fetus and mother. Early identification and treatment are imperative for the survival of both clients.

10. **The nurse cares for a client in labor diagnosed with placenta previa. Which degree of previa should the nurse anticipate as the least likely to result in the need for cesarean delivery?**
    a. Total placenta previa.
    b. Partial placenta previa.
    c. Marginal placenta previa.
    d. Low-lying placenta.

Topic/Concept: Sexuality **Subtopic:** Placenta Previa **Bloom's Taxonomy:** Analyzing **Clinical Problem-Solving Process:** Planning **NCLEX-PN®:** Physiological Adaptation **QSEN:** Evidence-based Practice **CJMM:** Generate Solutions

Rationale: Low-lying placentas do not cover the cervical os and obstruct delivery, so cesarean delivery is unnecessary. Total placenta previa requires cesarean as it fully obstructs delivery. Partial previa is highly likely to result in cesarean as it carries a high risk of bleeding. Marginal is lower risk but still covers the os and can result in cesarean.

THIN Thinking: *Identify Risk to Safety* – It is important to differentiate between previa and abruption as these require very different treatments and carry different risks. If previa is suspected, vaginal examinations should not be done as the risk of bleeding is too high.

11. **The nurse prepares to care for their assigned postpartum clients. Which clients does the nurse consider to be at high risk for postpartum hemorrhage? *Select all that apply.***
    a. Multiple gestation delivery.
    b. Nulliparous.
    c. Prolonged labor.
    d. Induced labor.
    e. Hispanic heritage.

Topic/Concept: Sexuality **Subtopic:** Postpartum Hemorrhage **Bloom's Taxonomy:** Analyzing **Clinical Problem-Solving Process:** Data Collection **NCLEX-PN®:** Reduction of Risk Potential **QSEN:** Safety **CJMM:** Analyze Cues

Rationale: Increased risks for postpartum hemorrhage include grand multiparity, multiple gestation, Hispanic or Asian heritage, prolonged labor, and oxytocin-induced labor. Nulliparous labor is not at increased risk because they still have tonicity in their uterus.

THIN Thinking: *Identify Risk to Safety* – It is important to identify increased risks to ensure proper preventative care for those at higher risk of complications.

12. **The nurse reinforces breastfeeding education with a new mother. What does the nurse include in the education plan?**
    a. Avoid artificial nipples until breastfeeding is well established.
    b. Breastfeeding should be done five times in 24 hours.
    c. Breast milk should not be given to the infant for the first 24 hours.
    d. Education should only be addressed to the mother.

Topic/Concept: Sexuality **Subtopic:** Breastfeeding **Bloom's Taxonomy:** Applying **Clinical Problem-Solving Process:** Implementation **NCLEX-PN®:** Health Promotion and Maintenance **QSEN:** Patient-centered Care **CJMM:** Take Action

Rationale: Breastfeeding should be started at birth as soon as possible when milk comes in and encouraged 8-12 times in 24 hours. Education should include family members or significant others as they can help monitor and encourage the mother. Artificial nipples and pacifiers should be avoided until breastfeeding is well established, which can take 4-6 weeks.

THIN Thinking: *Top Three* – Breastfeeding mothers need a lot of education and encouragement to succeed in breastfeeding their infant. They also need to be able to measure the success of their breastfeeding to ensure the health of their infant.

13. **The nurse cares for a client diagnosed with pelvic inflammatory disease (PID) related to a sexually transmitted infection (STI). What STI does the nurse expect to see in the client's chart as the probable causative factor?**
    a. Syphilis.
    b. Yeast.
    c. Gonorrhea.
    d. Chlamydia.

Topic/Concept: Sexuality **Subtopic:** STI: Chlamydia **Bloom's Taxonomy:** Analyzing **Clinical Problem-Solving Process:** Data Collection **NCLEX-PN®:** Safety and Infection Control **QSEN:** Evidence-based Practice **CJMM:** Analyze Cues

Rationale: Chlamydia is the most common cause of PID as it is most frequently asymptomatic until it spreads to the fallopian tubes and uterus. It can result in infertility, ectopic pregnancy, or early miscarriage. Gonorrhea can result in PID but is less likely as it is symptomatic. Yeast is not an STI and is symptomatic, making it less likely to result in PID. Syphilis is a systemic infection and not a cause of PID.

THIN Thinking: *Clinical Problem-Solving Process* – A nurse should be aware of potential causes of diseases to identify other concerns needing treatment. Chlamydia can spread to many areas of the body and, if left untreated at the time of birth, can result in damage to a newborn's eyesight.

14. **The nurse evaluates a client for sexually transmitted diseases. Which client below does the nurse document as having human papillomavirus?**

Answer: d.

Topic/Concept: Sexuality **Subtopic:** STI: Human Papillomavirus (HPV) **Bloom's Taxonomy:** Applying **Clinical Problem-Solving Process:** Data Collection **NCLEX-PN®:** Coordinated Care **QSEN:** Teamwork and Collaboration **CJMM:** Recognize Cues

Rationale: The first image depicts a syphilis chancre. The second image is herpes simplex virus. The third image is of jock itch caused by a skin yeast infection. The last image depicts warts caused by human papillomavirus; they can form on the genitals, mouth, or any other area of the body in contact with the virus.

THIN Thinking: *Clinical Problem-Solving Process* – Human papillomavirus causes genital warts and is the cause of 99% of cervical cancers. The nurse needs to be able to differentiate between rash types to ensure the correct treatment is given.

15. The nurse cares for a client diagnosed with syphilis. What does the nurse expect to be included in the client's treatment plan? *Select all that apply.*

a. HIV testing.
b. Follow-up testing in 3 and 6 months.
c. Recommended abortion due to birth defects.
d. Sexual activity with condoms only.
e. Penicillin G injections.

Topic/Concept: Sexuality **Subtopic:** STI: Syphilis **Bloom's Taxonomy:** Applying **Clinical Problem-Solving Process:** Planning **NCLEX-PN®:** Safety and Infection Control **QSEN:** Evidence-based Practice **CJMM:** Generate Solutions

Rationale: The treatment plan should not include sexual activity; the client should abstain and then use condoms after cured. The client should be retested in three and six months after treatment and receive HIV testing as HIV has a higher incidence in those positive with syphilis. Penicillin G injections are the primary treatment for syphilis, with doxycycline used in cases of penicillin allergy. The provider will treat the women who are pregnant but not recommend abortion.

THIN Thinking: *Top Three* – The entire treatment plan needs to be explained and evaluated with the client. Especially when dealing with the treatment and prevention of STDs, the client must accept the treatment plans to be compliant as this is the most personal part of their life.

16. The nurse speaks with a client diagnosed with gestational diabetes about the associated risks. What potential risk is not associated with the client's diagnosis?

a. Macrocephaly.
b. Shoulder dystocia.
c. Macrosomia.
d. Cesarean birth.

Topic/Concept: Sexuality **Subtopic:** Gestational Diabetes **Bloom's Taxonomy:** Applying **Clinical Problem-Solving Process:** Planning **NCLEX-PN®:** Reduction of Risk Potential **QSEN:** Evidence-based Practice **CJMM:** Prioritize Hypotheses

Rationale: Gestational diabetes increases the risks of the fetus being larger than gestational age (macrosomia), putting it at higher risk of shoulder dystocia, birth trauma, and needing cesarean birth. There is no increased risk for macrocephaly.

THIN Thinking: *Identify Risk to Safety* – Even though an infant is large, it is not necessarily unhealthy, but its size increases the risk of issues during birth. When the increased size is related to gestational diabetes, there can be issues after birth with glucose metabolism that the nurse should closely monitor.

17. Which image depicts the most common nonnutritive pica substance related to iron deficiency anemia in pregnant women?

Answer: b.

Topic/Concept: Sexuality **Subtopic:** Prenatal Care **Bloom's Taxonomy:** Applying **Clinical Problem-Solving Process:** Data Collection **NCLEX-PN®:** Safety and Infection Control **QSEN:** Patient-centered Care **CJMM:** Recognize Cues

Rationale: Ice is the most commonly eaten pica substance in pregnant women and is associated with high rates of iron deficiency anemia. It is unknown if it causes the condition or whether having iron deficiency anemia causes the craving for ice, but there is a direct correlation between them.

THIN Thinking: *Top Three* – Educating a client on symptoms of illnesses will help them more quickly identify when they should seek help. This is extremely important when the client is pregnant.

18. The nurse cares for a pregnant adolescent client. When planning care, what does the nurse consider about adolescent pregnancies that differs from adult pregnancies?

a. Young adolescents under 15 need to gain more weight.
b. Adolescents require less caloric intake daily.
c. Young adolescents do not require as much calcium as adults.
d. Folic acid needs are higher for adults than adolescents.

Topic/Concept: Sexuality **Subtopic:** Pregnancy **Bloom's Taxonomy:** Applying **Clinical Problem-Solving Process:** Planning **NCLEX-PN®:** Health Promotion and Maintenance **QSEN:** Evidence-based Practice **CJMM:** Prioritize Hypotheses

Rationale: Young adolescents need to gain more weight to produce an adequate-sized baby as they have more immature reproductive organ sizes. To gain this weight, they will require more calories; more active adolescents will also require more caloric intake. Adolescents have the same folic acid needs regardless of age but require more calcium, vitamin A, D, B6, and iron than adults.

THIN Thinking: *Clinical Problem-Solving Process* – There are specific needs in every health condition that can vary based on the client's age, so the nurse needs to ensure they understand and address these for the best outcomes.

19. The nurse assists a new mother as she begins to breastfeed her newborn. Rank order the steps to breastfeeding as the nurse walks the mother through the process.

a. "Assume a comfortable position with arms supported."
b. "Lightly brush your baby's mouth with the breast."
c. "Expose the breast."
d. "Direct the nipple straight into the baby's mouth."
e. "Turn the baby's entire body toward you with their mouth adjacent to your nipple."

Answer: A, C, E, B, D

Topic/Concept: Sexuality **Subtopic:** Breastfeeding **Bloom's Taxonomy:** Applying **Clinical Problem-Solving Process:** Planning **NCLEX-PN®:** Basic Care and Comfort **QSEN:** Evidence-based Practice **CJMM:** Generate Solutions

Rationale: Brushing the cheek will stimulate sucking, but do not instruct them to brush both cheeks. The mother should ensure they are comfortable and supported, so they do not have to constantly readjust during feeding.

THIN Thinking: *Help Quick* – The more successful a mother is at breastfeeding, the healthier her infant will be. Providing proper education will help her have the best chance at success in this endeavor.

20. The nurse cares for a client in the postpartum period and documents this nursing note. What finding does the nurse report immediately to the health care provider?

a. Lochia rubra.
b. Abdominal cramping.
c. Fundus at station 2.
d. Perineum edematous.

Topic/Concept: Sexuality **Subtopic:** Postpartum Care **Bloom's Taxonomy:** Applying **Clinical Problem-Solving Process:** Implementation **NCLEX-PN®:** Reduction of Risk Potential **QSEN:** Safety **CJMM:** Take Action

Rationale: At 18 hours, the fundus should be firm and around the umbilicus at station 5 or less. Bogginess could indicate bleeding; a firm but sub involuted fundus, as reported here, could indicate infection and should be reported. Abdominal cramping or after pains, lochia rubra (dark red), and edema and bruising of the perineum are all expected findings at this time.

THIN Thinking: *Identify Risk to Safety* – There is a high risk for infection and hemorrhage in the postpartum period. The nurse must be vigilant in monitoring lochia and fundal height and tone to identify and address symptoms immediately.

CHAPTER

6

Circulation

Perfusion / Clotting

This chapter addresses conditions that impair or damage circulation, including perfusion and clotting disorders. The human body relies on the cardiovascular system to circulate blood through the body to provide oxygen and nutrients to the tissues and take away waste products.

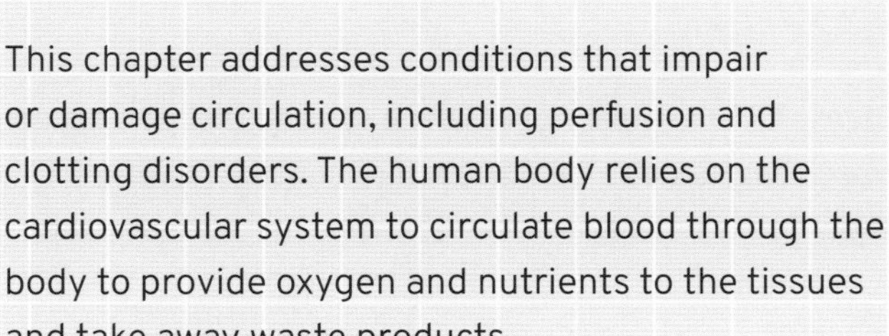

Next Gen Clinical Judgment

Priority focused data collection is an essential part of nursing practice and clinical judgment. Recognizing cues quickly and responding accordingly are central to nursing care. Find a mirror and note three data collection findings that indicate you have effective central perfusion (e.g. brain, heart, and renal). Observe two of your limbs for effective peripheral perfusion. Now try this out with a friend. Remembering these basics of perfusion can help with many exam questions.

Nurses play a significant role in collecting data on changes in circulation and perfusion, anticipating changes in clotting and circulation, and providing interventions to enhance or restore circulation.

Priority Exemplars:

- Hypertension
- Pulmonary embolism (PE)
- Stroke – cerebrovascular accident (CVA)
- Heart failure
- Shock
- Cardiomyopathy
- Coronary artery disease (CAD)
- Myocardial infarction (MI)/acute coronary syndrome
- Peripheral artery disease (PAD)
- Valvular heart disease
- Buerger's/Raynaud's
- Venous thromboembolism (VTE)
- Disseminated intravascular coagulation (DIC)

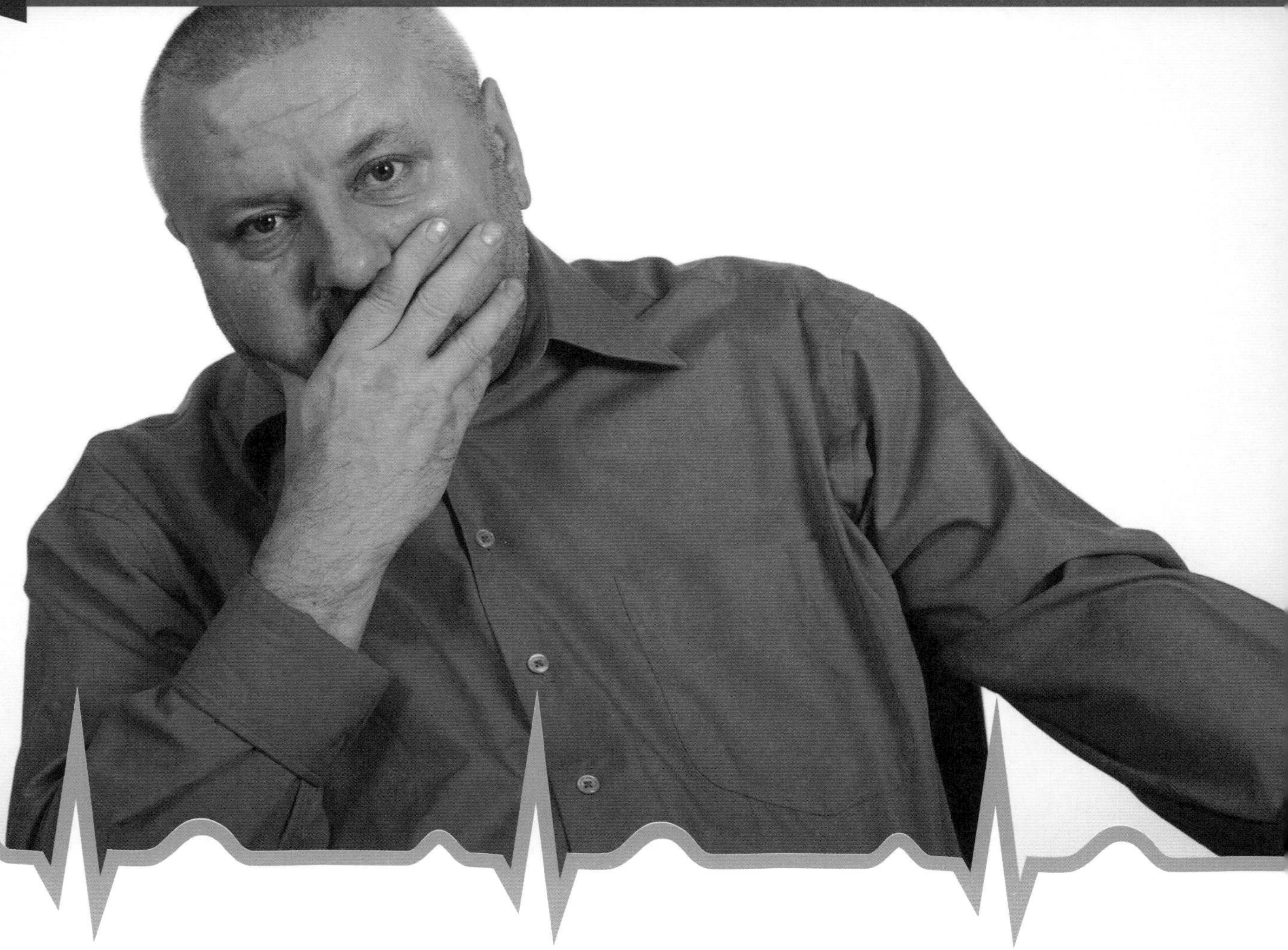

Go To Clinical

Go To Clinical Case 1

A 58-year-old male client is being admitted for observation. His current blood pressure is 190/110 mmHg. He had previously been advised to monitor his blood pressure but was never given an actual diagnosis. The client is a former smoker, as he quit about a year ago. He has a past medical history of diabetes mellitus and obesity (BMI of 28.8). His family medical history includes a grandfather diagnosed with heart disease in his early 50s, and his mother has a diagnosis of hypertension.

The client went to the doctor today for a routine physical exam. It had been a year since his last doctor's visit. He states, "he feels fine" and did not have any indication that anything was wrong. He currently lives with his wife and two teenage children. He works in a corporate setting, which he describes as "stressful". He does not follow a special diet and rarely exercises. He does take the stairs "once in a while" when going between floors at work. He typically eats out for lunch.

His additional vital signs include a temperature of 98.9°F, respirations at 14 breaths/ minute, and a pulse of 92 beats per minute. He states he is in no pain currently.

NurseThink® Time

Using the NurseThink® system, complete the priorities. Check your answers designated by in the Hypertension Priority Exemplar.

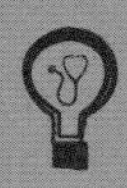

Priority Data Collection or Cues

1.

2.

3.

Priority Laboratory Tests/Diagnostics

1.

2.

3.

Priority Interventions or Actions

1.

2.

3.

Priority Potential & Actual Complications

1.

2.

3.

Priority Nursing Implications

1.

2.

3.

Priority Medications

1.

2.

3.

Reinforcement of Priority Teaching

1.

2.

3.

Hypertension

Pathophysiology/Description

- High blood pressure associated with genetic, physiological, and lifestyle factors
- May be primary or secondary
- Related to water and sodium retention, altered renin-angiotensin-aldosterone mechanism, stress and increased sympathetic nervous system activity, insulin resistance and hyperinsulinemia, and endothelium dysfunction

Priority Data Collection or Cues

- Check blood pressure in both arms and note differences. Check for orthostatic changes in blood pressure
- Use the correct size cuff, allow one minute between readings, and ensure that the arm is at the level of the heart
- Although associated with few symptoms, ask about headaches, epistaxis, fatigue, angina, dizziness, anxiety, visual disturbances, or dyspnea
- Determine client's age and ethnicity, ask about family history, stress, and related medical history (diabetes, hypercholesterolemia)
- Determine weight and BMI (Body mass index)
- Discuss lifestyle including cigarette smoking, sodium intake, alcohol intake, level of activity and exercise, sedentary habits, and usual diet

Priority Laboratory Tests/Diagnostics

- Routine urinalysis, BUN and creatinine/creatinine clearance
- Basic metabolic panel/CBC
- Lipid profile
- ECG

Priority Interventions or Actions

- Weight reduction, low sodium diet, DASH diet (high in fruits and vegetables, low-fat meats and milk products, few sweets and added sugars)
- Smoking cessation and reduction in alcohol and caffeine intake
- Physical activity and stress management
- Antihypertensive medications

Priority Potential & Actual Complications

- Coronary artery disease, left ventricular hypertrophy, and heart failure
- Cerebrovascular disease and CVA (stroke)
- Peripheral vascular disease, nephrosclerosis, and retinal damage
- Hypertensive crisis

Priority Nursing Implications

- Assist with major lifestyle changes
- Reinforce need for treatment despite absence of symptoms

Priority Medications

- Hydrochlorothiazide
  - May be given orally or intravenous
  - Determine potassium levels
  - Orthostatic hypotension
- Atenolol
  - May be given orally or intravenous
  - Monitor pulse and blood pressure
  - Contraindicated with asthma or COPD-bronchoconstriction
- Lisinopril
  - ACE inhibitors (end in -pril)
  - Usually taken orally
  - Dry, hacking cough
  - NSAIDs and ASA may reduce effectiveness
  - Not with K+ sparing diuretics
- Nifedipine, verapamil
  - Calcium channel blockers
  - Given orally or intravenous
  - Monitor for headache, edema, and hypotension

Reinforcement of Priority Teaching

- Watch for orthostatic hypotension and risk for falls
- Monitoring of blood pressure at home, using proper technique with automated device
- Life-long treatment, adherence to medication regimen, and life style changes
- Contact HCP before using OTC medications

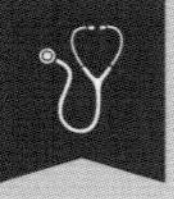

Go To Clinical Answers

Text designated by 💡 are the top answers for the Go To Clinical related to Hypertension.

Next Gen Clinical Judgment

Why is hypertension called the "silent killer?"

What are the complications of untreated hypertension?

How might the lack of symptoms of hypertension impact client adherence to medication regimens?

Pulmonary embolism (PE)

Pathophysiology/Description

- Occlusion of the pulmonary arteries by a thrombus, fat, or air embolus, or tumor
- Emboli are frequently mobilized from deep vein thrombosis (DVT), in the lower extremities, large emboli from the iliac and femoral veins are most lethal. May also originate in the heart secondary to atrial fibrillation
- Fat emboli are from long bone fractures and air emboli from intravenous administration
- Emboli may travel through the circulatory system until they become wedged in a vessel, obliterating blood flow to the area
- With PE, the embolus travels through venous systems and into the pulmonary circulation and cuts off the blood supply to the alveoli, most often in the lower lobes

Priority Data Collection or Cues

- Ask about risk factors including advanced age, pregnancy, oral contraceptives/hormone therapy, prolonged air travel, surgery, reduced activity, or immobility, tobacco use, heart failure, clotting disorders, DVTs, cancer, obesity, and trauma
- Determine respiratory status including dyspnea (may be associated with angina, increased on inspiration), hypoxemia, cyanosis, tachypnea, chest pain, cough, crackles, hemoptysis, wheezing, shallow respirations
- Monitor vital signs such as accentuated pulmonic heart sound, tachycardia, hypotension, pulse oximetry, and low-grade fever
- Monitor level of consciousness and for syncope, check for pain and anxiety, restlessness, or apprehension
- Check for petechiae in axillae or chest

Priority Laboratory Tests/Diagnostics

- D-Dimer-fibrin fragments-may not be specific nor sensitive to PEs
- Spiral CT scan with contrast
- Ventilation-perfusion (V/Q) scan-perfusion/ventilation scanning
- Pulmonary angiography
- Arterial blood gases, CXR, ECG

Priority Interventions or Actions

- Prophylaxis including pneumatic compression boots, early ambulation, anticoagulant medications
- Provide oxygen and ventilation, prevent atelectasis
- Anticoagulant therapy
- Surgical intervention if unstable or fibrinolytic therapy contraindicated
- Inferior vena cava filter, for at-risk clients

Priority Nursing Implications

- Nurses have a significant role in identifying those at risk and in the prevention of DVT
- Prognosis is better with early intervention
- When PE is a medical emergency, contact the Rapid Response Team as per agency protocol
- Elevate the head of the bed to ease respirations
- Ensure intravenous access
- Provide care to minimize effects of immobility including turning, positioning, pad pressure areas, frequent data collection
- Place at-risk clients on fall precautions
- Provide emotional support, clients may feel a sense of doom or anxiety

Priority Medications

- Enoxaparin
  - Anticoagulant–administered subcutaneously
  - Low-molecular weight heparin
  - Check for bleeding, hematomas, other sources of bleeding
- Heparin
  - Anticoagulant–administered subcutaneously
  - Monitor aPTT (normal 25-35 seconds, on heparin-1.5-2.5 times the normal)
  - Bleeding precautions
  - Antidote-protamine sulfate
- Warfarin
  - Anticoagulant–administered orally
  - Overlap with intravenous heparin
  - Warfarin for 3-6 months
  - Monitor INR (0.9-1.1 not on anticoagulants, 2-3 on warfarin, 2.5-3.5 for high-risk clients)
  - Antidote—Vitamin K (effects are not immediate)
- Tissue plasminogen activator (tPA)
  - Thrombolytic to dissolve current thrombi/emboli
  - Within 3 hours of event, check for contraindications
  - Given intravenously
- Rivaroxaban
  - Novel oral anticoagulant
  - No lab monitoring needed
  - Observe for bleeding

Reinforcement of Priority Teaching

- Education and support for clients on anticoagulants
- Ensure that client and support systems understand the risk for and means to prevent DVTs and future PEs
- Means and frequency of monitoring anticoagulants
- Encourage progressive activity and exercise program
- Limit Vitamin K foods while on warfarin

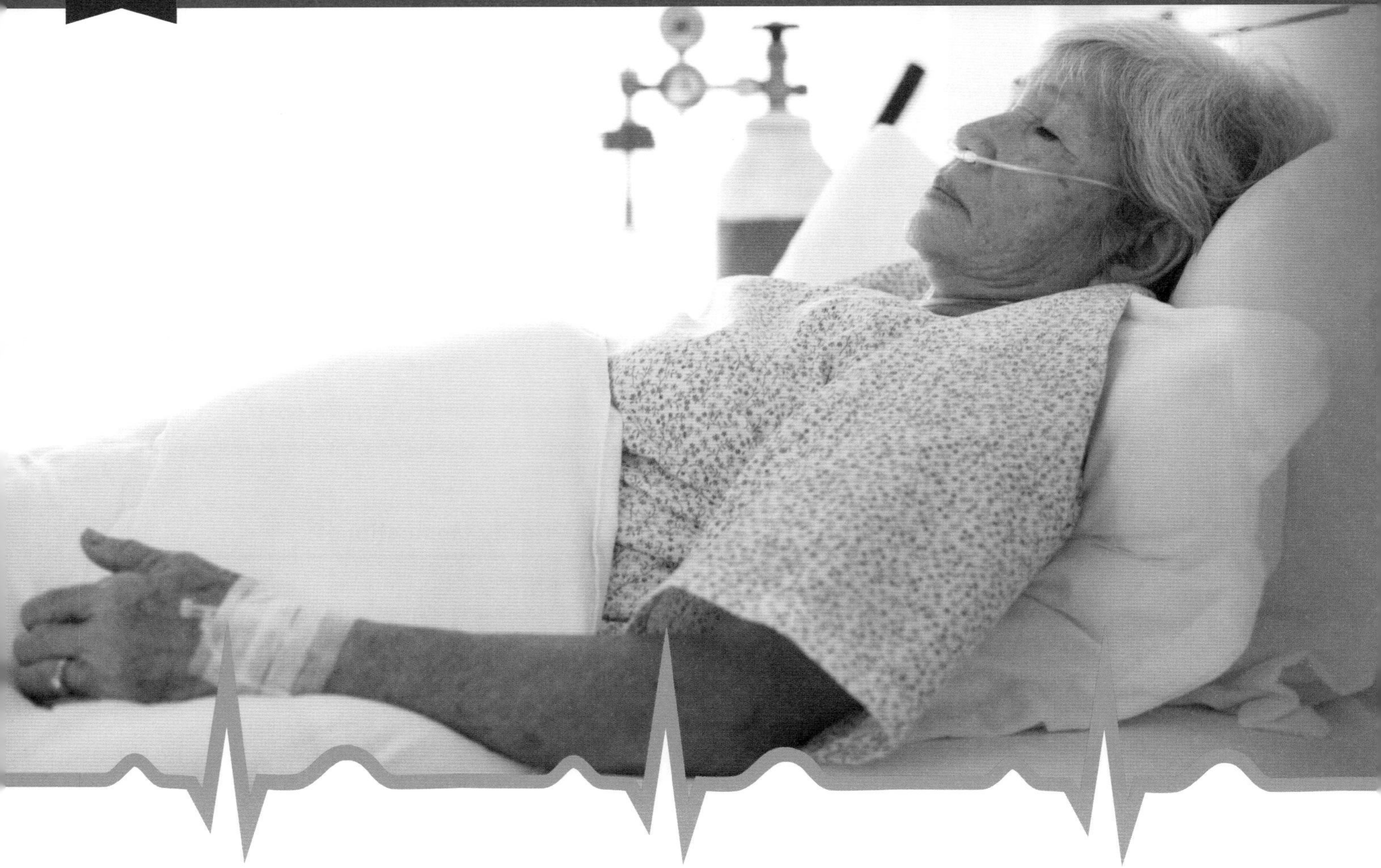

Go To Clinical Case 2

An 88-year-old female client, H.S., has been a resident at the long-term care facility for the past three years. She is historically independent in most ADLs, including ambulation. Today, she is having difficulty speaking and a loss of balance. Her face is drooping on the right side and she is complaining of a severe headache. Her right arm is also remarkably weaker compared to the left. These signs and symptoms appeared within the last hour.

She has a past medical history of hypertension, high cholesterol, and diabetes mellitus, type 2. She currently takes atenolol, simvastatin, insulin, and aspirin along with a multiple vitamin. She has no significant family history. She is a widow with one child who regularly comes to visit.

She was taken via ambulance to the local hospital. Her vital signs are blood pressure 178/98 mm Hg, pulse of 90 beats per minute, respirations 16 breaths per minute, oxygen saturation of 98% on 2L of oxygen via nasal cannula.

Next Gen Clinical Judgment

Describe how the words **BE FAST** are used to identify victims of stroke?

NurseThink® Time

Using the NurseThink® system, complete the priorities. Check your answers designated by 💡 in the Stroke Priority Exemplar.

NurseThink® Time

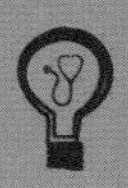

Priority Data Collection or Cues

1.

2.

3.

Priority Laboratory Tests/Diagnostics

1.

2.

3.

Priority Interventions or Actions

1.

2.

3.

Priority Potential & Actual Complications

1.

2.

3.

Priority Nursing Implications

1.

2.

3.

Priority Medications

1.

2.

3.

Reinforcement of Priority Teaching

1.

2.

3.

Pathophysiology/Description

- Also called brain attack (conveys the message of medical emergency), causes brain cell necrosis/infarction
- Effects and prognosis depends upon location and extent of brain damage
- Increasing incidence with the aging population
- Risk factors
  - Non-modifiable include age, gender, race/ethnicity, and family history/heredity
  - Modifiable include hypertension, heart disease, diabetes, hypercholesterolemia, smoking, alcohol abuse, cocaine, abdominal obesity, physical activity, high estrogen/progestin oral contraceptives, sickle cell disease, dysrhythmias (atrial fibrillation)
- Types:
  - Ischemic stroke
    - Thrombotic occlusion of a vessel-related to hypertension and diabetes, often preceded by a TIA (transient ischemic attack)
    - Embolic in which thrombus from heart or elsewhere travels to cerebral vessel and lodges, rapid progression
  - Hemorrhagic is bleeding into the brain tissues, intracerebral, subarachnoid, cerebral aneurysm–related to hypertension, poor prognosis
- Transient ischemic attacks (TIA) which are short-term changes in neurological function without brain infarction (1/3 TIA victims have a stroke, 1/3 have additional TIAs, 1/3 have no further effects)

Priority Data Collection or Cues

- Check vital signs and neurological status
- Check for motor changes contralateral to the site of brain cell death–visual changes, weakness, hemiparesis, numbness, loss of sensation, facial drooping, tinnitus, vertigo, darkened or blurred vision, diplopia, ptosis, dysphagia, dysarthria, ataxia, aphasia
- Additional signs and symptoms may include: headache ("the worst headache ever"), nausea/vomiting, loss of bowel/bladder function, change in level of consciousness, cognitive abilities, changes in affect, memory limitations, spatial/perceptual alterations

Priority Laboratory Tests/Diagnostics

- CT Scan or MRI (serial CT scans for progress)
- CT angiography or MR angiography/Intraarterial digital subtraction angiography
- Cardiac, carotid angiography
- Transcranial doppler, lumbar puncture (avoid with increased intracranial pressure [ICP])

Priority Interventions or Actions

- Prevention such as lifestyle changes and routine antiplatelet therapy
- Acute management with oxygenation, stabilize blood pressure, balance hydration: Maintain perfusion without increasing ICP (maintain normal ICP), check sodium and glucose levels
- Ischemic treated with fibrinolytic treatment
- Hemorrhagic stroke is managed by controlling hypertension and surgical evacuation of hemorrhage
- Rehabilitation includes the interprofessional team–physical/occupational/speech therapy for swallow therapy and speech therapy
- Place the client on fall prevention as indicated

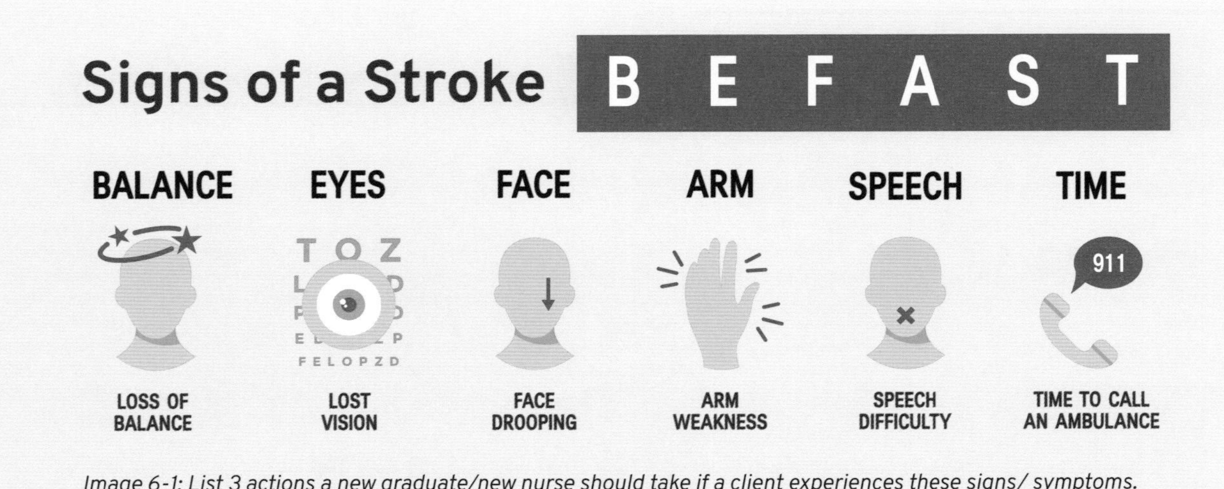

Image 6-1: List 3 actions a new graduate/new nurse should take if a client experiences these signs/ symptoms.

Priority Potential & Actual Complications

- About one-third of stroke victims have permanent disability, about one-fourth require long-term care
- Strokes are the 4th leading cause of death in adults
- Long-term consequences include hemiparesis, inability to walk, aphasia, lack of independence in personal care, and depression
- Other complications related to immobility, disuse, and treatment/lack of treatment (hemorrhage, neurological compromise, cerebral edema, urinary tract infection)

Priority Nursing Implications

- The significant role of nursing is prevention such as monitoring and managing modifiable risk factors-healthy diet, smoking cessation, regular exercise, weight control, limitation of alcohol, and routine screening
- Use evidence-based stroke scales
- During acute treatment, nurses maintain client safety. Watch for breathing and hydration status. Notify the charge nurse of any changes
- Provide strategies to prevent pneumonia (coughing, deep breathing, turning) and contractures/skin breakdown (positioning, splinting, passive and active ROM exercises)
- Provide support in communication, dealing with visual and functional changes (bowel and bladder retraining), unilateral neglect caused by visual field changes

Priority Medications

- Tissue plasminogen activator (tPA)
  - Thrombolytic
  - With ischemic strokes
  - 3-4.5 hours from onset of symptoms
  - Monitor closely for bleeding
  - Administered intravenously or intraarterially usually administered by RN
- Aspirin
  - Monitor for bleeding
  - Administered orally
- Clopidogrel
  - Antiplatelet
  - Hold prior to surgery or dental procedures
  - Administered orally
- Simvastatin
  - Antilipemic
  - Take orally at bedtime
  - Watch for rhabdomyolysis
- Labetalol
  - Beta-blocker
  - To control blood pressure
  - Given prior to tPA administration
  - May be given orally or intravenous

Reinforcement of Priority Teaching

- Provide client/family support related to changes in function
- Explore strategies to enhance self-esteem/self-care in all activities of daily living, dealing with frustration, fear, and emotional lability
- Provide referrals for rehabilitation-access adapted devices to promote self-care
- Provide community resources for client and family

Next Gen Clinical Judgment

From the Go To Clinical Case 2, answer the following:

1. What non-modifiable and modifiable risk factors did Ms. S demonstrate?
2. What are the symptoms that differentiate a right-sided stroke from a left-sided stroke?
3. When using an evidence-based stroke scale, what data would the nurse need to collect?
4. Based on Ms. S's current living situation, who should be included in the discharge planning?

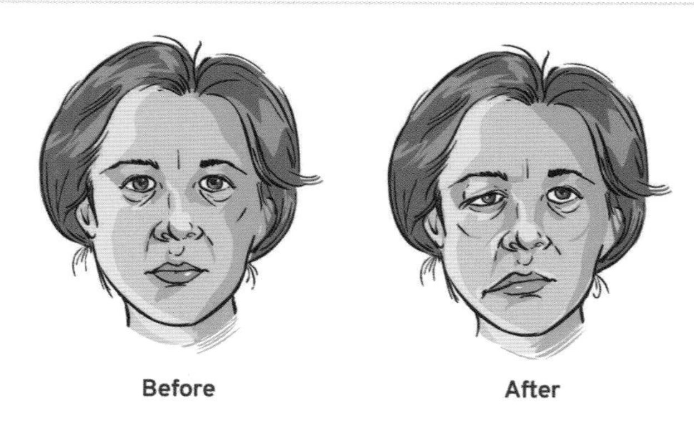

Image 6-2: A client in the outpatient clinic is sitting in the waiting room. You see the change depicted in the image. What is the next nursing action?

Go To Clinical Answers

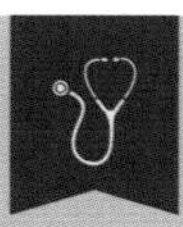

Text designated by 💡 are the top answers for the Go To Clinical related to Stroke.

Heart failure

Pathophysiology/Description

- Inadequate pumping/filling of the heart, insufficient blood to meet the oxygen needs of tissues. Impaired cardiac output from changes in preload, afterload, contractility, and heart rate
- Related to untreated or prolonged hypertension, coronary artery disease, myopathies and history of myocardial infarction, also age and health of the ventricles
- Related to advanced age, obesity, high serum cholesterol, and tobacco use
- Described as systolic, diastolic, or mixed failure or left and right failure
  - Left-sided failure-fluid in lung tissue/pleural circulation
  - Right-sided failure-fluid in the periphery/systemic circulation

Priority Data Collection or Cues

- Vital signs. Watch for increased respiratory rate, increased heart rate (compensate for clients on beta-blockers), monitor for hypotension (increased tissue perfusion or medication side effects) and hypertension (anxiety/history)
- Increased respiratory effort, cough (early sign), later-productive cough of blood-tinged sputum; breath sounds-decreased sounds, crackles, wheezes, sonorous wheeze
- Edema may be dependent/peripheral, ascites, pulmonary edema/pleural effusion, pitting edema (1 kg. weight/1 liter fluid), check perfusion in edematous extremities
- Health history may include: orthopnea (may experience paroxysmal nocturnal dyspnea), shortness of breath with exertion (dyspnea), levels of fatigue, history of nocturia, chest pain, or rapid fluid weight gain
- Appearance such as anxiety, pallor, cyanosis, confusion, restlessness

Priority Laboratory Tests/Diagnostics

- BNP (brain natriuretic protein levels)
- Chest X-ray/arterial blood gases in acute phase
- ECG may show hypertrophy
- Cardiac ultrasound/cardiac catheterization
- Endomyocardial biopsy
- Ejection fraction studies

Priority Interventions or Actions

- Oxygen, elevate head of bed to relieve dyspnea
- Monitor vital signs, ECG, oxygen saturation, urine output, daily or more frequent weights
- Cardiac rehabilitation, rest
- Low sodium diet, with possible fluid restrictions
- Support and counseling for depression and anxiety

Priority Potential & Actual Complications

- Respiratory Distress secondary to pleural effusion
- Cardiac dysrhythmias, Cardiogenic shock, Cardiopulmonary failure
- Skin breakdown with edema
- Left ventricular thrombus
- Hepatomegaly
- Renal failure

Priority Nursing Implications

- Monitor hydration status, provide fluid restrictions if prescribed
- Comfort interventions and skin care with edema, elevate legs to relieve edema, use of compression stockings
- Encourage a low-sodium, adequate potassium diet
- Provide a calm environment, reduce anxiety
- Manage other cardiac diseases as needed

Priority Medications

- Digoxin
  - Slows heart rate and strengthen contractility
  - Apical pulse for one minute prior to administration-hold for low heart rate (< 60 bpm for adults, <100 bpm for infants, as prescribed by health care provider for children)
  - Monitor for signs of digoxin toxicity
  - Administered orally
- Furosemide
  - Diuretic-reduce fluid volume
  - Monitor output-diuresis
  - Serum potassium level, supplement may be needed
  - Administered orally, IM or intravenous
- Potassium chloride
  - Potassium supplement–administered orally
  - Monitor lab work

Reinforcement of Priority Teaching

- Watch for FACES including fatigue, limitation of activity, cough and congestion, edema, and shortness of breath
- Using oxygen at home including safe oxygen use
- Eat a potassium–rich/low sodium food each day
- Plan for rest periods and spread out activities
- Monitor weigh daily using same scale and similar clothes at similar times of day. Report if weight increases 3+ lbs
- Check with health care provider when considering over-the-counter medications and herbal preparations
- Fall prevention and accessing emergency assistance

Shock

Pathophysiology/Description

- Shock is decreased perfusion yielding inadequate blood flow to the tissues with decreased oxygen and nutrients, impaired cellular metabolism, and buildup of CO_2
- Stages include compensatory, progressive, and irreversible
- Cardiogenic includes reductions in cardiac output, largely related to left ventricular failure (MI), inability of the heart to fill, dysrhythmias, and structural factors
- Hypovolemic includes a decrease in circulating blood flow related to loss of blood or other body fluids, fluid shifts, or internal bleeding (may be absolute or relative)
- Septic/Neurogenic/Anaphylactic are secondary to vasodilation related to infection, spinal cord injury/ anesthesia, or hypersensitivity

Priority Data Collection or Cues

- Identify early and manage clients at risk to prevent shock
- General shock signs/symptoms
    - Early signs include tachycardia, anxious appearance, confusion, tachypnea, restlessness, impaired end organ perfusion, hypoactive bowel sounds
    - Later signs include tachycardia, hypotension, changes in level of consciousness, changes in urine output, narrowing pulse pressure
- Cardiogenic
    - Crackles in the lung fields, may have chest pain, nausea or vomiting
- Hypovolemic
    - Tachypnea may progress to bradypnea
- Distributive: Septic/Neurogenic/Anaphylactic
    - Septic signs – bradycardia, skin warm and flushed
    - Neurogenic signs – dysfunction will correlate with level of insult or injury (bladder dysfunction)
    - Anaphylactic signs – shortness of breath, stridor, wheezing, incontinence, swelling

Priority Laboratory Tests/Diagnostics

- General: CBC, electrolytes, and arterial blood gases
- Cardiogenic
    - BNP (brain natriuretic protein levels)
    - ECG (dysrhythmias)
    - CXR
    - Echocardiogram
- Hypovolemic
    - Decreased Hgb and Hct
    - Elevated urine specific gravity
- Septic
    - Elevated white blood cell count, glucose, lactate levels
    - Positive blood cultures
    - Elevated urine specific gravity

Priority Interventions or Actions

- General: Early identification and eliminate cause
    - Provide high flow oxygen as prescribed
    - Intravenous access, nasogastric tube and urinary catheter
    - Warm fluids to prevent hypothermia and dysrhythmias
- Septic
    - Antibiotics
- Early initiation of enteral feedings and monitor client weight

Priority Potential & Actual Complications

- Systemic inflammatory response syndrome (SIRS)
- Multiorgan system failure
- Renal failure
- Dependence on mechanical ventilation
- Neurological changes secondary to anoxia
- May be fatal (high mortality rate)

Priority Nursing Implications

- Closely monitor neurological status that may be a result of poor perfusion, safety measures with changes in level of consciousness
- Monitor I & O and hydration status/perfusion status
- Check bowel sounds and abdominal girth
- Early nasogastric/enteral feedings are associated with improved prognosis
- Check client's temperature and manage environmental temperature closely
- Provide basic care (bathing, oral hygiene, and turning/ positioning) to avoid complications
- Ask about allergens in cases of anaphylactic shock

Priority Medications

- In most situations, the following medications will be administered intravenous by a RN
    - Dobutamine, dopamine, epinephrine, atropine, corticosteroids

Reinforcement of Priority Teaching

- Depending upon the etiology, reinforce education on:
    - Allergies/allergy bracelet, safety and injury prevention, hydration and monitoring of fluids, rest, and activity moderation with cardiac disease
- Engage multidisciplinary team to recondition the client after a critical illness
- Engage family and support systems to set goals and motivate client with long-term recovery

Pathophysiology/Description

- Affects myocardial structure and function
- Disease of the heart muscle that makes it less able to pump blood to meet the needs of the body
- May be subacute or chronic
- May be primary or secondary (related to myocardial infarction, drug toxicity, hypertension, or infections)
- Three major types: Dilated, hypertrophic, and restrictive

Priority Data Collection or Cues

- Ask client about fatigue, weakness, dyspnea, angina, palpitations, syncope, and exercise intolerance
- Listen to heart sounds to include: S3 and S4 gallops, murmurs, dysrhythmias, exaggerated or displaced apical impulse (hypertrophic)
- Ask about history of infectious myocarditis or alcohol abuse (dilated), being an athlete (hypertrophic)

Priority Laboratory Tests/Diagnostics

- CXR may show cardiomegaly, pleural effusion
- ECG may show hypertrophy or dysrhythmias
- BNP(brain natriuretic protein levels) (< 100 pg/mL–HF unlikely; >400 pg/mL–HF likely; 100-400 pg/mL–use clinical judgment)
- Doppler echocardiography
- Endomyocardial biopsy, nuclear imaging studies (MUGA scan) to determine ejection fraction, or cardiac catheterization

Priority Interventions or Actions

- Often palliative, rather than curative treatment including management of heart failure
- Surgery or medications may be indicated

Priority Potential & Actual Complications

- Varies with type including acute pulmonary edema (restrictive), emboli (dilated, restricted), sudden death (nonobstructed hypertrophic), atrial fibrillation (obstructed hypertrophic, ventricular dysrthythmias (dilated)
- Leads to cardiomegaly, heart failure, valvular incompetence, dysrhythmias, and decreased cardiac output; leading indication for heart transplantation

Priority Nursing Implications

- Monitor client related to activities and exercise–optimize positive effects but decrease stress on heart
- Reinforce education about medications and management strategies
- Often care is palliative and requires support and sensitivity to maximize quality of life and contentment

Priority Medications

- Metoprolol
  - Beta-blocker (-lol)–may be given orally or intravenous
  - Check pulse
  - Cautious use with asthma, kidney disease, and COPD
- Digitalis
  - Cardiac glycocide–given orally
  - Watch for toxicity
  - Hold for apical heart rate less than 60 bpm
- Nifedipine, verapamil
  - Calcium channel blockers–given orally or intravenous
  - Check blood pressure and pulse
- Lisinopril
  - Angiotensin-converting enzyme (ACE) inhibitors–administered orally
  - Ask about (benign) cough

Reinforcement of Priority Teaching

- Monitor for signs of heart failure including dyspnea, pedal edema, orthopnea, fatigue, weight gain
- Adequate hydration (unless fluid restricted) and a low sodium diet, avoid large meals
- Avoid alcohol, caffeine, and other stimulants
- Light exercise, avoiding heavy lifting or isometric exercises, and adequate rest
- Have caregivers learn CPR
- May be at risk for infective endocarditis–prophylactic antibiotics

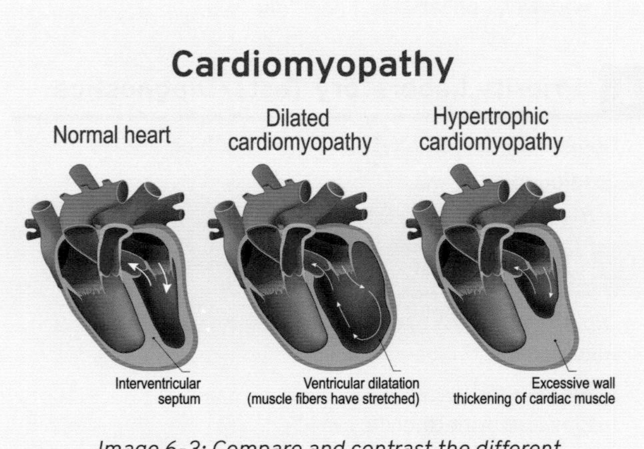

Image 6-3: Compare and contrast the different types of cardiomyopathies.

Coronary artery disease (CAD)

Pathophysiology/Description

- Deposits of lipids, endothelial injury, and inflammation within the intima of an artery
- Although known by many names, most symptomatic is atherosclerosis of the coronary arteries
- Progressive disease that develops in stages with fatty streaks (lipid deposits), fibrous plaques (changes in endothelium and reduction in blood flow), and complicated lesions (plaque ulceration and rupture, thrombus formation)
- Characterized by modifiable (elevated serum lipids, hypertension, tobacco use, physical inactivity, obesity), contributing/modifiable (diabetes mellitus, metabolic syndrome, stress/anger, high homocysteine levels, and substance abuse) and non-modifiable risk factors (age, gender, ethnicity, family history)

Priority Data Collection or Cues

- Collect family history and for nonmodifiable risk factors
- Determine if there are any symptoms of occlusion of a vessel (angina/MI) or poor perfusion
- Ask clients about modifiable risk factors and lifestyle

Priority Laboratory Tests/Diagnostics

- C-reactive protein is elevated with inflammation
- Serum cholesterol levels (Risk associated with total cholesterol >200 mg/dL; triglycerides >150 mg/dL; LDL >160 mg/dL; HDL <40 mg/dL in men; HDL <50 mg/dL in women)
- Fasting blood glucose >100 mg/dL increases risk

Priority Interventions or Actions

- Promote physical activity, optimal nutrition
- Smoking and substance use cessation
- Frequent monitoring of blood levels and risk determination

Priority Potential & Actual Complications

- Acute coronary syndrome-unstable angina, MI
- Sudden cardiac may be fatal

Priority Nursing Implications

- Role in screening and assisting clients to manage modifiable and contributing modifiable risk factors
- Omega-3 fatty acids, niacin, psyllium and soy have been associated with reductions in serum cholesterol levels
- Lifestyle changes may be difficult for clients and require information, goal setting, enhanced motivation, and ongoing support

Priority Medications

- Simvastatin
  - Antilipemic (statin)
  - Administered orally at night
  - May cause GI upset; avoid grapefruit and grapefruit juice
- Niacin
  - Antilipemic–administered orally
  - May cause significant flushing (may premedicate with NSAIDs or ASA)
  - May also cause GI side effects or orthostatic hypotension
- Low dose aspirin
  - Antiplatelet
  - Check for bleeding
  - Take orally with meals and monitor for GI upset, potential ulcerative
  - Clopidogrel may be considered
- Ezetimibe
  - Inhibit cholesterol absorption
  - Should be taken orally along with dietary revision
  - May be combined with statin medications
  - Considered a lifetime medication choice

Reinforcement of Priority Teaching

- Moderate exercise (30 minutes/day on most days)
- Modifying lifestyle-smoking cessation
- Diet- decreased saturated fats with adequate polyunsaturated fats

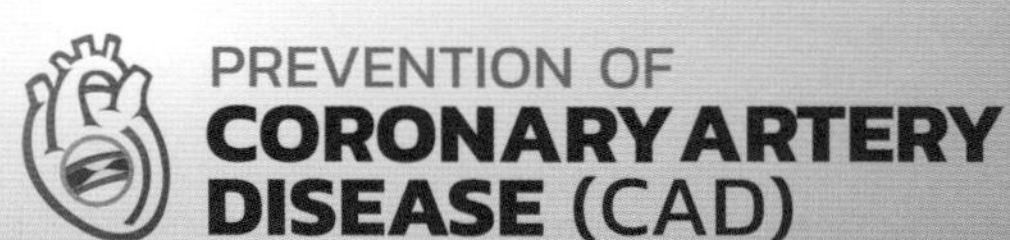

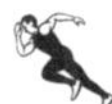 EXERCISING REGULARLY

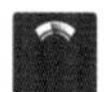 MAINTAINING A HEALTHY WEIGHT

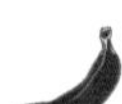 EATING A BALANCED DIET THAT'S LOW IN SODIUM AND HIGH IN FRUITS AND VEGETABLES

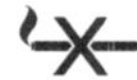 AVOIDING SMOKING

 DRINKING ONLY IN MODERATION

Image 6-4: What other recommendations could be made to prevent CAD?

Myocardial infarction (MI)/acute coronary syndrome

Pathophysiology/Description

- MI is Ischemia and necrosis of myocardial tissue, often related to thrombus blockage of a coronary vessel, described based on vessel/location of damage dictates severity, severity also impacted by extent of collateral circulation
- Acute coronary syndrome includes unstable angina, non-ST segment elevation MI, and ST elevation MI
- Unstable angina is a medical emergency when there is a change from previous, chronic angina, and significant chest pain with little exertion and fatigue

Priority Data Collection or Cues

- Check for vital signs and observe for elevated HR/RR, decreased or increased BP, decreased oxygen saturation
- Ask about chest pain. Determine if the chest pain is severe pain that is not relieved by rest, position change or nitrates, pain is described as heavy pressure on the chest or upper abdomen
- May include atypical presentations, for example, women may present with jaw or chin pain, fatigue, arm and chest pain, shortness of breath-leading to delays in treatment
- Observe perfusion in extremities, level of consciousness, urine output
- Ask about nausea/vomiting
- Observe for fever, diaphoresis, ashen/pale skin color, anxious appearance

Priority Laboratory Tests/Diagnostics

- ECG may show ST elevation, T wave inversion, abnormal Q waves
- Serum cardiac markers include cardiac specific troponin T/ cardiac specific troponin I (increase 4-6 hours after MI, peak 10-24 hours, baseline 10-14 days), creatine kinase/creatine kinase MB (rise 6 hours after MI, peak at 18 hours, baseline 10-14 days), Myoglobin (rise 2 hours after MI and peak 3-15 hours)
- Coronary angiography

Priority Interventions or Actions

- Bedrest with HOB elevated, ensure intravenous access is present, progressive activity
- Oxygen, Nitroglycerin, and chewable aspirin may be prescribed
- Unstable angina with negative cardiac markers: Antiplatelets and heparin
- Morphine to decrease sympathetic stimulation due to pain

Priority Potential & Actual Complications

- Dysrhythmias, heart failure, or cardiogenic shock
- Papillary muscle dysfunction (leading to mitral valve dysfunction), ventricular aneurysm, pericarditis, Dressler syndrome (antibody-antigen response post-MI- includes pericarditis with fluid/effusion and fever)
- May be fatal

Priority Nursing Implications

- Have client rate pain and describe location, radiation, relieving and precipitating factors
- Monitor pulse oximetry and vital signs closely
- Relieve client stress and provide analgesics as prescribed
- Lower head of bed with hypotension

Priority Medications

- Nitroglycerine
  - Various forms and routes
  - Watch for hypotension
  - May become tolerant
- Morphine
  - May be administered orally or intravenous
  - Decrease chest pain and anxiety
  - Watch for respiratory depression or hypotension
- Docusate sodium
  - Stool softeners–administered orally
  - Prevent straining-Valsalva induced bradycardia
- Other medications may include antiplatelets, anticoagulants, beta blockers, angiotensin-converting enzyme inhibitors, thrombolytics, and aspirin

Reinforcement of Priority Teaching

- Cardiac rehabilitation including progressive exercise, recommendations on sexual activity, and a diet low in cholesterol and sodium, high in fiber
- Avoid stressful situations, abrupt changes in environmental temperature and heavy meals
- Management of angina and emergency care
- Remind about home use and safe storage of NTG
- Risk factors and the benefits of cessation of smoking, weight management, moderation in alcohol, and a diet low in fat/sodium/cholesterol and high in fiber

Peripheral artery disease (PAD)

Pathophysiology/Description

- The peripheral arteries become narrowed and thickened in the upper and lower extremities, causing changes in perfusion
- Changes occur distal to the level of the obstruction
- Related to diabetes, other cardiovascular disease (atherosclerosis), and lifestyle choices
- May be acute or chronic

Priority Data Collection or Cues

- Ask about risk factors include tobacco use, diabetes, hyperlipidemia, and hypertension
- Consider family history, lifestyle (increased when sedentary), and levels of stress
- Check the affected extremities including intermittent claudication, paresthesias, skin may be shiny, tight, with loss of hair, thickening of toenails, pulses decreased or absent, elevation pallor/dependent rubor, prolonged capillary refill, rest pain, and cool extremities
- Check segmental blood pressures and note discrepancies

Priority Laboratory Tests/Diagnostics

- Elevated C-reactive protein, serum lipid levels
- Duplex doppler imaging and doppler pulse readings
- Serum blood glucose levels and glycosylated hemoglobin (HgbA1c)
- Arteriogram or ankle-brachial index to determine severity of PAD

Priority Interventions or Actions

- Risk modification including smoking cessation, management of diabetes and hypertension
- Control of serum lipid levels including diet and medications
- Exercise, weight reduction, and dietary modification-walking programs
- Skin care-clean and inspect feet regularly, do not soak feet
- Keep feet dependent and without constriction to increase blood flow
- Acute occlusions or ulcerations may require surgical or radiological intervention

Priority Potential & Actual Complications

- May progress to rest pain, ulceration, sepsis and/or gangrene, indicative of critical limb ischemia
- Gangrene and infection leading to potential amputation
- Acute arterial ischemia (sudden obstruction of blood flow caused by embolism, thrombosis, trauma, or atherosclerosis of artery)

Priority Nursing Implications

- Nurses should look at extremities thoroughly and frequently to detect changes early
- Provide skin care and refrain from soaking feet or hands to avoid maceration
- Position clients to avoid constriction; do not bend knees, use knee gatch, or cross legs
- Ask about pain and treat as appropriate

Priority Medications

- Aspirin (ASA)
  - Antiplatelet–administered orally
  - Watch for bleeding
  - Monitor for GI upset
- Clopidogrel
  - Antiplatelet–administered orally
  - Watch for bleeding
- Cilostazol
  - Administered orally
  - Inhibits platelet aggregation and is a vasodilator
  - Used for intermittent claudication
  - May require additional antiplatelet therapy (clopidogrel, dipyridamole)

Reinforcement of Priority Teaching

- Vigilant foot care, to wear white, all-cotton socks and to avoid extremes in temperature
- Provide client with a complete list of changes to watch for in circulation—appearance of feet and for changes in sensation or function
- Optimal diet, to include: High fiber, high protein, low-fat, low refined sugars, reduce sodium intake and drink plenty of water; avoid caffeine
- Relieve extremity pain by placing limb dependent; if edema exists, legs may be elevated but not above level of the heart

Valvular heart disease

Pathophysiology/Description

- Determined on which valve is affected (mitral, pulmonic, aortic, or tricuspid) and alteration (stenosis [constriction] or regurgitation [insufficiency]), or prolapse
- Occurs in children and teens from congenital heart defects or rheumatic heart disease; older adults from cardiovascular disease (previous MI, cardiomyopathy)
- Rheumatic heart disease from untreated streptococcal infections-represents key prevention strategy
- Degenerative valve disorder is most commonly seen in geriatric patients

Priority Data Collection or Cues

- Listen to heart sounds for abnormalities (a murmur may be heard with auscultation)
- Monitor extremities for pulses, skin color, and temperature
- Monitor level of consciousness and urine output
- Ask about history of chest pain, hemoptysis, shortness of breath, fatigue, palpitations, weakness, orthopnea, paroxysmal nocturnal dyspnea, peripheral edema, dizziness, and fever

Priority Laboratory Tests/Diagnostics

- Chest x-ray (may indicate cardiomegaly)
- CT of chest
- CBC
- ECG – Report any abnormalities
- Cardiac ultrasound-transesophageal echocardiography/catheterization

Priority Interventions or Actions

- Medications to prevent or treat heart failure, anticoagulants, antidysrhythmia agents
- Percutaneous valve replacement or percutaneous transluminal balloon valvuloplasty
- Potential for surgical intervention (valve repair or replacement)
- Sodium restricted diet, sometimes limit caffeine
- Anticoagulation therapy with valve replacement (for life with mechanical valve, 3-6 months for bioprosthetic valve)

Priority Potential & Actual Complications

- Mitral stenosis-atrial fibrillation, emboli (stroke)
- Mitral regurgitation-left ventricular hypertrophy, pulmonary hypertension/edema
- Aortic stenosis-aortic dissection, sudden cardiovascular collapse
- Infective endocarditis
- Operative mortality, especially with older adults

Priority Nursing Implications

- Monitor client safety with medications, including medication precautions and fall precautions
- Encourage communication and provide support to clients suffering chronic illness

Priority Medications

- Nitroglycerine
  - Various methods of administration
  - Vasodilator
  - For angina
  - Watch for hypotension-risk for syncope, falls
- Antibiotics
  - Administered orally or intravenous
  - To prevent subacute bacterial endocarditis
- Atenolol
  - Administered orally
  - Beta blocker
  - Check pulse and blood pressure
  - Avoid use with asthma or COPD (bronchoconstriction)
- Warfarin
  - Oral anticoagulant
  - Monitor bleeding times
  - Maintain normal intake of Vitamin K rich foods

Reinforcement of Priority Teaching

- Smoking cessation and moderate exercise regimens
- Follow health care providers' recommendations for antibiotic prophylaxis for dental and surgical procedures
- Adequate hydration and, in some cases, limit caffeine
- Monitor for signs of heart failure: Shortness of breath, pedal edema, orthopnea, fatigue
- If discharged on warfarin, encourage the client to monitor for bleeding and have regular lab work as prescribed

Pathophysiology/Description

- Thromboangiitis obliterans (Buerger's Disease)
  - Recurrent arterial inflammation in arms and legs when thrombus blocks the vessel—causes thrombosis, fibrosis, and ischemia
  - More in men with histories of smoking tobacco or marijuana
  - Associated with chronic periodontal infections
- Raynaud's Phenomenon
  - Spastic, episodic inflammation of small, cutaneous arteries
  - More common in women
  - May occur alone or with arthritis or systemic lupus erythematosus
  - Increased with chronic exposure to cold, vibrating machinery, or heavy metals

Priority Data Collection or Cues

- Thromboangiitis obliterans (Buerger's Disease)
  - Ask about intermittent claudication, pain at rest/aching pain most severe at night, paresthesias, cold sensitivity, and skin ulcerations
  - Monitor for changes in perfusion, pulses, skin temperature, lesions, and color--may be cool and red in dependent position
- Raynaud's Phenomenon
  - Determine perfusion in fingers, toes, nose, ears and cheeks-for temperature and color-pale to blue to purple
  - Monitor for recirculation after spasm for redness (rubor)
  - Client description of coldness and numbness/tingling followed by throbbing, aching pain, and swelling
  - Ask about changes in skin and nails, monitor for ulcers and lesions

Priority Laboratory Tests/Diagnostics

- Both conditions diagnosed based on symptoms, skin changes, and risk behaviors

Priority Interventions or Actions

- Thromboangiitis obliterans (Buerger's Disease)
  - Smoking cessation of tobacco and marijuana (nicotine replacement not an option)
  - Avoid triggers (tobacco, marijuana) progressive exercise, symptom management of skin lesions, and pain management
- Raynaud's Phenomenon
  - Avoid precipitating factors
  - Warm water soaks during vasoconstriction

Priority Potential & Actual Complications

- Thromboangiitis obliterans (Buerger's Disease)
  - Vascular occlusion, gangrene, and amputation
- Raynaud's Phenomenon
  - Ischemia requiring surgical debridement
  - In advanced cases surgical intervention may be indicated

Priority Nursing Implications

- Check for skin breakdown and infections in clients at high-risk for peripheral vascular conditions
- Assist clients with smoking cessation or participation in vasoconstrictive activities

Priority Medications

- Cilostazol
  - Oral antiplatelet and vasodilator improve circulation (more effective with vasospasm than vessel occlusion)
  - Causes orthostatic hypotension
  - Not with alcohol-increases hypotension
- Pentoxifylline
  - Administered orally
  - Decreases viscosity of blood
- Nifedipine
  - Relax smooth muscles of the arterioles
  - Calcium channel blockers–administered orally

Reinforcement of Priority Teaching

- Thromboangiitis obliterans (Buerger's Disease)
  - Permanent cessation of vasoconstrictive chemicals
  - Avoid trauma/infection
- Raynaud's Phenomenon
  - Triggers for episodes including avoiding emotional upset, exposure to cold, caffeine, cocaine, and tobacco
  - Avoid restrictive clothing, extreme changes in exposure, and vasoconstrictive chemicals, to wear warm clothes when exposed to cold
  - Soak toes and fingers in warm water during "attacks"
  - Stress management strategies

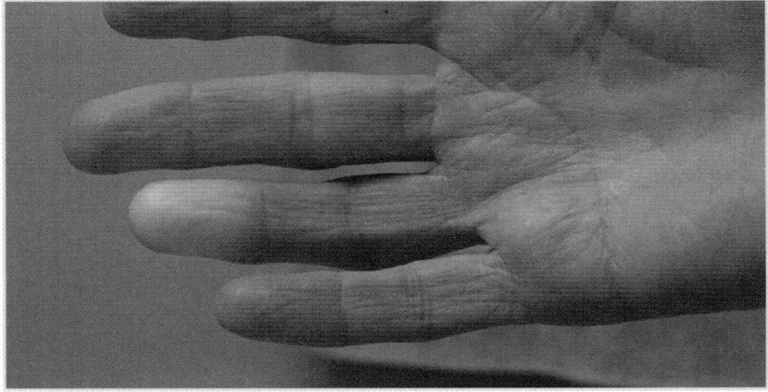

Image 6-5: What action would the nurse take for this client?

Venous thromboembolism (VTE)

Pathophysiology/Description

- Forming of a thrombus (clot) with inflammation of the vein
- May be superficial (SVT) or deep (VTE)
- Occur as the result of venous stasis, damage to the internal lining of the vein, and increased coagulability of the blood
- May become an embolus when it breaks off and goes through the bloodstream

Priority Data Collection or Cues

- Note calf, thigh, or groin pain with or without swelling, warmth and tenderness superficial to the area of pain
- Measure calves and thighs for comparison and baseline
- Homan's sign is controversial and may yield false positives and may mobilize the clot, not recommended in at risk clients
- With SVT, vein may be itchy, swollen, red or warm
- With VTE, symptoms of SVT plus paresthesias, may be febrile, marked edema or cyanosis of extremity

Priority Laboratory Tests/Diagnostics

- Venous compression/Duplex ultrasound
- D-Dimer-elevated results suggest VTE (normal <250 ng/mL)
- Fibrin monomer complex-thrombin>antithrombin (normal < 6.1 mg/L)
- CT/MRI
- APTT, INR, Hgb, Hct

Priority Interventions or Actions

- With SVT, larger clots may require anticoagulants, smaller clots may be treated with oral and topical NSAIDs, anti-embolic stockings, and light ambulation
- With Acute VTE, bed rest with elevation of extremity, promote deep vein circulation with anti-embolic stockings, pneumatic compression boots, and progressive activity
- May need thrombolytic therapy to dissolve clot
- Anticoagulation therapy to prevent enlargement of clot or new clot formation
- Provide warm, moist compresses

Priority Potential & Actual Complications

- If superficial thrombi are not managed, may progress to VTE
- Pulmonary embolism
- Post-thrombotic syndrome-20-50% of clients with VTE-venous stiffening, hypertension, and scarring-symptoms include pain, swelling, tingling, venous ulceration

Priority Nursing Implications

- Monitor at-risk clients and provide preventive reinforcement of teaching and care of/need for exercise and refraining from constrictive clothing
- Monitor for bleeding on hemorrhage in clients on anticoagulant therapy (bleeding precautions)
- Avoid massaging of clot site and avoid pneumatic compression devices with actual VTE (may mobilize clot)
- Avoid antiplatelets or NSAIDs with anticoagulants
- Encourage clients on bed rest to turn frequently
- Change position every two hours and perform leg exercises every two hours while awake

Priority Medications

- Heparin
  - Anticoagulant
  - Subcutaneously (or continuous intravenous infusion)
  - Monitor aPTT (normal 25-35 seconds, on heparin-1.5-2.5 times the normal)
  - Antidote is protamine sulfate
  - With subcutaneous injection, deep into the tissue, do not aspirate or rub site
  - Watch for heparin-induced thrombocytopenia
- Warfarin
  - Oral Anticoagulant
  - Monitor INR (International normalized ratio) (0.9-1.1 not on anticoagulants, 2-3 on warfarin, 2.5-3.5 for high-risk clients)
  - Vitamin K is antidote—not immediate
- Enoxaparin
  - Anticoagulant–administered subcutaneously
  - Low molecular weight heparin
  - Monitor CBC at regular intervals
  - Clients may be taught self-administration
  - Rotate injection sites

Reinforcement of Priority Teaching

- Women about the risk of VTE with oral contraceptives or hormone replacement, especially when combined with smoking
- Encourage prevention for those at risk including leg exercises, increased activity, early ambulation, elastic stockings (must be fitted and worn correctly), sequential compression boots (while in hospital), avoid restrictive clothing or crossing legs when sitting
- Some herbs (ginger, garlic, ginseng, gingko) increase bleeding
- Clients should avoid smoking or vasoconstrictive activities

Disseminated intravascular coagulation (DIC)

Pathophysiology/Description

- Uncontrolled bleeding/hemorrhage from disturbances in bleeding (hemorrhagic manifestations), coagulation, and thrombosis (thrombotic manifestations)
- Caused by systemic clot formation with depletion of coagulation factors and platelets
- Many risk factors including shock, septicemia, transfusion of incorrect blood type, obstetric procedures (abruptio placentae, HELLP syndrome), malignancies, burns or severe injury, liver disease, and lupus

Priority Data Collection or Cues

- Monitor vital signs for tachycardia, hypotension, and for deteriorating neurological status
- Check for profuse bleeding including petechiae, purpura, pallor, hematomas, occult blood, and bleeding not responding to pressure, abdominal distension, blood in urine
- Monitor respiratory status including hemoptysis, tachypnea, orthopnea
- Check skin for cyanosis, ischemic tissue necrosis, reductions in kidney function, paralytic ileus, and abdominal pain

Priority Laboratory Tests/Diagnostics

- Complete blood count
- Bleeding times prolonged (prothrombin time, partial thromboplastin time, activated partial thromboplastin time, thrombin time), reduced platelets and fibrinogen
- Elevated D-dimer levels (normal < 250 ng/dl)

Priority Interventions or Actions

- Stabilize the client with oxygenation, ventilation, fluids
- Treat underlying cause
- Monitor blood transfusion, if prescribed
- With thrombosis, assist with the administration of heparin or enoxaparin as prescribed

Priority Potential & Actual Complications

- Hemorrhage
- Renal failure/multiorgan system failure
- Death

Priority Nursing Implications

- Be aware of conditions that may lead to DIC
- Ensure intravenous access
- Conduct frequent checks for bleeding and skin changes associated with thrombosis

Priority Medications

- Heparin
  - Anticoagulant
  - Subcutaneous or intravenous infusion
  - Monitor bleeding times
  - Antidote: Protamine sulfate
- Enoxaparin
  - Low-molecular weight heparin
  - Administered subcutaneously

Reinforcement of Priority Teaching

- Assist clients and family to cope with and rehabilitate from critical illness
- Provide information about the disorder and underlying conditions that precipitate DIC

List 5 common side effects of:
HEPARIN
1. ____________________
2. ____________________
3. ____________________
4. ____________________
5. ____________________

Table 6-3: List the priority nursing action with each listed side effect.

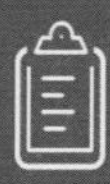

NurseThink® Quiz Questions

1. **The nurse cares for a client with right-sided heart failure. What finding indicates that the client now has secondary left-sided heart failure?**
   a. Jugular vein distention.
   b. Ascites.
   c. Crackles in the lung bases.
   d. Fatigue.

2. **What exercise and activity level does the nurse implement in a client diagnosed with early heart failure?**
   a. Total bedrest with little activity.
   b. Moderate exercise with progressive activity.
   c. Little exercise with minimal activity.
   d. Intense exercise with little other activity.

3. **The nurse reviews a client's health history. What data will increase their risk for developing restrictive cardiomyopathy?**

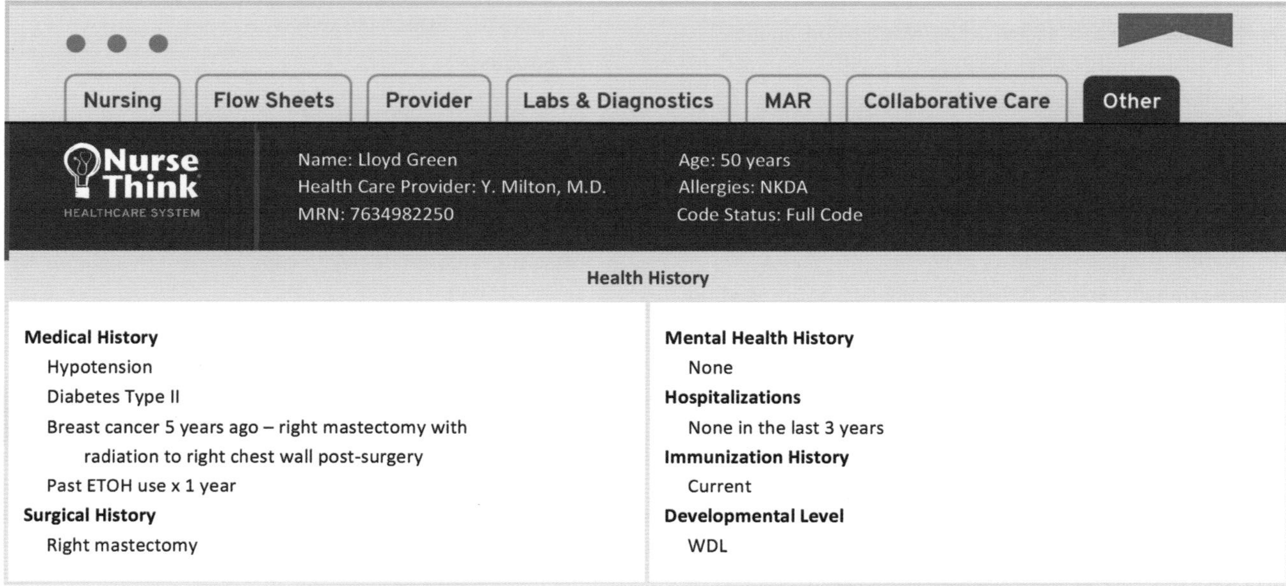

Nursing | Flow Sheets | Provider | Labs & Diagnostics | MAR | Collaborative Care | Other

NurseThink HEALTHCARE SYSTEM

Name: Lloyd Green
Health Care Provider: Y. Milton, M.D.
MRN: 7634982250

Age: 50 years
Allergies: NKDA
Code Status: Full Code

Health History

Medical History	**Mental Health History**
Hypotension	None
Diabetes Type II	**Hospitalizations**
Breast cancer 5 years ago – right mastectomy with radiation to right chest wall post-surgery	None in the last 3 years
Past ETOH use x 1 year	**Immunization History**
Surgical History	Current
Right mastectomy	**Developmental Level**
	WDL

   a. Radiation therapy.
   b. Past ETOH use.
   c. Hypotension.
   d. Diabetes type II.

4. **The nurse assists a client with coronary artery disease with meal planning. Which client choice does the nurse approve?**
   a. Microwavable low-sodium meals.
   b. Canned vegetable soup.
   c. Grilled cheese made with salted butter.
   d. Oatmeal with bananas.

5. **The nurse administers medications for coronary artery disease to a client who has also just been diagnosed with rhabdomyolysis. Which medication does the nurse hold and discuss with the health care provider?**

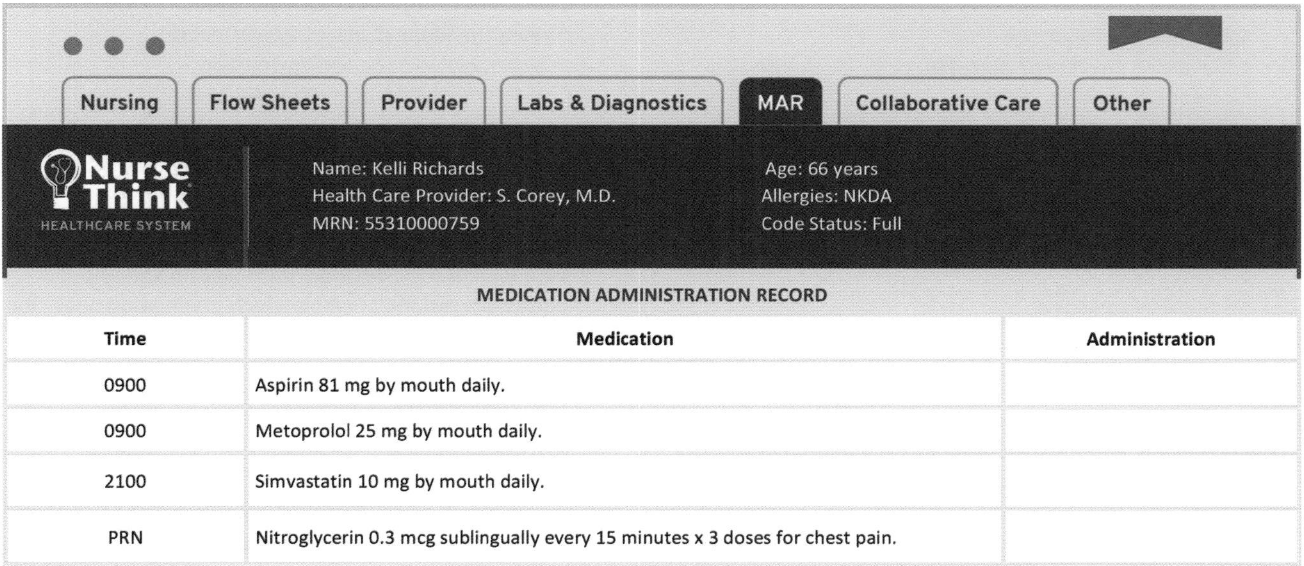
Nursing | Flow Sheets | Provider | Labs & Diagnostics | MAR | Collaborative Care | Other

Nurse Think HEALTHCARE SYSTEM

Name: Kelli Richards
Health Care Provider: S. Corey, M.D.
MRN: 55310000759

Age: 66 years
Allergies: NKDA
Code Status: Full

MEDICATION ADMINISTRATION RECORD

Time	Medication	Administration
0900	Aspirin 81 mg by mouth daily.	
0900	Metoprolol 25 mg by mouth daily.	
2100	Simvastatin 10 mg by mouth daily.	
PRN	Nitroglycerin 0.3 mcg sublingually every 15 minutes x 3 doses for chest pain.	

a. Simvastatin.
b. Nitroglycerin.
c. Metoprolol.
d. Aspirin.

6. **The nurse interviews a client with angina about the nature of their chest pain. What finding indicates the client will be evaluated for an acute myocardial infarction?**
   a. They have chest pain with exercise.
   b. The client is short of breath when climbing stairs.
   c. They have chest pain at rest that does not stop.
   d. They should not need evaluation as all chest pain is expected.

7. **What finding alerts the emergency department nurse that the client will most likely need to go to the heart catheterization lab for treatment?**
   a. Chest pain that is worse on inspiration.
   b. Troponin level that decreases on the second result.
   c. EKG with ST segment elevation in all inferior leads.
   d. Heart rate of 210 on telemetry diagnosed as SVT.

8. **A client with peripheral artery disease (PAD) asks the nurse how to relieve the pain in their lower extremities. What recommendation does the nurse provide?**
   a. Dangle the legs downward.
   b. Elevate the legs.
   c. Apply ice or cold therapy.
   d. Massage if unilateral edema is present.

9. **The nurse reinforces medication education for a client with peripheral artery disease. Which medication does the nurse identify that will inhibit platelet aggregation and vasodilate to improve blood flow?**
   a. Pentoxifylline.
   b. Clopidogrel.
   c. Aspirin.
   d. Cilostazol.

10. **What action does the nurse implement to relieve pain in the affected digits of a client experiencing Raynaud's phenomenon?**
   a. Applying a warm compress.
   b. Elevating the extremity.
   c. Administering ordered PRN analgesic.
   d. Massaging the affected digits.

11. **What does the nurse prioritize in the treatment plan for a client with Buerger's disease?**
   a. Warming affected digits.
   b. Smoking cessation.
   c. Infection prevention.
   d. High-fiber diet.

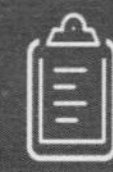

NurseThink® Quiz Questions

12. **A client with stroke is prescribed tissue plasminogen activator alteplase. What finding does the nurse report immediately to the health care provider?**
    a. Positive CT scan of the head.
    b. Symptom onset two hours ago.
    c. History of atrial fibrillation.
    d. Chronic hypertension.

13. **What findings cause the nurse to suspect a client is having an active stroke? *Select all that apply.***
    a. Chest pain.
    b. Slurred speech.
    c. Unilateral weakness.
    d. Sudden confusion.
    e. Expressive/receptive aphasia.

14. **The nurse reviews education for a client with secondary hypertension. What instruction does the nurse not plan to include?**
    a. Sodium restriction diet.
    b. Management of the primary disease.
    c. Activity restriction.
    d. Weight management.

15. **Which statement by the client with hypertension illustrates an understanding of the lifestyle changes in their plan of care?**
    a. "I will cut back on smoking and increase my daily milk consumption."
    b. "I will exercise every day to lose 10 pounds in the next week and stop smoking."
    c. "I will increase my fresh vegetables and limit to one 8-ounce glass of wine a day."
    d. "I will eat whole grain foods and have at least two servings of whole milk daily."

16. **What treatment will best address the lower extremity edema in a client with peripheral vascular disease?**
    a. Elevate the legs.
    b. Apply ice to the legs.
    c. Allow the legs to dangle while sitting.
    d. Instruct them to walk barefoot as much as they can.

17. **The nurse considers prophylactic treatments for the prevention of venous thromboembolism in a bedbound client. Which intervention does the nurse identify as having the highest risk of side effects?**
    a. Sequential compression devices.
    b. Passive range-of-motion exercises.
    c. Anti-embolism stockings.
    d. Low-molecular-weight heparin.

18. **The health care provider prescribes pharmacologic therapy for a client newly diagnosed with deep vein thrombosis. Because there are no specific contraindications present, which medication does the nurse expect the client to receive?**
    a. Heparin.
    b. Enoxaparin.
    c. Warfarin.
    d. Argatroban.

19. **Which new finding in a client being treated for a deep vein thrombus causes the nurse to suspect pulmonary embolism has occurred?**
    a. Bradycardia.
    b. Sharp chest pain.
    c. Positive Homan's sign.
    d. Rapid breathing and decreased pulse rate.

20. **While caring for a client with sepsis, what finding alerts the nurse of the possible need to implement treatment plans for disseminated intravascular coagulation (DIC)?**
    a. Blood oozing from the intravenous access site.
    b. Foul-smelling urine in the Foley catheter.
    c. Confusion and a decreased oxygen saturation.
    d. Hypertension and bradycardia.

NurseThink® Quiz Answers

1. **The nurse cares for a client with right-sided heart failure. What finding indicates that the client now has secondary left-sided heart failure?**
   a. Jugular vein distention.
   b. Ascites.
   c. Crackles in the lung bases.
   d. Fatigue.

   Topic/Concept: Circulation **Subtopic:** Heart Failure **Bloom's Taxonomy:** Analyzing **Clinical Problem-Solving Process:** Data Collection **NCLEX-PN®:** Basic Care and Comfort **QSEN:** Evidence-based Practice **CJMM:** Analyze Cues

   Rationale: Ascites, jugular vein distention, and fatigue are expected findings in right-sided heart failure. Crackles in the lung bases are expected in left-sided heart failure and not right-sided heart failure, so this could indicate advancement in the client's condition to left side involvement.

   THIN Thinking: *Top Three* – When collecting data on findings in a client with heart failure, the nurse must distinguish the right-sided symptoms from the left-sided ones. Left-sided heart failure is more serious since this is the workhorse of the heart that pushes blood to the body. When it fails, there will be severely decreased cardiac output.

2. **What exercise and activity level does the nurse implement in a client diagnosed with early heart failure?**
   a. Total bedrest with little activity.
   b. Moderate exercise with progressive activity.
   c. Little exercise with minimal activity.
   d. Intense exercise with little other activity.

   Topic/Concept: Circulation **Subtopic:** Heart Failure **Bloom's Taxonomy:** Applying **Clinical Problem-Solving Process:** Implementation **NCLEX-PN®:** Health promotion and maintenance **QSEN:** Patient-centered care **CJMM:** Take Action

   Rationale: The client will benefit from moderate exercise 3-7 days a week with 10-15 minute warm-up sessions, 20-30 minutes of moderate aerobic exercise, and a cool-down period. They should listen to their bodies and not push themselves beyond their limitations, but they should not stay on prolonged bedrest. This limited activity should only be implemented during exacerbation periods.

   THIN Thinking: *Clinical Problem-Solving Process* –To optimize compliance, the nurse needs to ensure the client understands the importance of the requirements and limitations of their activity expectations. With heart failure, there is a balance that needs to be reached in their activity levels. They must exercise enough to keep their heart strong and slow down the failure's progression while not overworking their heart and speeding the progression.

3. **The nurse reviews a client's health history. What data will increase their risk for developing restrictive cardiomyopathy?**
   a. Radiation therapy.
   b. Past ETOH use.
   c. Hypotension.
   d. Diabetes type II.

   Topic/Concept: Circulation **Subtopic:** Cardiomyopathy **Bloom's Taxonomy:** Applying **Clinical Problem-Solving Process:** Planning **NCLEX-PN®:** Reduction of Risk Potential **QSEN:** Evidence-based Practice **CJMM:** Prioritize Hypotheses

   Rationale: Hypertension increases risks for hypertrophic cardiomyopathy. ETOH chronic abuse increases risks for dilated cardiomyopathy. Diabetes type II does not increase risks directly but could contribute to hypertrophy by increasing hypertension risks and complications. Radiation and amyloidosis both increase the risk of restrictive cardiomyopathy.

   THIN Thinking: *Identify Risk to Safety* – The nurse needs to identify risk factors and inform clients of any preventative factors that can be put into place. If there is no prevention available, the nurse should then review symptoms of a disease so the client will report the earliest symptoms and get treatment as soon as possible.

4. **The nurse assists a client with coronary artery disease with meal planning. Which client choice does the nurse approve?**
   a. Microwavable low-sodium meals.
   b. Canned vegetable soup.
   c. Grilled cheese made with salted butter.
   d. Oatmeal with bananas.

   Topic/Concept: Circulation **Subtopic:** Coronary artery disease **Bloom's Taxonomy:** Applying **Clinical Problem-Solving Process:** Planning **NCLEX-PN®:** Health Promotion and Maintenance **QSEN:** Evidence-based Practice **CJMM:** Generate Solutions

   Rationale: Low-fat, low-sodium, high-fiber diets are going to be the most beneficial for a client with coronary artery disease (CAD). Microwavable meals (even low-sodium versions) and canned soups (no matter the flavor) are excessively high in sodium and should be avoided. Cheeses and salted butter are high in both fat and sodium content and should be avoided. Oatmeal and bananas are the best options as they are high in fiber which helps lower cholesterol.

   THIN Thinking: *Clinical Problem-Solving Process* –The nurse should evaluate what the client is eating to ensure it is the safest option based on their diagnosis. Many things can be deceptive in their presentation and are not as appropriate as they may claim.

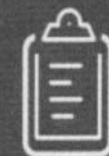

NurseThink® Quiz Answers

5. **The nurse administers medications for coronary artery disease to a client who has also just been diagnosed with rhabdomyolysis. Which medication does the nurse hold and discuss with the health care provider?**
   a. Simvastatin.
   b. Nitroglycerin.
   c. Metoprolol.
   d. Aspirin.

   Topic/Concept: Circulation **Subtopic:** Coronary artery disease **Bloom's Taxonomy:** Analyzing **Clinical Problem-Solving Process:** Evaluation **NCLEX-PN®:** Pharmacological Therapies **QSEN:** Quality Improvement **CJMM:** Take Action

   Rationale: A major side effect of statins is rhabdomyolysis, so the nurse would hold this medication and alert the provider. The other medications listed do not cause this side effect and do not interact with the diagnosis in a way that requires them to be held.

   THIN Thinking: *Identify Risk to Safety* – The nurse should be vigilant and evaluate the medications a client is taking to ensure they do not develop serious side effects. The nurse must be prepared to protect the client by holding a medication if there is a serious adverse reaction.

6. **The nurse interviews a client with angina about the nature of their chest pain. What finding indicates the client will be evaluated for an acute myocardial infarction?**
   a. They have chest pain with exercise.
   b. The client is short of breath when climbing stairs.
   c. They have chest pain at rest that does not stop.
   d. They should not need evaluation as all chest pain is expected.

   Topic/Concept: Circulation **Subtopic:** Myocardial infarction **Bloom's Taxonomy:** Analyzing **Clinical Problem-Solving Process:** Data Collection **NCLEX-PN®:** Coordinated Care **QSEN:** Teamwork and Collaboration **CJMM:** Analyze Cues

   Rationale: Stable angina occurs with exercise or other strenuous activity like climbing stairs and can include shortness of breath. The client should be concerned and be evaluated for possible acute MI if they start noticing chest pain at rest that does not subside; this is unstable angina that could indicate an MI.

   THIN Thinking: *Identify Risk to Safety* – The nurse needs to be aware of complications and when a client needs to be evaluated for those complications in order to prevent injury. Understanding that an angina diagnosis is stable as long as it stays within the symptomology of being aggravated by exercise and activity is important to the safety of the client.

7. **What finding alerts the emergency department nurse that the client will most likely need to go to the heart catheterization lab for treatment?**
   a. Chest pain that is worse on inspiration.
   b. Troponin level that decreases on the second result.
   c. EKG with ST segment elevation in all inferior leads.
   d. Heart rate of 210 on telemetry diagnosed as SVT.

   Topic/Concept: Circulation **Subtopic:** Myocardial infarction **Bloom's Taxonomy:** Analyzing **Clinical Problem-Solving Process:** Data Collection **NCLEX-PN®:** Coordinated Care **QSEN:** Evidence-based Practice **CJMM:** Prioritize Hypotheses

   Rationale: The heart catheterization lab is needed in the treatment of acute MI. A troponin that lowers does not indicate a heart problem. Chest pain on inspiration can indicate pneumonia, rib damage, or pericarditis which are not treated in the cath lab. An elevated heart rate to that magnitude in SVT should be cardioverted, not taken to the cath lab for treatment. The ST segment elevation indicates STEMI that should be treated in the cath lab immediately.

   THIN Thinking: *Help Quick* – Distinguishing between treatment types and symptoms is crucial when getting appropriate and timely treatment for the client.

8. **A client with peripheral artery disease (PAD) asks the nurse how to relieve the pain in their lower extremities. What recommendation does the nurse provide?**
   a. Dangle the legs downward.
   b. Elevate the legs.
   c. Apply ice or cold therapy.
   d. Massage if unilateral edema is present.

   Topic/Concept: Circulation **Subtopic:** Peripheral artery disease **Bloom's Taxonomy:** Applying **Clinical Problem-Solving Process:** Planning **NCLEX-PN®:** Basic Care and Comfort **QSEN:** Patient-centered care **CJMM:** Generate Solutions

   Rationale: In PAD, the client has blockages in their arterial blood flow, so dangling their legs will help direct blood flow to the extremity and help with tissues that are hurting due to lack of oxygen. Elevating and ice or cold application will restrict blood flow and increase pain. The client should never massage a leg displaying unilateral edema as this could indicate DVT that may break free and embolize if massaged.

   THIN Thinking: *Top Three* – Understanding the mechanism of a disease process will help the nurse reinforce appropriate interventions to lessen symptoms and discomfort associated with their disease.

9. **The nurse reinforces medication education for a client with peripheral artery disease. Which medication does the nurse identify that will inhibit platelet aggregation and vasodilate to improve blood flow?**
   a. Pentoxifylline.
   b. Clopidogrel.
   c. Aspirin.
   d. Cilostazol.

   Topic/Concept: Circulation **Subtopic:** Peripheral artery disease **Bloom's Taxonomy:** Applying **Clinical Problem-Solving Process:** Evaluation **NCLEX-PN®:** Pharmacological Therapies **QSEN:** Evidence-based Practice **CJMM:** Evaluate Outcomes

   Rationale: Cilostazol is the only medication with both effects. Clopidogrel and aspirin only work to inhibit platelet aggregation. Pentoxifylline decreases blood viscosity and increases RBC flexibility to increase circulation.

   THIN Thinking: *Clinical Problem-Solving Process* –Knowing what effect a medication is expected to have is imperative when evaluating whether or not it is having an unintended effect.

10. **What action does the nurse implement to relieve pain in the affected digits of a client experiencing Raynaud's phenomenon?**
   a. Applying a warm compress.
   b. Elevating the extremity.
   c. Administering ordered PRN analgesic.
   d. Massaging the affected digits.

   Topic/Concept: Circulation **Subtopic:** Raynaud's Phenomenon **Bloom's Taxonomy:** Applying **Clinical Problem-Solving Process:** Implementation **NCLEX-PN®:** Basic Care and Comfort **QSEN:** Evidence-based Practice **CJMM:** Take Action

   Rationale: Because cold and stress trigger the reaction, warmth is likely to reverse the response, alleviating the pain the severe vasoconstriction is causing. Elevating and massage will aggravate the pain and worsen the vasoconstriction. An analgesic may slightly help but will not be as effective as alleviating the cause and reversing the condition with heat application.

   THIN Thinking: *Help Quick* – A nursing intervention to reverse a condition is better than symptom-based treatment because alleviating the causative factor for pain alleviates the pain more effectively.

11. **What does the nurse prioritize in the treatment plan for a client with Buerger's disease?**
   a. Warming affected digits.
   b. Smoking cessation.
   c. Infection prevention.
   d. High-fiber diet.

   Topic/Concept: Circulation **Subtopic:** Buerger's disease **Bloom's Taxonomy:** Applying **Clinical Problem-Solving Process:** Planning **NCLEX-PN®:** Reduction of Risk Potential **QSEN:** Safety **CJMM:** Prioritize Hypotheses

   Rationale: Almost all clients with Buerger's disease smoke or use tobacco, and cessation is the only way to stop the disease. Raynaud's can be secondary, and warming digits is effective when this occurs, but it is not the priority. Infection prevention is necessary as sores often form but stopping tobacco use stops the disease making sores no longer an issue. A high-fiber diet does not impact this disease.

   THIN Thinking: *Top Three* – If the cause of a disease can be stopped, the action to do so will be the highest priority over symptomatic treatments.

12. **A client with stroke is prescribed tissue plasminogen activator alteplase. What finding does the nurse report immediately to the health care provider?**
   a. Positive CT scan of the head.
   b. Symptom onset two hours ago.
   c. History of atrial fibrillation.
   d. Chronic hypertension.

   Topic/Concept: Circulation **Subtopic:** Stroke/CVA **Bloom's Taxonomy:** Applying **Clinical Problem-Solving Process:** Implementation **NCLEX-PN®:** Pharmacological Therapies **QSEN:** Patient-centered care **CJMM:** Take Action

   Rationale: A positive head CT scan is indicative of a hemorrhagic stroke which is an absolute contraindication for the administration of this medication as it will severely worsen the acute bleeding. Atrial fibrillation and hypertension are not contraindications for therapy. Symptom onset up to 4.5 hours is within the window for administration.

   THIN Thinking: *Identify Risk to Safety* – Thrombolytics are dangerous medications that need to be managed closely. Any contraindication identified should be reported immediately to prevent serious injury or death.

13. What findings cause the nurse to suspect a client is having an active stroke? *Select all that apply.*

a. Chest pain.
b. Slurred speech.
c. Unilateral weakness.
d. Sudden confusion.
e. Expressive/receptive aphasia.

Topic/Concept: Circulation **Subtopic:** Stroke/CVA **Bloom's Taxonomy:** Analyzing **Clinical Problem-Solving Process:** Data Collection **NCLEX-PN®:** Safety and Infection Control **QSEN:** Evidence-based Practice **CJMM:** Recognize Cues

Rationale: Sudden confusion, expressive/receptive aphasia, slurred speech, and unilateral weakness are signs of active stroke. Chest pain can be a sign of acute MI and not stroke.

THIN Thinking: *Help Quick* – Time is tissue, and stroke needs to be identified as soon as possible to prevent permanent disability.

14. The nurse reviews education for a client with secondary hypertension. What instruction does the nurse not plan to include?

a. Sodium restriction diet.
b. Management of the primary disease.
c. Activity restriction.
d. Weight management.

Topic/Concept: Circulation **Subtopic:** Hypertension **Bloom's Taxonomy:** Applying **Clinical Problem-Solving Process:** Planning **NCLEX-PN®:** Coordinated Care **QSEN:** Teamwork and Collaboration **CJMM:** Generate Solutions

Rationale: Activity is encouraged with secondary hypertension as it will strengthen the heart muscle, help in weight management, and decrease stress levels. Sodium should be restricted, the primary disease that causes secondary hypertension should be managed, and weight needs to be managed.

THIN Thinking: *Clinical Problem-Solving Process* –Proper education is imperative in preventative maintenance for chronic illness to prevent injury, disease progression, and morbidity.

15. Which statement by the client with hypertension illustrates an understanding of the lifestyle changes in their plan of care?

a. "I will cut back on smoking and increase my daily milk consumption."
b. "I will exercise every day to lose 10 pounds in the next week and stop smoking."
c. "I will increase my fresh vegetables and limit to one 8-ounce glass of wine a day."
d. "I will eat whole grain foods and have at least two servings of whole milk daily."

Topic/Concept: Circulation **Subtopic:** Hypertension **Bloom's Taxonomy:** Analyzing **Clinical Problem-Solving Process:** Evaluation **NCLEX-PN®:** Coordinated Care **QSEN:** Evidence-based Practice **CJMM:** Generate Solutions

Rationale: The client should increase exercise slowly and develop realistic expectations of that routine. It is not healthy to lose more than two pounds a week regardless of the end goal weight. Smoking should be stopped, not just decreased. Whole grains are good, but whole milk is too high in fat. The client should use 2%, 1%, or skim instead. Fresh vegetables are high in fiber which helps lower cholesterol, and a glass of wine a day is heart healthy as long as it does not exceed that daily.

THIN Thinking: *Clinical Problem-Solving Process* –When reinforcing expectations of a client's treatment plan, the nurse should carefully evaluate their understanding and expectations to ensure proper education has been received for the most optimal outcomes.

16. What treatment will best address the lower extremity edema in a client with peripheral vascular disease?

a. Elevate the legs.
b. Apply ice to the legs.
c. Allow the legs to dangle while sitting.
d. Instruct them to walk barefoot as much as they can.

Topic/Concept: Circulation **Subtopic:** Vascular heart disease **Bloom's Taxonomy:** Applying **Clinical Problem-Solving Process:** Planning **NCLEX-PN®:** Health promotion and maintenance **QSEN:** Evidence-based Practice **CJMM:** Prioritize Hypotheses

Rationale: Clients with PVD should never walk barefoot; decreased sensation increases the risk of injury. Ice will constrict blood flow and increase pain and edema. In PVD, they will have dependent edema, so dangling the legs will increase the edema and should be avoided. Elevating the legs will promote venous return and help reduce pain and edema.

THIN Thinking: *Help Quick* – Understanding the anatomy of a disease will better equip the nurse to make the appropriate treatment plan. PVD allows for pooling as the venous system is failing and blood pools in extremities in dependent positions. PAD is a failure in the arterial system which restricts blood flow to the extremity itself, so dependent positions are more advantageous as they allow blood into the extremity more easily.

17. **The nurse considers prophylactic treatments for the prevention of venous thromboembolism in a bedbound client. Which intervention does the nurse identify as having the highest risk of side effects?**
    a. Sequential compression devices.
    b. Passive range-of-motion exercises.
    c. Anti-embolism stockings.
    d. Low-molecular-weight heparin.

Topic/Concept: Circulation **Subtopic:** Venous thromboembolism **Bloom's Taxonomy:** Analyzing **Clinical Problem-Solving Process:** Planning **NCLEX-PN®:** Reduction of Risk Potential **QSEN:** Patient-centered care **CJMM:** Prioritize Hypotheses

Rationale: SCDs, passive ROM, and anti-embolism stockings (TED hose) are all non-invasive, localized, and in most cases, nurse-driven treatments that have minimal risk of side effects or harm. Low-molecular-weight heparin is an injectable, systemic invasive therapy that requires a provider's prescription and has a high risk of side effects.

THIN Thinking: *Help Quick* – The least invasive and lowest risk treatments should be implemented as the first-choice regimens in prophylactic treatments.

18. **The health care provider prescribes pharmacologic therapy for a client newly diagnosed with deep vein thrombosis. Because there are no specific contraindications present, which medication does the nurse expect the client to receive?**
    a. Heparin.
    b. Enoxaparin.
    c. Warfarin.
    d. Argatroban.

Topic/Concept: Circulation **Subtopic:** Venous thromboembolism **Bloom's Taxonomy:** Applying **Clinical Problem-Solving Process:** Planning **NCLEX-PN®:** Pharmacological Therapies **QSEN:** Evidence-based Practice **CJMM:** Generate Solutions

Rationale: Heparin is the standard initial treatment for DVT unless specifically contraindicated. Enoxaparin is used as prophylaxis. Warfarin is used after breaking down the DVT to prevent the formation of new clots as an ongoing anticoagulant therapy. Argatroban is used during heart catheterization only.

THIN Thinking: *Clinical Problem-Solving Process* –Heparin is the only medication listed that can be given as a continuous intravenous therapy to prevent the DVT from getting larger. It does not break down the clot; it prevents its enlargement and the formation of others while the body breaks down and absorbs the clot.

19. **Which new finding in a client being treated for a deep vein thrombus causes the nurse to suspect pulmonary embolism has occurred?**
    a. Bradycardia.
    b. Sharp chest pain.
    c. Positive Homan's sign.
    d. Rapid breathing and decreased pulse rate.

Topic/Concept: Circulation **Subtopic:** Pulmonary embolism **Bloom's Taxonomy:** Analyzing **Clinical Problem-Solving Process:** Data Collection **NCLEX-PN®:** Physiological Adaptation **QSEN:** Evidence-based Practice **CJMM:** Recognize Cues

Rationale: Rapid breathing and rapid pulse rate is a sign of PE not decreased pulse rate. Tachycardia, not bradycardia, is a symptom. Positive Homan's sign is a symptom of the DVT, not a PE. Sudden, sharp, and stabbing chest pain is a symptom of PE.

THIN Thinking: *Help Quick* – The nurse needs to monitor closely for complications with every disease process. Pulmonary embolism is a serious risk with DVT. Half of the deaths that result from this condition occur within the first two hours of onset, making early recognition imperative.

20. **While caring for a client with sepsis, what finding alerts the nurse of the possible need to implement treatment plans for disseminated intravascular coagulation (DIC)?**
    a. Blood oozing from the intravenous access site.
    b. Foul-smelling urine in the Foley catheter.
    c. Confusion and a decreased oxygen saturation.
    d. Hypertension and bradycardia.

Topic/Concept: Circulation **Subtopic:** Disseminated intravascular coagulation **Bloom's Taxonomy:** Applying **Clinical Problem-Solving Process:** Implementation **NCLEX-PN®:** Safety and Infection Control **QSEN:** Safety **CJMM:** Take Action

Rationale: Hypertension and bradycardia indicate fluid overload, which may be related to blood loss. Foul-smelling urine points to infection. Confusion and decreased oxygen saturation could indicate other respiratory issues like ARDS. Irregular bleeding is a symptom of DIC, and it should be addressed as soon as possible to prevent injury and death.

THIN Thinking: *Clinical Problem-Solving Process* –DIC occurs when micro-clotting exhausts the clotting factors in a client, leading to hemorrhage. Sepsis is a major trigger for this syndrome, so monitoring for it closely is a priority.

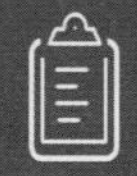

CHAPTER

7

Protection

Immunity / Inflammation / Infection

The immune system is the body's first line of defense. When functioning properly, the immune system prevents or limits the risk of infections in our bodies. Through intricate processes, it recognizes and disposes of substances that it identifies as foreign and potentially detrimental to the body's health. However, when there are problems with the immune system and it does not function as it should, there is the risk of diseases occurring in the body.

When there is injury of any type in the body inflammation is likely to occur. This is the body's way of attempting to defend itself against the cause of the injury and restore the tissue to functionality. However, pathogens often pose challenges to the immune system and invade our bodies causing a myriad of infections. Nurses must be knowledgeable about the role immunity plays in the body and skilled when caring for clients with all types of infections, as new strains of bacteria are emerging constantly.

Priority Exemplars:

- Urinary Tract Infection
- Influenza
- Polycystic kidney
- Meningitis
- Pancreatitis
- Appendicitis/peritonitis
- Cellulitis/wound infection/septicemia
- Gout
- Systemic lupus erythematosus
- Rheumatoid arthritis
- HIV/AIDS
- Hypersensitivity reactions
- Pyelonephritis
- Methicillin-resistant Staphylococcus aureus/ Vancomycin resistant Enterococcus

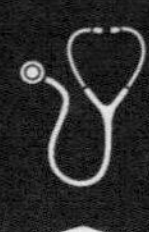

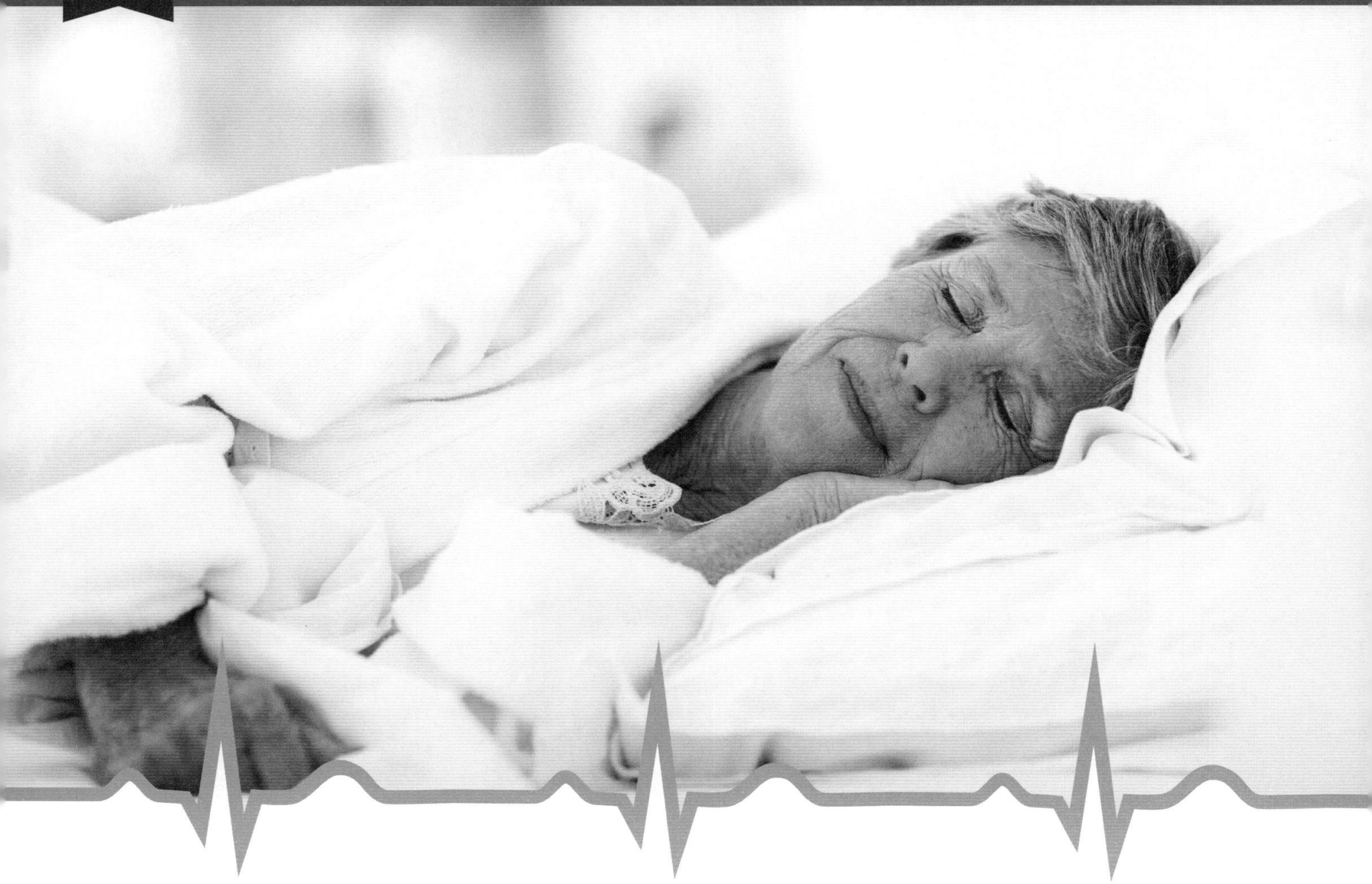

Go To Clinical

Go To Clinical Case 1

Ms. F. is an 82-year-old female resident of the Long-Term Care facility. Ms. F. has a history of coronary artery disease and diabetes mellitus type 2. Usually, Ms. F. is alert and orientated, friendly, and loves roaming the hallways of the facility visiting with the staff and other residents of the facility. Two days ago, she suddenly fell in the hallway while walking, with no reported injuries. Since her fall, Ms. F. has remained in bed and has noted to be lethargic, agitated, and confused. Also, the unlicensed assistive personnel reported that Ms. F. has had two episodes of urine incontinence in the last two days and has started to complain of lower abdominal discomfort. Vital signs are temperature 98.4°F (36.9°C), heart rate 106 beats/minute; respirations 22 breaths/minute; blood pressure 120/62 mmHg, oxygen saturation 96% on room air.

NurseThink® Time

Using the NurseThink® system, complete the priorities. Check your answers designated by 💡 in the Urinary Tract Infection Priority Exemplar.

Clinical Hint

Older adults with a UTI may not present with the usual symptoms of the condition. A UTI may be manifested with falls, incontinence, and an alternation in mental status, such as agitation and confusion. When an older adult client presents with new onset of confusion, the nurse should anticipate obtaining a urine culture.

NurseThink® Time

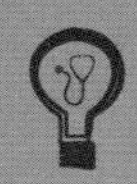

Priority Data Collection or Cues

1.

2.

3.

Priority Laboratory Tests/Diagnostics

1.

2.

3.

Priority Interventions or Actions

1.

2.

3.

Priority Potential & Actual Complications

1.

2.

3.

Priority Nursing Implications

1.

2.

3.

Priority Medications

1.

2.

3.

Reinforcement of Priority Teaching

1.

2.

3.

Urinary tract infection

Pathophysiology/Description

- A urinary tract infection is an inflammation of the bladder that results from bacteria, obstruction of the urethra or other factors
- Of all possible causes of a UTI, bacterial infection is the most prevalent
- The most common bacteria related to urinary tract infections is Escherichia coli, commonly called E. coli
- Urinary tract infections can also be caused by parasitic and fungal infections, but these causes are rare. When seen, they are usually in clients who are immunosuppressed
- Urinary tract infections are more common in women than men due to the close proximity of the urethra to the rectum
- Classification
  - Upper UTI: Occurring in the ureters, pelvic area or renal parenchyma
  - Lower UTI: Occurring in the urethra and bladder
- Types of UTI based on location
  - Urethritis inflammation occurring in the urethra
  - Cystitis inflammation occurring in the bladder
  - Pyelonephritis inflammation occurring in collecting system and renal parenchyma
- Urinary tract infection can be complicated or uncomplicated
  - With uncomplicated UTI, there are no other conditions complicating the infection
  - With complicated UTI, there are other co-existing conditions impacting the UTI, such as diabetes, renal stones among others
- Sexual intercourse and urinary catheterization increase the risk of getting a UTI because of possible introduction of bacteria

Priority Data Collection or Cues

- Monitor for fever, chills and flank pain, indicating upper UTI
- Monitor for burning and pain with urination
- Ask client about difficulty starting urine stream or delay between start and beginning of the urine flow, may be because urethral sphincter has relaxed
- Ask about interruption of stream once started or voiding in small amounts
- Ask about incomplete emptying of bladder and dribbling of urine after voiding
- Look at color of urine, cloudiness may indicate UTI
- Monitor for bladder spasms
- Ask about frequency of urinating, usually multiple times in a 24-hour period, with insignificant amounts each time (less than 200 mL)

Priority Laboratory Tests/Diagnostics

- Urine dipstick, shows nitrites, leukocyte esterase, white blood cells
- Microscopic urinalysis shows elevated white blood cell count, usually greater than 11,000 mm^3 as well as pus in the urine (pyuria)
- Urine culture and sensitivity will show the causative bacteria and the most effective antibiotic to treat the bacteria

Priority Interventions or Actions

- Collect a clean-catch urine sample. Reinforce teaching on the correct way to collect the sample to prevent contamination of the sample if the client is collecting their own specimen
- Administer antibiotic as ordered and monitor for side effects
- Administer analgesic as ordered for pain
- If a urinary catheter must be inserted, ensure sterile technique is used
- Provide client with adequate fluids and encourage intake of up to 3000 mL/day, if not contraindicated, help to flush the urinary tract of the bacteria
- Allow client to use sitz bath or heat to abdomen if discomfort is unbearable
- Re-culture urine after completion of antibiotic therapy to determine resolution of the infection

Priority Potential & Actual Complications

- Urosepsis
- Septicemia
- Sepsis

Priority Nursing Implications

- Understand that older adults with a UTI may not present with the usual symptoms of the condition. Quite often a UTI is manifested as an alteration in mentation, such as agitation and confusion

Clinical Hint

Current practice indicates that catheters should be used only in necessary circumstances and should be removed as soon as they are no longer needed due to Catheter-Associated Urinary Tract Infection (CAUTI).

Priority Medications

- There are several antibiotics from various classes that can be used to treat a UTI. The ones below are the first- choice drugs to treat uncomplicated and complicated UTI
- Trimethoprim/sulfamethoxazole given orally
  - First choice antibiotic to treat UTI
- Nitrofurantoin given orally
  - First choice antibiotic to treat UTI
- Fosfomycin given orally
  - First choice antibiotic to treat UTI
- Ciprofloxacin given orally and intravenous
  - Used to treat complicated UTI
- Levofloxacin given orally and intravenous
  - For complicated urinary tract infection
  - Has a serious adverse effect of tearing or rupture of a tendon, primarily Achilles' tendon
- Phenazopyridine given orally
  - Urinary analgesic and anesthetic, so it anesthetizes and reduces pain and discomfort
  - Should not be used for more than 2 days

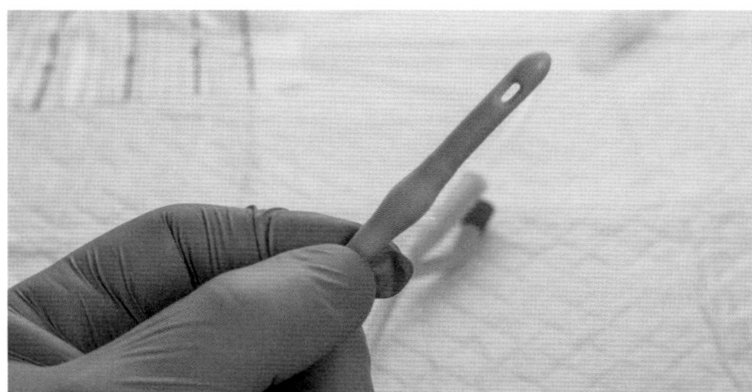

Image 7-1: Identify 3 priority interventions in preventing UTI's in clients with a Foley catheter.

____

____

____

Reinforcement of Priority Teaching

- Encourage women to urinate after sexual intercourse to prevent possible infection from bacteria that may be on the genitals
- Encourage women to wipe from front to back to prevent tracking bacteria from the rectum to the urethra
- Keep the genital area clean to minimize the risk of bacterial growth
- Recommend client to clean perineal area with warm water and soap after bowel movements, to decrease risk of bacterial growth and tracking into the urethra
- Advising women that cotton underwear and loose-fitting clothing help to keep the area around the urethra dry
- Signs and symptoms of urinary tract infection and when to contact a health care provider
- Complete the full course of antibiotics prescribed, even if the symptoms resolve, to ensure the infection is fully gone
- Empty bladder at least every 3-4 hours to prevent urinary stasis that can foster growth of bacteria
- Instruct client on foods that will help to maintain an acidic urine (pH of 5.5 or below), such as blueberries, prunes or cranberries. Drinking cranberry juice daily reduces the risk of a UTI
- Avoid or decrease intake of caffeinated beverages, such as coffee and cola, as both can cause bladder irritation
- Explain to client the importance of returning for follow-up urine culture once the course of antibiotic is finished
- Recognize clients at risk for a UTI and reinforce how to minimize risk

Next Gen Clinical Judgment

1. How does having a co-existing condition such as diabetes impact the development of a UTI?
2. In a client such as Ms. F., how can UTIs be prevented?
3. What information should be reinforced with Ms. F. about the current treatment and means to prevent future bladder infections?
4. What dietary recommendations would be included in instructions to Ms. F.?
5. In addition to antibiotics, what other medications may be used to manage the symptoms of a UTI?

Go To Clinical Answers

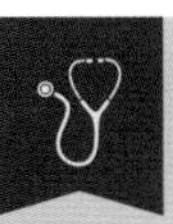

Text designated by the icon are the top answers for the Go To Clinical related to Urinary tract infection.

Go To Clinical

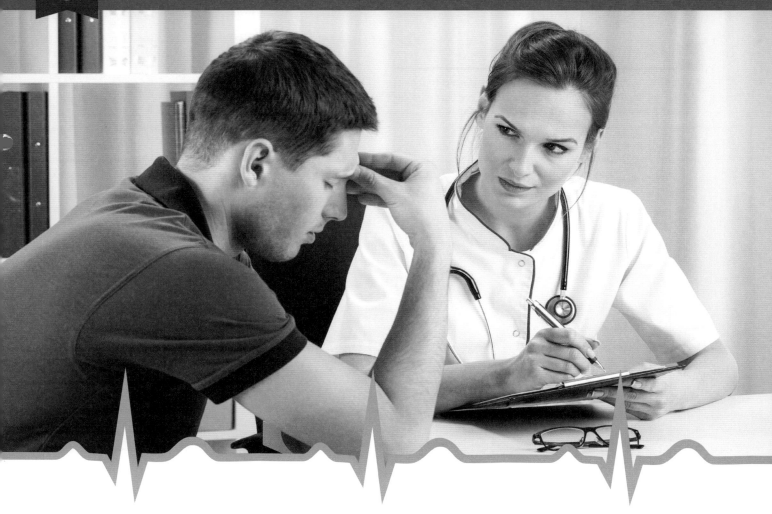

Go To Clinical Case 2

A.P. is a 33-year-old school teacher who presents to the clinic with increased coughing, runny nose, difficulty breathing, and muscle soreness. A.P. has a medical history of hypertension for which he takes amlodipine besylate 5 mg and losartan potassium 100 mg daily. A.P. reports receiving the influenza vaccine three days ago as a requirement for his job.

Vital Signs: temperature 101°F (38.3°C); heart rate 98 beats/minute; respirations 22 breaths/minute; blood pressure 126/78 mmHg; oxygen saturation 93% on room air. A.P. states he feels weak and complains of new-onset headache and chills.

He states these symptoms just started this morning, although he has been more tired than usual for the last few weeks.

NurseThink® Time

Using the NurseThink® system, complete the priorities. Check your answers designated by in the Influenza Priority Exemplar.

Clinical Hint

Nurses must work with clients to dispel the common myth that the influenza vaccine causes influenza. The truth is the vaccine is made from inactivated particles that cannot infect a person. The vaccine can take 1-2 weeks to be effective so a person can catch influenza before the antibodies can fight it off.

NurseThink® Time

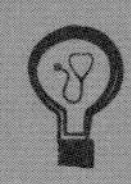

Priority Data Collection or Cues

1.

2.

3.

Priority Laboratory Tests/Diagnostics

1.

2.

3.

Priority Interventions or Actions

1.

2.

3.

Priority Potential & Actual Complications

1.

2.

3.

Priority Nursing Implications

1.

2.

3.

Priority Medications

1.

2.

3.

Reinforcement of Priority Teaching

1.

2.

3.

Pathophysiology/Description

- Influenza is a highly contagious viral respiratory illness that may be caused by several different types of viruses
- Classified as types A, B and C—A is the most common and virulent, affects humans and animals. Example is the swine flu (H1N1 influenza). B and C affect humans only
- Influenza is particularly troublesome because several strains exist, and the viruses can mutate. This is the reason the flu vaccine is administered every year
- Transmission by human to human via inhalation of infected particles or contact with infected droplets and from animals to humans when contact is made with animals that are infected
- There are two types of influenza that are common to animals but have impacted humans in recent years, swine influenza (H1N1) and avian influenza (H5N1)
    - Swine influenza is a strain of influenza that originated in pigs but is spread from human to human. It emerged in 2009 as a pandemic
    - Avian flu is a strain of influenza that affects birds, including chickens and turkeys. Avian flu is not common to humans but there have been sporadic human cases

Priority Data Collection or Cues

- Ask client about onset of muscle aches and fever, onset of influenza symptoms is usually abrupt. Also, antiviral treatment should ideally begin within 2 days of onset of symptoms
- Monitor for chills, headache, sore throat, cough, fatigue and malaise, expected with influenza
- May find crackles and dyspnea if pulmonary involvement
- Monitor for lethargy and weakness especially with an older adult
- Ask if client had an influenza vaccine
- Collect vital signs

Priority Laboratory Tests/Diagnostics

- Viral cultures done with swab from throat, nasopharyngeal, sputum or bronchial washing will identify the virus and the particular strain. Results can delay care as it takes 3-10 days so quite often diagnosis is made based on the client's clinical findings and history
- Rapid influenza test: Swab from nasal secretions gives result within minutes and will show influenza virus

Priority Interventions or Actions

- Perform viral culture or rapid influenza test
- Place client on droplet precautions, in acute care setting
- Treat complications of influenza, as prescribed
- Allow client to get adequate rest to relieve fatigue
- Administer antiviral medications as ordered
- Administer antitussives to alleviate cough
- Administer antipyretics to reduce fever
- Monitor lung sounds, to determine pulmonary compromise
- Encourage adequate fluids to liquefy secretions and prevent problems in pulmonary system

Priority Potential & Actual Complications

- Pneumonia, severe sinus and ear infections, and dehydration in older clients

Priority Nursing Implications

- For maximum effectiveness of antiviral therapy for influenza, treatment should start within 2 days of the onset of influenza symptoms
- There is a higher dose influenza vaccine for older adults to compensate for their weaker immune systems, caused by the aging process

Priority Medications

- Zanamivir
    - Reduce the duration of influenza by several days
    - Administered as inhalation therapy
- Oseltamivir
    - Reduce the duration of influenza by several days
    - Administered orally
- Peramivir
    - New drug for treating influenza
    - Administered intravenous
- Influenza vaccines
    - Must be administered yearly
    - Administered as an intramuscular injection that contains killed influenza virus
    - Administered intranasally and contains weakened live influenza virus

Reinforcement of Priority Teaching

- Importance of taking the influenza vaccine each year
- The best time to take the influenza vaccine is before exposure to the virus, which is usually in September
- Dispel the common myth that the influenza vaccine causes influenza
- Warn client to expect soreness at vaccination site
- Preventive measures such as covering cough, washing hands

Go To Clinical Answers

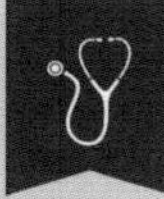

Text designated by the icon are the top answers for the Go To Clinical related to Influenza.

Polycystic kidney

Pathophysiology/Description

- Polycystic kidney disease (PKD) is formation of cysts and hypertrophy of the kidneys. It is considered a very common genetic condition worldwide
- The sequelae of the condition start with many tiny cysts in the medulla and cortex of the kidney. The cysts contain pus and fluid. They grow large and compress the surrounding tissue. These cysts usually rupture causing scar formation, infection, and nephrons that cannot function because of damage
- Forms of polycystic kidneys
  - Genetic in childhood, which is a rare inherited autosomal recessive disorder. The infant usually does not survive and dies within months
  - Adult onset, which is an autosomal dominant disorder, manifested in the third to fourth decade of life
- Both kidneys are usually involved. The condition is not gender specific
- Polycystic kidney disease can also affect other organs in the body
- By age 60, about half of clients with PKD have end-stage renal disease, needing either dialysis or transplant

Priority Data Collection or Cues

- Ask client about recurrent urinary tract infections
- Ask about feelings of heaviness in the side, abdomen or back, from enlarged cysts
- Monitor for proteinuria, pyuria and hematuria, which occur from ruptured cysts
- Monitor for chronic pain, usually described as a constant pain
- Monitor for headaches and hypertension
- Monitor for fever and chills, which might indicate infection
- Palpate kidneys usually felt as enlarged on both sides
- Abdominal girth, usually enlarged
- Gather data on body systems to determine signs and symptoms of PKD's impact on other organs, such as cysts in liver or diverticulosis in the intestines

Priority Laboratory Tests/Diagnostics

- Ultrasound and computed tomography (CT) scan of the kidneys and surrounding structures show evidence of the disease

Priority Interventions or Actions

- Monitor for signs of urinary tract infection and treat as prescribed, if present
- Prevent urinary tract infection, if client does not already have an infection
- Monitor for hematuria
- Encourage bed rest if bleeding occurs from ruptured cysts
- Administer medications to treat fever
- Use dry heat to abdomen and flanks for comfort when cysts are infected
- Increase fluid and sodium intake as sodium is usually lost with PKD
- Administer pain medications as needed
- Administer antihypertensive medications, if client is hypertensive
- Assist in preparing the client for procedure to drain cyst if obstruction or abscess is present
- Assist in preparing the client for dialysis or renal transplantation, if client is at that stage of the disease

Priority Potential & Actual Complications

- Diverticulosis
- Cerebral aneurysm
- Liver cysts
- Abnormal heart valves
- Dialysis
- Renal transplantation

Priority Nursing Implications

- Do not use non-steroidal anti-inflammatory drugs to treat pain with PKD because of the risk of bleeding if cysts rupture
- A cyst may need to be punctured and drained if it is abscessed or if there is obstruction

Priority Medications

- There are no medications to treat PKD. Medications are used to treat symptoms that may arise from complications

Reinforcement of Priority Teaching

- Explain the progression of PKD to client
- Education on future treatment options
- Explain to client and family the importance of seeking genetic counseling
- Strategies to prevent infection
- Signs and symptoms of urinary tract infection and ruptured cyst
- Signs and symptoms of worsening PKD and when to notify health care provider

Pathophysiology/Description

- Inflammation of the membranes surrounding the brain and spinal cord
- Cause is often times related to a viral infection but can be caused by viral or bacterial infections
- Viral meningitis is caused by enteroviruses and usually resolves without requiring treatment
- Bacterial meningitis is serious and can be fatal in a few days if not treated early
- Bacterial meningitis travels via the bloodstream to the brain and spinal cord. Bacteria can also invade the meninges of the brain directly because of sinus and ear infections, as well as skull fracture
- Risk factors for meningitis include
  - Community environments where large groups of people gather
  - Travelers to certain parts of the world where conditions are ideal for the disease, like sub-Saharan Africa
  - Pregnant women who contract listeriosis, a condition caused by the bacteria Listeria Monocytogenes
- The disease is spread from person to person in several ways
  - Breathing in the bacteria when a carrier coughs or sneezes
  - Sharing respiratory secretions, as in kissing
  - Eating food contaminated from infected persons who did not wash their hands properly
  - Mothers passing the bacteria to their infants during birth
- Bacteria commonly associated with meningitis
  - Streptococcus pneumoniae (most common cause)
  - Neisseria meningitidis
  - Haemophilus influenzae
  - Group B Streptococcus
  - Listeria monocytogenes

Priority Data Collection or Cues

- Complete history and physical. Monitor for nuchal rigidity, severe headache, vomiting and fever, all key indicators of meningitis
- Look for positive Brudzinski's sign, which is involuntary flexion of the hip and knee when the neck is bent forward and positive Kernig's sign, which is the inability to extend the leg while the hip is flexed to 90 degrees
- Monitor neurologic status, looking for decreased level of consciousness, signs of increased intracranial pressure and seizures
- Ask about intolerance to light, called photophobia
- Monitor vital signs for increased temperature and respirations and changes in blood pressure
- Monitor intake and output. Look for dehydration that can be caused by insensible fluid loss due to high fever
- Monitor nutritional status and ensure supplemental feeding as needed, to maintain nutritional status
- Additional data collection in a newborn/infant
  - Excessive sleepiness, fussiness, sluggishness, constant crying, difficult to comfort
  - Stiffness not just in the neck as with adults, but in the body as well, a bulging fontanel

Priority Laboratory Tests/Diagnostics

- Blood culture shows the causative bacteria
- Lumbar puncture shows cerebrospinal fluid (CSF) with low glucose level, increased protein, increased white blood cells and a cloudy color
- Computed tomography and magnetic resonance show inflammation and swelling and rule out an obstruction in the foramen magnum
- Xpert EV test is used to test for viral meningitis. CSF is placed on a single-use disposable cartridge, which is then loaded into an instrument that provides quick results
- With viral meningitis, the CSF usually appears cloudy or clear and is positive for white blood cells

Priority Interventions or Actions

- Immediate interventions
  - Place client on isolation for bacterial meningitis
  - Assist in preparing client for lumbar puncture procedure
  - Administer antibiotics and intravenous fluid
  - Administer antipyretics for fever
  - Initiate seizure precautions and administer antiseizure drugs, if needed
  - Maintain ongoing monitoring of neurologic status

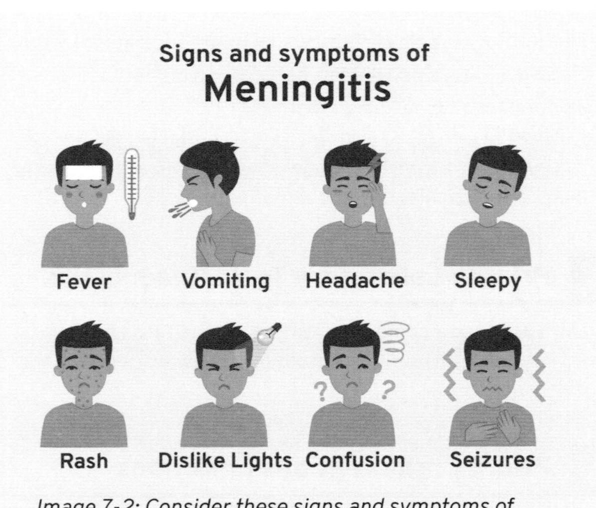

Image 7-2: Consider these signs and symptoms of meningitis. Which would be the most troublesome for the client? What nurse actions are required for clients experiencing this findings?

- Maintain safety as client will likely experience mental distortion
- Decrease environmental stimuli. Keep client in a darkened room and cover eyes with a cool cloth to relieve the effects of photophobia and to keep client calm
- Keep head of bed elevated to 30 degrees to increase comfort for the client. Avoid flexion of the hip and neck
- Use cooling blanket or a tepid sponge bath if fever persists after use of antipyretics
- Monitor client for adverse effects of antibiotics and manage accordingly. For vancomycin, slow the rate of infusion if flushing and itching occurs

Priority Potential & Actual Complications

- Seizures, brain damage
- Hearing loss, memory difficulty, learning disabilities
- May be fatal

Priority Nursing Implications

- A lumbar puncture is done after a CT scan rules out a foramen magnum obstruction. If lumbar puncture is done in the presence of a foramen magnum obstruction, a fluid shift can occur, causing herniation
- Viral meningitis cannot be treated with antibiotics. It is resolved with fluids, rest and over-the-counter medications for aches and pain
- Monitor vancomycin levels. Levels greater than 50 mcg/dL may cause toxicity, resulting in hearing loss and kidney damage. Itching and flushing to trunk, neck, head and face (red man syndrome) is another adverse effect of vancomycin

Priority Medications

- Antibiotics
  - Penicillin, ampicillin. Tricyclic glycopeptide like vancomycin
  - Cephalosporins such as cefuroxime, ceftriaxone, ceftazidime, cefotaxime, ceftizoxime
  - Administered oral, intravenous or intramuscular
- Corticosteroids
  - Administered orally, intravenous, and intramuscular
  - Dexamethasone
  - Given to prevent neurological complications, like cerebral edema
- Anti-seizure medications
  - Phenytoin, levetiracetam, used to treat seizures that can occur with meningitis
  - Phenytoin is administered as oral chewable tablets, oral suspension, extended-release capsules, intravenous, intramuscular
  - Levetiracetam is administered oral and intravenous
- Antipyretics
  - Aspirin, acetaminophen common ones used
  - Used to treat pain. Administered oral, rectal and now intravenous (new medication)
  - Maximum daily dosage for acetaminophen should not exceed 4 grams. Antidote for overdose of acetaminophen is acetylcysteine
- Medications specific to encephalitis
  - Acyclovir is an antiviral agent used to treat encephalitis when herpes simplex virus is the cause
  - Administered oral or intravenous

Reinforcement of Priority Teaching

- Types of meningococcal vaccines currently available
- Once discharged from acute care, it may take several weeks before client feels well enough to resume normal activities
- Increase exercise gradually but take rest breaks as needed
- Importance of proper nutrition, consuming a high-calorie and high-protein diet
- Client may still experience rigidity in the neck and that taking warm baths and doing range of motion exercises will relieve the stiffness
- Complications of meningitis and when to call the health care provider
- The importance of keeping all follow-up health care provider appointments

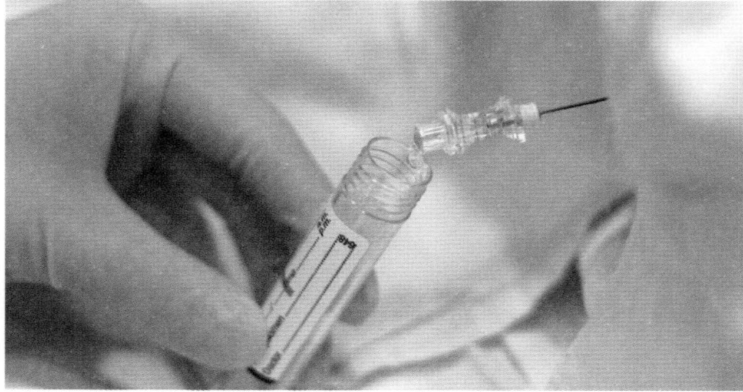

Image 7-3: List the priority nursing concerns for a client before, during, and after a lumbar puncture.

____

____

____

____

Pancreatitis

Pathophysiology/Description

- Inflammation of the pancreas
- Two categories of pancreatitis
  - Acute, occurring suddenly and usually lasts for days
  - Chronic, occurring over months to years
- If pancreatitis is mild, it may not require treatment but when severe, it can cause serious complications
- Main presenting symptoms for acute pancreatitis
  - Severe pain is the main symptom. It is sudden abdominal pain that usually radiates to the back and worsens with food
  - Fever, nausea, vomiting
  - Tenderness to abdomen. Client will guard the abdomen
- Symptoms for chronic pancreatitis
  - Weight loss that occurs without trying to lose weight
  - Stools that are foul smelling and oily, termed steatorrhea
  - Pain in upper abdomen
- Recurring acute pancreatitis can result in scar tissue formation in the pancreas. This can cause the pancreas to function poorly, leading to diabetes and digestion problems
- Common causes of pancreatitis
  - Gallstones
  - Alcoholism
  - Abdominal surgery
  - Biliary sludge comprised of calcium salts and cholesterol crystals
  - Cigarette smoking
  - High triglycerides, usually levels greater than 100 mg/dL
  - Pancreatic cancer

Priority Data Collection or Cues

- Assist in complete full system assessment as well as focused assessment
- Ask about abdominal pain. Pain usually occurs suddenly in the left upper quadrant and radiates to the back. Ask for a description of the pain. Pain with acute pancreatitis is often described as piercing, deep and severe
- Ask about alcohol intake and type of meal last consumed. Alcohol and fatty foods can increase the pain
- Monitor for fever, nausea and vomiting, decreased or absent bowel sounds. Observe for guarding of the abdominal area. Look for bowel distention, caused by paralytic ileus
- Monitor for Cullen's sign (bluish discoloration around the umbilicus) and Grey Turner's sign (bluish discoloration on the flanks), caused by bloody exudate seeping from the pancreas
- Measure vital signs, client is usually tachycardic and hypotensive
- In severe pancreatitis, monitor respiratory system for complications such as pleural effusion, atelectasis or acute respiratory distress syndrome
- Look for foul smelling, fatty stools in chronic pancreatitis

Priority Laboratory Tests/Diagnostics

- Blood test
  - Serum amylase and lipase, urinary amylase, glucose, triglycerides will be elevated
  - Serum calcium will be decreased
- Computed tomography (CT) scan will show gallstones, abscess or pseudocyst
- Stool test will show fat, indicating poor absorption of nutrients (mostly for chronic pancreatitis)
- Abdominal ultrasound will show pancreatic inflammation and gallstones
- Magnetic resonance imaging (MRI) reveals gallbladder, pancreatic and pancreatic duct abnormalities

Priority Interventions or Actions

- Withhold oral intake and initiate intravenous fluids. Insert nasogastric tube to prevent vomiting and gastric distention. Assist in administering parenteral nutrition to supplement nutrition
- Administer oxygen to keep oxygen saturation greater than 95%
- Assist in managing pain with intravenous morphine. Encourage client to lie on the side with head up to 45 degrees. This helps to ease the pain by decreasing abdominal tension
- Monitor glucose levels
- Administer medications that decrease production of hydrochloric acid to prevent pancreatic enzymes from being activated
- Ongoing monitoring of vital signs as fever, tachypnea and hypotension can cause compromise in hemodynamic stability
- Monitor fluid and electrolytes
- In severe acute pancreatitis, vasoactive medications may be administered to correct hypotension
- Monitor client for pancreatic necrosis and administer antibiotic as prescribed
- Prepare client for surgery if pancreatitis is caused by gallstones that must be removed
  - An endoscopic retrograde cholangiopancreatography (ERCP) is done using general anesthesia or sedative to examine internal structures and confirm gallstones and may include a sphincterotomy
  - Cholecystectomy may be performed to prevent recurrence
  - Monitor surgical site for bleeding and infection. Manage drainage tube
- When client can eat, provide meals in small amounts and at frequent intervals
- Carefully monitor client's toleration of dietary advancement

Priority Potential & Actual Complications

- Pseudocyst, the formation of a pocket in the pancreas that is filled with debris and fluid. If the cyst ruptures, bleeding and infection can occur
- Kidney failure
- Diabetes
- Pancreatic cancer
- Respiratory problems such as acute respiratory distress syndrome (ARDS), pleural effusion and atelectasis

Priority Nursing Implications

- For the client who has alcohol use disorder, assistance may be needed to get support for the client to quit drinking, to minimize the likelihood of a future pancreatitis exacerbation from alcohol intake
- Remember that pain is excruciating with acute pancreatitis, so pain management must be a priority
- With acute pancreatitis, it is crucial to prevent all actions that can stimulate the pancreas as this will only aggravate the condition. Clients must not be fed any foods by mouth until the acute condition is resolved

Priority Medications

- Pancrelipase
  - Administered orally
  - Pancreatic enzyme replacement
  - Used for chronic pancreatitis
- Morphine
  - Administered intravenously for pain
- Proton pump inhibitors
  - Used to decrease acid secretion, which acts as a stimulus for pancreatic activity
  - Omeprazole is given daily initially, then administered in multiple or single doses
  - Pantoprazole administered via oral or intravenous routes
- Antispasmodics
  - Dicyclomine (common one used in the class), used to decrease motility and pancreatic outflow
  - Administered orally

Reinforcement of Priority Teaching

- Avoid the triggers of pancreatitis, such as alcohol intake and cigarette smoking
- The condition may cause weakness and loss of strength so physical therapy to increase muscle strength may be needed when discharged
- Avoid fatty foods as they stimulate the pancreas and can cause an attack of pancreatitis
- Encourage clients to monitor the quality of stools and report increased foul-smelling stools that contain fat (steatorrhea) to the health care provider
- Signs and symptoms of diabetes
- For client with chronic pancreatitis, instruct on intake of pancreatic enzymes with meals
- The importance to keeping all follow-up medical appointments

Next Gen Clinical Judgment

List 3 health promotion statements made by a client to help prevent pancreatitis.

1. ______________________
2. ______________________
3. ______________________

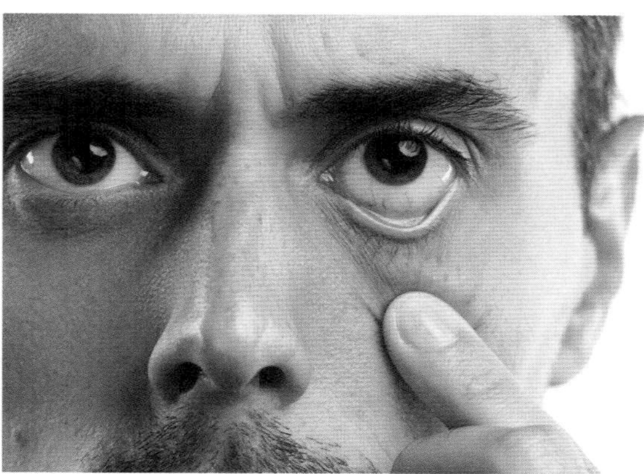

Image 7-4: Identify causes of jaundice in clients with pancreatitis. How is jaundice treated?

____

____

____

____

____

____

____

____

Appendicitis/peritonitis

Pathophysiology/Description

- Appendicitis is inflammation of the narrow tube of tissue that extends from the cecum, called the appendix
- Appendicitis accounts for many emergency visits and is the most common reason for abdominal surgery
- The goal is to remove the inflamed appendix before it ruptures but rupture often occurs, causing peritonitis. Appendicitis is a medical emergency
- The condition is commonly seen in ages 10-30
- Common cause of appendicitis is accumulated fecal deposits causing obstruction
- Clinical manifestations
  - Dull, persistent pain around the umbilicus that frequently moves to the right lower quadrant
  - The pain usually localizes between the right iliac crest and the umbilicus, known as McBurney's point
  - Nausea, vomiting and low-grade fever
  - Rebound tenderness (when pressure is applied to the abdomen and released, the pain is more intense) and client guards the abdomen
  - Client often lies on side with legs flexed to guard abdomen

Priority Data Collection or Cues

- Monitor for abdominal pain to umbilical area and right lower quadrant
- Monitor for nausea and vomiting
- Look to see if the client can deep breathe, cough or sneeze without increase in pain. With appendicitis, these actions will worsen that pain
- Monitor for rebound tenderness, which is indicative of appendicitis
- Monitor for abdominal distention, tachycardia and fever if peritonitis is suspected
- Monitor nasogastric tube to ensure proper functioning
- Monitor vital signs, if losing of blood from peritonitis, client may be hypotensive with tachycardia trying to compensate for hypotension

Clinical Hint

Sudden relief of pain and then an increase in pain accompanied by right guarding of the abdomen is an indication of a perforated appendix.

Priority Laboratory Tests/Diagnostics

- White blood cell count is expected to be elevated
- Computed tomography (CT) scan, magnetic resonance imaging and ultrasound used for appendicitis and peritonitis to examine the degree of damage as well as determine cause of either condition
- Urinalysis, to determine if appendicitis is being mimicked by a genitourinary condition
- Abdominal X-ray may show loops of dilated bowels, indicating conditions such as obstruction or paralytic ileus. Used when peritonitis is suspected
- Peritoneoscopy can allow direct view of the peritoneum. Used when peritonitis is suspected

Priority Interventions or Actions

- Keep the client NPO (nothing by mouth) until a decision regarding surgery is made
- Monitor for signs that indicate appendix has ruptured
- Monitor bowel sounds
- Ongoing monitoring of status and vital signs to determine change in condition
- Prepare client for emergency appendectomy
- Administer pain medications
- Administer medications for nausea and vomiting
- Administer antibiotic therapy and monitor for side effects
- Provide comfort measures, such as positioning client in a right side-lying position
- Administer antibiotics for peritonitis
- With peritonitis, insert nasogastric tube and connect to low-intermittent suction to decrease gastric distention
- With peritonitis, monitor intake, output and electrolytes level to guide fluid replacement
- Monitor surgical drain if one was used

Priority Potential & Actual Complications

- Complication of appendicitis
  - Perforation, with resulting peritonitis
- Complications of peritonitis
  - Hypovolemic shock
  - Paralytic ileus
  - Sepsis
  - Abscess formation in the abdomen
  - Acute respiratory distress syndrome

Priority Nursing Implications

- Note that with appendicitis, peritonitis is a significant complication. However, peritonitis can be caused by other factors as well, such as perforated duodenal or gastric ulcers, abdominal trauma, liver cirrhosis and ascites, infections of the genital tract or blood-borne pathogens
- When there is peritonitis from a ruptured appendix, intravenous fluids given for 6-8 hours prior to an appendectomy aids in the prevention of dehydration and sepsis
- With appendicitis, do not apply heat of any type to the abdomen as heat can cause the appendix to rupture

Priority Medications

- Analgesics
  - Used to manage pain
  - There are numerous analgesic medications from which to choose
  - Available via all routes. The choice of route and medication is dependent on the health care provider's assessment of the client and the severity of the pain. There is no one specific analgesic that is used in appendicitis and/or peritonitis
- Antiemetic medications
  - Used to treat nausea and vomiting
  - There are many in this class of drugs from which a prescriber can choose. Some common ones are ondansetron, prochlorperazine and dolasetron
  - Available oral, intravenous, intramuscular and rectal. For the client with appendicitis and or peritonitis it will most likely not be administered via the intravenous route
- Antibiotics
  - Cephalosporins most commonly used. Treat infection from a ruptured appendix, peritonitis or as prophylaxis
  - Several in the class of cephalosporins. Few common ones are cefuroxime, ceftriaxone, ceftazidime
  - Administer intravenous or intramuscular

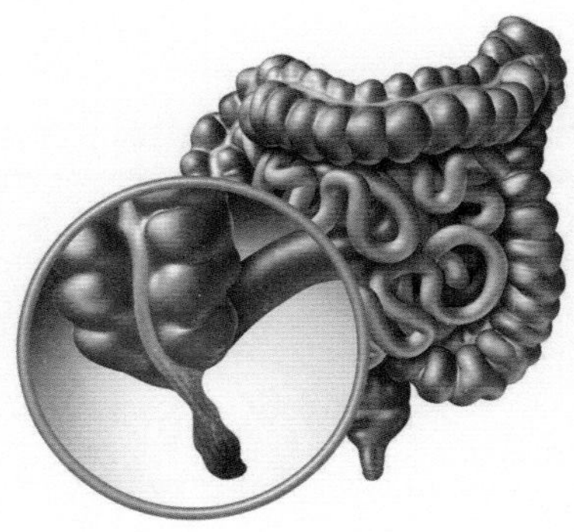

Image 7-5: What are the dangers of a ruptured appendix?

Reinforcement of Priority Teaching

- Discharge instruction to clients and explain that after 2-3 weeks they should be able to resume normal activities
- If discharged with antibiotics, reinforce the importance of, and rationale for taking all the medication and not stopping when they feel better
- Signs and symptoms of a wound infection and when to notify the health care provider
- The importance of keeping follow-up medical appointments

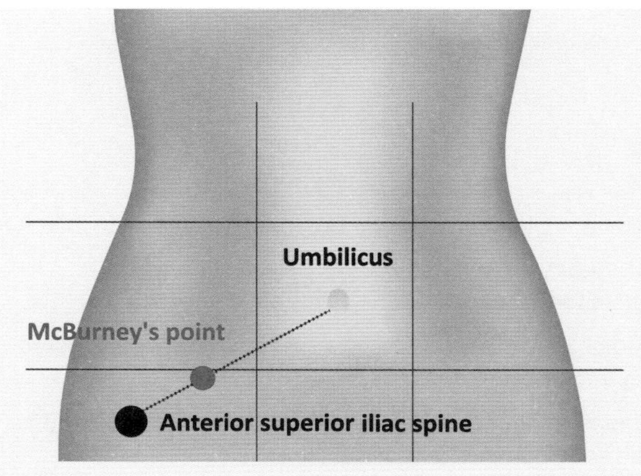

Image 7-6: Palpate a client's right lower quadrant over the McBurney's point. A positive McBurney's sign indicates appendicitis.

Complete this MNEMONIC
Early signs and symptoms of appendicitis
B ______________________
R ______________________
A ______________________
I ______________________
N ______________________

Table 7-1: Feel free to search the Internet or create your own.

Cellulitis/wound infection/septicemia

Pathophysiology/Description

- A wound infection occurs when bacteria invades an open wound
- Causes
  - Surgical complication
  - Poor aseptic technique
  - Certain medical conditions predispose to infections, such as diabetes mellitus
- Wound infections must be treated quickly and appropriately to foster healing and prevent complications. One of the more serious complications is septicemia, which is bacteria in the bloodstream

Priority Data Collection or Cues

- Monitor client for fever and chills, indicative of an infection
- Monitor wound for tenderness, swelling, warmth, malodorous and purulent drainage
- Monitor pain level. There is usually pain with an infected wound and with cellulitis
- Examine wound for dead tissue as necrotic tissue is often present in infected wounds
- Review complete blood count, expect increase in white blood cells due to infection and fever
- Monitor vital signs, expect temperature elevation
- Look for cellulitis, manifested as inflammation to surrounding skin and soft tissues under the skin, and red streaking to the skin
- If there is cellulitis, perform ongoing data collection to determine if fever, tachycardia and tachypnea are resolving with treatment
- Monitor for septicemia, manifested as chills, fever, tachycardia and tachypnea. Confusion, reduced urine output and shock are likely if septicemia progresses without treatment
- Assist in performing a complete physical assessment
- Complete a detailed health history

Priority Laboratory Tests/Diagnostics

- Complete blood count will show elevated white blood cell count
- Wound culture will show the causative bacteria
- X-ray or computed tomography (CT) scan to look for foreign objects in wound (as in an object left in a surgical wound) or examine deep tissues for signs of infection

Priority Interventions or Actions

- Collect wound samples for culture and sensitivity and send to the lab promptly
- Administer prompt treatment of septicemia, if present, to prevent progression to sepsis and septic shock
- Administer antibiotics promptly as prescribed and monitor for effectiveness
- Administer wound treatment as prescribed
- Monitor wound to determine effectiveness of treatment
- Monitor blood tests to determine decrease in white blood cell count
- Monitor skin with cellulitis to determine if inflammation is resolving
- Administer analgesics for pain, especially before performing wound care
- Assist with wound debridement procedure to remove dead tissue from wound
- If foreign body in wound, prepare client for procedure to remove the object
- Apply wound vacuum to assist with wound healing, if prescribed, and monitor wound drainage

Priority Potential & Actual Complications

- Chronic infection
- Loss of limb as a result of untreated infected wound
- Septicemia, which is bacteria in the blood that can result in sepsis. Some still refer to septicemia as blood poisoning or bacteremia. Septicemia occurs when bacteria gets into the bloodstream from another part of the body, as in an infected wound
- Sepsis is a widespread and potentially fatal inflammation of the body in response to bacteria in the bloodstream. Both septicemia and sepsis must be treated promptly
- May be fatal

Priority Nursing Implications

- Cellulitis can occur as a result of a wound infection, but it can also be seen in other conditions such as a foreign body in the skin, a tear to the skin, or chronic conditions such as eczema. Cellulitis must be treated promptly
- Cellulitis may progress to more severe infections in clients who are at risk

Priority Medications

- Cephalexin given orally
  - Antibiotic
  - First generation cephalosporin that is commonly used to treat bacterial and skin infections
- Amoxicillin given orally
  - Antibiotic in the penicillin family
  - Commonly prescribed for skin infections
- Augmentin given orally
  - Antibiotic
  - Used when amoxicillin and cephalexin are not effective
- Analgesics
  - Used to manage pain
  - There are numerous analgesic medications from which to choose
  - Available via all routes. The choice of route and medication is dependent on the health care provider's assessment of the client and the severity of the pain. There is no one specific analgesic that is used for the client with a wound infection, septicemia or cellulitis

Reinforcement of Priority Teaching

- How to care for wound at home to prevent re-infection
- Explain signs and symptoms of septicemia
- Signs and symptoms of wound infection and when to contact the health care provider
- The importance of follow-up medical care
- Healthy nutrition to promote wound healing
- Management of other health conditions the client has, especially those associated with poor wound healing, like diabetes
- The effects of smoking on wound healing. It causes poor wound healing
- Assist client to schedule visits to a wound care clinic if client is unable to care for wound

Clinical Hint

To treat cellulitis, the health care provider will prescribe antibiotics. Nurses must inform clients to complete the entire antibiotic regimen as prescribed.

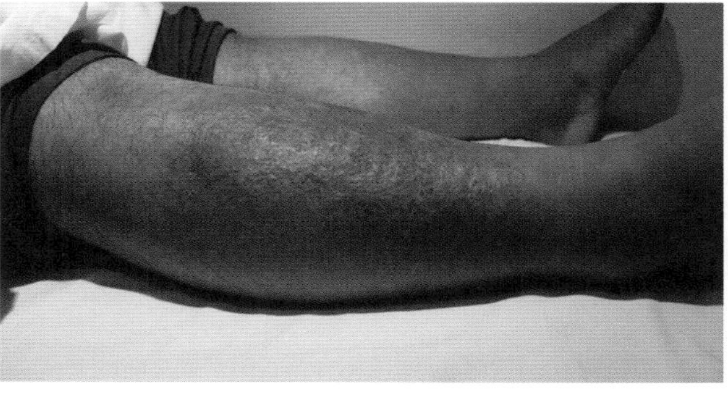

Image 7-7: This client has cellulitis and a deep vein thrombosis. What nursing actions should the nurse anticipate?

Complete this MNEMONIC
SEPSIS Symptoms
S ______
E ______
P ______
S ______
I ______
S ______

Table 7-2: Feel free to search the Internet or create your own.

______

______

______

______

______

______

Gout

Pathophysiology/Description

- Gout is a systemic condition characterized by high levels of uric acid (called hyperuricemia) and deposits of uric acid crystals in joints
- Gout is not a continuous condition but one that presents with long intervals of remission and periods of exacerbation
- There are two forms of gout
    - Primary, which occurs as a result of a problem with purine metabolism in the body. This is the most common type of gout
    - Secondary, which results from some other condition in the body, such as renal insufficiency, sickle cell anemia, hyperlipidemia, and medications
- Causes of primary gout
    - Kidney reduced capacity to excrete uric acid
    - Increased production of uric acid
    - Dietary increase in purine rich foods, such as shellfish, red meat, drinks with fructose
- There are 4 phases to gout
    - Asymptomatic phase, where there is hyperuricemia, but the individual has no symptoms
    - Acute phase, where one or more small joints is inflamed, causing excruciating pain. Pain is usually in the great toe
    - Intermittent phase, where the individual experiences intermittent periods with no symptoms between acute exacerbations or attacks
    - Chronic phase that is characterized by repeated attacks. With chronic gout, there can be deposits of urate crystal in major organs

Priority Data Collection or Cues

- Monitor for swelling and inflammation of joints, expect joints to be very tender and painful. Clients usually state that the affected area is very sensitive when touched lightly
- Examine great toe as this is the most common location where gout first manifests
- Monitor color of affected joints (cyanotic and dusky in color)
- Monitor range of motion limitation
- Ask client about family history. Complete a thorough health history
- Ask about risk factors for gout. This will help with client education on prevention of exacerbations
- Ask about onset of pain. Gout typically starts at night with swelling that occurs suddenly, followed by excruciating pain
- Monitor vital signs, a low-grade temperature is usually present
- Monitor joint for presence of tophi which appear as hard nodules in the skin. Tophi occur from deposits of sodium urate crystals
- Ask client about itching (pruritus) to skin. Urate crystals in skin causes itching

Priority Laboratory Tests/Diagnostics

- Serum uric acid will usually be elevated above 6 mg/dL
- 24-hour urine uric acid. This determines if gout is related to overproduction of uric acid or decreased excretion of uric acid from the kidneys
- Synovial fluid aspiration. This is the gold standard for diagnosis and will show urate crystals
- X-ray of the affected area will show tophi in chronic gout but may be normal in the early stages of gout

Priority Interventions or Actions

- Use a bed cradle to prevent the bed linens from touching the affected lower extremity. Handle extremity carefully to avoid direct touching of the affected area
- Administer anti-inflammatory, uricosuric drugs and analgesic medications as prescribed, to treat the condition. Monitor for desired, and side effects
- Monitor intake and output to ensure uric acid is not being precipitated in the renal tubules. Encourage fluid intake of 2000 mL/day
- Ensure client has a diet low in purine. Encourage client to eat foods that help to increase the pH of urine (above 6), called alkaline ash foods. Most vegetables and fruits fall in this category
- Encourage bedrest initially to immobilize affected joint, until condition has started to resolve
- Monitor for common adverse effect of NSAIDs, gastrointestinal bleeding

Priority Potential & Actual Complications

- Deformity to joints
- Urate deposits in organs causing organ dysfunction
- Renal calculi

Priority Nursing Implications

- Bedrest may be needed in initial stage of acute gout when it is most painful. However, be mindful of problems that can occur when clients are immobilized, such as pressure ulcers. Use strategies to prevent complications
- Note that even though the gold standard for diagnosing gout is synovial fluid aspiration, it is only done in a small percentage of clients. This is because clinical symptoms alone can usually diagnose gout

Priority Medications

- Colchicine given orally
  - The oldest drug used to treat acute gout
  - Reduces the inflammatory response. Provides excellent pain relief in 12 -24 hours
- Non-steroidal anti-inflammatory drugs (NSAIDs)–given orally
  - For acute treatment of inflammatory process
  - There are several that can be used but indomethacin, naproxen and sulindac are quite often used for gout
  - Most significant adverse effect of NSAIDs is gastrointestinal bleeding
- Allopurinol given orally
  - Used as maintenance therapy
  - Prevents uric acid production
- Probenecid given orally
  - Used to increase the kidney's excretion of uric acid in urine
  - Probenecid is ineffective if client has renal impairment
- Febuxostat given orally
  - This is the first new drug for gout in recent years
  - Used for chronic gout to manage high levels of uric acid in the blood
- Pegloticase given intravenous
  - Used when clients do not respond to other drugs that decrease uric acid level in the blood
  - Pre-medicate client with corticosteroids or antihistamines before pegloticase to prevent infusion reactions
- Corticosteroids
  - Can be used to treat attacks, especially for clients who cannot take NSAIDs and/or colchicine
  - Administered oral or intraarticular (into the joints)
  - Several used at various dosages, but most common are dexamethasone, prednisone, triamcinolone, hydrocortisone, methylprednisolone

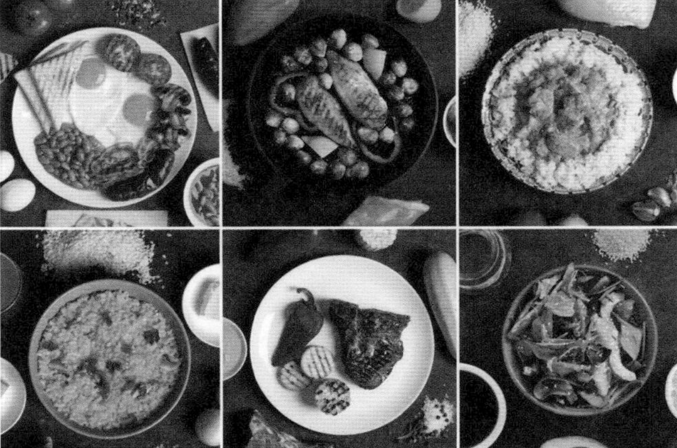

Image 7-8: What foods should the nurse recommend that a client avoid to prevent a flare-up of gout?

Reinforcement of Priority Teaching

- The importance of adhering to the treatment plan. Take medications as prescribed
- The importance of getting uric acid in the blood checked periodically
- The importance of keeping follow-up medical appointments
- Signs and symptoms of gout attack
- Factors that can precipitate a gout attack such as overeating foods that are rich in purine. These include organ meat, anchovies, and shellfish
- Avoidance of alcoholic drinks as alcohol precipitates gout attacks
- Adverse effects of maintenance drugs such as allopurinol. Allopurinol has the following serious adverse effects
  - Aplastic anemia
  - Toxic epidermal necrolysis
  - Agranulocytosis
  - Stevens-Johnson syndrome

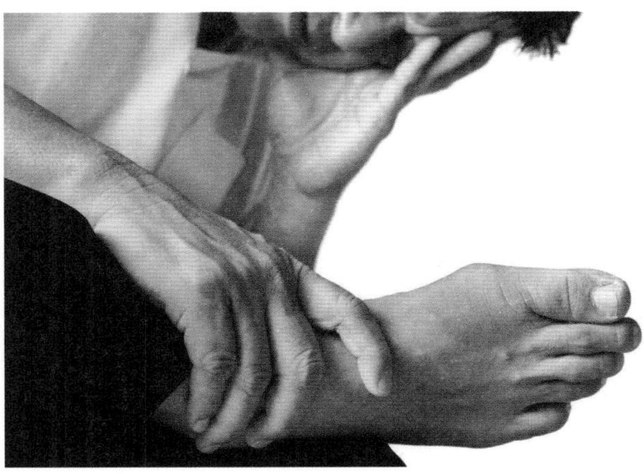

Image 7-9: List 3 Health Promotion statements made by the client in the prevention of the reoccurrence of gout.

____

____

____

____

____

____

Systemic lupus erythematosus

Pathophysiology/Description

- Systemic lupus erythematosus is a chronic, autoimmune, progressive multisystem disease that causes failure to major organ systems of the body
- Occurs most frequently in women of child-bearing age and generally seen most often in Hispanics, Native Americans, African Americans and Asian Americans
- The disease is characterized by exacerbations and remissions
- Cause
  - Even though the etiology is unknown, it is observed that SLE usually runs in families, so genetics is suspected as a causative factor
  - The disease worsens with menstruation, during and immediately after pregnancy and when oral contraceptives are used
  - Environmental factors such as sunlight, chemical exposure and stress have been known to exacerbate SLE
  - Several medications have been identified as triggers for SLE such as isoniazid, hydralazine, procainamide, minocycline and quinidine
- In SLE, the immune system attacks the body's own tissues causing major damage to many organs. Fibrin deposits and connective tissue collect on collagen fibers and inside the blood vessels, causing widespread inflammation and necrosis
- All body systems are affected with SLE
- There is no cure for SLE but clients experience periods of remission

Priority Data Collection or Cues

- Assist in collecting a complete history and physical assessment
- Monitor signs and symptoms such as joint pain
- Ask about excessive fatigue, weight loss and fever as these symptoms usually occur before SLE activity worsens
- Monitor for redness to the face with classic "butterfly" rash over cheeks and bridge of nose, scaly rash to face and upper torso. Palms for erythema
- Monitor for general feeling of malaise, weakness and anorexia
- Look for ulcers to the mouth and nose, these are common with SLE
- Examine hair for balding and lesions to scalp
- Note infections due to increased susceptibility to infections
- Cough and difficulty breathing, suggestive of lung involvement
- Monitor for cardiac dysrhythmias due to fibrosis of atrioventricular nodes
- Monitor for polyarthralgia (pain in many joints) and stiffness in the morning (this is a common complaint). Look for stiffness to joints
- Renal involvement, shows SLE impact on renal system
- Monitor for neurological involvement such as seizures, disordered thinking, impaired memory and peripheral neuropathy. Monitor for photosensitivity
- Monitor for anxiety, depression and psychosis due to the stress of a major life-altering illness

Priority Laboratory Tests/Diagnostics

- Labs, looking for hematologic conditions such as thrombocytopenia, anemia, leukopenia and clotting issues
- Antinuclear antibody (ANA), a type of antibody directed against the nuclei of the cell: will be positive in about 97% of clients with SLE
- Antiphospholipid Antibodies (ALPs), antibodies that are directed at phospholipids: will be positive in about 30% of clients with SLE
- Anti-Smith antibody, a protein found in cell nucleus called Sm, will be positive in about 30% of clients with SLE
- C-Reactive Protein (CRP), a protein in body that can suggest inflammation, will be elevated: not used to diagnose the disease but is used to determine therapy effectiveness and activity of the disease
- Erythrocyte sedimentation rate is elevated in SLE and is used to monitor SLE activity and effectiveness of therapy

Priority Interventions or Actions

- Monitor for signs of organ involvement, such as peritonitis, hypertension, arrhythmias, nephritis, pericarditis, anemia and coronary artery disease (this is not an exhaustive list since all systems are impacted)
- Monitor skin integrity and provide meticulous skin care
- Apply creams and ointments for skin rash, as prescribed
- Administer medication as prescribed to manage pain and decrease the inflammatory response
- Perform client care activities, to include rest periods due to fatigue
- Ensure client is provided with proper nutrients due to weight loss
- Provide appropriate respiratory care if respiratory system involvement, such as oxygen
- Measure intake and output, primarily if the client is receiving corticosteroids. Corticosteroids can cause fluid retention
- Monitor neurologic functioning to determine change in neurologic symptoms, such as memory deficits, personality changes and seizures. Administer anti-seizure medications if seizure involvement
- Monitor for bleeding or bruising due to hematologic involvement
- Monitor hands and feet to determine improvement in numbness, tingling and weakness. Peripheral neuropathy is an issue in SLE
- Provide diet high in iron, protein, folic acid and vitamins, if there are no contraindications to any of these, such as kidney disease that would prevent intake of a high-protein diet

- Provide emotional support for client and family
- Provide supportive environment for client to verbalize feelings about the disease

Priority Potential & Actual Complications

- Complications of SLE are many and affect all systems. This is not an all-inclusive list of possible complications
  - Stroke, seizure, memory impairment
  - Psychological problems, usually from coping with the myriad of complications
  - Heart attack, dysrhythmias, pericarditis, cardiac failure
  - Pleurisy, difficulty breathing
  - Kidney failure
  - Severe arthralgia, impaired mobility, paralysis, may be fatal

Priority Nursing Implications

- Focus of care will be on all body systems
- Monitor for depression and ensure appropriate referrals to address the issue
- Hydroxychloroquine causes retinopathy so client taking the drug should have an eye examination every 6-12 months
- Methotrexate has serious side effects of hepatoxicity and bone marrow suppression, so CBC must be monitored frequently

Priority Medications

- Non-steroidal anti-inflammatory drugs (NSAIDs)– given orally
  - NSAIDs are frequently used interventions for arthralgia and arthritis seen with SLE
  - There are several that can be used but indomethacin, naproxen and sulindac are quite often used for systemic lupus erythematosus
  - Most significant adverse effect of NSAIDs is gastrointestinal bleeding
- Hydroxychloroquine–given orally
  - Antimalarial drugs
  - Used to treat fatigue and joint and skin problems
- Dapsone–given orally
  - Antileprosy drug
  - Administered if client cannot tolerate an antimalarial drug
- Corticosteroids (several in the class)
  - Corticosteroids use should be limited
  - Methylprednisolone used intravenously and in tapering doses may be effective in managing the flare-up from polyarthritis
  - High doses of corticosteroids are effective in treating severe cutaneous problems from SLE
- Methotrexate–given orally, subcutaneous, and intramuscular
  - Steroid-sparing immunosuppressant. Considered a standard treatment
  - Used as an alternate to corticosteroids
- Azathioprine, cyclophosphamide
  - Immunosuppressants, used to treat severe organ involvement with SLE
  - Prevents the need for long-term corticosteroid therapy
  - Both drugs given orally or intravenous
- Warfarin–given orally
  - Anticoagulant
  - Used to thin the blood and prevent blood clotting, which is a complication of SLE
  - Dosage is dependent on desired therapeutic range of the drug. Labs must be drawn to determine the international normalized ratio (INR)
- Tacrolimus, pimecrolimus
  - Topical immunomodulators that suppress immune activity of the skin
  - Used instead of corticosteroids to manage skin rashes
  - Dosage of these creams depend on the severity of the rash. Results are usually seen in 8-15 days
- Belimumab–given subcutaneous
  - First approved immunosuppressant drug for specific treatment of systemic lupus
  - Works by specifically targeting immune cells

Reinforcement of Priority Teaching

- Disease and long-term expectations
- Explain the triggers for SLE and how the client can avoid these triggers
- Proper skin care at home, wash with mild soap and do not apply perfumed or harsh emollients to skin
- Instruct client to avoid sun or ultraviolet light
- Provide client with information for SLE support groups
- Provide client with a list of community resources
- Medication therapy, to include why the drugs are being used, how to use them and the side effects
- Foods to eat that will provide essential nutrients needed

Clinical Hint

One of the classic characteristics in SLE is the butterfly rash. This is when lesions appear on the cheeks and the bridge of the nose, creating a butterfly pattern. This rash may vary in severity.

Rheumatoid arthritis

Pathophysiology/Description

- Rheumatoid arthritis is a chronic systemic immune disease
- It is characterized by inflammation and destruction of connective tissue and membranes within the synovial joints
- The disease is characterized by exacerbations and remissions and can occur at any point in an individual's life. However, incidence of RA peaks between 30 and 50 years and affect women more than men
- Even though the etiology is unknown, it is thought to result from genetic as well as environmental factors
- The condition is life-altering and without treatment, many with the condition will have significant functional impairment, such as required replacement of joints, use of mobility aids and loss of ability to perform activities of daily living without assistance
- There are 4 stages to RA. Stage 1 is characterized by mild symptoms, such as swelling of synovial membrane and soft tissue, and elevated white blood cell count in the synovial fluid. As the client progresses to the final stage (end-stage), there will be loss of joint function and formation of nodules in subcutaneous tissue
- Definitive diagnostic criteria for RA is based upon scores the client receives from four specific categories: joint involvement, serology, acute phase reactants and duration of symptoms. Possible scores range from 0-10. A score greater than or equal to 6 is definitive for RA

Priority Data Collection or Cues

- Joint pain, warmth, limited range of motion, deformity, nodules at joints and muscle atrophy. Focus data collection on small and large joints as large peripheral joints may also be involved
- Signs of inflammation manifested as heat, swelling and tenderness to area
- Ask about excessive fatigue, weight loss, anorexia and generalized stiffness as these usually signify the start of joint symptoms
- Ask about severity and duration of pain in the morning. Pain and stiffness usually occur in the morning and last for more than 30 minutes, sometimes all day
- Monitor vital signs, expect a low-grade temperature, because of the inflammatory process
- Ask client to grasp objects. RA may affect the extensor and flexor tendons in the wrist, making grasping objects difficult
- Monitor for specific deformities of RA
    - Swan neck deformity: the middle joint of a finger is extended (bent back) more than normal. The end joint is flexed (bent down)
    - Ulnar drift: a hand deformity where swelling of the metacarpophalangeal joints (the knuckles at the base of the fingers) causes the fingers to become displaced towards the little finger
    - Hallux valgus (bunion): lateral deviation of the hallux (great toe) on the first metatarsal
    - Boutonniere deformity: the finger permanently bends down at the middle joint and the end joint bends backwards
- Monitor all body systems as RA can impact all systems
- Monitor for Sjogren's syndrome manifested by decreased secretion of saliva and tears, resulting in dry eyes, photosensitivity and dry-mouth
- Monitor for felty syndrome, especially if client's RA is long-standing, manifested by low white blood cell count and splenomegaly
- Monitor for signs of infection as felty syndrome predisposes client to infection
- Be aware of client and family's psychosocial needs

Priority Laboratory Tests/Diagnostics

- White blood cell count (WBC) in synovial fluid will be elevated with decreased viscosity
- X-ray will show erosion and narrowing of joint space, bony growths and osteoporosis because of corticosteroid usage
- Rheumatoid Factor (RH) will be positive in up to 90% of clients with RA
- Antinuclear antibody (ANA), a type of antibody directed against the nuclei of the cell, will be positive in up to 30% of clients with RA
- C-Reactive Protein (CRP), a protein in body that can suggest inflammation, will be elevated, showing active inflammation
- Erythrocyte sedimentation rate will be elevated showing active inflammation
- Anti-cyclic citrullinated peptide (ant-CCP), autoantibodies that are directed against certain peptides and proteins, will be positive in more than 80% of clients with RA

Priority Interventions or Actions

- Administer drug therapy as prescribed
- Assist with completion of activities of daily living, being mindful of morning stiffness
- Provide range of motion exercises to client's tolerance to maintain functioning of joint
- Avoid weight bearing to inflamed extremity
- Apply cold and heat applications to joints as prescribed
- Administer medication as prescribed to manage pain and decrease the inflammatory response
- Perform client care activities, to include rest periods due to fatigue and joint discomfort
- Ensure client is provided with proper nutrients due to loss of appetite from pain and fatigue
- Ensure client gets assistance from physical and occupational therapies, if needed
- Use splints on affected extremities to prevent contractures
- Measure intake and output, primarily if the client is receiving corticosteroids. Corticosteroids can cause fluid retention
- Provide supportive environment for client to verbalize feelings about the disease

Priority Potential & Actual Complications

- Complications mostly relate to rheumatoid nodules forming in body parts
  - Scleritis
  - Sjögren's Syndrome
  - Heart complications such as pericarditis and myocarditis
  - Lung problems such as pleural effusion, collapsed lung
- Physical immobility due to deformity of extremities

Priority Nursing Implications

- Hydroxychloroquine causes retinopathy so client taking the drug should have an eye examination every 6-12 months
- Leflunomide is teratogenic, so this drug must not be administered to women of child-bearing age unless pregnancy is ruled out
- For clients who are administered aspirin, serum salicylate levels must be checked if dosage is more than 3600 mg daily to avoid the complications of aspirin toxicity
- RA is common in older adults and they often use several medications to treat their health conditions. It is important that polypharmacy be considered and addressed with the older client
- Methotrexate has the serious side effects of hepatoxicity and bone marrow suppression so CBC must be monitored frequently

Priority Medications

- Non-steroidal anti-inflammatory drugs (NSAIDs)–given orally
  - There are several NSAIDs that can be used. celecoxib and aspirin are ones commonly used
  - Most significant adverse effect of NSAIDs is gastrointestinal bleeding
- Hydroxychloroquine–given orally
  - Antimalarial drug
  - Used to treat fatigue and joint problems
- Leflunomide, sulfasalazine–given orally
  - Antirheumatic drugs
  - Leflunomide blocks immune cell overproduction and sulfasalazine decreases the pain and swelling of inflammatory arthritis, but may also prevent damage to joints
- Corticosteroids (several in the class)
  - Low-dose corticosteroids are usually administered until the antirheumatic drugs can start to take effect
  - Used to manage symptoms during acute RA flare-up
  - When administered as intraarticular injections, may decrease pain and inflammation
- Methotrexate–given orally, subcutaneous, and intramuscular
  - Steroid-sparing immunosuppressant
  - Used as an alternate to corticosteroids
- Tofacitinib–given orally
  - Antirheumatic drug
  - Interferes with certain enzymes (JAK enzymes) that cause joint inflammation
- Tumor necrosis factor inhibitors–given intravenous
  - Used in clients who have not responded to the antirheumatic drugs
  - Decrease immune and inflammatory response
- Interleukin-1 receptor antagonists
  - Interleukin inhibitor. There are several in the class
  - Mostly used to treat clients who have not responded to, or cannot tolerate other drugs used for RA
  - Administered via various routes

Reinforcement of Priority Teaching

- Disease and long-term expectations
- Instruction on protection of small joints such as avoiding repetitive movements, using strongest joint for tasks and modifying activities to decrease stress on joints
- Provide client with information for RA support groups and a list of community resources
- Medication therapy, to include why the drugs are being used, how to use them and the side effects
- Assist clients in identifying foods to eat that will provide essential nutrition needed
- Instructions for the client and/or caregiver about modifications that may need to be made to the home to maintain a safe environment, if client has functional deficits from RA
- Assist clients on safe use of assistive devices
- The effects of corticosteroid therapy to client, the fact that it causes weight gain. Encourage a weight loss program and tolerable exercise regimen. Reinforce teaching on minimizing overexertion, which may worsen RA
- Engage in aquatic exercises in warm water, this will make the joints move easier
- Use of cold and heat therapy to relieve stiffness, muscle spasms and pain
- Stress the importance for client to keep follow-up appointments

Next Gen Clinical Judgment

Why is it important to monitor weight in clients with rheumatoid arthritis?

Pathophysiology/Description

- Human immunodeficiency (HIV) is a retrovirus that damages the immune system and renders the host susceptible to infections that would otherwise be prevented because of the body's immune response
- Even though the infection is seen in both men and women, in the United States, it is more prevalent in men who are sexually active with other men
- Transmission
  - Can occur when contact is made with infected vaginal secretions, blood, semen, breast milk, sexual intercourse
  - Exposure to HIV infected blood or blood products
  - Sexual intercourse with infected partner
  - Through birth or breastfeeding
- The target cell for HIV in the body is the CD4 T cell. HIV binds with receptors on the outside of the cell and RNA from HIV enters the cell. Several processes occur ending in destruction of the CD4 T cell. The rate that HIV kills CD4 T cells exceeds the rate at which CD4 T cells can replicate
- With inadequate CD4 T cells, immune function is impaired. Problems with immune function starts to occur when CD4 T cell count drops below 500 CD4 T cells/uL. With CD4 T cell count below 200 CD4 T cells/uL, severe immune function problems occur. When CD 4 T cells are destroyed to a point where not enough are left to maintain immune function, the host becomes susceptible to opportunistic infections
- When HIV progresses, and the individual meets at least one of the diagnostic conditions delineated by the following criteria, acquired immune deficiency syndrome (AIDS) is diagnosed
  - One significant opportunist infection, whether bacterial, fungal, viral or protozoal
  - CD 4 T cell count below 200 cells/uL
  - Wasting syndrome, an ideal body mass loss of more than 10%
  - An opportunistic cancer such as immunoblastic lymphoma, Burkitt's lymphoma (and others)

Priority Data Collection or Cues

- Determine engagement in risky behaviors
- Monitor for symptoms that resemble mononucleosis, such as nausea, headache, malaise, swollen lymph nodes, sore throat, fever, joint pain, rash. These symptoms usually present about 2-3 weeks after infection with HIV
- Monitor eyes for papilledema and presence of exudates
- Monitor for cardiac problems such as pericardial friction rubs or a murmur
- Monitor neuro status for neurological impairment such as memory loss, slurred speech, tremors, agitation, seizures, paralysis
- May find dyspnea, tachypnea, wheezing, cough
- The gastrointestinal system, may see a myriad of impairments such as, candida patches, blisters and other lesions in mouth, tooth decay, gingivitis, white patches in throat, white lesions on sides of tongue, diarrhea, vomiting rectal lesions
- Assist in performing a system assessment to detect presence of opportunistic infections
- Gather data of the skin, may find pallor, cyanotic areas, alopecia, poor skin turgor, lesions and other skin eruptions, bruises to mucous membranes
- The genitourinary system, may see lesions and discharge from genitals and excoriation to vagina or perianal area
- Monitor client's access to social support
- Monitor client's mindset regarding end-of-life care

Priority Laboratory Tests/Diagnostics

- Rapid HIV screening test: A device is placed in the mouth against the gum and fluid is drawn into the pad, the pad is placed in a solution and if client has the HIV antibodies, the corresponding change is noted. Results are available in 20 minutes. If positive, a follow-up blood test is needed
- In home testing for HIV: A drop of blood is placed on a test card and the card is mailed to a laboratory for testing. The card has a code number. Result is received when the client calls a special telephone number and enters the code
- P24 antigen assay detects the amount of HIV viral core protein in the client's blood. Blood is drawn in a lab. Can detect HIV about 2-3 weeks after infection occurs. Result is usually available hours to days
- CD 4 T cell count is used to monitor progression of HIV. Normal CD4 T cell count is 800-1200 cells/uL. The CD4 T cell count decreases as the disease progresses
- Viral load provides information on progression of HIV. Higher viral load indicates more disease activity
- Complete blood cell count (CBC) will likely show low white blood cell count due to opportunistic infections. Anemia and thrombocytopenia may be present due to effects of drug therapy or antiplatelet antibodies

Priority Interventions or Actions

- Administer ART therapy. Monitor for, and treat side effects
- Allow client time to process the news of being HIV positive, if new diagnosis
- Provide adequate oxygenation if client has pneumonia
- Provide other appropriate system care if client has AIDS
- Treat client with dignity and respect
- Provide safe care environment if client has neurological impairments from HIV/AIDS
- Provide gentle but meticulous skin care, as diarrhea and incontinence may be copious
- Be gentle when providing care as client may be emaciated and hurting from muscle wasting

- Protect bony prominences to prevent pressure ulcer formation
- Support client through process of taking multiple medications several times daily
- Provide case management to client to manage social and post discharge plans
- Allow client time to verbalize emotions and end-of-life wishes

Priority Potential & Actual Complications

- Opportunistic infections
- Progression of HIV to AIDS
- Social isolation
- Severe depression
- Coma
- May be fatal

Priority Nursing Implications

- The main cause of disability, disease and death of persons with HIV is opportunistic diseases
- It is important to note that ART interacts with many over-the-counter drugs and alternative therapies. Clients must understand that when on ART, they must seek advice from health care providers and pharmacists before taking OTC drugs and herbal remedies
- Think about the implication when older adults have HIV. They may be ashamed and not want to speak about it, which delays treatment. Nursing implication is that as nurses, a discussion about sexually transmitted diseases must be had when assisting in admissions of any client, regardless of age

Priority Medications

- Non-nucleoside reverse transcriptase inhibitors (NNRTIs)
  - Given orally
  - Stops the action of a protein needed by HIV to make copies of itself
  - There are many drugs in this class
- Nucleoside or nucleotide reverse transcriptase inhibitors (NRTIs)
  - Stops the action of reverse transcriptase
  - There are many drugs in this class
  - This drug is also given in pregnancy orally until labor begins, then is administered intravenously until the umbilical cord is clamped
- Protease inhibitors (PIs)
  - Given orally
  - Inactivate another protein that HIV needs to make copies of itself called HIV protease
  - There are many drugs in this class
- Entry or fusion inhibitors
  - Given orally and intravenous
  - Block entry of HIV in CD4 T cells, thus decreasing replication
  - There are many drugs in this class
- Integrase inhibitors
  - Given orally
  - Disables a protein called integrase, which HIV uses to insert its genetic material into CD4 T cells
  - There are many drugs in this class
- Fixed dose combination drugs
  - These are more than one drug that may come from various classes that are combined into a single tablet

Reinforcement of Priority Teaching

- Preventative measures, in terms of not infecting future partners. Encourage alternate safe sex activities, such as mutual masturbation
- HIV, the susceptibility to infection and treatment options
- Signs and symptoms to report to healthcare team
- Provide community resources and support for psychosocial, financial and spiritual need
- Slowing or preventing progression of HIV to AIDS
- Not sharing drug equipment, such as needles, syringes and cookers, as they may be contaminated with blood
- Use of a needle and syringe exchange program, if the client's community has one
- Proper nutrition to ensure adequate intake of nutrients
- How to reduce risk of getting opportunistic infections
- Stay current with vaccines
- The preexposure prophylaxis drug therapy (tenofovir and emtricitabine) in event client may want to provide this information to loved ones
- How to manage end-of-life issues, especially for the client with AIDS

Next Gen Clinical Judgment

You are caring for a client who is HIV positive and their sexual partner is HIV negative. What recommendations can you provide to keep them both safe?

Hypersensitivity reactions

Pathophysiology/Description

- Hypersensitivity reactions are undesirable reactions that occur as a result of the immune response acting against foreign antigens or against its own tissue
- Hypersensitivity reactions are considered over-reaction of the body's immune system
- Can result in outcomes as simple as being uncomfortable, to as severe as death
- Classified based on the source of the antigen, whether the reaction is immediate or delayed and the way the injury is caused
- There are four types of hypersensitivity reactions
  - Type I: IgE mediated reactions: an allergic reaction that occurs because of re-exposure to a specific type of antigen called an allergen. Includes allergic reactions such as anaphylaxis and atopic reactions, such as rashes
  - Type II: Cytotoxic and cytolytic reactions: the antibodies produced by the immune response bind to antigens on the individual's own cell surfaces. Common antigens involved in type II reactions are Rh factor and the ABO blood group
  - Type III: Immune-complex reactions: Antigen-antibody complexes cause tissue damage in immune complex reactions. Type III reactions may be immediate or delayed, localized or systemic. Type III reactions are seen in autoimmune conditions such as rheumatoid arthritis and systemic lupus erythematosus
  - Type IV: Delayed hypersensitivity reactions: is referred to as delayed type hypersensitivity meaning that the reaction takes several days to develop. It is not an antibody-mediated reaction but a type of cell-mediated response. Example is transplant rejections, reaction to bacterial infections, contact dermatitis

Priority Data Collection or Cues

- Ask about exposure to allergens
- Look for pale wheal on the skin that is edematous, contains fluid and is surrounded by a red flare (called wheal and flare reaction), indicating an anaphylactic reaction that is localized. A mosquito bite is an example of such a reaction
- Assist in data collection of the cause of hypersensitivity reaction
- Monitor for systemic anaphylactic reaction, manifested by initial edema and pruritus to exposure site, followed by respiratory and cardiac involvement such as, constriction of bronchioles, airway obstruction and shock
- Monitor for symptoms indicating atopic reactions such as angioedema, asthma, atopic dermatitis, hay fever and hives
- Monitor for sneezing, nasal drainage, swelling of mucosa that obstructs airway, itching around the eyes and throat and excessive tearing from eyes, indicating hay fever
- Monitor for wheezing, tightness in chest, thick sputum production and dyspnea, indicating asthma reaction
- Examine skin for lesions that are edematous and contain vesicle formation, indicating atopic dermatitis
- Ask client about swelling that started in the face and then progressed to other parts of the body and look for lesions on the body that client describes as itching, burning or stinging, indicating angioedema reaction
- Monitor for areas on the body that are raised, edematous, pink in color and described by client as itching, which may indicate urticaria reaction
- Monitor for signs and symptoms of Type II hypersensitivity reaction as in Goodpasture's Syndrome and hemolytic blood transfusion reaction. Manifestations relate to kidney injury, pulmonary hemorrhage
- Monitor for reaction to immunotherapy, if injection was initiated

Priority Laboratory Tests/Diagnostics

- Sputum, nasal and bronchial secretions: will show presence of eosinophils
- Pulmonary function test: if asthma reaction, will show poor pulmonary functioning
- Complete blood count with white blood cell differential, shows immunodeficiency if lymphocyte count is below 1200/μL
- Skin test for allergens (the preferred test) is done via different methods
  - A patch test, where allergen is put on a patch that is then placed on skin. Reaction is delayed because the patch must be worn for 48-72 hours
  - A scratch or prick test, where allergen is placed on the skin and a pricking device allows the allergen to enter the skin. Reaction is seen in 5-10 minutes
  - An intradermal test, where the allergen is injected under the skin. Reaction is seen in 10 minutes
  - Positive reaction to the tests is indicated by the presence of a wheal-and-flare response

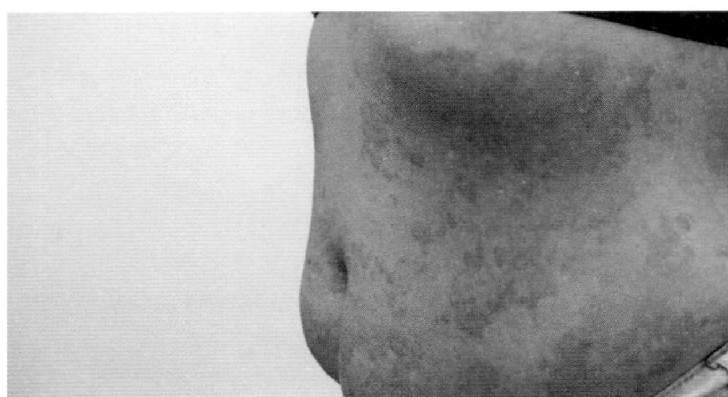

Image 7-10: The client arrives to the clinic with complaints of a rash on his abdomen. List top 3 components of data collection.

Priority Interventions or Actions

- Ensure a list of all client's allergies are on the health record
- Observe for allergy to latex, as many clients do not know they have this allergy
- Use latex free gloves and supplies when caring for clients with known latex allergy
- Administer antihistamines as prescribed
- Administer decongestants as prescribed
- Administer anti-itch medications as prescribed
- Administer corticosteroids as prescribed
- Administer leukotriene receptor agonists as prescribed
- Monitor for adverse effects of prescribed medications
- Treat skin rashes and lesions as prescribed
- Assist in managing hypovolemic shock if severe anaphylaxis
- Administer immunotherapy injections
- Rotate site for allergen injections
- Monitor client for anaphylactic or other reaction to immunotherapy
- Observe client for 20-30 minutes after immunotherapy injections to ensure no adverse reaction

Priority Potential & Actual Complications

- Anaphylactic shock
- May be fatal

Priority Nursing Implications

- When skin testing occurs to diagnose allergens, some clients may be highly sensitive and may develop an anaphylactic reaction to the skin tests. Do not leave the client alone during testing
- With an anaphylactic reaction, the key is to act quickly as death will occur if immediate care is not rendered

Priority Medications

- Antihistamines
  - Given orally and intramuscular
  - Several in the class so dosage is dependent on drug used
  - Most common drugs for treating urticaria and allergic rhinitis
  - Relieve acute symptoms of allergic response. Cause drowsiness
- Antipruritic(anti-itch) drugs
  - Given topical
  - Applied to skin to relieve itching
  - Should not be used if skin is broken
  - Several in the class but common ones are coal tar solutions and calamine lotion
- Sympathomimetic drugs
  - Given intramuscular
  - Main drug of choice in class is epinephrine
  - Used to treat anaphylactic reaction
  - Do not use epinephrine if solution is cloudy or contains particles
- Decongestants
  - Given orally
  - Used primarily to treat allergic rhinitis
  - Main one in class is pseudoephedrine
- Leukotriene receptor antagonists
  - Given orally
  - Blocks leukotriene, a major mediator of allergic inflammatory process
  - Used to treat asthma and allergic rhinitis
- Mast cell stabilizer
  - Used to inhibit the release of histamine and leukotriene
  - Treat allergic rhinitis. Only one used in the class is cromolyn
  - Used as a nasal spray
- Corticosteroids
  - Treat allergic rhinitis
  - Not for long-term use but for cases of severe reaction
  - Administered as nasal spray
- Immunotherapy
  - Used when usual drug therapy is ineffective or when the client cannot avoid the allergen
  - Injections with titrated amounts of allergen administered subcutaneously for 1-2 years to reach maximum effect
  - Allergen placed under the tongue, and administered by the client at home until hyposensitivity to the allergen is achieved

Reinforcement of Priority Teaching

- Importance of avoiding the allergen that caused the client's reaction
- Identify with the client the signs and symptoms of hypersensitivity reaction specific to the client's condition
- Proper administration of medications, such as nasal sprays
- Delayed reaction to immunotherapy injections and what to do if a reaction occurs
- Seek medical assistance at the first sign of anaphylaxis
- Report all allergies on medical visits, including allergy to latex

Next Gen Clinical Judgment

Why is it so important to access every client's allergy history prior to providing care?

Pyelonephritis

Pathophysiology/Description

- Pyelonephritis is inflammation of the collecting ducts, renal parenchyma and pelvis
- Bacteria is the most common cause, but it can also be caused by parasitic and fungal infections
- The etiology of pyelonephritis is that it starts with bacteria and infection in the lower urinary tract or it occurs after invasive procedures. The renal medulla is usually first affected then it moves to the renal cortex
- Pyelonephritis usually occurs in the presence of a pre-existing condition such as diabetes, retrograde flow of urine or presence of urinary stones, catheter-associated urinary tract infections, to name a few
- As with lower urinary tract infection, Escherichia coli (E.coli) is the most common causative agent
- When pyelonephritis is recurrent in the presence of chronic conditions that cause obstruction, it ensues in chronic pyelonephritis
- Chronic pyelonephritis
  - Kidneys shrink in size
  - Ureter narrowed by strictures
  - Scarring occurs
  - End-stage renal disease occurs
  - Dialysis and/or transplantation is needed if both kidneys are affected

Priority Data Collection or Cues

- Monitor for flank pain on side that is affected, indicates inflamed kidney
- Monitor for costovertebral angle tenderness, which indicates inflamed kidneys
- Monitor for nausea, fever and chills, vomiting indicative of infection
- Monitor for blood in urine
- Ask about dysuria, urine frequency and urgency
- Monitor color and smell of urine. Foul-smelling, cloudy urine is usually present with pyelonephritis
- Ask about recurring urinary tract infections, can help to determine chronic pyelonephritis
- Ask about usage of a urinary catheter, which is associated with chronic pyelonephritis
- Ongoing data collection of vital signs, primarily to determine decrease in temperature

Next Gen Clinical Judgment

Why are clients with infections of the kidneys prone to progressing to sepsis?

Priority Laboratory Tests/Diagnostics

- Urinalysis shows elevated white blood cell count, hematuria, pyuria and bacteriuria in the urine. Proteinuria and azotemia may be present in the urine with chronic pyelonephritis, because the kidneys may not be able to filter protein properly or get rid of nitrogen waste
- With involvement of the renal parenchyma, WBC casts may be seen in urinalysis
- Urine culture and sensitivity will show the causative bacteria and the most effective antibiotic to treat the bacteria
- Complete blood count (CBC) shows immature neutrophils and leukocytes
- Blood cultures for clients who are severely ill is done to determine if infection is more systemic and may show septicemia
- Ultrasound to look for obstructions and/or other abnormalities of the urinary system
- Computed tomography (CT) scan to look for complications of the condition, such as renal abscess
- Renal biopsy may be used in chronic pyelonephritis to determine infiltration of the renal parenchyma and functionality of nephrons

Priority Interventions or Actions

- Collect a clean catch urine sample. Reinforce with client the proper way to collect the sample to prevent contamination of the sample if the client is collecting the specimen
- Administer antibiotic as ordered and monitor for side effects
- Administer analgesic as ordered for pain
- If a urinary catheter must be inserted, ensure sterile technique is used
- Administer intravenous fluids in acute setting until client can tolerate oral fluids
- Monitor intake and output
- Provide client with adequate oral fluids and encourage intake of up to 3000 mL/day, if not contraindicated, help to flush the urinary tract of the bacteria and prevent dehydration
- Monitor client for urosepsis and septicemia, complications of pyelonephritis
- Apply warm, moist heat to the client's flank area to minimize discomfort caused by pain
- Monitor for signs of progression of chronic pyelonephritis to chronic kidney disease
- Re-culture urine after completion of antibiotic therapy to determine resolution of the infection

Priority Potential & Actual Complications

- Urosepsis
- Septicemia
- Chronic kidney disease
- Dialysis
- Renal transplantation

Priority Nursing Implications

- Understand that for older adults living in long-term and skilled nursing facilities, a common cause of pyelonephritis is catheter-associated urinary tract infections (CAUTI)
- If vancomycin is administered too quickly itching of the head, face neck and upper torso, along with flushing (called red man syndrome), is likely to occur. The rate of infusion will need to be decreased if this syndrome occurs

Priority Medications

- Ampicillin–given intravenous
  - Broad-spectrum antibiotic
  - Started immediately before result of urine culture is received
- Vancomycin–given intravenous
  - Combined with tobramycin or gentamycin
  - Started immediately before result of urine culture is received
  - Drug levels of vancomycin must be monitored for therapeutic range. Trough drug level should be 10-20 mcg/mL. Peak level is no longer monitored
- Tobramycin–given intravenous
  - Combine with vancomycin
  - Start immediately before urine culture received
- Gentamycin–given intravenous
  - Combine with vancomycin
  - Start immediately before urine culture received
- Trimethoprim/sulfamethoxazole–given orally
  - Switch to this drug once urine culture results are received
- Ciprofloxacin–given orally and intravenous
  - Switch to this drug once urine culture result is received
- Levofloxacin–given orally and intravenous
  - Switch to this drug once urine culture result is received
  - Has a serious adverse effect of tearing or rupture of a tendon, primarily Achilles' tendon
- Ofloxacin–given orally
  - Switch to this drug once urine culture result is received
  - Has a serious adverse effect of tearing or rupture of a tendon, primarily Achilles' tendon
- Non-steroidal anti-inflammatory drugs (NSAIDs)–given orally
  - For outpatient management of mild pain and discomfort
  - There are several that can be used but indomethacin, naproxen and sulindac are quite often used
  - Most significant adverse effect of NSAIDs is gastrointestinal bleeding

Reinforcement of Priority Teaching

- Encourage women to urinate after sexual intercourse to prevent possible infection from bacteria that may be on the genitals
- Encourage women to wipe from front to back to prevent tracking bacteria from the rectum to the urethra
- Keep the genital area clean to minimize the risk of bacterial growth
- Clean perineal area with warm water and soap after bowel movements, to decrease risk of bacterial growth and tracking into the urethra
- Women that cotton underwear and loose-fitting clothing help to keep the area to the urethra dry
- Empty bladder at least every 3-4 hours to prevent urinary stasis that can foster growth of bacteria
- Signs and symptoms of pyelonephritis and when to contact a health care provider
- Known urinary tract abnormalities to seek regular medical care
- Complete the full course of antibiotics prescribed, even if the symptoms resolve, to ensure the infection is fully gone
- Foods that will help to maintain an acidic urine (pH of 5.5 or below), such as blueberries, prunes or cranberries. Drinking cranberry juice daily reduces the risk of a UTI that can progress to pyelonephritis
- Avoid or decrease intake of caffeinated beverages, such as coffee and cola, as both can cause bladder irritation
- Explain to client the importance of returning for follow-up urine culture once the course of antibiotic is finished
- Recognize clients at risk for pyelonephritis and show client how to minimize risk

Next Gen Clinical Judgment

Compare and contrast the differences between cystitis, urethritis, and pyelonephritis.

Methicillin-resistant Staphylococcus Aureus/vancomycin resistant Enterococcus

Pathophysiology/Description

- Resistance to antibiotics has become a major issue as more and more bacteria are becoming resistant to antibiotics normally used to treat them
- Pathogens have become smarter and have discovered that they can become adaptable and modify themselves to make it more difficult for drugs to kill them
- Methicillin-resistant Staphylococcus (MRSA) and vancomycin-resistant Enterococcus (VRE) are two strains of bacteria that have become resistant to many antibiotics and so when clients have infections where these are the causative agents, treatment modalities must be used that are effective in killing these resistant pathogens
- Even though both strains are serious and can cause serious complications, VRE can cause more serious disease and infection (more virulent) than MRSA
- These resistant strains were once only localized to the healthcare setting but in recent years, MRSA has been identified in community settings such as fitness centers and sports locker rooms
- Community-acquired methicillin-resistant Staphylococcus aureus (CA-MRSA) occurs in healthy individuals in the community and usually causes severe systemic diseases
- Some Risk factors for CA-MRSA
    - Prisoners
    - Athletes
    - Crowded living conditions
    - Individuals who get tattoos
    - Day care workers
    - Persons using shared items at fitness centers
    - Persons who abuse intravenous drugs
    - Persons who are immunocompromised
- The problem of medication over-use and misuse is thought to have contributed significantly to the emergence of resistant strains of bacteria

Priority Data Collection or Cues

- Monitor for nausea, fever and chills and vomiting which are suggestive of infection, regardless of where in the body the infection is located
- Perform focused system data collection based on location of infection to determine effectiveness of treatment
- Ask about onset of symptoms and history of recent activity to try and isolate where infection occurred, important information to have if infection is CA-MRSA
- Ongoing data collection of vital signs, primarily to determine decrease in temperature
- Determine client's understanding of disease and preventative measures while hospitalized and upon discharge

Priority Laboratory Tests/Diagnostics

- Culture and sensitivity of infected area will show the causative bacteria and the most effective antibiotic to treat the bacteria
- Complete blood count (CBC) shows immature neutrophils and leukocytes, indicating infection
- Blood cultures for clients who are severely ill is usually done to determine if infection is more systemic and may show blood involvement (septicemia)

Priority Interventions or Actions

- Collect and send culture of affected area to lab in a timely manner to facilitate early treatment
- Practice good hand hygiene
- Change gloves when moving from one task to another, even while caring for the same client, to minimize cross contamination
- Use standard, as well as transmission-based precautions for client admitted with MRSA and VRE and ensure use of the correct personal protective equipment (PPE)
- Ensure client is not taken off isolation until cleared of the infection
- Administer antibiotics as ordered
- Administer intravenous fluids in acute setting until client can tolerate oral fluids
- Monitor intake and output
- Provide client with adequate oral fluids and encourage intake of up to 3000 mL/day, help to flush the bacteria from the body and prevent dehydration
- Re-culture wound after completion of antibiotic therapy to determine resolution of the infection

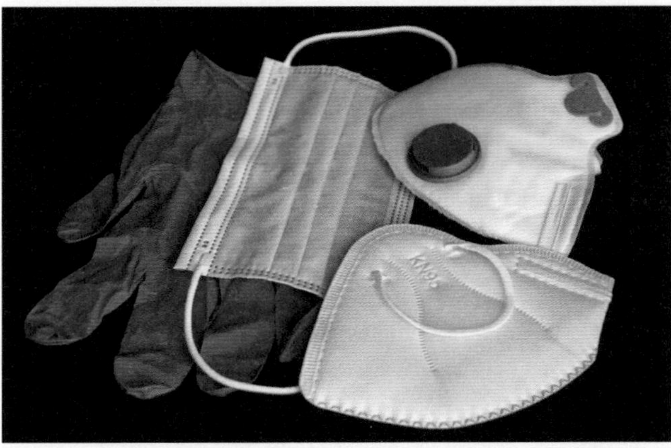

Image 7-11: What PPE is appropriate for clients admitted with MRSA or VRE?

Priority Potential & Actual Complications

- Septicemia
- Sepsis
- May be fatal

Priority Nursing Implications

- If vancomycin is administered too quickly itching of the head, face neck and upper torso, along with flushing (called red man syndrome), is likely to occur. The rate of infusion will need to be decreased if this syndrome occurs
- Because linezolid is a monoamine oxidase inhibitor (MAOI), it must not be taken within 14 days of a client taking an MAOI. If this precaution is not taken, the level of these compounds in the system may be increased, causing increased side effects

Priority Medications

- Ampicillin
  - Given intravenous
  - Treat VRE
- Vancomycin
  - Given intravenous
  - Treat MRSA
  - Drug levels of vancomycin must be monitored for therapeutic range. Trough drug level should be 10-20 mcg/mL. Peak level is no longer monitored
- Linezolid
  - Given intravenous
  - Treat VRE
  - Should not be started if client used a Monoamine oxidase inhibitor (MAOI) in the past 14 days

Reinforcement of Priority Teaching

- Complete the full course of antibiotics prescribed, even if the symptoms resolve, to ensure the infection is fully gone
- Explain to client the importance of returning for follow-up culture once the course of antibiotic is finished
- Provide reinforcement education to client about the infection (VRE or MRSA) and preventative measures while hospitalized
- Inform client that MRSA and VRE can be transmitted to family members in the community setting. Reinforce teaching on preventive measures, to include proper handwashing and personal hygiene practice
- Encourage client to not save old antibiotics and reuse them as needed, as antibiotic overuse contributes to drug resistance
- Only take antibiotics that have been prescribed
- Encourage client not to request antibiotics from health care providers to treat a cold or influenza
- Signs and symptoms of recurring infection and when to contact the health care provider
- Explain the importance of returning to the health care provider for a follow-up culture to ensure the infection is all gone
- For prevention of C-MRSA
  - Encourage client to not share towels or other personal items at home, at the gym or in the sports locker room
  - Clean gym and daycare equipment before use
  - Avoid crowded environments as best as possible
  - Do not share drug paraphernalia

Next Gen Clinical Judgment

Consider these questions:

1. Identify risk factors for community associated MRSA.
2. Identify 3 behaviors that can potentially increase the development of resistant strains.
3. What can nurses do to prevent health-care associated MRSA?
4. What policies exist at your current clinical agency related to VRE or MRSA?

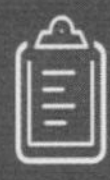

NurseThink® Quiz Questions

1. **The nurse monitors a client with acute pancreatitis. Where in the abdomen is the client most likely to indicate pain?**
   a. Left lower quadrant.
   b. Left upper quadrant.
   c. Right lower quadrant.
   d. Right upper quadrant.

2. **A client with chronic pancreatitis is asking the nurse for clarification on their recommended diet. What does the nurse advise the client to avoid to reduce the likelihood of recurring symptoms? *Select all that apply.***
   a. Alcohol.
   b. Foods high in fat.
   c. Foods high in sodium.
   d. Foods high in protein.
   e. Foods high in carbohydrates.
   f. Caffeine.

3. **The nurse collects a sample for a wound culture to identify the cause of the client's cellulitis. After gently cleansing the wound with normal saline, where does the nurse swab?**

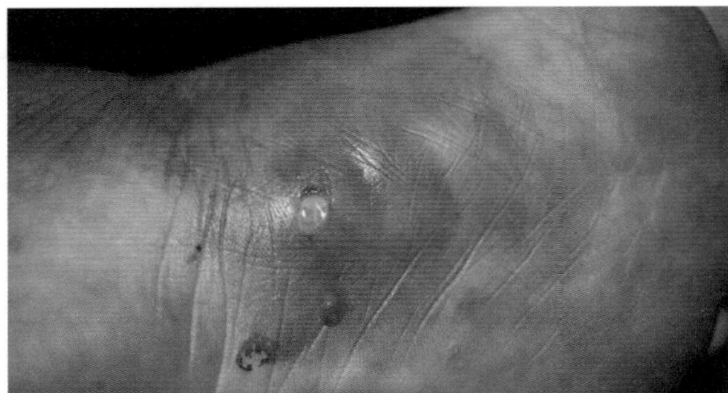

   a. The outer edges of the wound.
   b. The tissue surrounding the wound.
   c. Only on the wound opening and drainage.
   d. At or near the center of the wound.

4. **When caring for a client with septicemia, what safety measure does the nurse implement?**
   a. Droplet precautions.
   b. Negative air pressure isolation.
   c. Strict aseptic technique.
   d. Strict no-visitor policy.

5. **The nurse overhears a 16-year-old with appendicitis talking to their parents. Which statement by the client warrants follow-up by the nurse?**
   a. "I have a fever because I have an infection."
   b. "I can't go home until after I have surgery."
   c. "A heating pad would help my pain."
   d. "It's important not to eat or drink anything."

6. **While caring for a client with appendicitis, the nurse notes a change in the client's condition. What change prompts the nurse to notify the health care provider immediately?**
   a. Temperature of 100.2°F.
   b. Rigid, board-like abdomen.
   c. Rebound tenderness.
   d. Pulse of 98 beats/minute.

7. **The nurse reviews laboratory results of a client with gout who is currently receiving treatment with corticosteroids. Which lab value does the nurse monitor closely during this treatment?**
   a. Serum glucose.
   b. Serum sodium.
   c. Serum potassium.
   d. White blood cell count.

8. **A client with systemic lupus reports common manifestations of the disease, worsening over the last six months. Which problem in the client's plan of care does the nurse identify as the priority?**
   a. Decreased self-image due to alopecia.
   b. Fatigue related to chronic inflammation.
   c. Decreased mobility related to fatigue.
   d. Pain related to chronic inflammation.

9. **The nurse cares for a client with rheumatoid arthritis who has many identified problems in their care plan. Rank order the problems in order of priority.**
   a. Altered self-image related to joint nodules.
   b. Chronic pain related to disease process.
   c. Self-care deficit related to decreased range of motion.
   d. Ineffective sleep patterns related to pain.
   e. Social isolation related to decreased activity.

10. The nurse reviews recent laboratory values for a client with rheumatoid arthritis. Which lab value best indicates significant inflammation?

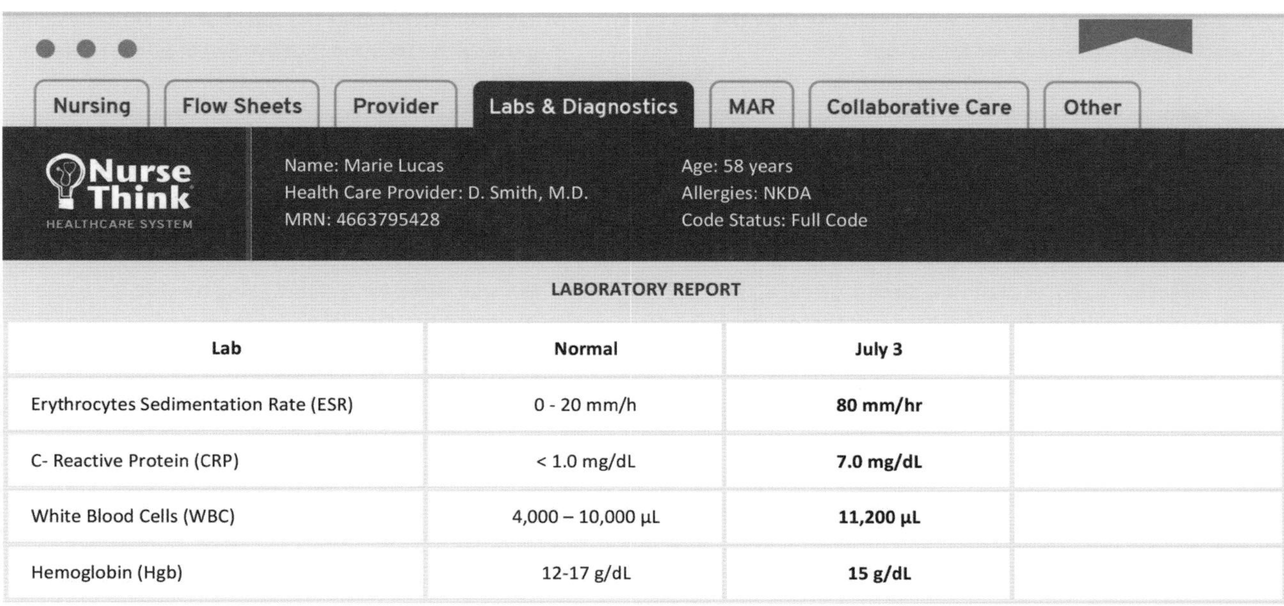

Nursing | Flow Sheets | Provider | Labs & Diagnostics | MAR | Collaborative Care | Other

Nurse Think HEALTHCARE SYSTEM

Name: Marie Lucas
Health Care Provider: D. Smith, M.D.
MRN: 4663795428

Age: 58 years
Allergies: NKDA
Code Status: Full Code

LABORATORY REPORT

Lab	Normal	July 3	
Erythrocytes Sedimentation Rate (ESR)	0 - 20 mm/h	**80 mm/hr**	
C- Reactive Protein (CRP)	< 1.0 mg/dL	**7.0 mg/dL**	
White Blood Cells (WBC)	4,000 – 10,000 µL	**11,200 µL**	
Hemoglobin (Hgb)	12-17 g/dL	**15 g/dL**	

a. Erythrocyte sedimentation rate.
b. C-reactive protein.
c. White blood cells.
d. Hemoglobin.

11. The nurse initiates a plan of care with the priority concern of avoiding opportunistic infections. Which client is the nurse most likely caring for?
a. A client with disseminated intravascular coagulation (DIC).
b. A client with advanced AIDS.
c. A client with Type 1 Diabetes.
d. A client with chronic obstructive pulmonary disease (COPD).

12. A client recently diagnosed with HIV informs the nurse that they feel overwhelmed by so many instructions. What information does the nurse highlight to prevent the most common complications of HIV? *Select all that apply.*
a. "Travel as much as possible when you feel well."
b. "Wash fresh fruits and vegetables carefully."
c. "Keep your skin well moisturized."
d. "Avoid exposure to others who have colds or viruses."
e. "Avoid overheating your food."

13. Upon arrival at the urgent care clinic, a mother states that her child is having an "allergic reaction." What does the nurse expect to find when evaluating the child? *Select all that apply.*
a. Wheezing or stridor.
b. Red raised rash.
c. Angioedema.
d. Peripheral edema.
e. Tachycardia.
f. Bradypnea.

14. A client presents to the emergency room with a rash and itching to the back. Inspection of the back reveals a rash as pictured. What medication does the nurse anticipate administering first?

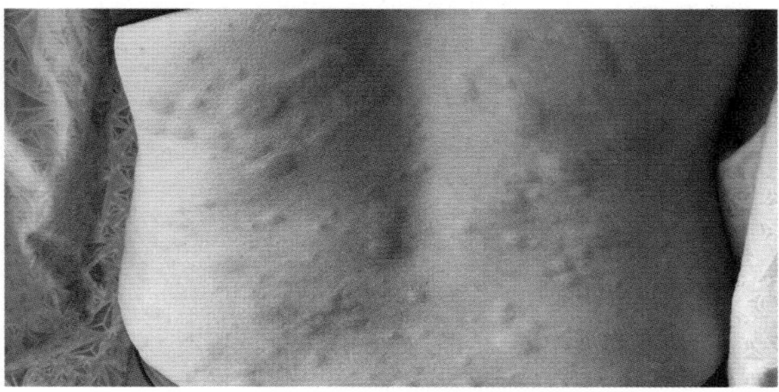

a. Intramuscular epinephrine.
b. Inhaled bronchodilators.
c. Oral diphenhydramine.
d. Intramuscular corticosteroids.

15. An older adult with influenza requires hospitalization for influenza. What interventions does the nurse plan to implement in the client's care? *Select all that apply.*
a. Administer antipyretics as ordered.
b. Limit fluid intake to < 1000 mL/day.
c. Initiate droplet precautions.
d. Administer supplemental oxygen as needed.
e. Position the client with HOB < 30 degrees.
f. Administer analgesics as needed for pain.

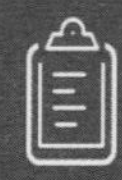

NurseThink® Quiz Questions

16. **The nurse provides nutritional information to a client diagnosed with polycystic kidney disease and mild impairment of renal function. Which statement by the client indicates the need for follow-up?**
    a. "It is important that I limit how much fluid I drink daily."
    b. "I should avoid cooked spinach, broccoli, and leafy greens."
    c. "This diet will work well with my taste for seafood."
    d. "I should avoid organ foods, such as brain and liver."

17. **The nurse cares for a female client with a urinary tract infection (UTI). In planning discharge care, the nurse prepares the client to reduce risk factors for UTI recurrence. What risk factors for UTI does the nurse include? *Select all that apply.***
    a. Sexual intercourse.
    b. Smoking.
    c. Feminine products.
    d. Wet bathing suits.
    e. Synthetic undergarments.
    f. Excessive water intake.

18. **The urgent care nurse administers antibiotics and oral phenazopyridine to a client with a urinary tract infection. What information does the nurse share with the client regarding the treatment plan? *Select all that apply.***
    a. Courses of antibiotics should be completed in full.
    b. Pyridium may turn urine a reddish-orange color.
    c. Increase fluid intake while taking these medications.
    d. Stop taking the antibiotics once you feel better.
    e. Nausea, vomiting, and flank pain are typical side effects.

19. **The nurse cares for a client being treated for acute pyelonephritis after failed treatment of a urinary tract infection. Which action does the nurse prioritize?**
    a. Monitoring nutritional status.
    b. Monitoring fluid intake and output.
    c. Administering antibiotics as prescribed.
    d. Preparing for discharge and home treatment.

20. **Based on the client's history and current status of the wound, what does the nurse do first?**

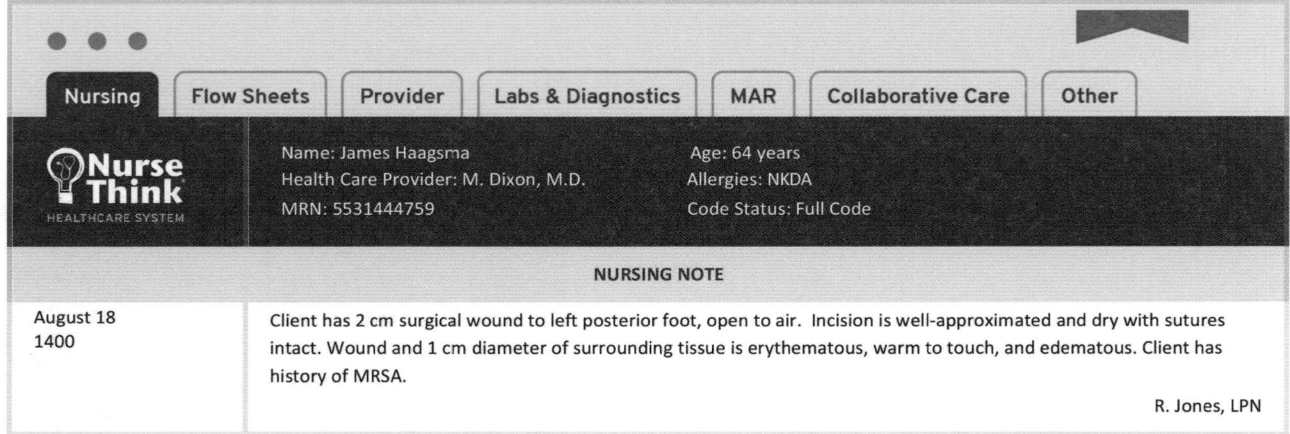

Nursing
Flow Sheets
Provider
Labs & Diagnostics
MAR
Collaborative Care
Other
Nurse Think
HEALTHCARE SYSTEM
Name: James Haagsma
Health Care Provider: M. Dixon, M.D.
MRN: 5531444759
Age: 64 years
Allergies: NKDA
Code Status: Full Code
NURSING NOTE
August 18
1400
Client has 2 cm surgical wound to left posterior foot, open to air. Incision is well-approximated and dry with sutures intact. Wound and 1 cm diameter of surrounding tissue is erythematous, warm to touch, and edematous. Client has history of MRSA.
R. Jones, LPN

a. Initiate contact isolation precautions.
b. Administer oral clindamycin.
c. Swab the wound for culture.
d. Apply wet-to-dry dressing to the wound.

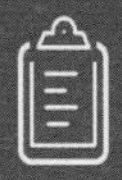

NurseThink® Quiz Answers

1. **The nurse monitors a client with acute pancreatitis. Where in the abdomen is the client most likely to indicate pain?**
   a. Left lower quadrant.
   b. Left upper quadrant.
   c. Right lower quadrant.
   d. Right upper quadrant.

   Topic/Concept: Protection **Subtopic:** Pancreatitis **Bloom's Taxonomy:** Applying **Clinical Problem-Solving Process:** Data Collection **NCLEX-PN®:** Basic Care and Comfort **QSEN:** Evidence-based Practice **CJMM:** Recognize Cues

   Rationale: Pancreatitis manifests as sudden onset epigastric or LUQ pain, radiating to the flank or shoulder blades. The pain may be constant and persistent. Clients often report worsening pain when sitting forward or in the supine position. Pain in other areas of the abdomen is not specific to pancreatitis.

   THIN Thinking: *Clinical Problem-Solving Process* –When collecting data related to this client's pain, the nurse notes the client has upper left quadrant or mid-abdominal pain described as boring, deep, sharp, and increased with consumption of high-fat content or alcohol. The nurse should know common signs/symptoms and report concerning or unexpected findings to the provider.

2. **A client with chronic pancreatitis is asking the nurse for clarification on their recommended diet. What does the nurse advise the client to avoid to reduce the likelihood of recurring symptoms? *Select all that apply.***
   a. Alcohol.
   b. Foods high in fat.
   c. Foods high in sodium.
   d. Foods high in protein.
   e. Foods high in carbohydrates.
   f. Caffeine.

   Topic/Concept: Protection **Subtopic:** Pancreatitis **Bloom's Taxonomy:** Applying **Clinical Problem-Solving Process:** Planning **NCLEX-PN®:** Health promotion and maintenance **QSEN:** Patient-centered care **CJMM:** Generate Solutions

   Rationale: The nurse should instruct the client to avoid high-fat and high-protein foods, caffeine, and alcohol as these are all pancreatic stimulants. The client should also avoid large meals, smoking, and stress. Carbohydrate and sodium consumption is not restricted with pancreatitis.

   THIN Thinking: *Clinical Problem-Solving Process* – When instructing this client on reducing pain related to pancreatitis, the nurse should advise the client to avoid foods that stimulate the pancreas.

3. **The nurse collects a sample for a wound culture to identify the cause of the client's cellulitis. After gently cleansing the wound with normal saline, where does the nurse swab?**
   a. The outer edges of the wound.
   b. The tissue surrounding the wound.
   c. Only on the wound opening and drainage.
   d. At or near the center of the wound.

   Topic/Concept: Protection **Subtopic:** Cellulitis **Bloom's Taxonomy:** Applying **Clinical Problem-Solving Process:** Planning **NCLEX-PN®:** Physiological Adaptation **QSEN:** Evidence-based Practice **CJMM:** Generate Solutions

   Rationale: After cleaning the wound to remove old drainage, the nurse should swab at or near the center of the wound, which may also include new wound drainage. The further away the swab is from the center of the wound, the greater chance that findings will not be consistent with the wound itself. The nurse should obtain a culture of the wound before initiating antibiotics.

   THIN Thinking: *Clinical Problem-Solving Process* –When planning care, the nurse should obtain the wound culture before initiating antibiotics. The culture can be obtained at or near the center of the wound and with a sample of drainage from the lesion.

4. **When caring for a client with septicemia, what safety measure does the nurse implement?**
   a. Droplet precautions.
   b. Negative air pressure isolation.
   c. Strict aseptic technique.
   d. Strict no-visitor policy.

   Topic/Concept: Protection **Subtopic:** Septicemia **Bloom's Taxonomy:** Applying **Clinical Problem-Solving Process:** Implementation **NCLEX-PN®:** Safety and Infection Control **QSEN:** Safety **CJMM:** Take Action

   Rationale: Septicemia is a bacterial infection in the blood caused by various organisms from one or more sources. To prevent additional complications or infections, the nurse should maintain strict aseptic technique with all procedures and sterile technique as indicated. Droplet precautions, negative air pressure isolation, and strict restrictions on visitors are unnecessary for septicemia, though visitors may be limited to avoid exposing the client to infection risks.

   THIN Thinking: *Identify Risk to Safety* – Aseptic technique will prevent the introduction of new or additional organisms into the body. Droplet precautions, negative-pressure isolation, and no visitors are client-specific and dependent on the type of infection present.

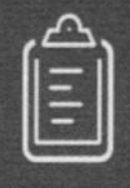

NurseThink® Quiz Answers

5. The nurse overhears a 16-year-old with appendicitis talking to their parents. Which statement by the client warrants follow-up by the nurse?

a. "I have a fever because I have an infection."
b. "I can't go home until after I have surgery."
c. "A heating pad would help my pain."
d. "It's important not to eat or drink anything."

Topic/Concept: Protection **Subtopic:** Appendicitis (peds) **Bloom's Taxonomy:** Analyzing **Clinical Problem-Solving Process:** Planning **NCLEX-PN®:** Reduction of Risk Potential **QSEN:** Patient-centered care **CJMM:** Prioritize Hypotheses

Rationale: Avoid applying heat to the abdomen as it may cause the appendix to rupture. The client is correct that the fever is due to inflammation/infection of the appendix. NPO status must be maintained in preparation for surgery, and surgical intervention is the only resolution for appendicitis.

THIN Thinking: *Help Quick* – The nurse should intervene and explain to the client that heat is contraindicated in appendicitis. It may increase blood flow and inflammation in the area, causing the appendix to rupture and leading to peritonitis.

6. While caring for a client with appendicitis, the nurse notes a change in the client's condition. What change prompts the nurse to notify the health care provider immediately?

a. Temperature of 100.2°F.
b. Rigid, board-like abdomen.
c. Rebound tenderness.
d. Pulse of 98 beats/minute.

Topic/Concept: Protection **Subtopic:** Peritonitis **Bloom's Taxonomy:** Applying **Clinical Problem-Solving Process:** Implementation **NCLEX-PN®:** Safety and Infection Control **QSEN:** Evidence-based Practice **CJMM:** Take Action

Rationale: The nurse should recognize the presence of a rigid, board-like abdomen as a hallmark sign of peritonitis. This is a medical emergency indicating rupture of the appendix and spilling of its contents into the peritoneal cavity. A mild fever and rebound tenderness are not uncommon with appendicitis and would not warrant notification as a change in condition. A pulse between 60-99 is considered normal.

THIN Thinking: *Top Three* – When caring for a client with appendicitis, the nurse needs to monitor the client for deterioration continually. An increasing temperature, significant change in vital signs, or major change in a client with an acute inflammatory process (board-like abdomen) warrants immediate notification of the provider for further evaluation.

7. The nurse reviews laboratory results of a client with gout who is currently receiving treatment with corticosteroids. Which lab value does the nurse monitor closely during this treatment?

a. Serum glucose.
b. Serum sodium.
c. Serum potassium.
d. White blood cell count.

Topic/Concept: Protection **Subtopic:** Gout **Bloom's Taxonomy:** Applying **Clinical Problem-Solving Process:** Data Collection **NCLEX-PN®:** Pharmacological Therapies **QSEN:** Evidence-based Practice **CJMM:** Analyze Cues

Rationale: The nurse should closely monitor the serum glucose of clients receiving corticosteroids, as these medications are likely to increase blood glucose levels. Sodium, potassium, and WBCs are not necessarily impacted by gout or the use of corticosteroids.

THIN Thinking: *Top Three* – Uric acid is the laboratory value most noted with gout, but it is important to monitor blood glucose levels of clients receiving corticosteroids as these medications can increase serum glucose. This monitoring is critical in diabetic clients.

8. A client with systemic lupus reports common manifestations of the disease, worsening over the last six months. Which problem in the client's plan of care does the nurse identify as the priority?

a. Decreased self-image due to alopecia.
b. Fatigue related to chronic inflammation.
c. Decreased mobility related to fatigue.
d. Pain related to chronic inflammation.

Topic/Concept: Protection **Subtopic:** Systemic Lupus **Bloom's Taxonomy:** Applying **Clinical Problem-Solving Process:** Planning **NCLEX-PN®:** Physiological Adaptation **QSEN:** Patient-centered care **CJMM:** Prioritize Hypotheses

Rationale: The care plan for the client with lupus is likely to include pain, fatigue, reduced mobility, and alopecia. However, the priority problem is pain control.

THIN Thinking: *Top Three* – The nurse should plan the client's care in order of priority. There are no life-threatening risks listed, so pain takes the greatest precedence.

9. The nurse cares for a client with rheumatoid arthritis who has many identified problems in their care plan. Rank order the problems in order of priority.

a. Altered self-image related to joint nodules.
b. Chronic pain related to disease process.
c. Self-care deficit related to decreased range of motion.
d. Ineffective sleep patterns related to pain.
e. Social isolation related to decreased activity.

Answer: B, D, C, E, A

Topic/Concept: Protection **Subtopic:** Rheumatoid arthritis **Bloom's Taxonomy:** Applying **Clinical Problem-Solving Process:** Planning **NCLEX-PN®:** Reduction of Risk Potential **QSEN:** Evidence-based Practice **CJMM:** Prioritize Hypotheses

Rationale: The nurse should always address life-threatening issues first. There are no specific problems related to airway, breathing, circulation, neurological deficits, or safety. The care plan for the client with rheumatoid arthritis often focuses on pain management, rest, maintenance of ADLs and self-care, and psychosocial needs, in that order.

THIN Thinking: *Clinical Problem-Solving Process* –The nurse should implement according to priority, beginning with airway, breathing, and circulation concerns and moving in the order of those posing the greatest risk to the client.

10. The nurse reviews recent laboratory values for a client with rheumatoid arthritis. Which lab value best indicates significant inflammation?

a. Erythrocyte sedimentation rate.
b. C-reactive protein.
c. White blood cells.
d. Hemoglobin.

Topic/Concept: Protection **Subtopic:** Rheumatoid Arthritis **Bloom's Taxonomy:** Analyzing **Clinical Problem-Solving Process:** Data Collection **NCLEX-PN®:** Physiological Adaptation **QSEN:** Evidence-based Practice **CJMM:** Analyze Cues

Rationale: ESR measures the speed at which red blood cells settle at the bottom of the test tube sample. Inflammation can cause RBCs to clump, settling to the bottom quickly. A faster than normal rate may indicate inflammatory activity. This client's ESR is approximately 3-4 times the normal range for men and women, indicating a high level of inflammation.

THIN Thinking: *Clinical Problem-Solving Process* –The nurse familiar with lab values knows that the Hgb and CRP are within normal ranges and the WBC count is only slightly elevated. The ESR, however, is significantly elevated.

11. The nurse initiates a plan of care with the priority concern of avoiding opportunistic infections. Which client is the nurse most likely caring for?

a. A client with disseminated intravascular coagulation (DIC).
b. A client with advanced AIDS.
c. A client with Type 1 Diabetes.
d. A client with chronic obstructive pulmonary disease (COPD).

Topic/Concept: Protection **Subtopic:** HIV/AIDS **Bloom's Taxonomy:** Applying **Clinical Problem-Solving Process:** Planning **NCLEX-PN®:** Reduction of Risk Potential **QSEN:** Safety **CJMM:** Prioritize Hypotheses

Rationale: Clients in advanced stages of AIDS have a significant risk of contracting an opportunistic infection. Maintaining asepsis should be the priority. Care for COPD and DM should also reduce the risk of infection, but that is not the priority concern. DIC can be caused by infection but does not necessarily increase the risk of infection.

THIN Thinking: *Identify Risk to Safety* – The nurse should first address life-threatening needs and client safety. For the client with a reduced immune system, opportunistic infections can be life-threatening. It is essential to maintain asepsis (and sterility when appropriate) in all procedures.

12. A client recently diagnosed with HIV informs the nurse that they feel overwhelmed by so many instructions. What information does the nurse highlight to prevent the most common complications of HIV? *Select all that apply.*

a. "Travel as much as possible when you feel well."
b. "Wash fresh fruits and vegetables carefully."
c. "Keep your skin well moisturized."
d. "Avoid exposure to others who have colds or viruses."
e. "Avoid overheating your food."

Topic/Concept: Protection **Subtopic:** HIV/AIDS **Bloom's Taxonomy:** Applying **Clinical Problem-Solving Process:** Planning **NCLEX-PN®:** Health promotion and maintenance **QSEN:** Patient-centered care **CJMM:** Generate Solutions

Rationale: The client with HIV should be instructed to avoid risks for infection. They should avoid undercooked meat and eggs, bathe daily with antimicrobial soap, wash dishes in hot water, and practice good hygiene and handwashing to reduce the overall risk for infection. Clients at a higher risk for infection should avoid travel, exposure to crowds and strangers, and maintain good hygiene. Dry skin may crack, opening up wounds for possible infection.

THIN Thinking: *Identify Risk to Safety* – The nurse should identify best practices and instruct the client with HIV in preventing infection and maintaining an optimum level of wellness.

13. Upon arrival at the urgent care clinic, a mother states that her child is having an "allergic reaction." What does the nurse expect to find when evaluating the child? *Select all that apply.*

a. Wheezing or stridor.
b. Red raised rash.
c. Angioedema.
d. Peripheral edema.
e. Tachycardia.
f. Bradypnea.

Topic/Concept: Protection **Subtopic:** Hypersensitivity reaction (peds) **Bloom's Taxonomy:** Analyzing **Clinical Problem-Solving Process:** Data Collection **NCLEX-PN®:** Safety and Infection Control **QSEN:** Evidence-based Practice **CJMM:** Analyze Cues

Rationale: A hypersensitivity or allergic reaction often results in airway tightness resulting in stridor, SOB, wheezing, and tachypnea. A pruritic rash and angioedema to the face, lips, and tongue are often present with a hypersensitivity response, not peripheral edema. Tachycardia, not bradycardia, is expected during a hypersensitivity response and may be worsened with epinephrine administration.

THIN Thinking: *Clinical Problem-Solving Process* – Hypersensitivity reactions result in a release of histamine that results in smooth muscle contraction, vasodilation, and decreased venous return. The manifestations of hypersensitivities are in response to these physiologic changes. Severe symptoms that indicate a compromised airway or breathing difficulties should be reported to the provider immediately.

14. A client presents to the emergency room with a rash and itching to the back. Inspection of the back reveals a rash as pictured. What medication does the nurse anticipate administering first?

a. Intramuscular epinephrine.
b. Inhaled bronchodilators.
c. Oral diphenhydramine.
d. Intramuscular corticosteroids.

Topic/Concept: Protection **Subtopic:** Hypersensitivity reactions (Adult) **Bloom's Taxonomy:** Applying **Clinical Problem-Solving Process:** Implementation **NCLEX-PN®:** Coordinated Care **QSEN:** Teamwork and Collaboration **CJMM:** Take Action

Rationale: The client is currently experiencing a rash and itching, indicating a local reaction. IM epinephrine, bronchodilators, and IM steroids are not always necessary to manage a local reaction. Oral diphenhydramine will likely be ordered.

THIN Thinking: *Help Quick* – The client is experiencing a local reaction, and antihistamine administration is the best approach. The nurse should monitor the client closely for signs of systemic involvement.

15. An older adult with influenza requires hospitalization for influenza. What interventions does the nurse plan to implement in the client's care? *Select all that apply.*

a. Administer antipyretics as ordered.
b. Limit fluid intake to < 1000 mL/day.
c. Initiate droplet precautions.
d. Administer supplemental oxygen as needed.
e. Position the client with HOB < 30 degrees.
f. Administer analgesics as needed for pain.

Topic/Concept: Protection **Subtopic:** Influenza **Bloom's Taxonomy:** Applying **Clinical Problem-Solving Process:** Planning **NCLEX-PN®:** Basic Care and Comfort **QSEN:** Evidence-based Practice **CJMM:** Generate Solutions

Rationale: Clients with influenza should be placed on droplet precautions to prevent the spread of infection. Additional interventions include providing antipyretics, antiemetics, and analgesics as ordered and PRN; maintaining adequate fluid and nutritional intake; administering oxygen PRN; keeping HOB >30 degrees to facilitate sinus drainage, prevent aspiration, and facilitate lung expansion. Fluid intake is typically increased with influenza to maintain hydration.

THIN Thinking: *Clinical Problem-Solving Process* –Influenza is a virus; the nurse should plan treatment that includes reducing symptoms, maintaining adequate fluid and nutritional intake, and preventing the spread of infection.

16. The nurse provides nutritional information to a client diagnosed with polycystic kidney disease and mild impairment of renal function. Which statement by the client indicates the need for follow-up?

a. "It is important that I limit how much fluid I drink daily."
b. "I should avoid cooked spinach, broccoli, and leafy greens."
c. "This diet will work well with my taste for seafood."
d. "I should avoid organ foods, such as brain and liver."

Topic/Concept: Protection **Subtopic:** Polycystic kidney **Bloom's Taxonomy:** Analyzing **Clinical Problem-Solving Process:** Evaluation **NCLEX-PN®:** Reduction of Risk Potential **QSEN:** Evidence-based Practice **CJMM:** Evaluate Outcomes

Rationale: The PKD diet is similar to the diet for impaired renal function. The client should avoid excessive fluids, sodium, phosphorous, potassium, and protein as the kidneys may have impaired elimination of these substances. Seafood is often high in phosphorous and should be limited. The nurse should follow up with the client who indicates a misunderstanding of which foods to avoid.

THIN Thinking: *Identify Risk to Safety* – When providing reinforcement of client teaching related to PKD, the client must modify dietary intake to be consistent with impaired renal function.

17. **The nurse cares for a female client with a urinary tract infection (UTI). In planning discharge care, the nurse prepares the client to reduce risk factors for UTI recurrence. What risk factors for UTI does the nurse include? *Select all that apply.***
    a. Sexual intercourse.
    b. Smoking.
    c. Feminine products.
    d. Wet bathing suits.
    e. Synthetic undergarments.
    f. Excessive water intake.

    Topic/Concept: Protection **Subtopic:** Urinary Tract Infection **Bloom's Taxonomy:** Applying **Clinical Problem-Solving Process:** Planning **NCLEX-PN®:** Safety and Infection Control **QSEN:** Patient-centered care **CJMM:** Prioritize Hypotheses

    Rationale: Urinary Tract Infections (UTIs) are more common in females, primarily due to the short urethra and proximity of the urethra to the rectum. Exposure to bacteria through sexual intercourse, feminine hygiene products, and exposure to conditions conducive to bacterial growth (dark, warm, moist environments) increase the risk for UTI. Smoking is not a specific risk factor for UTI, and water consumption is encouraged to prevent UTI.

    THIN Thinking: *Identify Risk to Safety* – To prevent the recurrence of UTIs, the nurse should inform the client of the risk factors and provide alternatives.

18. **The urgent care nurse administers antibiotics and oral phenazopyridine to a client with a urinary tract infection. What information does the nurse share with the client regarding the treatment plan? *Select all that apply.***
    a. Courses of antibiotics should be completed in full.
    b. Pyridium may turn urine a reddish-orange color.
    c. Increase fluid intake while taking these medications.
    d. Stop taking the antibiotics once you feel better.
    e. Nausea, vomiting, and flank pain are typical side effects.

    Topic/Concept: Protection **Subtopic:** Urinary Tract Infection **Bloom's Taxonomy:** Applying **Clinical Problem-Solving Process:** Implementation **NCLEX-PN®:** Basic Care and Comfort **QSEN:** Evidence-based Practice **CJMM:** Generate Solutions

    Rationale: Treatment of Urinary Tract Infection includes antibiotics, analgesics, and bladder analgesics (phenazopyridine). Key information to provide for all antibiotics includes finishing the entire course of medications even if symptoms resolve or improve and increasing fluid intake. Phenazopyridine does turn urine red/orange, so clients should be aware of this to avoid concern.

    THIN Thinking: *Top Three* – The nurse should inform the client of common signs/symptoms of Urinary Tract Infection and specific instructions related to the medications given.

19. **The nurse cares for a client being treated for acute pyelonephritis after failed treatment of a urinary tract infection. Which action does the nurse prioritize?**
    a. Monitoring nutritional status.
    b. Monitoring fluid intake and output.
    c. Administering antibiotics as prescribed.
    d. Preparing for discharge and home treatment.

    Topic/Concept: Protection **Subtopic:** Pyelonephritis **Bloom's Taxonomy:** Applying **Clinical Problem-Solving Process:** Implementation **NCLEX-PN®:** Physiological Adaptation **QSEN:** Evidence-based Practice **CJMM:** Take Action

    Rationale: The greatest risks to the client with pyelonephritis are renal damage and sepsis. Antibiotic treatment is the priority with acute pyelonephritis. The other actions are necessary but are not the priority.

    THIN Thinking: *Help Quick* – The nurse should plan the client's care in the order of priority. Preventing organ damage and advancement of infection are the priority.

20. **Based on the client's history and current status of the wound, what does the nurse do first?**
    a. Initiate contact isolation precautions.
    b. Administer oral clindamycin.
    c. Swab the wound for culture.
    d. Apply wet-to-dry dressing to the wound.

    Topic/Concept: Protection **Subtopic:** Methicillin-Resistant Staphylococcus Aureus **Bloom's Taxonomy:** Applying **Clinical Problem-Solving Process:** Implementation **NCLEX-PN®:** Reduction of Risk Potential **QSEN:** Safety **CJMM:** Take Action

    Rationale: Many institutions consider a client with a history of MRSA to be indefinitely colonized. Regardless, based on the data collection and the client's history, it is vital to prevent the spread of MRSA, so contact isolation precautions should be implemented as soon as possible. The provider will specify dressings and antibiotics, and the wound will be swabbed before initiating antibiotics. The priority, however, is the implementation of contact precautions.

    THIN Thinking: *Identify Risk to Safety* – The priority here is to reduce the spread of MRSA. Contact isolation precautions are indicated in the case of MRSA.

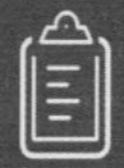

NurseThink® Quiz Answers

CHAPTER

8

Homeostasis

Acid-base Balance / Electrolyte Imbalance / Fluid Imbalance

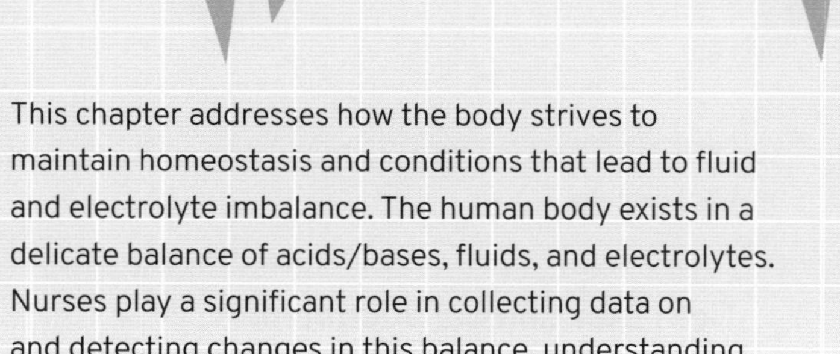

This chapter addresses how the body strives to maintain homeostasis and conditions that lead to fluid and electrolyte imbalance. The human body exists in a delicate balance of acids/bases, fluids, and electrolytes. Nurses play a significant role in collecting data on and detecting changes in this balance, understanding conditions that require vigilant monitoring, and implementing strategies to promote homeostasis.

Next Gen Clinical Judgment

Although many clinical agencies provide norms and designate abnormal values for various laboratory values, the nurse should be familiar with some of the more common values. Go to the inside back cover of this book and consider which are the values you need to know. Develop a NurseThink® flashcard of those laboratory values, the normal ranges, the implications, of high and low values, and potential nursing interventions/ management of these abnormal values. Use this chapter and other resources to develop these cards.

Clinical Hint

The body is primarily made up of water. The water in the body, when it is out of balance, requires measures to achieve equilibrium. This validates the importance of the material covered in this chapter!

Priority Exemplars:

- Overhydration/Fluid overload
- Dehydration/Fluid deficit
- Hyper/Hypocalcemia
- Hyper/Hypokalemia
- Hyper/Hypomagnesemia
- Hyper/Hyponatremia
- Hyper/Hypophosphatemia
- Metabolic acidosis
- Metabolic alkalosis
- Respiratory acidosis
- Respiratory alkalosis

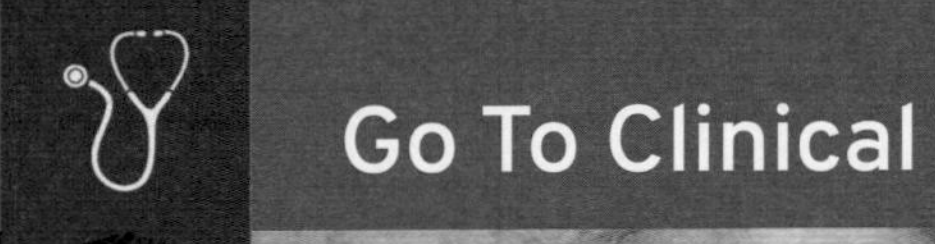

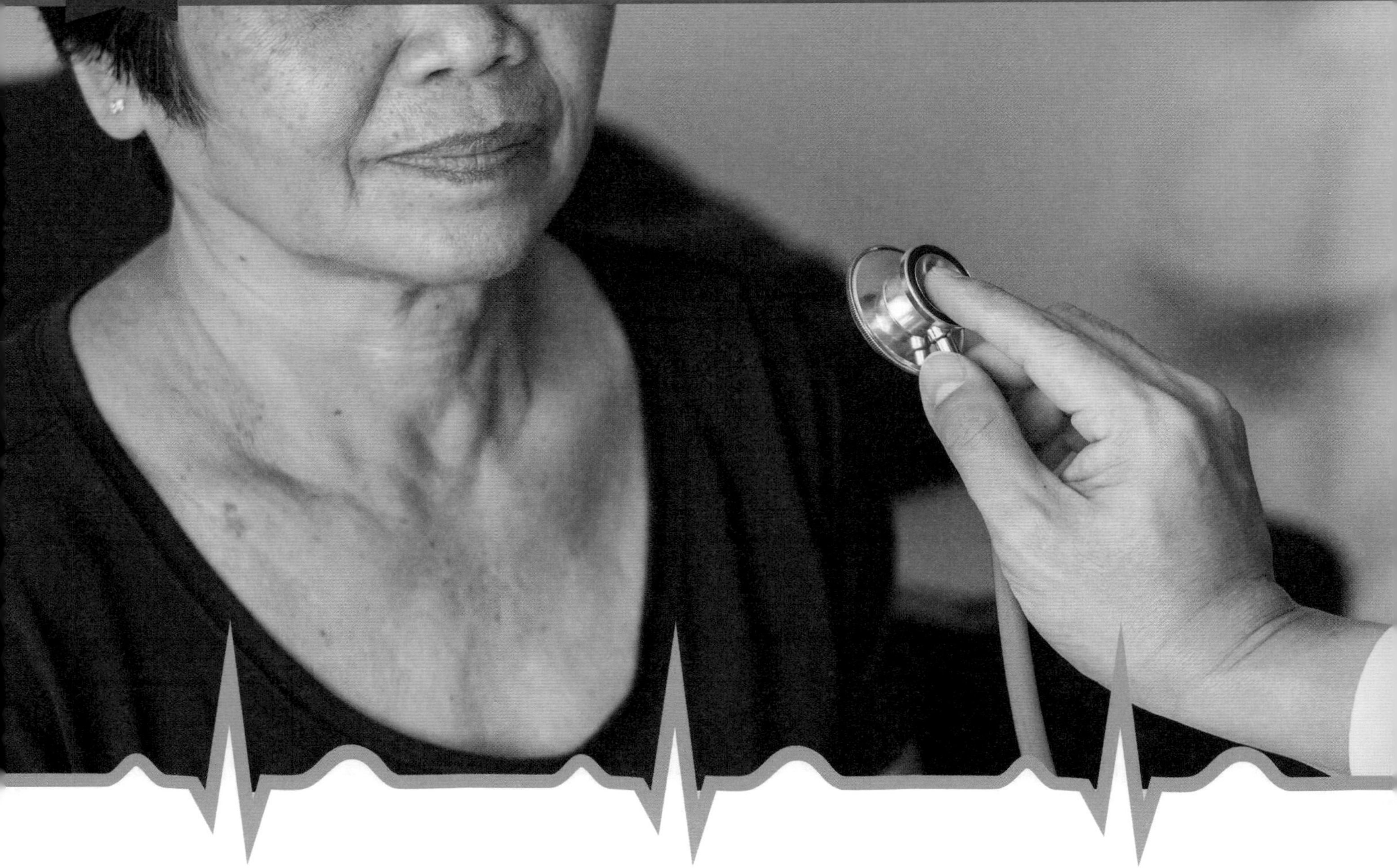

Go To Clinical

Go To Clinical Case 1

S.O. presents to the walk-in clinic with her son. The son reports that S.O. is 72-years-old, speaks little English, and S.O. told her son that she has been increasingly short-of-breath over the last 3 days. S.O.'s son reports that his mother usually is active and independent but today was short of breath after walking a short distance to the car. S.O. has a history of heart failure and hypertension. S.O.'s son reports that his mother's feet are "so swollen, he can't get her shoes on." The shortness-of-breath is worse at night such that S.O. slept in her recliner chair for the last two nights. When her son came to visit her this morning, he noticed she also had a "wet cough" and so he brought her to the clinic this morning. He also brought her medication bottles with him.

The nurse takes the client vital signs and allows S.O. to sit in the chair. S.O.'s vital signs are: 99.2°F (37.2°C), 132 beat/minute, 38 breaths/minute, 154/90 mmHg.

Next Gen Clinical Judgment

When caring for a client with heart failure:

1. What is the significance of pedal edema?
2. What is the significance of shortness of breath and a "wet cough?"
3. What is the significance of orthopnea?
4. What interventions should the nurse anticipate for this condition?

NurseThink® Time

Using the NurseThink® system, complete the priorities. Check your answers designated by 💡 in the Overhydration/fluid overload Priority Exemplar.

NurseThink® Time

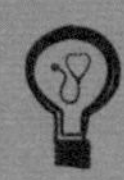

Priority Data Collection or Cues

1.

2.

3.

Priority Laboratory Tests/Diagnostics

1.

2.

3.

Priority Interventions or Actions

1.

2.

3.

Priority Potential & Actual Complications

1.

2.

3.

Priority Nursing Implications

1.

2.

3.

Priority Medications

1.

2.

3.

Reinforcement of Priority Teaching

1.

2.

3.

Pathophysiology/Description

- Fluids and electrolytes exist in homeostasis in the body in the intravascular, intracellular, and interstitial compartments
- Diffusion, osmosis, filtration, and hydrostatic pressure maintain fluids and ensure fluids move throughout the body and meet the metabolic needs
- About 60% of adults, 55% of older adults, and 80% of infants are made up of fluids/water; decreased organ function (cardiac) may lead to overhydration
- Intake of fluids comes from water, solid foods mixed with liquids, food oxidation, and medications such as those administered via the parenteral routes
- Output of water is lost via measurable sources (urine, emesis, drainage/drains) and insensible sources (perspiration, exhale air, water in stool)
- The kidneys maintain homeostasis of fluids within the body such that increased intake, increases output; water is conserved with decreased intake and increased body needs (diaphoresis, diarrhea, vomiting)
- An elaborate system of aldosterone secretion (adrenals), antidiuretic hormone (pituitary gland), and the kidneys assist the body to maintain homeostasis
- Overload of fluids/fluid volume excess occurs when fluid intake or availability is more than needed for body functioning
- Types of overhydration
  - Isotonic overhydration/hypervolemia
    - Excessive fluid in the extracellular spaces (does not enter the cells)
    - Yields circulatory overload and interstitial edema
    - Causes include excessive intravenous fluids, kidney disease/failure, fluid retention secondary to steroid use/Cushing's syndrome
  - Hypertonic overhydration
    - Too much sodium intake, rarely occurs
    - Extracellular volume expands, intracellular volume contracts
    - Causes include increased sodium ingestion, high volume/rapid infusion of hypertonic intravenous solutions, high dose sodium bicarbonate replacement
  - Hypotonic overhydration/water intoxication
    - Fluid moves into the cells
    - Dilutional electrolyte deficiencies
    - Causes include early kidney impairment, heart failure, syndrome of inappropriate antidiuretic hormone (SIADH), excessive intravenous hypotonic or oral fluids, irrigation with hypotonic fluids, primary polydipsia, inappropriate dialysis, rapid correction of hyperglycemia with large infusions of hypotonic fluids
- May be characterized by "third-spacing" and edema (excessive fluids in interstitial spaces)

Priority Data Collection or Cues

- Determine risk related to age and diagnosis (older adults, infants with immature kidney function in response to overhydration, heart failure, kidney disease)
- Take vital signs and watch for bounding tachycardia, hypertension, dysrhythmias, tachypnea
- Auscultate breath sounds for crackles, shallow/rapid respirations
- Observe jugular vein distension
- Monitor weight—obtain accurate weight, compare to baseline
- Observe level of consciousness including level of alertness, confusion and restlessness. The client may report muscle weakness/spasms, visual changes and a headache
- Monitor skin/extremities/abdomen for edema (pitting), pale/cool skin, hepatomegaly, ascites
- Monitor perfusion—edema may impair perfusion to extremities. Check peripheral and central pulses, capillary refill, skin color and temperature, sensory and motor function
- Observe for urine output (requires adequate kidney function to excrete excess fluids)

Next Gen Clinical Judgment

Seek out breath sounds on the Internet. Find recordings of crackles.

1. How do crackles differ from clear breath sounds?
2. How would your interpretation of crackles differ based on where they were present over the client's lung fields?
3. What are the traditional management strategies for clients who have crackles?
4. What other signs and symptoms would you anticipate in a client with crackles?
5. What healthcare problems or disorders would you anticipate when a client has crackles?

Priority Laboratory Tests/Diagnostics

- Decreased serum osmolality normal 275-295 mOsm/kg; decreased found in overhydration (< 275 mOsm/kg); < 265 mOsm/kg is a critical finding
- CBC—decreased hemoglobin and hematocrit
- Decreased BUN (blood urea nitrogen)
- Decreased serum sodium (may occur with other electrolyte shifts due to dilution)
- Decreased urine specific gravity <1.005

Priority Interventions or Actions

- Goal: Reduce excess body fluids, promote desired elimination
- Manage underlying cause
- Restrict dietary sodium intake
- Monitor I&O
- Administer diuretics to remove excess fluids
- Monitor client signs and electrolyte values
- Restrict oral and other fluid intake as prescribed

Priority Potential & Actual Complications

- Isotonic overhydration
    - Heart failure
    - Pulmonary edema
- Seizure
- Coma

Priority Nursing Implications

- Closely monitor intravenous fluid infusions and avoid potential fluid overload
- Provide appropriate skin care to edematous tissues
- Collect data of pitting edema depression—2 mm (+1), 4 mm (+2), 6 mm (+3), 8 mm (+4)
- Nurses should be vigilant for signs of cerebral edema (secondary to overhydration, stroke, trauma, infections) and report to health care provider
- Monitor and maintain comfort measures for clients with edema and ascites, including easing work of breathing, skin care, and treating underlying cause

Priority Medications

- Furosemide
    - Loop diuretic
    - Rapid removal of excess fluid
    - Potassium-wasting—monitor serum potassium levels
    - High ceiling medication-increased doses may be given to achieve diuresis
    - Oral and intravenous route (also IM/subcutaneous when oral/intravenous not available)
- Mannitol
    - Osmotic diuretics
    - Stimulate diuresis
    - Used to decrease peripheral, intracranial, and intraocular edema, prevent renal failure
    - Potassium-wasting—monitor serum potassium levels
    - May exacerbate heart failure and pulmonary edema
    - Only given in inpatient settings as an emergency intervention
    - Administered via intravenous route

Reinforcement of Priority Teaching

- Counsel parents of infants that intake of high volumes of free water or incorrectly mixed formula may cause fluid overload
- Advise parents/guardians to ensure infants do not drink water during swimming or in baths
- Ensure client/family understands the care of edematous tissues-elevation, skin care, avoid crossing legs, avoid constrictive clothing
- Clients understand causative factors of overhydration and means of prevention

Clinical Hint

One kilogram (2.2 pounds) equals 1 liter of fluid. Loss/gain of weight is an excellent indicator dehydration/overhydration.

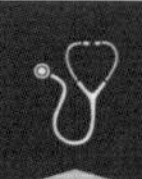

Go To Clinical Answers

Text designated by are the top answers for the Go To Clinical related to Overhydration/fluid overload.

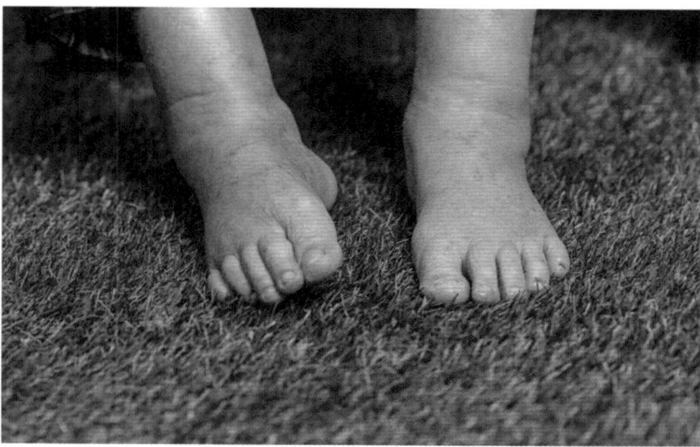

Image 8-1: How would you describe the appearance of this client's ankles and feet? How do the right and left leg compare? What treatments would you anticipate for this client?

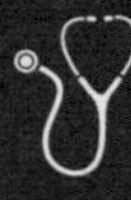

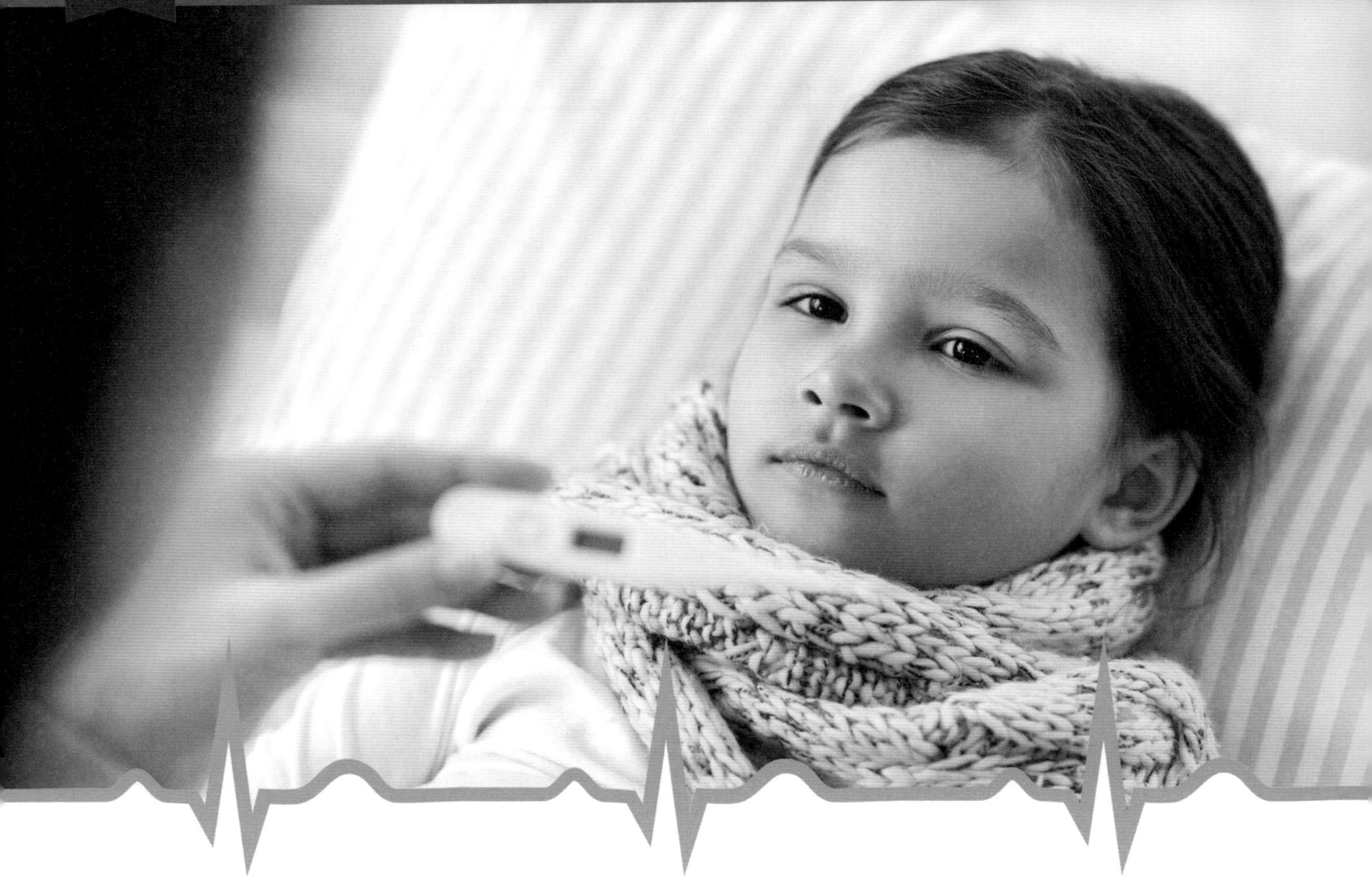

Go To Clinical

Go To Clinical Case 2

F.V. is a 5-year-old child of Hispanic origin regularly seen in the pediatric endocrine clinic for Type 1 diabetes diagnosed three months ago. Her mother calls the clinic and states, "F.V. is just not herself. She has been vomiting and had some diarrhea for the last few days. Since she hasn't been eating, I cut down on her usual dose of insulin. She's been so cranky, and I haven't had the heart to prick her finger. Her blood sugar was normal yesterday. I figure since she is still in her honeymoon period that it wouldn't be a problem. Now she is just so listless. I think she is getting worse rather than better. She was peeing a lot yesterday and the day before, but not so much today. She won't drink at all. Now I think she has a low fever. What should I do?"

The nurse advises the mother to bring the child to the clinic. When the client arrives, the nurse begins to collect data and establish priorities.

NurseThink® Time

Using the NurseThink® system, complete the priorities. Check your answers designated by in the Dehydration/fluid deficit Priority Exemplar.

Please check the exemplars on Type 1 diabetes mellitus and diabetic ketoacidosis to assist in completing this NurseThink® Time!

NurseThink® Time

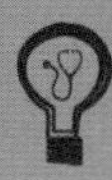

Priority Data Collection or Cues

1.

2.

3.

Priority Laboratory Tests/Diagnostics

1.

2.

3.

Priority Interventions or Actions

1.

2.

3.

Priority Potential & Actual Complications

1.

2.

3.

Priority Nursing Implications

1.

2.

3.

Priority Medications

1.

2.

3.

Reinforcement of Priority Teaching

1.

2.

3.

Dehydration/fluid deficit

Pathophysiology/Description

- Fluids and electrolytes exist in homeostasis in the body in the intravascular, intracellular, and interstitial compartments
- Diffusion, osmosis, filtration, and hydrostatic pressure maintain fluids and ensure fluids move throughout the body and meet the metabolic needs
- About 60% of adults, 55% of older adults, and 80% of infants are made up of fluids/water, indicating the risk associated with fluid loss in older adults and infants
- Intake of fluids comes from water, solid foods mixed with liquids, food oxidation, and medications such as those administered via the parenteral routes
- Output is water lost via measurable sources (urine, emesis, drainage/drains) and insensible sources (perspiration, exhaled air, water in stool)
- The kidneys maintain homeostasis of fluids within the body with increased intake, increasing output; water is conserved with decreasing intake and increased body needs (examples include diaphoresis, diarrhea, vomiting)
- An elaborate system of aldosterone secretion (adrenals), antidiuretic hormone (pituitary gland), and the kidneys assist the body to maintain homeostasis
- Dehydration occurs when fluid intake is insufficient to meet the metabolic needs of the body
- Types of dehydration
  - Isotonic/hypovolemia
    - Water and electrolytes are lost, with decreased circulating blood volume and poor tissue perfusion (most common form)
    - Causes are inadequate intake of fluid/electrolytes, increased loss of fluids/electrolytes, fluid shifts
  - Hypertonic
    - More water is lost than electrolytes, excesses in electrolytes change the homeostatic balance, leading to fluid leaching into the vascular and interstitial spaces, resulting in cellular dehydration
    - Causes are increased fluid loss, as in diabetes insipidus, hyperventilation, profuse diaphoresis, ketoacidosis/osmotic diuresis, early phases of kidney failure
  - Hypotonic
    - More electrolytes are lost than water, plasma leaves the intravascular compartment into the cells, yielding low intravascular fluids and cellular swelling
    - Causes are chronic illness, hypotonic/water replacement deficient in electrolytes, kidney disease, malnutrition

Priority Data Collection or Cues

- Monitor for risk related to age including infants, older adults
- Take vital signs, watch for tachycardia/weak pulse (dysrhythmias evident in late dehydration), tachypnea/dyspnea, low-grade temperature. Blood pressure may be normal or low—dramatic reductions in blood pressure are a late sign of dehydration/fluid deficit
- Determine weight—obtain accurate weight, compare to baseline
- Monitor level of consciousness—alertness, reports of dizziness/syncope, orthostatic hypotension, muscle weakness, restlessness
- Collect data on perfusion—peripheral/central pulses, capillary refill (< 3 seconds), skin temperature, skin color, peripheral motor and sensory function, later sign: decreased urine output
- Determine hydration status—skin turgor, intake and output, moisture in mucous membranes of mouth, nose, and eyelids, decreased bowel sounds/constipation, thirst
- Consider conditions leading to dehydration—diarrhea, poor intake, vigorous exercise, vomiting, polyuria, fluid losses (burns, trauma), clients with drains/nasogastric tube, burns/fluid shifts, overuse of diuretics
- Determine potential for injury—falls, aspiration, alterations in skin integrity

Priority Laboratory Tests/Diagnostics

- Serum electrolytes—depending upon type of dehydration, often hypernatremia
- Increased serum osmolality—Normal: 275-295 mOsm/kg; Elevated: > 295 mOsm/kg found in dehydration; >320 mOsm/kg is a critical finding
- CBC—elevated hemoglobin and hematocrit
- Elevated urine specific gravity >1.030
- Increased BUN (blood urea nitrogen)
- Monitor serum blood glucose levels; norms 70-100 mg/dl

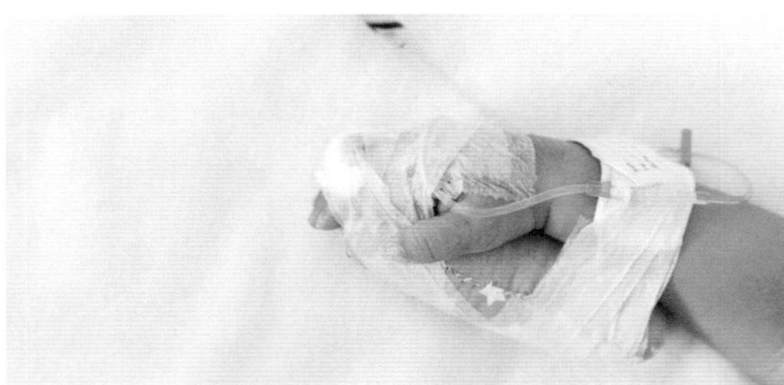

Image 8-2: What are the indicators for oral versus intravenous rehydration?

Priority Interventions or Actions

- Goal of interventions—replace fluid and electrolytes to achieve homeostasis
- Closely monitor client's status and rehydration, avoid overcorrection
- Monitor I&O and body weight
- Identify and manage cause—diarrhea, vomiting, blood loss, poor intake
- Oral rehydration is priority if tolerating PO fluids
- Intravenous fluid resuscitation/replacement, general guidelines:
  - Hypertonic dehydration—hypotonic fluids-D5W (once dextrose is metabolized), 0.45% NaCl (½ normal saline)
  - Isotonic dehydration—isotonic fluids (normal saline solution, lactated ringers)
  - Hypotonic dehydration—hypertonic fluids (3% or 5% saline solutions)
  - Blood products in increased blood loss/trauma
- Medications to treat cause—antidiarrheals, antiemetics, antibiotics, antipyretics
- Ingestion of food—to replace electrolytes

Priority Potential & Actual Complications

- Hypovolemia
- Hypovolemic shock
- Seizures/coma
- Multiorgan system failure

Priority Nursing Implications

- Nurses at the bedside may detect subtle changes in client's behavior that indicates dehydration and poor perfusion
- Nurses should consider clients at risk (children, older adults) and watch for dehydration
- Clients with nasogastric tubes should not drink water. This will leach out electrolytes as they are suctioned out of the stomach
- Encourage older adults to drink oral fluids. Due to decreased thirst, decreased mobility to access fluids, and reluctance to hydrate and need to urinate, older adults are often poorly hydrated
- Monitor for and prevent skin breakdown

Priority Medications

- Diphenoxylate with atropine
  - Oral and low-case for opiate antidiarrheal
  - Atropine causes less dependence
  - Less sedation
- Loperamide
  - Oral antidiarrheal
  - Less sedation and safety risk
- Promethazine HCl
  - Oral or rectal suppository antiemetic
  - Causes sedation and safety concerns
- Acetaminophen
  - Oral antipyretic
  - Treat high fevers to prevent fluid loss
  - Allow low-grade fevers to increase immune function

Reinforcement of Priority Teaching

- Advise clients/family to intervene early with clients with diarrhea and vomiting; encourage small, frequent fluid attempts of oral rehydration solution
- Add flavoring to oral electrolyte solutions to enhance palatability
- Plan for clients and families to know and report early signs of dehydration

Go To Clinical Answers

Text designated by the icon are the top answers for the Go To Clinical related to Dehydration/fluid deficit.

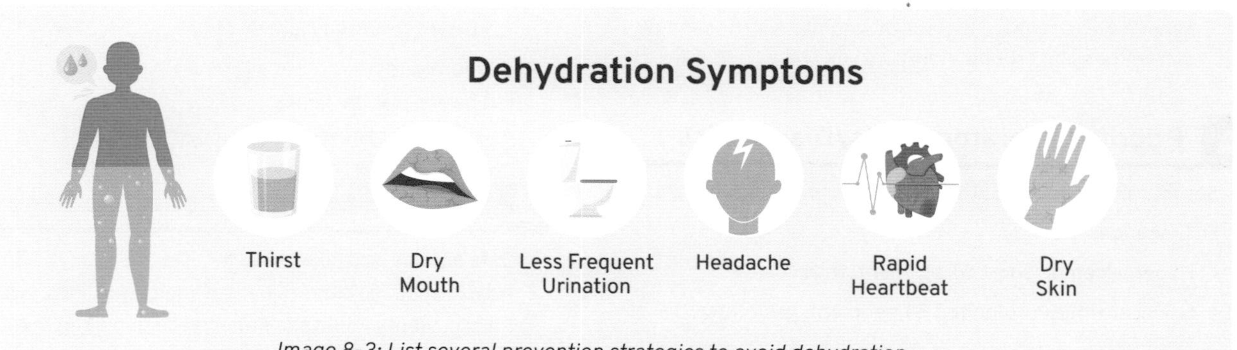

Image 8-3: List several prevention strategies to avoid dehydration.

Hyper/hypocalcemia

Pathophysiology/Description

- Calcium is an essential component of nerve/muscle/cardiac contractions, and blood clotting, along with the major element of bones and teeth
- Calcium required via daily intake, requires Vitamin D for metabolism, and requires parathormone and calcitonin to move calcium in and out of bone
- Hypercalcemia
  - High calcium levels may be associated with increased intake and mobilization from bones/metastatic processes
  - Causes include malignancies resulting in bone destruction, bone metastasis, hyperparathyroidism, decreased excretion with kidney disease, glucocorticoids, dehydration, immobilization, calcium and/or Vitamin D overdose, acidosis, milk-alkali syndrome, thiazide diuretics, and increased intake of calcium antacids
- Hypocalcemia
  - Low levels may be associated with decreased parathormone, decreased intake, and alkalosis
  - Causes include low calcium intake, lactose intolerance, parathyroidism, pancreatitis, multiple blood transfusions (citrate binds with calcium), alkalosis, laxative abuse, malabsorption syndromes, kidney disease, high phosphorus levels, Vitamin D deficiency, low magnesium levels, alcoholism, diarrhea, loop diuretics, wound drainage, and immobility

Priority Data Collection or Cues

- Hypercalcemia
  - Monitor clients at risk—vital signs for tachycardia, hypertension, bounding pulses
  - Observe for lethargy, weakness (may be profound), confusion, decreased reflexes, nausea/vomiting, bone pain, physiologic fractures, polyuria, and kidney stones
- Hypocalcemia
  - Monitor clients at risk—vital signs for bradycardia, hypotension, weak peripheral pulses
  - Observe for tetany, Chvostek sign, Trousseau sign, laryngeal stridor, dysphagia, fatigue, anxiety, depression, hyperreflexia, and muscle spasms numbness/tingling of extremities and around mouth

Priority Laboratory Tests/Diagnostics

- Serum calcium levels 8.6-10.2 mg/dL and 4.5-5.5 mEq/L
- ECG changes
  - Hypercalcemia—short ST segment, wide T wave
  - Hypocalcemia—prolonged ST segment, prolonged QT segment

Priority Interventions or Actions

- Hypercalcemia
  - Determine and manage underlying cause
  - Enhance calcium excretion with diuretics
  - Hydrate with isotonic saline solutions/oral hydration of 3000-4000 mL/day
  - Low calcium diet
  - Increase weight bearing exercises
- Hypocalcemia
  - Determine and manage underlying cause
  - Enhance dietary calcium and Vitamin D intake
  - Administer intravenous calcium gluconate-monitor ECG and patency of intravenous

Priority Potential & Actual Complications

- Hypercalcemia
  - Coma
- Hypocalcemia
  - Seizures
  - Laryngospasm
  - Ventricular tachycardia

Priority Nursing Implications

- High calcium levels may be associated with renal lithiasis—strain urine and check for kidney/flank pain
- High calcium may exacerbate digoxin toxicity
- Monitor clients with neck or thyroid surgery for potential parathyroid damage
- Manage pain and anxiety of clients at risk for hypocalcemia - respiratory alkalosis may exacerbate symptoms

Priority Medications

- Furosemide
  - Given orally or intravenous
  - Enhances renal excretion of calcium
- Calcitonin
  - Given IM/subcutaneous; calcitonin-salmon is intranasal
  - Lowers serum calcium level
- Pamidronate
  - Lowers calcium levels
  - Used with cancer-related hypercalcemia

Reinforcement of Priority Teaching

- Safe antacid and laxative use
- Advise about calcium-rich foods (dairy, sardines, canned fish)
- Inform clients about the importance of mobility and weight-bearing exercises

Hyper/hypokalemia

Pathophysiology/Description

- Potassium is involved in neuromuscular and cardiac function
- Potassium regulates intracellular osmolality and enhances cellular growth
- Allows glycogen to be deposited into muscle and liver cells
- Plays a role in acid-base balance
- Potassium ingested from dietary sources, excreted by the kidneys, lost also in stool and sweat
- Hyperkalemia
  - Increased K+ from impaired excretion, moving from ICF to ECF, and large intake of K+
  - Causes: Acidosis, cellular lysis (burns, injury, infection), medications maintain K+ in intravascular space, high oral intake of potassium, rapid or high dose infusion of intravenous potassium, renal failure, adrenal insufficiency, overuse of K+ salt substitute, tumor lysis syndrome, use of K+ sparing diuretics, and hyperuricemia
- Hypokalemia
  - Decreased K+ from loss of potassium via urine, movement of the K+ from ECF to ICF, or decreased intake
  - Causes: Diarrhea, vomiting, inadequate intake of potassium, overuse of laxatives, low magnesium levels, massive diuresis, hydration with fluids without KCl, side effect of insulin treatment with diabetic ketoacidosis, stress, delirium tremens, coronary muscle necrosis, alkalosis, wound drainage, diaphoresis, potassium-wasting diuretics, kidney disease, water intoxication, nasogastric suction

Priority Data Collection or Cues

- Hyperkalemia
  - Determine vital signs for irregular pulse, bradycardia
  - Determine clients at risk
  - Observe for irritability, anxiety, leg cramping and pain, weakness, abdominal cramps and diarrhea, cardiac dysrhythmias, and paresthesias
- Hypokalemia
  - Monitor vital signs for weak, irregular pulse, shallow respirations, orthostatic hypotension
  - Determine clients at risk
  - Observe for muscle weakness, leg weakness, paralytic ileus, hyperglycemia, paralysis, anxiety, confusion, lethargy, paresthesias, depressed deep tendon reflexes

Clinical Hint

Both high and low levels of serum potassium may cause dangerous or lethal cardiac rhythms. Monitor ECGs closely.

Priority Laboratory Tests/Diagnostics

- Serum potassium levels 3.5-5.0 mEq/L
- ECG
  - Hyperkalemia—peaked T waves, prolonged PR interval, ST depression, loss of p waves, prolonged QRS
  - Hypokalemia—ST depression, flattened T wave, prolonged QRS, premature ventricular contractions

Priority Interventions or Actions

- Hyperkalemia
  - Determine and manage underlying cause
  - Decrease oral or parenteral intake of potassium (restrict diet)
  - Increase excretion with diuretics (furosemide)
  - Potassium-binding medications
  - Intravenous infusion of insulin with glucose to force K+ into the cells and reduce serum K+
  - Intravenous infusion of calcium gluconate or NaHCO3 to decrease cellular cardiac excitability
  - Dialysis
- Hypokalemia
  - Oral and intravenous supplementation

Priority Potential & Actual Complications

- Hyperkalemia
  - Ventricular fibrillation
  - Complete respiratory arrest
  - Cardiac standstill/arrest
- Hypokalemia
  - Lethal cardiac dysrhythmias
  - Coma
  - Cardiac arrest

Priority Nursing Implications

- Observe for hypotension and provide safety interventions
- All potassium chloride, oral and intravenous, must be well diluted. Intravenous administration requires slow infusion in a well-mixed dilution via infusion pump
- Ensure renal function prior to administration of potassium
- Safety measures with hypotension
- Monitor ECG for rhythm changes

Priority Medications

- Furosemide
  - Potent loop diuretic
  - Lowers potassium levels
  - Usually given oral (IM/subcutaneously) only in selected cases
- Sodium styrene sulfonate
  - Administered orally or per rectum
  - Binds with potassium for excretion in feces
- Potassium chloride (KCl)
  - Given orally or intravenous
  - Oral or intravenous solutions must be well diluted
  - Check intravenous site for infiltration
  - Oral KCl causes nausea and vomiting, best if mixed with juice

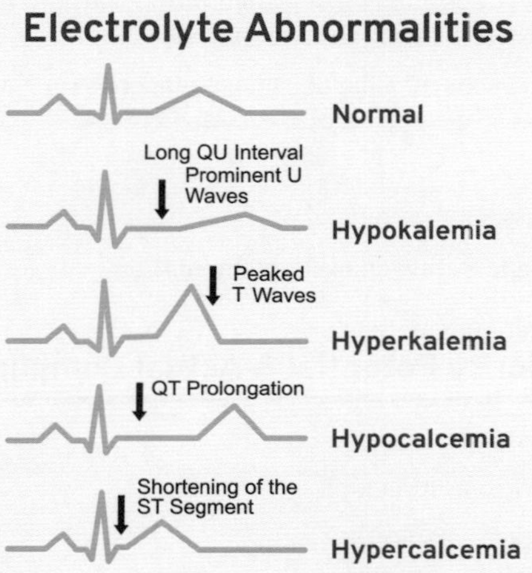

Electrolyte Abnormalities

Normal

Long QU Interval
Prominent U Waves

Hypokalemia

Peaked T Waves

Hyperkalemia

QT Prolongation

Hypocalcemia

Shortening of the ST Segment

Hypercalcemia

Image 8-4: Note the abnormal rhythms discussed in this image. What interventions would you anticipate for each of these conditions and these changes in heart rhythms?

Clinical Hint

Both oral and intravenous potassium chloride should be well diluted when administered.

Next Gen Clinical Judgment

A health care provider prescribes 40 mEg of KCl. oral solution per day. The nurse administers the medication and the client becomes nauseated. What actions should the nurse consider?

Reinforcement of Priority Teaching

- Inform clients about food high in potassium: fruits (bananas, oranges), dried fruits (raisins), vegetables, fish, pork, beef, veal
- Avoid overuse of sodium replacements that are high in potassium
- Hypokalemia potentiates digoxin toxicity–counsel clients to watch for signs and symptoms, especially if on a potassium-wasting diuretic
- Inform clients at risk about need to monitor potassium levels
- If client is changed from a potassium-wasting to a potassium sparing diuretic, make sure they are instructed to adjust diet accordingly

Clinical Hint

Potassium chloride should not be added to intravenous fluids in post-operative clients until renal function is confirmed through urine production.

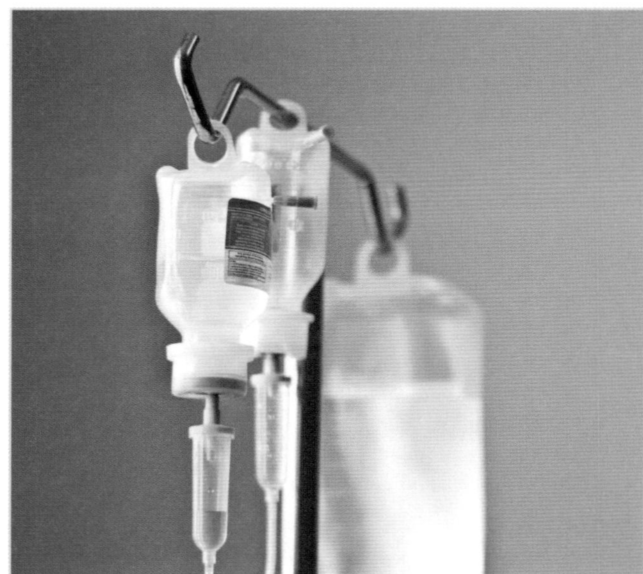

Image 8-5: A nurse cares for a client who is prescribed to receive a K rider to treat hypokalemia. The nurse receives the medication from the pharmacy and hangs the medication. About halfway through the infusion, the nurse notes that the dosage of the potassium is incorrect.

1. *What interventions do you anticipate?*
2. *What processes are required when a medication error is made?*
3. *What liability does a nurse incur when administering an incorrect medication or dosage?*
4. *How could this error have been prevented?*

Hyper/hypomagnesemia

Pathophysiology/Description

- Essential component of cellular processes and metabolism of carbohydrates and proteins, synthesis of nucleic acids and proteins, balance phosphorus and calcium levels, assist in the function of the sodium-potassium pump
- Influences neuromuscular excitability and contractility
- Hypermagnesemia
  - High magnesium levels > 2.5 mEq/L
  - Causes include increased magnesium intake along with renal insufficiency/failure, excess intake of magnesium sulfate during pregnancy in management of eclampsia, tumor lysis syndrome, and diabetic ketoacidosis
- Hypomagnesemia
  - Low magnesium levels < 1.5 mEq/L
  - Occurs with limited intake or increased renal losses
  - Causes include diarrhea, vomiting, alcoholism, malabsorption syndrome, malnutrition, high urine output, nasogastric tube with suction drainage system, hyperaldosteronism, diabetes mellitus, prolonged parenteral nutrition, and prolonged use of diuretics

Priority Data Collection or Cues

- Hypermagnesemia
  - Determine clients at risk (renal failure/insufficiency or pregnant woman receiving magnesium sulfate for eclampsia)
  - Take vital signs, observe for bradycardia, hypotension
  - Observe for lethargy, nausea/vomiting, decreased deep tendon reflexes, decreased level of consciousness, flushed warm skin, muscle weakness, dysphagia
- Hypomagnesemia
  - Determine clients at risk
  - Observe vital signs, observe for tachycardia, hypertension
  - Monitor for confusion, tremors, hyperactive deep tendon reflexes, insomnia, muscle cramps

Priority Laboratory Tests/Diagnostics

- Serum magnesium levels 1.5-2.5 mEq/L

Priority Interventions or Actions

- Hypermagnesemia
  - Determine and manage underlying cause
  - Focus is on prevention
  - Avoid magnesium containing foods (green vegetables, nuts, bananas, oranges, peanut butter, chocolate)
  - Emergency treatment for high magnesium levels-intravenous calcium gluconate or calcium chloride
  - With intact renal function promote urinary excretion with intravenous fluids, oral fluids, and intravenous furosemide
  - With impaired renal function, dialysis is used to draw off magnesium
- Hypomagnesemia
  - Determine and treat underlying cause
  - Dietary replacement of magnesium-supplements/magnesium containing foods
  - With significant deficits, provide intravenous magnesium

Priority Potential & Actual Complications

- Hypermagnesemia
  - Paralysis
  - Respiratory and cardiac arrest
- Hypomagnesemia
  - Seizures
  - Dysrhythmias—ventricular tachycardia, ventricular fibrillation

Priority Nursing Implications

- Magnesium, calcium, and potassium are balanced together in the body and require that nurses monitor all three in clients at risk of imbalance
- Nurses must carefully monitor intravenous infusions of magnesium—infusing too rapidly may lead to cardiac or respiratory arrest
- Monitor vital signs carefully when magnesium levels are abnormal
- Magnesium enhances digoxin toxicity

Priority Medications

- Furosemide
  - High ceiling, rapid acting diuretic
  - Removes excess magnesium
  - Monitor hydration and serum potassium levels
  - Administered orally or intravenous (subcutaneous/IM in special cases)

Reinforcement of Priority Teaching

- Counsel clients in chronic renal failure to avoid magnesium-containing drugs and limit magnesium containing foods
- Ensure that clients monitor their urine output as a reflection of renal function
- Depending upon excess or deficit, tell clients to eat or avoid magnesium-rich foods

Clinical Hint

As with many electrolyte disorders, it is critical to determine and manage the underlying cause of abnormal magnesium levels.

Pathophysiology/Description

- Sodium maintains extracellular volume and water distribution in extracellular/ intracellular compartments and changes in sodium levels create changes in osmolality
- Functions in nerve conduction, muscle contractility, and acid-base balance
- Changes in serum sodium levels may reflect changes in amount of sodium relative to water or water relative to sodium
- Sodium is acquired from dietary sources, usually in excess of needs
- Sodium excreted in urine, feces, and sweat, regulated by the kidneys
- Hypernatremia—elevated serum sodium levels > 145 mEq/L (water loss, sodium increases)
  - Hyperosmolality
  - Fluid shift from cells to extracellular space, causing dehydration
  - Causes include diabetes insipidus, hyperosmolar tube feedings, hyperglycemia/diabetes mellitus, excessive diaphoresis, sodium intake without water (ocean water, sodium tablets), primary aldosteronism, overdose with hypertonic saline intravenous solution, lack of free water with tube feedings, osmotic diuretics, and diarrhea
- Hyponatremia—decreased serum sodium levels < 135 mEq/L
  - Water excess relative to sodium levels related to sodium loss or loss of sodium containing fluids
  - Fluid shifts into cells from extracellular space, causing cellular edema
  - Causes include diaphoresis, diarrhea, draining wounds, vomiting, trauma with blood loss, infusion of low sodium or no sodium fluids, intravenous fluids with clients in renal failure, excessive water intake, and Syndrome of Inappropriate Antidiuretic Hormone (SIADH)

Priority Data Collection or Cues

- Monitor clients at risk
- Hypernatremia
  - Take vital signs, observe for hypotension/postural hypotension
  - Monitor for poor skin turgor and dry/swollen tongue
  - Observe level of consciousness for agitation, lethargy, weakness
  - Ask about thirst, sodium intake, water intake
  - Determine if client is exhibiting hypernatremia with decreased or increased extracellular volume
- Hyponatremia
  - Observe level of consciousness (changes in neurological function may be first symptoms from cerebral edema) for headache, confusion, irritability

Priority Laboratory Tests/Diagnostics

- Serum sodium levels 135-145 mEq/L

Priority Interventions or Actions

- Hypernatremia
  - Monitor serum electrolytes
  - Determine and treat underlying cause
  - Administer oral or intravenous hypotonic or isotonic fluids as prescribed
  - Limit sodium intake
  - Diuretics to pull off sodium
- Hyponatremia
  - Fluid restriction
  - Determine and treat underlying cause
  - If hyponatremia related to fluid loss, replace with sodium containing fluids
  - If seizures develop, administration of small volumes of hypertonic solutions titrated to serum osmolality and sodium levels
  - Close monitoring of serum sodium levels

Priority Potential & Actual Complications

- Hypernatremia/hyponatremia
  - Seizures
  - Coma
  - Neurological damage/coma

Priority Nursing Implications

- Hyper- and hyponatremia may occur from diarrhea—nurses need to monitor serum electrolyte levels of clients
- Carefully monitor intravenous fluid infusions

Priority Medications

- Hydrochlorothiazide diuretics (HCTZ)
  - Pull off excess fluids and sodium
  - Used with diabetes insipidus

Reinforcement of Priority Teaching

- Inform clients to avoid drinking seawater and prevent children from ingestion of seawater
- Discuss the decreased thirst mechanism with older clients and the need to drink when thirsty

Hyper/hypophosphatemia

Pathophysiology/Description

- Most phosphorus is in bones and teeth as calcium phosphate
- Also works in function of muscle, red blood cells, and the nervous system
- Functions in the acid-base balancing system, function of ATP, cellular uptake and use of glucose, and metabolism of carbohydrates, proteins, and fats
- Excretion requires adequate kidney function. Regulation in the body is controlled by the parathyroid hormone
- Hyperphosphatemia
  - Phosphorus levels > 4.5 mg/dL
  - Causes include acute kidney injury or chronic kidney disease, chemotherapy, excessive ingestion of cow's milk, excessive intake of phosphorus-based laxatives/enemas, large intake of Vitamin D, hypoparathyroidism, and sickle cell anemia
- Hypophosphatemia
  - Phosphorus levels < 3.0 mg/dL
  - Low levels are rare
  - Causes include malnutrition, malabsorption syndrome, alcohol withdrawal, use of phosphate-binding antacids, total parenteral nutrition with low phosphorus levels, recovery from diabetic ketoacidosis, respiratory alkalosis

Priority Data Collection or Cues

- Hyperphosphatemia
  - Determine clients at risk and monitor serum phosphorus levels
  - Clients may be asymptomatic
  - Monitor serum calcium levels
  - Symptoms of high levels of phosphorus often associated with hypocalcemia
  - Observe for tetany, muscle cramps, paresthesias, numbness and tingling of extremities and around mouth, and hyperreflexia
- Hypophosphatemia
  - Determine clients at risk and monitor serum phosphorus levels
  - Mild hypophosphatemia is asymptomatic
  - Monitor serum calcium levels
  - Observe for decreased level of consciousness, confusion, muscle weakness, pain, dysrhythmias, osteomalacia, rhabdomyolysis, and neuropathy

Priority Laboratory Tests/Diagnostics

- Serum phosphorus levels 3.0-4.5 mg/dL
- Serum calcium levels 9.0-10.5 mg/dL (exist in inverse proportions with phosphorus)

Priority Interventions or Actions

- Hyperphosphatemia
  - Determine and treat underlying cause
  - Restrict phosphorus-containing foods (dairy products, eggs, meats, nuts, legumes, grains, fish)
  - Phosphorus-binding medications
  - Dialysis
  - Insulin and glucose infusion
  - Ensure adequate hydration and monitor serum calcium and phosphorus levels
- Hypophosphatemia
  - Oral phosphorus supplements
  - Diet high in phosphorus
  - Intravenous sodium phosphate/potassium phosphate

Priority Potential & Actual Complications

- Seizures associated with hyperphosphatemia
- Calcium/phosphorus deposits may precipitate on major organs including joints, kidneys, skin, arteries, corneas, and may lead to organ dysfunction
- Severe hypophosphatemia may result in cardiomyopathy and be fatal

Priority Nursing Implications

- Clients receiving intravenous phosphorus infusions need to be carefully monitored for hypocalcemia
- Monitor intravenous site as phosphorus may be sclerotic and cause tissue necrosis

Priority Medications

- Calcium carbonate
  - Bind with phosphorus in hyperphosphatemia
  - Treats both hyperphosphatemia and hypocalcemia
  - May cause constipation and flatulence

Reinforcement of Priority Teaching

- Counsel clients to not take in excessive milk products or laxatives/enemas with phosphorus

Clinical Hint

Calcium and phosphorus exist in inverse levels in the human body—high levels of phosphorus yield low calcium levels and low levels of phosphorus yield high calcium levels.

Metabolic acidosis

Pathophysiology/Description

- Deficit of base bicarbonate
- When acids accumulate in the body or bicarbonate is lost
- Compensation occurs by the release of CO_2 via rapid respirations (Kussmaul respirations) and kidney excretion of acids
- Calculate anion gap to determine cause of metabolic acidosis Na – (Cl + HCO_3)
- May occur with respiratory acidosis, as in cardiopulmonary arrest
- Causes include diabetic ketoacidosis, lactic acid accumulation when in shock or after a trauma, loss of HCO_3 from diarrhea, starvation, renal tubular necrosis, gastrointestinal fistulas, aspirin overdose, high-fat diets, ineffective metabolism of carbohydrates, and renal disease that impairs ability to reabsorb HCO_3

Priority Data Collection or Cues

- Monitor for signs and symptoms of respiratory distress
- Take vital signs and observe for hypotension, tachypnea, dysrhythmias
- Observe for symptoms of drowsiness, confusion, headache, warm flushed skin, nausea, vomiting, diarrhea, abdominal pain

Priority Laboratory Tests/Diagnostics

- Normal anion gap is 10-14 mEq/L (increased with acid gains related to metabolic acidosis, it is normal with bicarbonate loss)
- Arterial blood gases
  - Normal values
    - pH 7.35-7.45
    - $PaCO_2$ 35-45 mmHg
    - HCO_3 22-26 mEq/L
  - Metabolic Acidosis
    - pH decreased
    - $PaCO_2$ normal (uncompensated)
    - $PaCO_2$ decreased (compensated)
    - HCO_3 decreased
- Monitor serum potassium levels 3.5-5.0 mEq/L

Priority Interventions or Actions

- Determine and manage underlying cause
- Establish seizure precautions, as indicated
- Monitor intake and output
- Provide $NaHCO_3$ via intravenous
- Treat DKA with insulin and hydration
- Clients with kidney disease are treated with dialysis and a low protein/high calorie diet

Priority Potential & Actual Complications

- Seizures
- Coma
- Polyuria/osmotic diuresis/diarrhea may lead to hypovolemia and shock

Priority Nursing Implications

- Read and interpret arterial blood gas findings, watching for trends and change
- Establish seizure precautions and observe/describe seizures

Reinforcement of Priority Teaching

- Clients with diabetes about sick day care and means to avoid DKA
- Clients with renal disease to report signs/symptoms out of the ordinary to health care provider

Next Gen Clinical Judgment

A client sustains a seizure from metabolic acidosis due to a history of renal dysfunction. Create the ABG values for this client.

	ABG VALUES
pH	
$PaCO_2$	
HCO_3	

Table 8-1:

1. *How is metabolic acidosis managed?*
2. *Why are clients experiencing metabolic acidosis at risk for seizures?*
3. *What specific nursing care is required because the client had a seizure?*
4. *What precautions are required when a client is at risk for seizure?*

Metabolic alkalosis

Pathophysiology/Description

- Base bicarbonate excess
- Loss of acid (vomiting or nasogastric suction) or gain in bicarbonate (eating baking soda)
- Compensation includes renal excretion of HCO_3
- May also compensate with reduction in the respiratory rate to retain carbon dioxide, this is limited by body's natural impulse to take the next breath/ventilate
- Causes include vomiting, nasogastric suctioning, diuretics, hypokalemia, increased mineral corticoids, eating baking soda/infusion of excess Na HCO_3, hyperaldosteronism, large blood transfusions wherein citrates bind with HCO_3
- May occur with respiratory acidosis (client with COPD on thiazide diuretic)
- May occur with respiratory alkalosis (hypoventilating and losing gastric acids via nasogastric drainage)

Priority Data Collection or Cues

- Determine clients at risk
- Monitor for increased work of breathing or respiratory distress
- Take vital signs and observe for tachycardia, bradypnea, dysrhythmias
- Observe for dizziness, drowsiness, confusion, headache, nausea/vomiting, anorexia, tetany, muscle cramps, tremors, hypotonicity

Priority Laboratory Tests/Diagnostics

- **Arterial blood gases**
    - Normal values
        - pH 7.35-7.45
        - $PaCO_2$ 35-45 mmHg
        - HCO_3 22-26 mEq/L
    - Metabolic alkalosis
        - pH increased
        - $PaCO_2$ normal (uncompensated)
        - $PaCO_2$ elevated (compensated)
        - HCO_3 increased
- Monitor serum potassium levels 3.5-5.0 mEq/L
- Monitor serum calcium levels 8.6-10.2 mg/dL and 4.5-5.5 mEq/L

Priority Interventions or Actions

- Determine and manage underlying cause
- Implement seizure precautions, as indicated
- Replace potassium
- Medications to increase excretion of bicarbonate

Priority Potential & Actual Complications

- Seizures

Priority Nursing Implications

- Read and interpret arterial blood gas findings, watching for trends and change
- Maintain safety precautions with change in sensorium
- Monitor clients with profuse vomiting/gastric suctioning for changes in level of consciousness

Reinforcement of Priority Teaching

- Adequate hydration
- Signs and symptoms that warrant reporting to health care provider

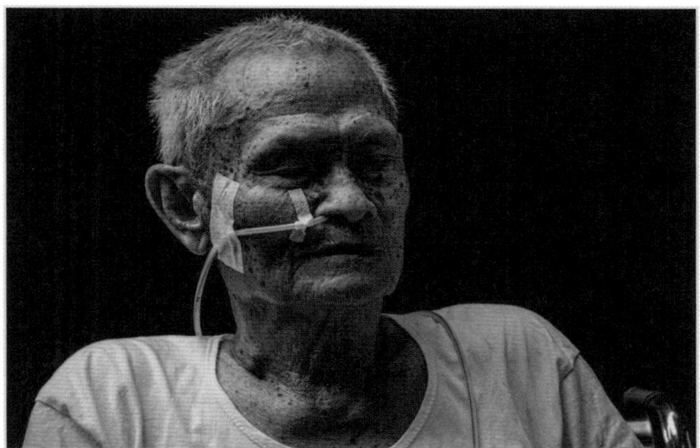

Image 8-6: A nurse caring for this client notes that the client experiences metabolic alkalosis from loss of gastric acids. Create the ABG values for this client.

	ABG VALUES
pH	
$PaCO_2$	
HCO_3	

Table 8-2: How should metabolic alkalosis be prevented? How is metabolic acidosis managed?

Respiratory acidosis

Pathophysiology/Description

- Occurs from carbonic acid excess (CO_2 and H_20 combine, high hydrogen ion concentration)
- Generally due to hypoventilation and CO_2 retention —lowers the pH
- Kidneys compensate with conservation of HCO_3 —renal compensation occurs within 24 hours
- May occur with metabolic alkalosis (client with COPD on thiazide diuretic)
- May occur with metabolic acidosis, as in cardiopulmonary arrest
- Causes include COPD, barbiturate/CNS depressant/opioid overdose, pneumonia, asthma, atelectasis, low respiratory rate on a mechanical ventilator/hypoventilation, conditions causing respiratory muscle weakness (Guillain-Barré, myasthenia gravis), high oxygen provision to CO_2 retainers, pulmonary edema, and pulmonary embolism

Priority Data Collection or Cues

- Determine clients at risk
- Monitor for respiratory depression or obstructed airway
- Take client vital signs and observe for hypotension, bradypnea, oxygen saturation-hypoxia
- Observe for dizziness, drowsiness, confusion, headache, warm flushed skin

Priority Laboratory Tests/Diagnostics

- Arterial blood gases
  - Normal values
    - pH 7.35-7.45
    - $PaCO_2$ 35-45 mmHg
    - HCO_3 22-26 mEq/L
  - Respiratory Acidosis
    - pH decreased
    - $PaCO_2$ increased
    - HCO_3 normal (uncompensated)
    - HCO_3 increased (compensated)
- Monitor serum potassium levels 3.5-5.0 mEq/L

Priority Interventions or Actions

- Determine and treat underlying cause and manage respiratory distress
- Provide oxygen as prescribed
- Position in semi-Fowler's position
- Encourage client to turn, cough, and deep breath
- Encourage fluids to liquefy secretions, suction as needed
- Avoid medications that cause respiratory depression
- Provide respiratory treatments and antibiotics as prescribed
- Monitor for rising CO_2 and need for intubation and mechanical ventilation
- Implement seizure precautions as indicated

Priority Potential & Actual Complications

- Seizures
- Coma
- Ventricular fibrillation
- May be fatal

Priority Nursing Implications

- Monitor clients at risk for and symptoms of increasing respiratory distress
- Read and interpret arterial blood gas findings, watching for trends and change
- Respiratory distress is very frightening for clients requiring nurses to provide support and remain calm

Reinforcement of Priority Teaching

- Inform client and family about signs of deteriorating respiratory condition
- Inform clients about means to prevent respiratory infections

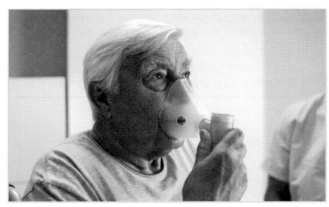

Image 8-7: This client has COPD and chronically retains carbon dioxide. Create the ABG values for this client.

	ABG VALUES
pH	
$PaCO_2$	
HCO_3	

Table 8-3: How is respiratory acidosis managed?

Pathophysiology/Description

- Carbonic acid deficit with increased carbon dioxide excretion
- Occurs with client hyperventilation
- Related to hypoxia from respiratory distress
- Compensation usually does not occur, it may include HCO_3 being excreted or transferred into the cells
- Associated with anxiety, CNS conditions, overventilation/overstimulation of respiratory system
- Causes include hyperventilation, hypoxia, pulmonary embolism, fear, pain, fever, anxiety, overventilation during exercise, brain injury/encephalitis, septicemia, salicylate poisoning, and overventilation via mechanical ventilator
- May occur with metabolic alkalosis (hypoventilating and losing gastric acids via nasogastric drainage)

Priority Data Collection or Cues

- Determine clients at risk including those in respiratory distress
- Take client vital signs and observe for tachycardia, tachypnea, dysrhythmias
- Observe for confusion, lethargy, headache, dizziness, nausea/vomiting, epigastric pain, tetany, numbness, tingling, and hyperreflexia

Priority Laboratory Tests/Diagnostics

- Arterial blood gases
  - Normal values
    - pH 7.35-7.45
    - $PaCO_2$ 35-45 mmHg
    - HCO_3 22-26 mEq/L
  - Metabolic alkalosis
    - pH increased
    - $PaCO_2$ decreased
    - HCO_3 normal (uncompensated)
    - HCO_3 decreased (compensated)
- Monitor serum potassium levels 3.5-5.0 mEq/L
- Monitor serum calcium levels 8.6-10.2 mg/dL and 4.5-5.5 mEq/L

Priority Interventions or Actions

- Determine and manage underlying cause
- Provide emotional support
- Encourage normal breathing patterns
- Advise clients on means to retain CO_2
  - Holding breath
  - Use of a rebreathing mask
  - Breathing into a paper bag
- Alleviate hypoxemia to lower respiratory rate, ensure adjustment of ventilator settings
- Implement seizure precautions, as indicated

Priority Potential & Actual Complications

- Seizures

Priority Nursing Implications

- Read and interpret arterial blood gas findings, watching for trends and change
- Monitor and manage a client on mechanical ventilation
- Provide education and emotional support as indicated

Priority Medications

- Calcium carbonate
  - Treats respiratory alkalosis, hyperphosphatemia, and hypocalcemia
  - May cause constipation and flatulence
  - Intravenous infusion
  - Monitor for tetany

Reinforcement of Priority Teaching

- Breathing techniques to manage breathing pattern
- Provide referrals for emotional support as needed

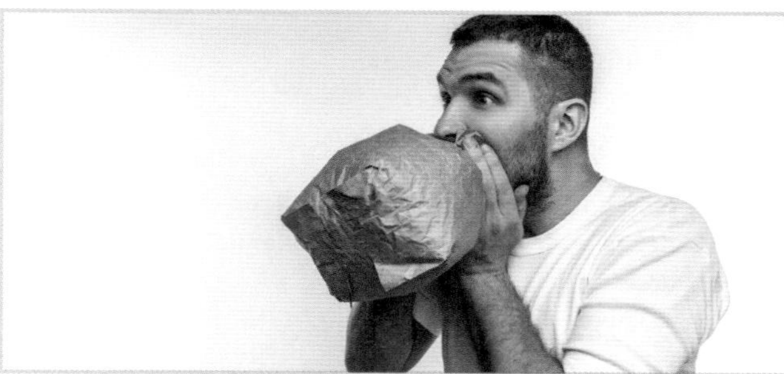

Image 8-8: A man coaches his partner through childbirth. He proceeds to hyperventilate for a prolonged period of time. Create the ABGs for this client.

	ABG VALUES
pH	
$PaCO_2$	
HCO_3	

Table 8-4: How is respiratory alkalosis managed?

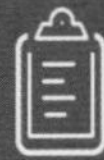

NurseThink® Quiz Questions

1. **When collecting data on a dehydrated client, which finding indicates the most severe dehydration?**
   a. Dry cracked lips.
   b. Poor skin turgor.
   c. Little urinary output.
   d. Dry mucous membranes.

2. **What does the nurse expect to implement in the care of a client with mild dehydration?**
   a. Intravenous fluid replacement therapy.
   b. Oral rehydration.
   c. Sodium restriction.
   d. NPO status.

3. **What action should the nurse implement when trying to prevent respiratory alkalosis in a hyperventilating client?**
   a. Constantly reassure the client so they will calm down and breathe deeply.
   b. Give the client a high dose of antianxiety medication.
   c. Hyperventilation causes acidosis, not alkalosis.
   d. Have the client breathe in and out into a paper bag.

4. **When reviewing lab results, which lab value does the nurse correlate with the client's hypocalcemia?**
   a. Phosphorus 12.2 mg/dL.
   b. Calcium 9.3 mg/dL.
   c. Sodium 132 mEq/L.
   d. Potassium 4.5 mEq/L.

5. **What does the nurse prioritize when caring for a client with hyperkalemia?**
   a. Monitoring telemetry.
   b. Monitoring blood pressure.
   c. Monitoring temperature.
   d. Monitoring oxygen saturation.

6. **What food does the nurse encourage the client to add to their diet to address chronic hypokalemia?**
   a. Apples.
   b. Oranges.
   c. White rice.
   d. Eggplant.

7. **What finding is consistent with the client's diagnosis of hypermagnesemia?**
   a. Muscle cramps.
   b. Confusion.
   c. Dyspnea.
   d. Seizures.

8. **The nurse monitors telemetry for a client with hypomagnesemia. What telemetry finding indicates the condition is worsening, and the client will require immediate intravenous administration of supplemental magnesium to reverse its life-threatening effects?**
   a. Atrial fibrillation.
   b. Ventricular fibrillation.
   c. Junctional tachycardia.
   d. Torsades de pointes.

9. **When evaluating a client with hypernatremia, what factor does the nurse expect to address as the probable cause of their condition?**
   a. Severe, watery diarrhea.
   b. Severe indigestion.
   c. Fluid overload.
   d. Hypertension.

10. **What statement by the client illustrates an understanding of their education on preventing the reoccurrence of hyponatremia?**
   a. "I will be sure to increase my dietary intake of sodium to 4000 mg daily."
   b. "I will drink at least 2 gallons of water daily to prevent dehydration."
   c. "I will take an extra water pill when I notice swelling in my legs."
   d. "I will drink a sports drink after extensive exercise instead of water."

11. **Which client would the nurse identify as being at the highest risk of hyperphosphatemia?**
   a. Kidney failure on dialysis.
   b. Heart failure on beta-blockers.
   c. Older adult with dementia.
   d. Pregnant with advanced age.

12. **What finding does the nurse understand is related to the client's diagnosis of hypophosphatemia?**
   a. Chronic alcoholism.
   b. Dehydration.
   c. Seizure disorder.
   d. Hyperlipidemia.

13. **When planning client care, which client does the nurse consider to be at the highest risk of developing metabolic acidosis?**
   a. Bulimic client.
   b. Child with hypokalemia.
   c. Hyperventilating client.
   d. Older adult client on diuretics.

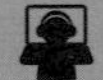

14. What medications does the nurse anticipate being used to correct a client's metabolic acidosis? *Select all that apply.*

a. Sodium bicarbonate.
b. Hypertonic sodium.
c. Tris-hydroxymethyl aminomethane.
d. 0.45% sodium chloride.
e. Furosemide.

15. The nurse evaluates several clients and their lab results. Which data prompts the nurse to plan interventions to address metabolic acidosis?

a. Glucose 635 mg/dL.
b. Glucose 60 mg/dL.
c. Sodium 140 mEq/L.
d. Sodium 125 mEq/L.

16. Which prescription does the nurse question when implementing the treatment plan for a client with metabolic alkalosis?

a. Administer potassium intravenously.
b. Administer sodium bicarbonate intravenously.
c. Discontinue supplemental oxygen therapy.
d. Infuse sodium chloride 0.9% intravenously at 80 mL per hour.

17. Which lab result indicates to the nurse that the client will need interventions to treat metabolic alkalosis?

a. HCO3 32 mEq/L.
b. pH 7.20.
c. PO2 42 mmHg.
d. PCO2 38 mmHg.

18. What finding suggests a causative factor for a client diagnosed with respiratory acidosis?

a. Hyperventilation.
b. Severe anxiety disorder.
c. Overdose of oxycodone.
d. Mechanical ventilation.

19. A nurse receives these arterial blood gas results from the lab. Which nursing actions should the nurse anticipate?

a. Provide high-flow oxygen via face mask.
b. Elevate the head of the bed to 90 degrees.
c. Administer prescribed intravenous anxiolytic.
d. Provide a bag for the client to breath in and out.

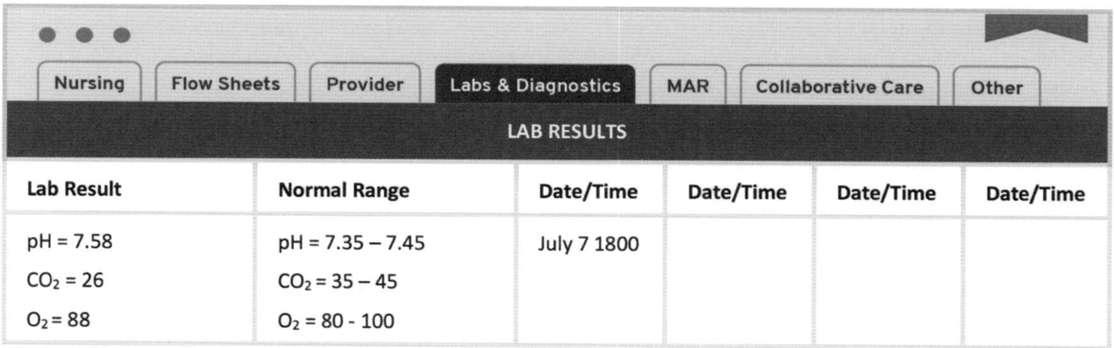

Lab Result	Normal Range	Date/Time	Date/Time	Date/Time	Date/Time
pH = 7.58 CO_2 = 26 O_2 = 88	pH = 7.35 – 7.45 CO_2 = 35 – 45 O_2 = 80 - 100	July 7 1800			

20. What finding does the nurse attribute to the client's diagnosis of chronic respiratory acidosis?

a. Blurred vision.
b. Personality changes.
c. Decreased level of consciousness.
d. Tachycardia.

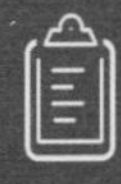

NurseThink® Quiz Answers

1. **When collecting data on a dehydrated client, which finding indicates the most severe dehydration?**
   a. Dry cracked lips.
   b. Poor skin turgor.
   c. Little urinary output.
   d. Dry mucous membranes.

   Topic/Concept: Homeostasis **Subtopic:** Dehydration **Bloom's Taxonomy:** Applying **Clinical Problem-Solving Process:** Data Collection **NCLEX-PN®:** Coordinated Care **QSEN:** Teamwork and Collaboration **CJMM:** Recognize Cues

   Rationale: Dry lips and mucous membranes and poor skin turgor all show dehydration is at least moderate. However, little urinary output illustrates systemic dehydration and probable kidney damage, making it the most severe symptom.

   THIN Thinking: *Clinical Problem-Solving Process* – When dehydration gets to the point of oliguria, this is the body's attempt to hold on to any water it can as it is severely volume depleted. Monitoring urine output is an accurate way to determine the severity of fluid loss in a dehydrated client.

2. **What does the nurse expect to implement in the care of a client with mild dehydration?**
   a. Intravenous fluid replacement therapy.
   b. Oral rehydration.
   c. Sodium restriction.
   d. NPO status.

   Topic/Concept: Homeostasis **Subtopic:** Dehydration **Bloom's Taxonomy:** Applying **Clinical Problem-Solving Process:** Planning **NCLEX-PN®:** Reduction of Risk Potential **QSEN:** Safety **CJMM:** Generate Solutions

   Rationale: Sodium restriction is inappropriate in most cases, as it is only retained in the body's attempt to hold in water with dehydration. The best and safest course of action in mild dehydration is oral rehydration, allowing the client to rehydrate naturally. Intravenous fluids are only needed in more severe levels of dehydration.

   THIN Thinking: *Help Quick* – Least invasive measures should be employed first as they have the lowest risks.

3. **What action should the nurse implement when trying to prevent respiratory alkalosis in a hyperventilating client?**
   a. Constantly reassure the client so they will calm down and breathe deeply.
   b. Give the client a high dose of antianxiety medication.
   c. Hyperventilation causes acidosis, not alkalosis.
   d. Have the client breathe in and out into a paper bag.

   Topic/Concept: Homeostasis **Subtopic:** Respiratory Alkalosis **Bloom's Taxonomy:** Applying **Clinical Problem-Solving Process:** Evaluation **NCLEX-PN®:** Physiological Adaptation **QSEN:** Evidence-based Practice **CJMM:** Take Action

   Rationale: Because hyperventilation causes too much oxygen consumption and too much release of carbon dioxide, having the client breathe into a paper bag will cause them to breathe in their carbon dioxide and prevent alkalosis. High doses of antianxiety medication may cause respiratory depression and eventual acidosis. Having the client breathe in deeply to calm down will increase oxygen consumption and worsen the alkalosis.

   THIN Thinking: *Help Quick* – Understanding the cause of a condition can also help the nurse prevent or anticipate the need to treat the condition before injury or harm occurs.

4. **When reviewing lab results, which lab value does the nurse correlate with the client's hypocalcemia?**
   a. Phosphorus 12.2 mg/dL.
   b. Calcium 9.3 mg/dL.
   c. Sodium 132 mEq/L.
   d. Potassium 4.5 mEq/L.

   Topic/Concept: Homeostasis **Subtopic:** Hypocalcemia **Bloom's Taxonomy:** Analyzing **Clinical Problem-Solving Process:** Data Collection **NCLEX-PN®:** Coordinated Care **QSEN:** Patient-centered care **CJMM:** Analyze Cues

   Rationale: Calcium and phosphorus have an inverse relationship, so if calcium is low, phosphorus is expected to be high. Sodium and potassium have a minimal direct relationship with calcium, so abnormalities are not expected to be related.

   THIN Thinking: *Top Three* – The nurse can anticipate the symptoms a client will have and the lab values expected when they understand the relationships present between electrolytes.

5. **What does the nurse prioritize when caring for a client with hyperkalemia?**
   a. Monitoring telemetry.
   b. Monitoring blood pressure.
   c. Monitoring temperature.
   d. Monitoring oxygen saturation.

   Topic/Concept: Homeostasis **Subtopic:** Hyperkalemia **Bloom's Taxonomy:** Applying **Clinical Problem-Solving Process:** Planning **NCLEX-PN®:** Safety and Infection Control **QSEN:** Safety **CJMM:** Prioritize Hypotheses

   Rationale: High potassium levels can lead to fatal dysrhythmias making monitoring of telemetry a high priority. Blood pressure, temperature, and oxygen saturation are not as much a priority because if these are affected, it would only be indirectly due to poor perfusion from a dysrhythmia.

   THIN Thinking: *Top Three* – Close monitoring is critical in electrolyte imbalances of all kinds, but potassium is the most crucial imbalance to watch as this most highly impacts the heart's electrical conduction.

6. **What food does the nurse encourage the client to add to their diet to address chronic hypokalemia?**
   a. Apples.
   b. Oranges.
   c. White rice.
   d. Eggplant.

   Topic/Concept: Homeostasis **Subtopic:** Hypokalemia **Bloom's Taxonomy:** Applying **Clinical Problem-Solving Process:** Planning **NCLEX-PN®:** Health Promotion and Maintenance **QSEN:** Patient-centered care **CJMM:** Generate Solutions

   Rationale: Oranges are high in potassium and should be added. Apples, eggplant, and white rice are all low in potassium.

   THIN Thinking: *Clinical Problem-Solving Process* – Dietary supplementation can prevent and treat many conditions. Knowing which foods are high and low in particular substances will give the nurse the best opportunity to inform their clients properly.

7. **What finding is consistent with the client's diagnosis of hypermagnesemia?**
   a. Muscle cramps.
   b. Confusion.
   c. Dyspnea.
   d. Seizures.

   Topic/Concept: Homeostasis **Subtopic:** Hypermagnesemia **Bloom's Taxonomy:** Analyzing **Clinical Problem-Solving Process:** Data Collection **NCLEX-PN®:** Coordinated Care **QSEN:** Teamwork and Collaboration **CJMM:** Analyze Cues

   Rationale: Muscle cramps, seizures, and confusion are related to low magnesium; dyspnea can be caused by hypermagnesemia.

   THIN Thinking: *Clinical Problem-Solving Process* – Distinguishing between symptoms of low or high electrolyte levels will help the nurse identify expected findings and help them identify the effectiveness of treatment and identify if the treatment has lowered or raised a level too much.

8. **The nurse monitors telemetry for a client with hypomagnesemia. What telemetry finding indicates the condition is worsening, and the client will require immediate intravenous administration of supplemental magnesium to reverse its life-threatening effects?**
   a. Atrial fibrillation.
   b. Ventricular fibrillation.
   c. Junctional tachycardia.
   d. Torsades de pointes.

   Topic/Concept: Homeostasis **Subtopic:** Hypomagnesemia **Bloom's Taxonomy:** Applying **Clinical Problem-Solving Process:** Implementation **NCLEX-PN®:** Pharmacological Therapies **QSEN:** Evidence-based Practice **CJMM:** Take Action

   Rationale: Ventricular fibrillation, junctional tachycardia, and atrial fibrillation are not related to low magnesium as a causative factor; only torsades de pointes is caused by this condition. Also, AFib and junctional tach are not life-threatening.

   THIN Thinking: *Help Quick* – Understanding dysrhythmias and their causes is imperative when preserving life. Torsades de pointes is caused by hypomagnesemia and corrected by intravenous administration of this supplement.

9. **When evaluating a client with hypernatremia, what factor does the nurse expect to address as the probable cause of their condition?**
   a. Severe, watery diarrhea.
   b. Severe indigestion.
   c. Fluid overload.
   d. Hypertension.

   Topic/Concept: Homeostasis **Subtopic:** Hypernatremia **Bloom's Taxonomy:** Applying **Clinical Problem-Solving Process:** Evaluation **NCLEX-PN®:** Safety and Infection Control **QSEN:** Safety **CJMM:** Evaluate Outcomes

   Rationale: Hypernatremia occurs with dehydration, so vomiting and diarrhea need to be addressed to reduce hypernatremia. Indigestion, hypertension, and fluid overload are not risk for hypernatremia.

   THIN Thinking: *Clinical Problem-Solving Process* – Treatment of an underlying cause will often correct a problem and prevent the need for further treatments. The nurse should know how to identify the causative factor related to electrolyte imbalances.

10. **What statement by the client illustrates an understanding of their education on preventing the reoccurrence of hyponatremia?**
   a. "I will be sure to increase my dietary intake of sodium to 4000 mg daily."
   b. "I will drink at least 2 gallons of water daily to prevent dehydration."
   c. "I will take an extra water pill when I notice swelling in my legs."
   d. "I will drink a sports drink after extensive exercise instead of water."

   Topic/Concept: Homeostasis **Subtopic:** Hyponatremia **Bloom's Taxonomy:** Analyzing **Clinical Problem-Solving Process:** Evaluation **NCLEX-PN®:** Health promotion and maintenance **QSEN:** Patient-centered care **CJMM:** Evaluate Outcomes

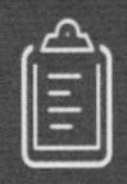

Rationale: Excessive sweating can cause the release of large amounts of sodium, and sports drinks will help replace that when plain water won't. A dietary intake of sodium should not be more than 2000 mg daily, or hypernatremia, heart problems, and fluid overload may become issues. Excessive water intake of 2 gallons a day can cause deadly levels of hyponatremia. Extra dosing of diuretics can cause severe dehydration and sodium imbalances.

THIN Thinking: *Clinical Problem-Solving Process* – Nurses need to evaluate the client's understanding of their treatment plan and be sure they understand how to implement that plan correctly to ensure they treat themselves appropriately.

11. **Which client would the nurse identify as being at the highest risk of hyperphosphatemia?**
    a. Kidney failure on dialysis.
    b. Heart failure on beta-blockers.
    c. Older adult with dementia.
    d. Pregnant with advanced age.

Topic/Concept: Homeostasis **Subtopic:** Hyperphosphatemia **Bloom's Taxonomy:** Applying **Clinical Problem-Solving Process:** Planning **NCLEX-PN®:** Reduction of Risk Potential **QSEN:** Evidence-based Practice **CJMM:** Prioritize Hypotheses

Rationale: Clients with kidney failure, even if they are on dialysis, are at the highest risk of hyperphosphatemia as the kidneys do not function to pull out excess phosphorus. All others listed do not have significantly increased risks.

THIN Thinking: *Top Three* – Clients in renal failure can be educated on lowering hyperphosphatemia risks by managing their diet. They may also be prescribed phosphorus binding medications or calcium baths on dialysis to help lower their levels when diet management is not enough.

12. **What finding does the nurse understand is related to the client's diagnosis of hypophosphatemia?**
    a. Chronic alcoholism.
    b. Dehydration.
    c. Seizure disorder.
    d. Hyperlipidemia.

Topic/Concept: Homeostasis **Subtopic:** Hypophosphatemia **Bloom's Taxonomy:** Applying **Clinical Problem-Solving Process:** Data Collection **NCLEX-PN®:** Coordinated Care **QSEN:** Patient-centered care **CJMM:** Analyze Cues

Rationale: Chronic alcohol use can cause hypophosphatemia. Dehydration can raise levels. Low levels can cause seizures. Hyperlipidemia has no identified relation.

THIN Thinking: *Clinical Problem-Solving Process* – Phosphorus levels need to be maintained as they are inversely related to calcium levels and can affect bone integrity. Management of levels starts with identifying factors that affect the levels and addressing those factors.

13. **When planning client care, which client does the nurse consider to be at the highest risk of developing metabolic acidosis?**
    a. Bulimic client.
    b. Child with hypokalemia.
    c. Hyperventilating client.
    d. Older adult client on diuretics.

Topic/Concept: Homeostasis **Subtopic:** Metabolic acidosis **Bloom's Taxonomy:** Analyzing **Clinical Problem-Solving Process:** Planning **NCLEX-PN®:** Reduction of Risk Potential **QSEN:** Evidence-based Practice **CJMM:** Prioritize Hypotheses

Rationale: Hypokalemia, hyperventilation, and self-induced vomiting can all increase the risk of alkalosis. Older adult clients on diuretics are at the highest risk of metabolic acidosis.

THIN Thinking: *Identify Risk to Safety* – Understanding risk factors and addressing them is an excellent preventative practice to reduce morbidity and mortality.

14. **What medications does the nurse anticipate being used to correct a client's metabolic acidosis? *Select all that apply.***
    a. Sodium bicarbonate.
    b. Hypertonic sodium.
    c. Tris-hydroxymethyl aminomethane.
    d. 0.45% sodium chloride.
    e. Furosemide.

Topic/Concept: Homeostasis **Subtopic:** Metabolic acidosis **Bloom's Taxonomy:** Applying **Clinical Problem-Solving Process:** Planning **NCLEX-PN®:** Pharmacological Therapies **QSEN:** Evidence-based Practice **CJMM:** Generate Solutions

Rationale: Sodium bicarbonate and tris-hydroxymethyl aminomethane are used to reverse acidosis. Hypertonic solution and diuretics may worsen acidosis. Sodium chloride 0.45% will also not be effective in the treatment of this imbalance.

THIN Thinking: *Top Three* – Proper treatment regimens must be anticipated to ensure safety. The nurse should know what is and isn't used to treat a specific condition to reduce potential treatment errors.

15. **The nurse evaluates several clients and their lab results. Which data prompts the nurse to plan interventions to address metabolic acidosis?**
   a. Glucose 635 mg/dL.
   b. Glucose 60 mg/dL.
   c. Sodium 140 mEq/L.
   d. Sodium 125 mEq/L.

Topic/Concept: Homeostasis **Subtopic:** Metabolic acidosis **Bloom's Taxonomy:** Analyzing **Clinical Problem-Solving Process:** Data Collection **NCLEX-PN®:** Safety and Infection Control **QSEN:** Safety **CJMM:** Analyze Cues

Rationale: Low to normal sodium levels and low glucose levels will not cause metabolic acidosis. High glucose levels can cause metabolic acidosis and states like diabetic ketoacidosis.

THIN Thinking: *Help Quick* – Being aware of specific conditions clients are at risk for helps the nurse plan and monitor the clients to avoid complications from these conditions.

16. **Which prescription does the nurse question when implementing the treatment plan for a client with metabolic alkalosis?**
   a. Administer potassium intravenously.
   b. Administer sodium bicarbonate intravenously.
   c. Discontinue supplemental oxygen therapy.
   d. Infuse sodium chloride 0.9% intravenously at 80 mL per hour.

Topic/Concept: Homeostasis **Subtopic:** Metabolic alkalosis **Bloom's Taxonomy:** Applying **Clinical Problem-Solving Process:** Implementation **NCLEX-PN®:** Reduction of Risk Potential **QSEN:** Evidence-based Practice **CJMM:** Take Action

Rationale: Sodium bicarbonate will worsen alkalosis and should not be administered to this client. All other orders are appropriate for a client in metabolic alkalosis.

THIN Thinking: *Identify Risk to Safety* – Proper treatment regimens must be anticipated to ensure safety. The nurse should know what is and isn't used to treat a specific condition to reduce potential treatment errors.

17. **Which lab result indicates to the nurse that the client will need interventions to treat metabolic alkalosis?**
   a. HCO3 32 mEq/L.
   b. pH 7.20.
   c. PO2 42 mmHg.
   d. PCO2 38 mmHg.

Topic/Concept: Homeostasis **Subtopic:** Metabolic alkalosis **Bloom's Taxonomy:** Analyzing **Clinical Problem-Solving Process:** Data Collection **NCLEX-PN®:** Physiological Adaptation **QSEN:** Patient-centered care **CJMM:** Analyze Cues

Rationale: The Ph is acidic, so this is not indicative of metabolic acidosis. The pO2 and pCO2 are both indicators of respiratory status and not metabolic status. The HCO3 indicates metabolic function, and since it is alkaline, it will be elevated in alkalosis.

THIN Thinking: *Clinical Problem-Solving Process* – Understanding the effects that conditions have on lab values will help the nurse prepare proper interventions for the treatment of clients.

18. **What finding suggests a causative factor for a client diagnosed with respiratory acidosis?**
   a. Hyperventilation.
   b. Severe anxiety disorder.
   c. Overdose of oxycodone.
   d. Mechanical ventilation.

Topic/Concept: Homeostasis **Subtopic:** Respiratory acidosis **Bloom's Taxonomy:** Analyzing **Clinical Problem-Solving Process:** Data Collection **NCLEX-PN®:** Safety and Infection Control **QSEN:** Safety **CJMM:** Analyze Cues

Rationale: Hyperventilation, which may be caused by severe anxiety, causes excess oxygen consumption and respiratory alkalosis. Mechanical ventilation will also put the client at risk for respiratory alkalosis. Overdose of oxycodone or other narcotics will depress respirations, causing increased retainment of CO2 and respiratory acidosis.

THIN Thinking: *Identify Risk to Safety* – Understanding the cause of a condition can also help the nurse prevent or anticipate the need to treat the condition before injury or harm occurs.

19. **A nurse receives these arterial blood gas results from the lab. Which nursing actions should the nurse anticipate?**
    a. Provide high-flow oxygen via face mask.
    b. Elevate the head of the bed to 90 degrees.
    c. Administer prescribed intravenous anxiolytic.
    d. Provide a bag for the client to breath in and out.

Topic/Concept: Homeostasis **Subtopic:** Acid-base balance **Bloom's Taxonomy:** Applying **Clinical Problem-Solving Process:** Implementation **NCLEX-PN®:** Reduction of Risk Potential **QSEN:** Safety **CJMM:** Take Action

Rationale: The arterial blood gas results reflect respiratory alkalosis, with a low carbon dioxide level associated with hyperventilation. The nurse would use a paper bag or mask to allow for rebreathing of carbon dioxide.

THIN Thinking: *Help Quick* – This is an action that can be rapidly implemented to increase carbon dioxide levels.

20. **What finding does the nurse attribute to the client's diagnosis of chronic respiratory acidosis?**
    a. Blurred vision.
    b. Personality changes.
    c. Decreased level of consciousness.
    d. Tachycardia.

Topic/Concept: Homeostasis **Subtopic:** Respiratory acidosis **Bloom's Taxonomy:** Applying **Clinical Problem-Solving Process:** Data Collection **NCLEX-PN®:** Basic Care and Comfort **QSEN:** Patient-centered care **CJMM:** Recognize Cues

Rationale: Tachycardia, decreased LOC, and blurred vision are all symptoms of acute respiratory acidosis. Personality changes are indicative of chronic respiratory acidosis.

THIN Thinking: *Clinical Problem-Solving Process* – Long-term respiratory acidosis causes chronic symptoms and a reversed respiratory drive compelled by high carbon dioxide levels instead of low oxygen levels.

CHAPTER

9

Respiration

Oxygenation / Gas Exchange

This chapter addresses conditions that impair or damage respiration, including oxygenation and gas exchange disorders. We have learned the importance of airway patency and breathing in sustaining and living a quality life. Nurses play a significant role in monitoring for changes in oxygenation and ventilation, anticipating changes in gas exchange, and providing interventions to enhance or restore respiration.

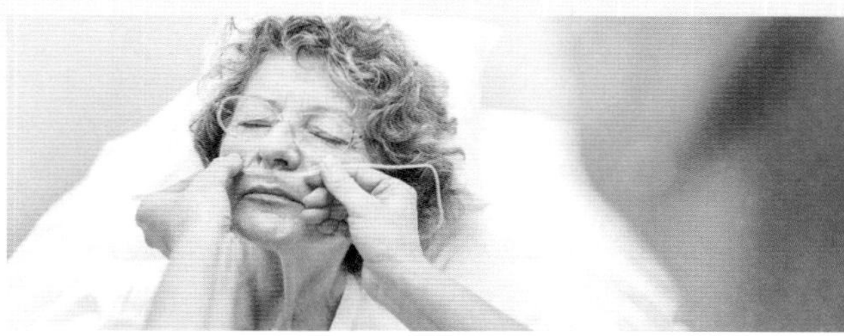

Image 9-1: In addition to monitoring airway patency and breathing, what other nursing actions do you anticipate for a client receiving oxygen via nasal cannula?

Priority Exemplars:

- Asthma
- Pneumonia
- Tuberculosis
- Bronchiolitis/lower airway infections
- Upper airway infections
- Croup syndromes/epiglottitis
- Chronic obstructive pulmonary disease (COPD)
- Cystic fibrosis (CF)
- Sickle cell anemia (SSA)
- Iron-deficiency anemia
- Pulmonary hypertension
- Acute respiratory distress syndrome (ARDS)
- Chest trauma/pneumothorax

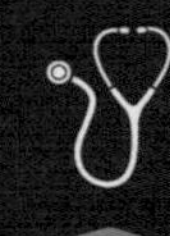

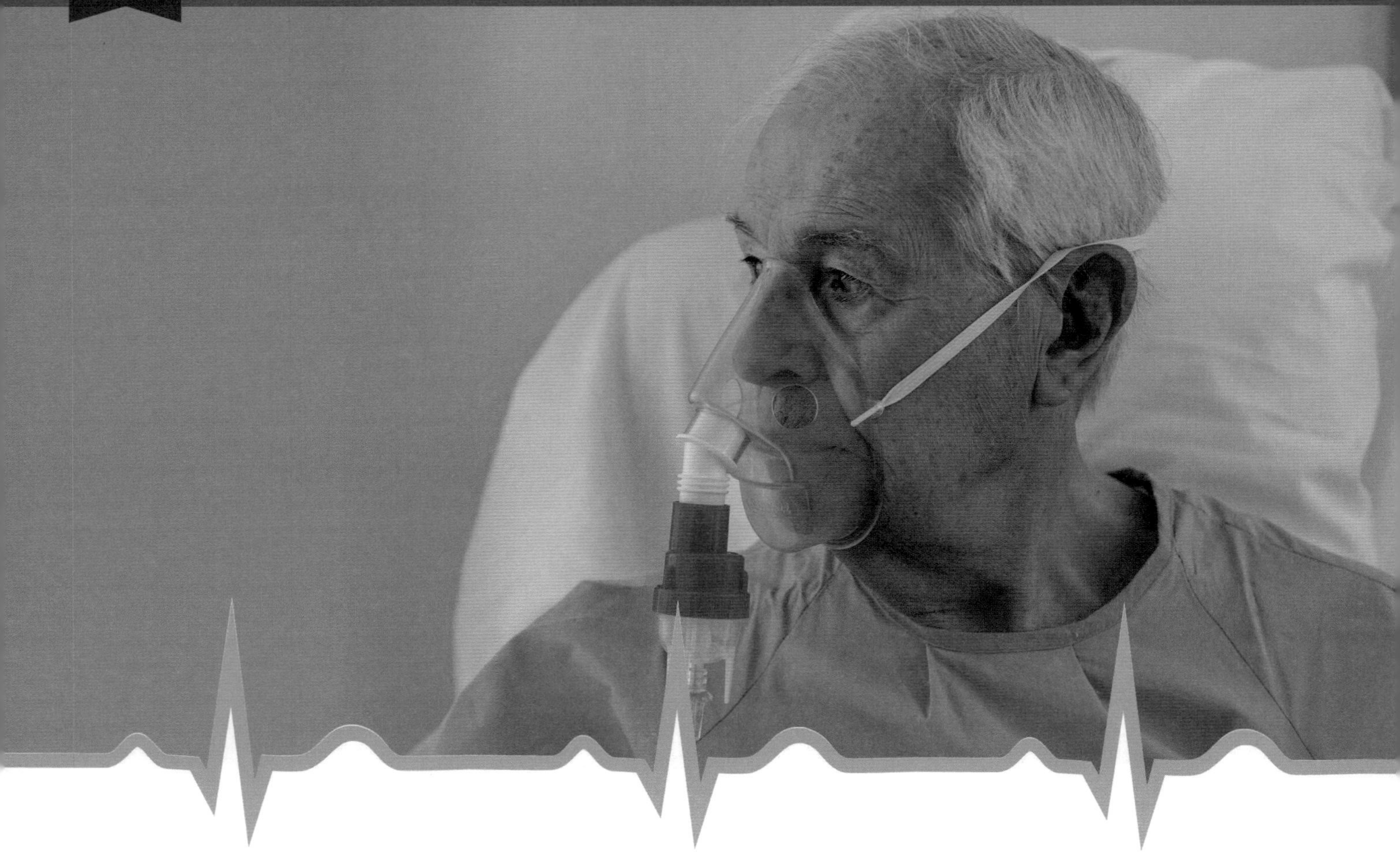

Go To Clinical

Go To Clinical Case 1

E.W. is a 70-year-old man admitted to the acute care unit from the emergency department. His wife brought him to the ED due to coughing throughout the night, wheezing, and shortness of breath that was unresponsive to omalizumab (Xolair) and ipratropium bromide (Atrovent). The nurse notes that he is unable to lie down on the stretcher, is using accessory muscles to breath, and appears anxious.

E.W.'s wife states he had been doing so well on his current treatment regimen; she thinks his asthma may have been triggered due to the housecleaning they did together last week. She states E.W. is highly allergic to dust. The nurse notes the client feels hot and auscultates the client's lungs. There are wheezes in the upper lobes and decreased breath sounds in the lower lobes.

The nurse notes that the client's vital signs are: Temperature 104.1°F (40.1°C), 122 beats/minute, 32 breaths/minutes, 136/88 mmHg. His oxygen saturation is 87%. He is receiving oxygen at 2 liters/minute.

NurseThink® Time

Using the NurseThink® system, complete the priorities. Check your answers designated by 💡 in the Asthma and Pneumonia Priority Exemplars.

Clinical Hint

When a client with asthma has a decrease in the volume or presence of breath sounds, it may be an ominous sign known as the "silent chest."

NurseThink® Time

Priority Data Collection or Cues

1.

2.

3.

Priority Laboratory Tests/Diagnostics

1.

2.

3.

Priority Interventions or Actions

1.

2.

3.

Priority Potential & Actual Complications

1.

2.

3.

Priority Nursing Implications

1.

2.

3.

Priority Medications

1.

2.

3.

Reinforcement of Priority Teaching

1.

2.

3.

Pathophysiology/Description

- Allergen/antigen mediated hypersensitive reaction
- Results in decreased airflow due to inflammation, bronchoconstriction, hyperresponsiveness, airway obstruction, airway edema, and mucus production and/or stasis
- Types include exercise-induced, allergic, infantile as manifested by eczema, food intolerance, allergic rhinitis
- Known as a chronic disease with acute exacerbations, classified based on severity of symptoms: Severe persistent, moderate persistent, mild persistent, and intermittent
- Increased risk factors include exposure/responses to allergens, hereditary factors; exposure to smoking or maternal smoking during pregnancy, low birth weight (LBW), obesity

Priority Data Collection or Cues

- Monitor vital signs and oxygen saturation
- Respiratory effort including increased work of breathing, non- or productive cough, forced expiration, retractions, nasal flaring
- Breath sounds may include a wheeze, coarse breath sounds, prolonged expiration, decreased breath sounds (lack of air movement-ominous sign), may have dyspnea with speech
- Ask about tightness of chest, chest pain, itching around neck, headache, fatigue, coughing at night
- Observe for restlessness, air hunger, tripod positioning, pursed lips, irritability, apprehension, cyanosis

Priority Laboratory Tests/Diagnostics

- Chest X-ray for infiltrates and hyperexpansion/pneumonia
- Pulmonary function tests/spirometry-presence and degree of pulmonary involvement/evaluate response to treatment
- Bronchoprovocation testing-exposure to antigens/skin testing
- Peak expiratory flow rate-peak flow meter-establish personal best and compare to peak flow at times of respiratory distress
- White blood cell count to determine infection
- Arterial blood gases for hypercapnia and respiratory acidosis

Priority Interventions or Actions

- Position client to aid in breathing-tripod or sitting with head forward, 100% oxygen therapy unless contraindicated
- Identify and alleviate triggers—environmental and lifestyle control; use of air conditioners/filters and dehumidifiers
- Medications—a combination of preventer/long-term and rescue/quick relief agents. Intravenous access during acute attack

Priority Potential & Actual Complications

- Airway remodeling/damage to structure that is nonresponsive to anti-inflammatory and other treatments
- Hypoxemia, respiratory acidosis, respiratory failure, death

Priority Nursing Implications

- Reinforce teaching about use of metered-dose inhalers, dry powder inhalers, spacers, nebulizers, abdominal breathing, and pursed-lip breathing, stress management
- Discuss with clients about environmental and trigger control
- Advise clients about benefits of breathing exercises and physical exercises as ways to enhance conditioning
- Monitor for status asthmaticus/, "silent chest", medical emergencies, or deterioration of status requiring intubation and ventilatory support

Priority Medications

- Rescue/quick-relief medications
    - Short-acting beta-agonists—albuterol (caution with heart disease-tachycardia); inhaler or nebulizer
    - Anticholinergics-ipratropium inhaler or nasal spray
    - Systemic steroids-methylprednisolone; oral or intravenous
- Maintenance/long-term control medications
    - Inhaled steroids/encourage mouth care after use
    - Cromolyn and nedocromil-maintenance therapy-via nebulizer and metered-dose inhaler
    - Long-acting beta-agonists—salmeterol powder inhaler
    - Methylxanthines-theophylline oral (only when not responsive to other treatments) or Aminophylline
    - Leukotriene modifiers; oral
- Omalizumab-monoclonal antibodies for use in clients resistant to inhaled corticosteroids; subcutaneous injection

Reinforcement of Priority Teaching

- Advise clients to avoid personal triggers such as animal dander, pollen, mold, food additives/foods, strong emotions, cold air, exercise, aspirin, upper respiratory infection (URI), exposure to cold environmental temperatures, endocrine factors, dust, cockroach antigen/feces
- Avoid overuse of short-acting beta-agonists to avoid rebound bronchospasm or lack of effective bronchodilation during an attack
- Hydration to liquefy secretions
- Ensure that clients have an asthma action plan-monitor for symptoms, monitoring peak flow readings, and action steps
- Discuss personal early symptoms of asthma and means to intervene or seek emergency help early with clients

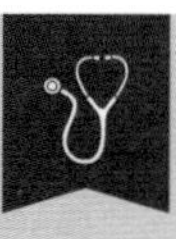

Go To Clinical Answers

Text designated by the icon are the top answers for the Go To Clinical related to Asthma.

Pneumonia

Pathophysiology/Description

- Infection of the lung parenchyma (bacterial, viral, or mycoplasma)
- Community-acquired pneumonia (CAP) is the leading cause of death in individuals 65 years and older
- Incompetent defense mechanism (air filtration, epiglottis, cough reflex, bronchoconstriction, or the mucociliary escalator mechanism) or virulent causative factors lead to pneumonia
- Three causative mechanisms include aspiration, inhalation, or hematogenous spread from other locations in the body
- Types include community-acquired pneumonia (CAP), medical care associated pneumonia (MCAP), healthcare-associated pneumonia (HCAP), hospital-acquired pneumonia (HAP), and ventilator-associated pneumonia (VAP)

Priority Data Collection or Cues

- Monitor for causative factors, including exposure to air pollution, cigarette smoking, upper respiratory infections, age (> 65 years), abdominal/chest surgery, altered levels of consciousness, immobility, chronic illness, inhalation injuries, immunosuppression, smoking, malnutrition, residence in long-term care, and endotracheal intubation
- Observe for risk factors for aspiration pneumonia, including decreased level of consciousness, dysphagia, nasogastric intubation, or decreased gag or cough
- Monitor for risk of opportunistic pneumonia including immunosuppression, malnutrition, or history of radiation and chemotherapy
- Observe for common symptoms including non-productive cough, chills, dyspnea, fever, tachypnea, pleuritic chest pain, green/yellow/rust sputum, fatigue, diaphoresis, anorexia, headache, and abdominal pain
- In older adults, initial and progressive symptoms may include decreased level of consciousness, confusion, and hypothermia
- Auscultate breath sounds for wheezes, crackles, decreased breath sounds, and increased fremitus

Priority Laboratory Tests/Diagnostics

- Chest X-ray may show consolidation, infiltrates, and effusions
- Thoracentesis and bronchoscopy may be done if infection is refractory to other treatments
- Sputum specimen
- Blood cultures
- Arterial blood cultures demonstrate hypoxia, hypercapnia, and acidosis
- Elevated white blood cell count (> 15,000/microliter)
- C-reactive protein levels may assist with antibiotic choice/ sensitivity

Priority Interventions or Actions

- Oxygen therapy
- Antibiotics
- Analgesics for chest pain/antipyretics
- Rest and activity as tolerated
- Adequate hydration and nutrition

Priority Potential & Actual Complications

- Pleurisy, pleural effusion, empyema, pneumothorax
- Atelectasis, lung abscess, pericarditis, meningitis
- Bacteremia and sepsis, acute respiratory failure

Priority Nursing Implications

- Do not delay use of antibiotics for culture results
- Implement preventative practices such as activity/ ambulation, checking nasogastric tube placement, aspiration precautions, oral care, coughing and deep breathing, turning, incentive spirometry, tracheostomy care

Priority Medications

- Levofloxacin; orally or intravenous
  - For clients with CAP with other health issues
  - For clients with HCAP/MCAP
- Erythromycin; orally, intravenous or IM (also topical and opthalmic for other indications)
  - For clients with CAP in otherwise healthy individuals

Reinforcement of Priority Teaching

- Avoid cigarette smoking
- Pneumococcal vaccine for at-risk individuals and older adults
- Adequate nutrition, hydration, mobility, and effective coughing in immobile, postoperative, and at-risk clients

Next Gen Clinical Judgment

How did E.W.'s diagnosis of asthma contribute to his contraction of pneumonia? How might E.W. and his wife prevent infections and control his asthma in the future?

Go To Clinical Answers

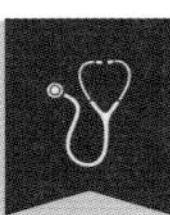

Text designated by 💡 are the top answers for the Go To Clinical related to Pneumonia.

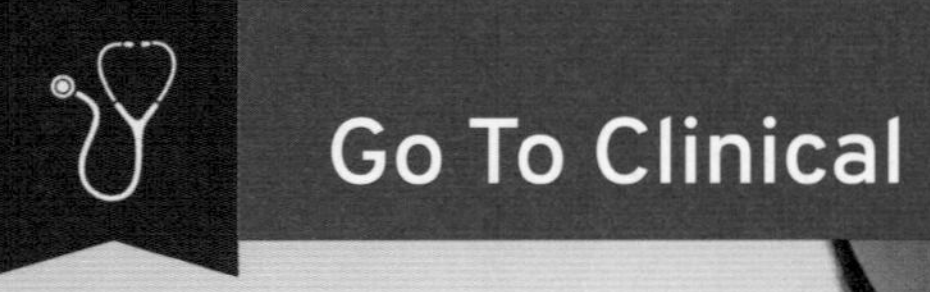

Go To Clinical

Go To Clinical Case 2

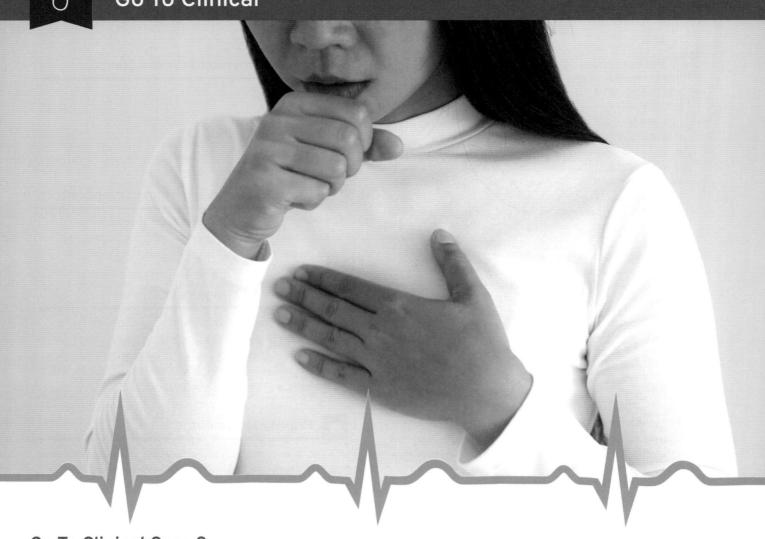

A nurse works at a local health department in the immunization clinic. A client needs to show proof of a negative purified protein derivative (PPD) test before starting her job in the healthcare field. The client is excited to start her new job at a healthcare agency and she recently immigrated to the United States. The client came to the clinic two days ago to obtain a PPD test. She returned to the clinic to have the results read. After looking at the results, it appears the client may have a positive result. Determine the priorities for the nurse.

Clinical Hint

Tuberculosis is a critical public health concern and nurses need to have a comprehensive knowledge of the signs, symptoms, and diagnostic procedures associated with this diagnosis.

NurseThink® Time

Using the NurseThink® system, complete the priorities. Check your answers designated by 💡 in the Tuberculosis Priority Exemplar.

Next Gen Clinical Judgment

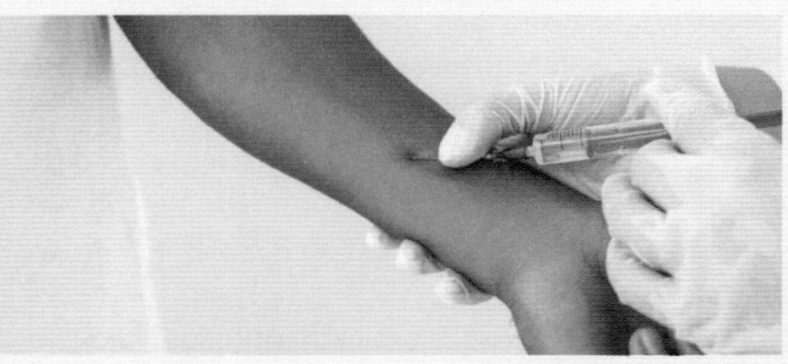

Image 9-2: What is the meaning of a positive ppd? What comments do you have about this practitioner's injection technique?

NurseThink® Time

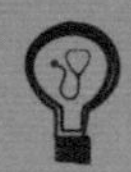

Priority Data Collection or Cues

1.

2.

3.

Priority Laboratory Tests/Diagnostics

1.

2.

3.

Priority Interventions or Actions

1.

2.

3.

Priority Potential & Actual Complications

1.

2.

3.

Priority Nursing Implications

1.

2.

3.

Priority Medications

1.

2.

3.

Reinforcement of Priority Teaching

1.

2.

3.

Pathophysiology/Description

- Tuberculosis (TB) caused by *Mycobacterium tuberculosis*
- Leading cause of death in world, high co-morbidity with HIV
- Previously eradicated in the US, increase in prevalence related to increased immunosuppressed populations, migration, and among those living in poverty
- Spread via airborne droplets, requires close, frequent exposure or decreased immunocompetence to contract
- May be primary, latent (asymptomatic/can't transmit), or reactivated; may be pulmonary or extrapulmonary

Priority Data Collection or Cues

- Monitor clients for risk factors related to social and occupational history/social determinants
- Observe for dry cough, fatigue, malaise, anorexia, weight loss, low-grade fevers, and night sweats
- Later in disease, dyspnea, hemoptysis, high fever, chills, flu-like symptoms, pleuritic pain, productive cough, decreased breath sounds, and afternoon temperature elevation
- Early symptoms in older adults-cognitive decline
- With extrapulmonary forms, monitor for dysuria/hematuria (renal), headache, vomiting, lymphadenopathy (tuberculin meningitis) or pain and decreased range of motion (bone and joint involvement)

Priority Laboratory Tests/Diagnostics

- Tuberculin skin test as purified protein derivative (PPD), site read 48 to 72 hours after injection for induration. A positive test indicates exposure to TB
- Interferon release assays
- Chest X-ray (CXR) for infiltrates
- Bacteriostatic studies including sputum for acid-fast bacillus. Three consecutive morning specimens recommended for disease confirmation

Priority Interventions or Actions

- Outpatient management optimal
- Long-term antimicrobials; multidrug therapy has changed the way disease is managed and increased prognosis; several first and second line regimens available
- Follow-up CXRs and bacterial studies
- Latent TB is treated for 6-9 months with isoniazid (INH)

Priority Potential & Actual Complications

- Pulmonary scarring/pulmonary effusions/pneumonia/ decreased pulmonary function
- Miliary TB with systemic spread
- Extrapulmonary may include peritonitis, meningitis, and vertebral degeneration
- May be fatal

Priority Nursing Implications

- Initiate and maintain airborne isolation including negative pressure room and high efficiency particulate air masks (HEPA)
- Isolate for two weeks after starting medications
- Reinforce importance with long-term/complex drug therapy to ensure eradication of disease. May initiate direct observing taking medication practices (DOT)
- BCG vaccine recommended for those who are continuously exposed to TB including healthcare workers
- Report TB to local health departments

Priority Medications

- Isoniazid (INH); orally or intravenous
  - No alcohol with medication, may increase hepatotoxicity
  - Periodic monitoring of liver function
- Rifampin; orally or intravenous
  - Causes orange discoloration of body fluids
  - Monitor for thrombocytopenia and/or hepatitis
  - Not with liver disease or during pregnancy
- Pyrazinamide; orally
  - May enhance uric acid buildup and symptoms of gout
  - Hepatotoxic, may cause arthralgia
- Ethambutol; orally
  - May decrease visual acuity, monitor frequently
  - May inhibit green red color differentiation

Reinforcement of Priority Teaching

- The importance of adherence to medication regimen and the reasons for treatment plans to prevent drug resistance and reactivation
- Screen contacts and determine need for treatment
- While at home encourage client to sleep alone, spend time outside, encourage adequate ventilation of living spaces, and hygiene with tissues, bed linens, and strict handwashing
- Advise clients about symptoms of relapse and the role of smoking in fostering relapse (cessation)

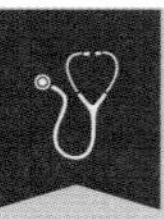

Go To Clinical Answers

Text designated by ⓖ are the top answers for the Go To Clinical related to Tuberculosis.

Pathophysiology/Description

- Inflammation of the bronchioles producing copious, thick mucus
- Most frequent origin is respiratory syncytial virus (RSV) which is highly virulent and communicable via contact with respiratory secretions
- Most often contracted in winter and spring
- Rare in children over 2 years of age, peak incidence at 6 months and in children at risk across childhood (risk associated with prematurity, congenital heart disease, chronic respiratory disorders, bronchopulmonary dysplasia, or immunosuppression)
- Most common cause for hospitalization of infants less than one year of age
- See also Pneumonia Priority exemplar

Priority Data Collection or Cues

- Monitor for early symptoms including nasal, eye, and ear drainage, copious nasal secretions, nasal crusting, pharyngitis, dry cough, sneezing, wheezing, fever, poor oral intake, and irritability
- Observe for symptoms as disease progresses including air hunger, tachypnea, retractions, crackles in the lung fields, and cyanosis
- Monitor for severe disease including a respiratory rate over 70 breaths/minute, decreased breath sounds and air movement, apneic periods, significant restlessness

Priority Laboratory Tests/Diagnostics

- Culture of nasal or nasopharyngeal (NP) secretions
- Pulse oximetry to determine oxygen saturation
- Rapid immunofluorescent antibody/direct fluorescent antibody staining
- Arterial blood gases if indicated

Priority Interventions or Actions

- Cool humidified oxygen
- Hydration
- Elevate head of bed
- Attempt small frequent feedings to encourage oral intake
- Suction as needed using bulb or nasopharyngeal suctioning
- Intravenous/nasogastric hydration or nasogastric feedings as indicated
- May require ventilatory support

Priority Potential & Actual Complications

- Pneumonia
- Respiratory failure from fatigue
- Electrolyte imbalance
- Apnea/respiratory arrest

Priority Nursing Implications

- Contact (gown/gloves) and/or droplet (gown/gloves/mask) isolation practices
- Ensure a private room or cohort with other children with RSV
- Do not assign nurses with RSV with other clients who may be at risk or who are immunosuppressed
- Encourage mothers who breastfeed to pump and preserve milk if infants taking no or low oral intake

Priority Medications

- Palivizumab
  - Monoclonal antibody therapy
  - Prevention of RSV in high-risk groups (including preterm children born earlier than 32 weeks gestation)
  - IM injection monthly for 5 months from November to March
  - Also available intravenous
- Ribavirin
  - Inhaled antiviral agent
  - Decreases duration and severity of viral infection
  - Potential toxic effects to exposed healthcare workers

Reinforcement of Priority Teaching

- Breastfeeding to increase immune function
- Strict handwashing
- Need for prevention of exposure to secondhand smoke
- Assist family to instill normal saline solution nose drops before meals and at bedtime to encourage sleep and oral intake
- Limiting exposure of affected clients to others who are at risk/may contract RSV

Clinical Hint

The airway of a child is approximately the same diameter as the small "pinkie" finger. This highlights the potential for compromise of infants' and children's airways due to mucus, bronchoconstriction, or edema.

Upper airway infections

Pathophysiology/Description

- Tonsillitis is inflammation of the tonsils/lymph tissue in the pharynx
- Adenoiditis is inflammation in the glands in the posterior pharynx
- Viral nasopharyngitis (NP) is often referred to as a "URI" or the "common cold"
- Acute streptococcal pharyngitis due to Group A beta-hemolytic streptococcus (GABHS) may lead to an acute or chronic issue in clients
- Tracheobronchitis is a mild viral infection that often occurs with a "URI"

Priority Data Collection or Cues

- Upper airway infections often characterized by a dry, hacking, non-productive cough which may be worse at night, rhinorrhea, chills, poor oral intake, open-mouth breathing, lethargy, nausea/vomiting, fever, and malaise
- Monitor for tonsillitis including sore throat, dysphagia, fever, mouth breathing, malodorous breath, and cough
- Observe for adenoiditis including nasal speech, snoring, sleep apnea, hearing difficulties, and mouth breathing

Priority Laboratory Tests/Diagnostics

- Diagnosis based on symptoms
- GABHS throat culture/rapid antigen testing

Priority Interventions or Actions

- Mild infections treated with cool, humidified air, increasing hydration, allowing rest, and antipyretics. These infections usually resolve in 4 to 10 days
- Warm salt-water gargles may relieve symptoms
- Bacterial infections treated symptomatically and with antibiotics
- Chronic tonsillitis/adenoiditis may indicate the need for surgical removal of tonsils and adenoids
- May develop secondary bacterial infections after viral infection which lower resistance

Priority Potential & Actual Complications

- With untreated GABHS, complications include acute glomerulonephritis, scarlet fever, rheumatic fever, and cardiac valve damage/rheumatic heart disease

Priority Nursing Implications

- For clients with URI, antitussives are only recommended in select situations. They may suppress the natural cough mechanism, are to be used only with a dry cough that disrupts sleep or is annoying. Instead, expectorants are encouraged to mobilize secretions
- Nursing care for clients having tonsillectomy/adenoidectomy (T & A) may include
    - Reinforce preoperative teaching plans to ensure preparation of child and to assist family to watch for infection and bleeding in the postoperative period
    - Postoperative care includes analgesics, use of an ice collar as tolerated, and watching for post-op bleeding/hemorrhage (bloody drool, frequent swallowing, pallor, or restlessness), discourage coughing/clearing throat/nose-blowing which may cause bleeding
    - Encourage client to lay on side to allow for drainage of secretions. Have suction available for emergencies
    - Postoperative fluids should be clear, non-citrus, and non-carbonated. Do not use red or brown fluids which may be mistaken for blood. Avoid milk or thick fluids that may cause clearing of the throat
    - Advance to a soft diet as tolerated, avoiding irritating foods

Priority Medications

- Analgesia after T & A
    - Morphine
        - Intravenous narcotic for severe pain
        - Watch for respiratory depression
    - Acetaminophen with codeine; orally
        - For moderate postoperative pain
        - Need to eat crackers or small snack to avoid nausea/vomiting
        - May cause constipation
- Nasopharyngitis/viral/URI
    - Acetaminophen; oral
        - Antipyretic
        - May be used for mild pain
    - Decongestants; oral or nasal spray/drops
        - Nasal more effective than systemic
        - Not with children less than 6 years of age
        - 2 drops per nares, wait 10 minutes, repeat
        - Use for less than 3 days to prevent rebound congestion
- GABHS
    - Amoxicillin via oral route
    - PCN G via intramuscular route
        - Used when adherence is difficult
        - May include procaine to decrease pain of injection

Reinforcement of Priority Teaching

- Advise family how to make saline/salt solution for home use
- Reinforce teaching plan with family about postoperative medication and feeding of clients after a T&A including the potential for the scab to slough up to 10 days postoperatively and to observe for bleeding, to avoid sharp objects in mouth, and monitor for fever
- After GABHS, get a new toothbrush 24 hours after beginning antibiotics
- Avoid spread of infections through handwashing, staying away from crowds, safe tissue handling, fluids, and rest

Croup syndromes/epiglottitis

Pathophysiology/Description

- Laryngitis is a common viral syndrome, often associated with the "common cold"
- Laryngotracheobronchitis (LTB) is the most common type of croup; most often associated with children < 5 years, may be bacterial or viral
- Epiglottitis is a bacterial form of croup, characterized by inflammation of the epiglottis and has a rapid onset
  - H. Flu immunizations (H. Influenzae type B-HIB) have decreased incidence
  - Most often in children 2-8 years but may be at any age
  - Medical emergency as may progress quickly to respiratory distress and edema of epiglottis may cause total airway obstruction

Priority Data Collection or Cues

- Observe for laryngitis including headache, malaise, nasal congestion, and hoarseness
- Monitor for LTB including low-grade temperature, brassy/barky cough, inspiratory stridor, retractions, cough, hoarseness, tachypnea, and restlessness. May progress to stridor, retractions, hypoxia/hypercapnia, cyanosis, and apnea
- Collect data related to epiglottitis including fever, drooling, pain with swallowing, dysphagia, dyspnea, restlessness, tachycardia, tachypnea, increased work of breathing, retractions, nasal flaring, and inspiratory stridor
- Observe client's position of choice/comfort. Client may tripod body position to breathe
- Monitor for progression to respiratory distress
- Observe client's level of consciousness

Priority Laboratory Tests/Diagnostics

- Treatment often based on symptoms
- For epiglottitis, neck X-rays may be done to confirm diagnosis
- ABGs to monitor for hypercapnia, hypoxia, and respiratory acidosis
- Pulse oximetry for oxygen saturation

Priority Interventions or Actions

- For laryngitis, treatment is symptomatic
- For LTB with mild croup/no stridor at rest, management may be at home using cool mist vaporizers. Counsel family to expose to cool air with respiratory distress (take child to basement, garage, open freezer door, go outside, cool shower). Encourage rest, oral hydration, elevate head of bed, analgesics, and antibiotics (if bacterial). Hospitalization indicated for increased respiratory distress or poor hydration status
- For epiglottitis
  - No oral temperatures, manipulation of mouth/visualization/no tongue depressors
  - Keep client calm/with caregivers, sitting up, in position of comfort, do not restrain
  - Cool mist oxygen therapy with least invasive method (blow-by mask held by family member)
  - Keep NPO
  - Determine ability to attain intravenous access, defer to airway management if child becomes upset. intravenous hydration and antibiotics if able
  - Analgesics and antipyretics
  - May require nasotracheal intubation/tracheostomy

Priority Potential & Actual Complications

- Airway occlusion and lack of access to airway (epiglottitis)
- Respiratory failure
- Respiratory arrest

Priority Nursing Implications

- Advocate for family participation in care to keep child calm. Allow child to sit in caregiver's lap for all care and provide age-appropriate distraction/instruction as indicated
- For epiglottitis, follow agency protocol for resuscitation equipment availability/transfer of client to the operating room for all assessments/care due to potential need for surgical intervention/tracheostomy
- Croup may require droplet isolation as a precaution in hospital until organism is specified or on antibiotics for 24 hours
- May use Heliox (helium/oxygen) to decrease edema and work of breathing

Priority Medications

- Methylprednisolone
  - Intravenous steroid
  - Decreases airway inflammation in epiglottitis
- Dexamethasone
  - Oral steroids
  - Single dose for inflammation of LTB
- Epinephrine
  - Nebulized, racemic
  - Reduces airway edema

Reinforcement of Priority Teaching

- Emergency procedures related to epiglottitis and provide support in efforts to keep child calm and resting during respiratory distress. Inform about comfort measures and the importance of cuddling
- Recommend that the family avoids antitussives which depress the cough reflex
- Client and family reinforcement of teaching about signs of deteriorating respiratory status
- HIB vaccine
- May provide prophylactic antibiotics for family/contacts depending upon infectious organism

Chronic obstructive pulmonary disease (COPD)

Pathophysiology/Description

- Airway obstruction secondary to emphysema (permanent enlargement of alveoli) or chronic bronchitis (consistent, unrelieved cough) and concurrent inflammatory changes
- Symptoms related to inflammation of central airways/ destruction of cilia, remodeling of peripheral airways, destruction of pulmonary parenchyma, and pulmonary vascular changes leading to ineffective gas exchange, mucus hypersecretion, hyperinflation of lungs, loss of recoil, alveolar destruction, and airflow limitation
- Generally associated with cigarette smoking/passive smoking/environmental tobacco smoke. Also related to occupational chemicals/dust, air pollution, and infections
- Genetic components associated with α1-antitrypsin deficiency
- Although symptoms present and increase with aging, it is not known if aging is a risk factor
- COPD may occur with asthma
- An increased number of women are now diagnosed with COPD (increased smoking) and may have poorer outcomes (smaller airways, decreased quality of life)
- COPD is progressive, with constant/non-fluctuating airway resistance, is not usually reversible

Priority Data Collection or Cues

- Monitor for risk factors including tobacco smoking, occupation, and environmental exposure
- Observe for cough, exertional dyspnea, sputum production, weight loss (monitor weight over time), later-dyspnea at rest
- Observe dyspnea during speech by counting the number of words a client can say between breaths is a measurable demonstration of dyspnea and responses to care
- Auscultate breath sounds for wheezing/crackles, prolonged expiration, decreased breath sounds
- Monitor vital signs for tachypnea, cardiac dysrhythmias
- Observe for barrel chest, use of accessory muscles
- Ask about orthopnea, number of pillows used in bed
- Collect data about confusion or changes in level of consciousness
- Observe and document characteristics of sputum including amount, color, thickness
- Determine client's ability to cough and expectorate sputum, provide suction as needed

Clinical Hint

Differentiate clients with emphysema (Pink Puffers) from chronic bronchitis (Blue Bloaters). Use these descriptors to consider your nursing care of each of these conditions.

Priority Laboratory Tests/Diagnostics

- Chest X-ray may show congestion and hyperinflation, flattening of diaphragm
- Arterial blood gases for hypoxemia, hypercapnia, and respiratory acidosis
- Pulmonary function tests for forced vital capacity/Forced expiratory volume (FEV_1/FVC) <70% (lower percentages = decreased capacity)
- CBC: Polycythemia
- Sputum culture and sensitivity

Priority Interventions or Actions

- Administer oxygen and titrate with pulse oximetry readings/ arterial blood gases. Use caution with oxygen administration and maintain low-flow to preserve hypoxic drive to breathe—may use CPAP or BiPAP
- Place client in sitting position and/or leaning forward—use overbed table or hands to knees (tripod)
- Treatment based on symptoms and severity as in GOLD (Global Initiative for Chronic Obstructive Lung Disease) classification of airway limitation
- Administer breathing treatments and strategies to clear the airway
- Encourage small, frequent meals and hydration to liquefy secretions; encourage high calorie/high-protein diet
- Provide antibiotics in case of infection/pneumonia
- Activity as tolerated and progress as able
- Advise client to employ diaphragmatic or abdominal breathing techniques and pursed-lip breathing to maintain end-expiratory pressure and exhale carbon dioxide

Priority Potential & Actual Complications

- COPD exacerbations with increased severity and frequency
- Creation of bullae (air spaces in the tissue) and blebs (air collection in open spaces)
- Deterioration in lung capacity/pulmonary hypertension and cor pulmonale (Right heart failure)
- Acute respiratory failure
- Depression and anxiety

Next Gen Clinical Judgment

Why is oxygen limited in some clients with COPD or clients with carbon dioxide retention? What are the consequences of high flow/concentration oxygen if used in clients with COPD/carbon dioxide retention?

Priority Nursing Implications

- Be aware of many administration devices including metered dose inhalers, dry powder inhalers, nebulizers, and the use of spacers
- Nurses may work at institutions that use standardized dyspnea and COPD scales
- Troubleshoot and use oxygen delivery devices safely. Observe for skin breakdown, airway dryness, client tolerance of device, need for humidity
- Medications for COPD are usually increased as the client's symptoms intensify
- Note that clients with COPD have lower baseline oxygen norms. Oxygen should not be increased above 2 liters/minute to avoid respiratory depression

Priority Medications

- Bronchodilators
  - To decrease dyspnea and increase FEV_1
  - Via inhaler or nebulizer
  - Adrenergic agonist-albuterol
  - Anticholinergics-ipratropium, tiotropium
  - May be as needed (PRN) or scheduled
- Mucolytics; oral inhaler, intratracheal, nebulizer
- Corticosteroids; nasal, inhaler, oral, nebulizer
  - Fluticasone with salmeterol
  - Oral steroids only used during exacerbations—prednisone
- Antibiotics; orally, intravenous, nebulizer
  - Recommended if client has dyspnea, has increased sputum volume, or sputum is purulent (or if client is on mechanical ventilation)

Reinforcement of Priority Teaching

- Try to avoid others with respiratory infections, crowds during high-risk periods, and ensure immunizations (influenza and pneumococcal vaccine)
- Encourage smoking cessation
- Safety aspects of oxygen therapy at home including continuous use improves prognosis, portability, maintaining oxygen supplies, battery backup, delivery mechanisms
- If dusting, use a wet cloth to avoid free-floating of dust and avoid environmental allergens/triggers such as open flames, feathers, extremes in temperatures, and dust
- Home oxygen therapy risk for combustion, oxygen toxicity, absorption atelectasis, infection

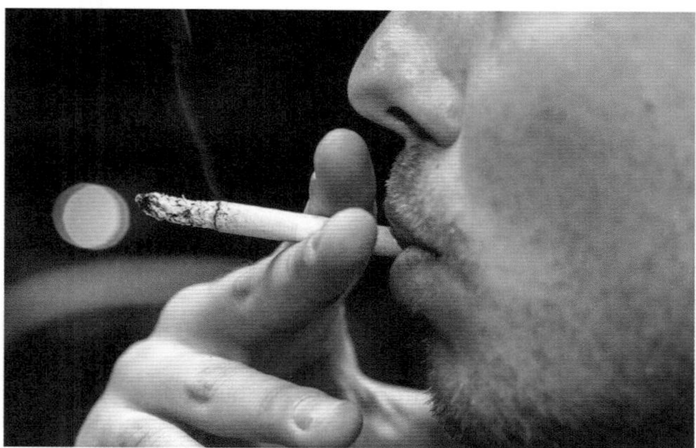

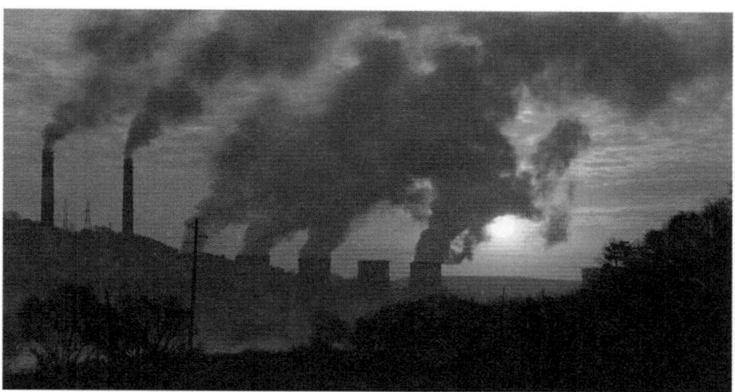

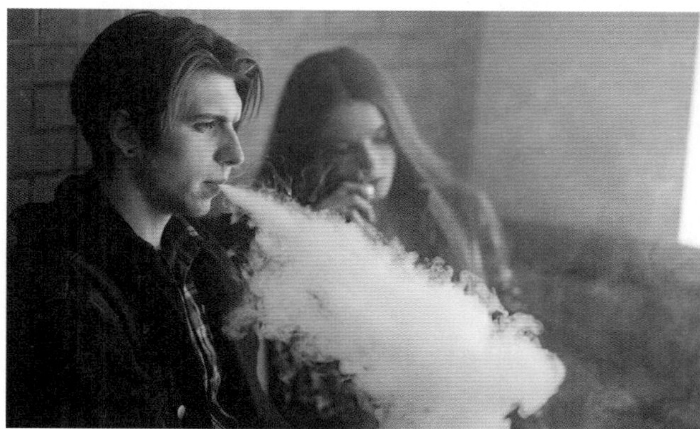

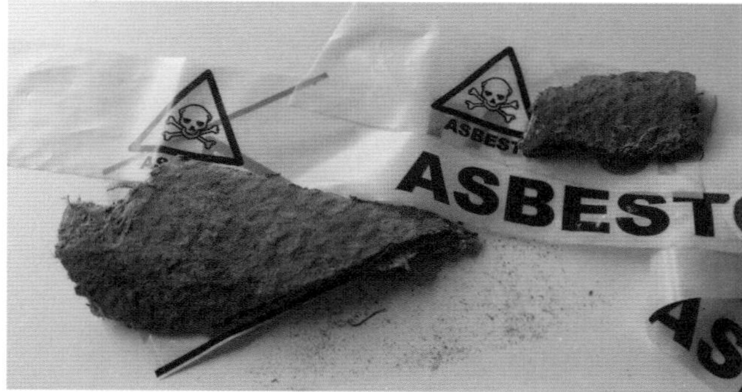

Image 9-3: Each of these images depicts a risk factor for COPD. How would you assist clients with COPD to understand the relationships of these images to their disease?

Cystic fibrosis (CF)

Pathophysiology/Description

- Dysfunction of the exocrine (mucus-producing) glands, effects many systems
- Most common lethal genetic disorder of Caucasians
- Inherited as an autosomal recessive trait (if both parents carry trait, each pregnancy as a 1:4 chance of the disease)
- Cystic fibrosis transmembrane regulator (CFTR) reduces cells' transporting of chloride
- Lungs most effected
  - Increased thick, tenacious mucus
  - Mucus retention/obstruction
  - Pneumonia, hypoxia, hypercapnia, acidosis
- Increased electrolytes in sweat, may yield electrolyte disturbances
- Increased viscosity of the pancreatic mucus producing glands
  - Pancreatic duct fibrosis
  - Enzymes unable to reach duodenum, impairing digestion
- Many males are sterile; females have copious uterine/cervical secretions. Women who conceive are at risk for preterm labor and low-birth-weight infants

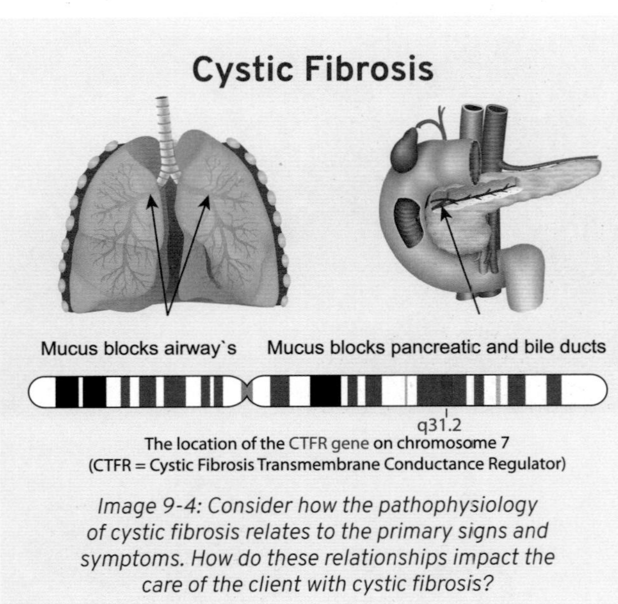

Image 9-4: Consider how the pathophysiology of cystic fibrosis relates to the primary signs and symptoms. How do these relationships impact the care of the client with cystic fibrosis?

Priority Data Collection or Cues

- Collect data on pulmonary signs/symptoms including wheezing, dry, non-productive chronic cough, dyspnea, signs of upper and lower airway respiratory infections/involvement, decreased breath sounds over areas of atelectasis
- Determine changes in appearance including barrel chest, clubbing of fingers and toes, cyanosis, lack of weight gain despite adequate intake/growth failure, signs of anemia (pallor, fatigue, shortness of breath, tachycardia)
- Ask about history of meconium ileus, frequent respiratory infections, or dry mouth
- Monitor for gastrointestinal signs/symptoms such as large/bulky frothy stools containing undigested food, volume of stools increased with solid food, steatorrhea (stools float in toilet) and azotorrhea (foul smelling due to protein)
- Parents may report the child "tastes salty" from elevated sodium in the sweat

Priority Laboratory Tests/Diagnostics

- Positive sweat chloride test (pilocarpine iontophoresis)—requires 75 grams of sweat—normal <40 mEq/L (mean 18 mEq/L); Diagnosed with 2 readings of >60 mEq/L
- Negative pancreatic enzyme lab findings
- Chest X-ray for pulmonary changes
- Pulmonary function testing
- Newborn screening is part of newborn panel-nonreactive trypsinogen analysis
- Genetic testing-mutations on CTR/Δ F508 gene (may be done in utero)
- Stool—72-hour samples for fats and enzymes
- Early diagnosis leads to better management
- Screening of parents may be done prenatally or prior to pregnancy

Priority Interventions or Actions

- Early treatment and prophylactic antibiotics
- Ensure airway clearance. Provide chest physiotherapy, percussion and postural drainage, high frequency chest compressions via vests, exercise, positive expiratory therapy (flutter mucus clearance device), huffing/forced expiration, handheld percussors, positive expiratory pressure mask
- Bronchodilators to break down mucus, inhaled powdered mannitol (rehydrate airway), nebulized hypertonic saline (hydrate secretions), aerosolized or intravenous antibiotics
- Long-term NSAIDs treatment (ibuprofen) to prevent inflammation
- Pancreatic enzymes that are titrated to food eaten and a high protein, high calorie, unrestricted fat diet is recommended (determine need for supplemental NaCl)

Priority Potential & Actual Complications

- Hyponatremia when profusely sweating or during fever
- Chronic respiratory infections (pneumonia)
- Acidosis with hypoxia and hypercapnia
- Pulmonary fibrosis or rupture of blebs causing pneumothorax
- Pulmonary hypertension and/or cor pulmonale; may indicate need for lung transplantation

- Chronic sinusitis and bone erosion
- Pancreatic fibrosis may lead to type 1 and type 2 diabetes mellitus
- Gastroesophageal reflux
- Prolapsed rectum
- Hypoalbuminemia and generalized edema
- Bleeding related to decreased Vitamin K absorption
- Liver and biliary cirrhosis or meconium ileus equivalent/ distal intestinal obstruction syndrome
- Respiratory failure
- May be fatal

Priority Nursing Implications

- Nurses are an important part of the multidisciplinary management of CF
- The family requires considerable support and assistance; despite many breakthroughs, a diagnosis with cystic fibrosis shortens the life expectancy and presents difficulty during exacerbations
- Clients are prone to infections. Nurses need to assist clients and families in balancing isolation from infectious sources and quality of life
- Nurses should be vigilant for early signs of respiratory infections (fever, tachypnea, increased dyspnea, characteristics of sputum)
- Nurses may provide home care to provide peripherally inserted catheter (PICC) or port medications and pulmonary care to prevent hospitalization and exposure to pathogens
- Clients are hypercapnic, therefore, oxygen must be administered carefully to prevent extinguishing the hypoxic drive to breath
- Children with CF metabolize medications differently and may need higher doses
- Pancreatic enzymes are enteric coated to be functional in the intestines. Do not crush or chew but capsule beads may be "sprinkled" over food. Enzymes may be inactivated in hot food

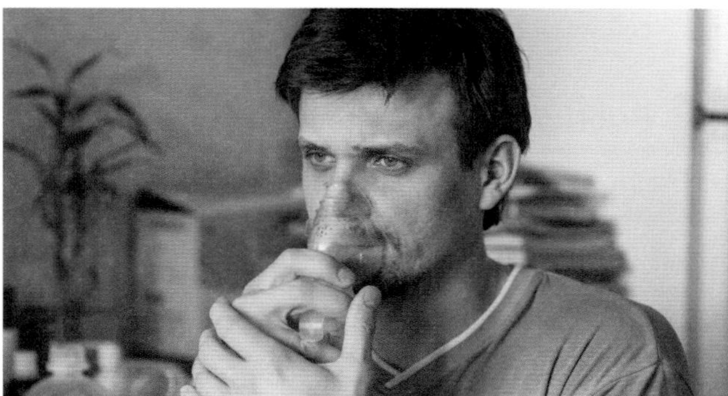

Image 9-5: Describe the procedure for administering a medication via nebulizer to a client. What data should the nurse collect before and after a nebulizer treatment?

Priority Medications

- Ibuprofen
  - Oral antiinflammatory
  - Monitor for GI erosion or bleeding
  - Monitor serum levels- maintain a blood level of 50-1000 mcg/mL
- Dornase alfa
  - Antibiotic
  - Decreases viscosity of the secretions
  - Given via nebulizer
- Tobramycin
  - Antibiotic
  - Given via nebulizer
  - Prevent infections
- Systemic antibiotics
  - Prevent or treat pulmonary infections
  - Nebulized or given intravenous via peripherally inserted central catheter (PICC) or port
- Oral water miscible solutions of vitamins A,D,E, & K

Reinforcement of Priority Teaching

- Parents and caregivers must consider the developmental age of the child—the regimen is rigorous and children/teens may not always adhere to procedures
- Nurses are often a key component of transitioning the child with cystic fibrosis to adult services, healthcare professionals, and support groups
- Family must learn to provide pulmonary/airway clearance care at least twice/day, often 4-6 times/day
- Nurses may offer resources to the teen/young adult with cystic fibrosis to become independent with personal healthcare. The regimen for cystic fibrosis is very rigorous and clients must learn to devote a significant amount of time and energy to staying healthy
- Client/family how to titrate pancreatic enzymes to achieve the optimal number of stools per day and for optimal growth; reinforce the importance of a high calorie/well-balanced diet
- Advise on nasal lavage to prevent/treat chronic sinusitis
- Assist client to establish an exercise program that is both fun and effective in mobilizing respiratory secretions
- Ensure that parents monitor their child for growth and achieving developmental milestones
- The need for routine immunizations and the annual influenza vaccination
- Inform parents about community and national resources to assist in coping with this diagnosis

Sickle cell anemia (SSA)

Pathophysiology/Description

- Inherited autosomal recessive disorders
- Sickled hemoglobin cells (Hgb S) with decreased oxygen carrying capacity cause vascular occlusion
- Sickled cells increase hemostasis which increases sickling
- Types include sickle cell anemia, Hgb C disease, sickle cell thalassemia, and sickle cell trait
- May not be apparent in newborn or younger infants due to the presence of functioning fetal hemoglobin
- Vaso-occlusive crisis (VOC) is severe and painful vessel blockage, characterized by plasma loss, tissue ischemia, necrosis, and shock
- Sequestration crisis is pooling of blood in liver
- Aplastic crisis occurs with increased destruction and decreased production of healthy red blood cells

Priority Data Collection or Cues

- Determine factors that increase cellular sickling, including fever, hypoxia, infections, emotional and physical stress, high altitude, blood loss, dehydration, acidosis, hypothermia, and surgery
- Monitor for a variety of symptoms depending on number of sickled cells, during remission may only have mild anemia and mild to moderate pain
- During exacerbation, pain may be moderate to severe
- Collect data related to fever, swelling of joints, tenderness around liver/spleen/joints, tachypnea, hypotension, nausea/vomiting, chest pain, dyspnea, pallor/gray skin/ mucous membranes, and jaundice
- Observe for priapism which is a sustained, painful, and engorged penile erection
- Monitor for splenomegaly/hepatomegaly

Priority Laboratory Tests/Diagnostics

- Peripheral blood smears for Hgb S
- Skeletal X-rays
- Chest X-ray
- Serum electrolytes as indicated
- Magnetic resonance imaging for cerebral vessels/ cerebrovascular accident
- Doppler studies for deep vein thromboses
- Newborn and other screening with sickle turbidity test

Clinical Hint

Anything that causes physical or emotional stress may exacerbate SSA symptoms or stimulate a crisis. Therefore, clients should be monitored carefully during illness or when they experience stressors.

Priority Interventions or Actions

- Avoid crisis-precipitating factors
- Provide rest and pain management
- Provide supplemental oxygen to relieve hypoxia
- Provide intravenous hydration and correct electrolyte imbalances
- For leg ulcers, treat with saline soaks and assist with debridement/grafting
- For priapism, provide fluids, pain medications, nifedipine, or penile injection of epinephrine
- Provide antibiotics to treat or prevent infection
- Monitor blood transfusions/red blood cell exchange transfusions to manage anemia
- Provide chelation therapy to reduce transfusion associated high iron levels
- Hematopoietic stem cell transplantation (research ongoing related to effectiveness/use)

Priority Potential & Actual Complications

- Vaso-occlusive/aplastic/sequestration crises
- Infection/pneumonia
- Leg ulcers
- Priapism
- Retinal detachment/blindness
- Osteoporosis/osteosclerosis
- Cholelithiasis/hepatomegaly
- Renal failure/hematuria
- Pulmonary failure/heart failure/cor pulmonale/pulmonary hypertension/pulmonary embolism
- Splenic scarring/functional autosplenectomy
- Acute chest syndrome including pneumonia, tissue infarction, and fat embolism
- Cerebrovascular accident (CVA)/stroke

Priority Nursing Implications

- Ensure clients with SSA receive immunizations (meningococcal/pneumococcal)
- Due to chronicity of pain, clients may become tolerant and dependent upon opiates. Nurses need to provide pain management and assist clients to deal with chronic pain
- Titrate pain medications and use client-controlled (PCA)/ continuous analgesia when available (meperidine is not suggested because high/sustained doses associated with seizures)
- Support newborn screening for SSA (standard in the US)

Priority Medications

- Morphine or hydromorphone
  - Intravenous narcotic for severe pain, may be used with PCA
  - Monitor for respiratory depression, tolerance, and dependency
- Nifedipine
  - Used to relieve priapism; oral
- Deferoxamine
  - Parenteral chelation therapy to remove excess iron
- Deferasirox
  - Oral iron chelation therapy
- Hydroxyurea; oral
  - Chemotherapy agent used to increase levels of fetal hemoglobin
  - Increases red blood cell volume/decreases sickled cells
  - Decreases sickled cell adhesion to blood vessel endothelium
  - May prevent CVA

Reinforcement of Priority Teaching

- Monitoring for and prevention of complications
- Requires ongoing monitoring and surveillance by healthcare professionals, including regular eye exams
- Intervene early with infections, signs/symptoms, and potential risk factors (hydration, stress, temperature/weather changes, infections)
- Provide support and referral to resources to assist in coping with the emotional burden of SSA, including depression, anxiety, and crisis intervention
- Refer to genetic counseling for children and subsequent pregnancies

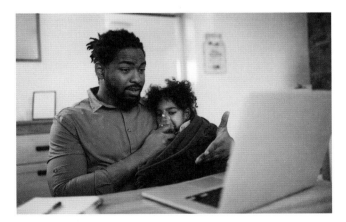

Image 9-6: A client with sickle cell anemia is treated at home with oxygen to prevent hypoxemia. What signs and symptoms would indicate the need for hospitalization or emergency care?

Symptoms of Sickle Cell Anemia

Fatigue and Decreased Hemoglobin

Eye Damage

Bacterial Infections

Bouts of Pain

Leg Ulcers

Pulmonary and Heart Diseases

Thrombosis in the Spleen and Liver

Swelling and Inflammation of the Fingers, Toes, Arthritis

Image 9-7: Consider how the pathophysiology of sickle cell anemia relates to the primary signs and symptoms.

Next Gen Clinical Judgment

You are a nurse caring for the following three clients. What concerns you most about each of these clients?

1. An infant with a respiratory rate of 50 breaths/minute, nasal flaring, and using his belly to breath.
2. A 12-year-old child with a history of asthma who uses his rescue inhaler 4-6 times per day.
3. A 5-year-old child who has not received immunizations presents with a high fever and is drooling.

Treatment of Sickle Cell Anemia

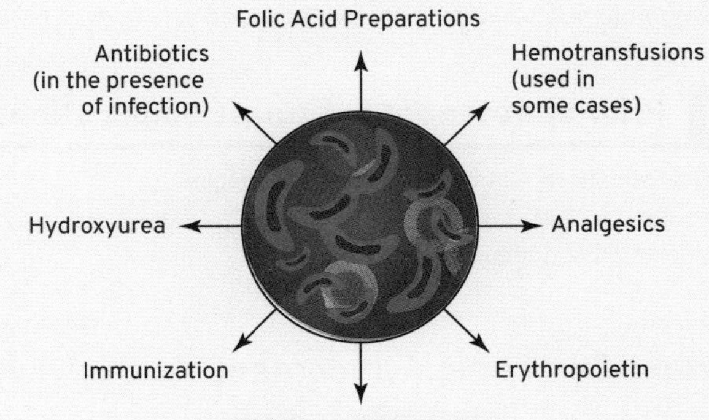

Image 9-8: Consider how the pathophysiology of sickle cell anemia relates to the primary treatment strategies.

Pathophysiology/Description

- Most common hematologic disorder, affects 2-5% of adult men and post-menopausal women, may be higher among very young clients and women in the reproductive years (menstruating, pregnant)
- Causes include inadequate dietary intake, blood loss, hemolysis, malabsorption, and nutritional deficiencies associated with alcoholism

Priority Data Collection or Cues

- Determine risk in pregnant and menstruating women, those with malabsorption (gastric bypass and removal), chronic blood loss (gastric bleed secondary to peptic ulcer, gastritis, hemorrhoids, and diverticulitis), chronic kidney disease (dialysis, frequent blood draws, or erythropoietin deficiencies)
- Observe for pallor, glossitis, cheilitis, headache, paresthesias, burning of tongue, fatigue, tachycardia (if severe)

Priority Laboratory Tests/Diagnostics

- Hemoglobin and hematocrit
- Red blood cells and reticulocytes
- Serum iron, ferritin, and transferrin levels
- Total iron-binding capacity (TIBC)
- Stool for occult blood (monitor for blood loss)

Priority Interventions or Actions

- Identify and treat underlying cause (malnutrition, blood loss, etc.)
- Nutritional therapy with foods high in iron
- Blood transfusions with severe deficiency symptoms
- Oral and parenteral iron supplements
- Ongoing monitoring of iron and red blood cell levels

Priority Potential & Actual Complications

- Complications from unexplained blood loss
- Prolonged, untreated anemia may lead to myocardial infarction and heart failure

Next Gen Clinical Judgment

A client on iron supplementation states they are "very constipated" from the medication. What recommendations might the nurse make to assist the client?

Priority Nursing Implications

- Counsel clients and monitor clients for constipation. Encourage clients to exercise, drink adequate fluids, eat high fiber diets, and take stool softeners as needed
- Encourage clients to take iron one hour before meals and with a vitamin C source (orange juice)
- If ingestion causes gastric upset, take with meals (but decreases absorption)
- Foods high in iron include liver and muscle meats, dried fruits, eggs, legumes, dark green leafy vegetables, whole grain breads, and potatoes
- Observe clients' skin color and mucous membranes with attention to baseline skin color and changes associated with iron-deficiency

Priority Medications

- Ferrous sulfate
  - Oral forms of iron should be enteric coated or sustained-release to ensure absorption in the duodenum for optimal absorption
  - Liquid oral forms of iron will stain the teeth so a straw and diluting the solution is recommended
- Ferrous gluconate
  - See above
- Iron dextran/sodium ferrous gluconate
  - Intramuscular and intravenous forms
  - Parenteral forms of iron may stimulate allergies or anaphylaxis
  - Intramuscular forms may stain and require needle changing or z-track method

Reinforcement of Priority Teaching

- Black stools are an expected side effect of iron treatment and are benign
- Client needs to take supplements for 2-3 months after a normal hemoglobin
- Clients who are recommended to take iron supplements for life should have liver enzymes monitored routinely

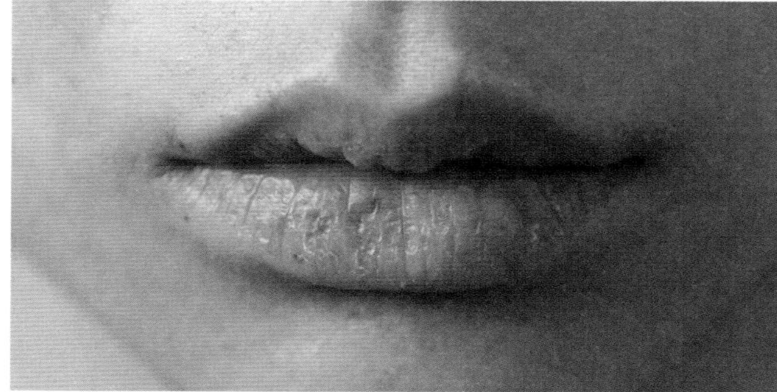

Image 9-9: How can the nurse determine pallor in clients who are Brown, African American/Black, or Caucasian/White?

Pulmonary hypertension

Pathophysiology/Description

- Elevated pulmonary artery pressure resulting in resistance to blood flow in the pulmonary circulation (normally low pressure/resistance)
- An insult (hormonal, mechanical, or other) leads to pulmonary endothelial injury (smooth muscle proliferation, vascular scarring) causing pulmonary hypertension
- May be idiopathic (primary) or secondary to other disorders such as heart failure or congenital heart defects
- Secondary often due to COPD with constriction of the pulmonary vessels secondary to hypoxia and acidosis
- Cor pulmonale is enlarged right ventricle secondary to pulmonary hypertension (usually related to COPD)

Priority Data Collection or Cues

- Monitor for dyspnea on exertion, shortness of breath, fatigue, exertional chest pain, dizziness, or exertional syncope
- May progress to dyspnea at rest or with feeding/eating
- May occur with early heart failure symptoms including peripheral edema, dyspnea, fatigue, increased pulmonic heart sounds, fourth heart sound, hepatomegaly, distended neck veins and full, bounding pulse
- Vigilantly monitor pulse oximetry

Priority Laboratory Tests/Diagnostics

- Right-sided cardiac catheterization
- Chest X-ray
- ECG
- CT scans
- Pulmonary function tests
- CBC to monitor for polycythemia secondary to chronic hypoxemia
- ABGs to determine hypoxemia

Priority Interventions or Actions

- In secondary pulmonary hypertension, treatment is most focused on management of the underlying disorder
- Low flow oxygen to keep saturations above 90%. O_2 may be long-term to correct hypoxemia
- Surgical intervention includes atrial septostomy, pulmonary thromboendarterectomy, or heart transplant
- Medications may include diuretics (reduce edema), anticoagulants (reduce production of thrombi), vasodilators (decrease pressure in vessels)
- Low sodium diet if cor pulmonale or heart failure develops
- Clients with pulmonary hypertension may be candidates for lung transplantation

Priority Potential & Actual Complications

- Right ventricular hypertrophy/cor pulmonale
- Right-sided heart failure
- May be fatal

Priority Nursing Implications

- Early intervention enhances effectiveness of treatment
- Many clients sustain significant damage prior to diagnosis
- Implement fall and safety precautions while on vasodilators and take BP frequently

Priority Medications

- Calcium channel blockers-diltiazem; intravenous
  - Vasodilates to reduce pressure in the pulmonary artery and on the right ventricle
  - Should not be used with right-sided heart failure
- Sildenafil; orally or intravenous
  - Smooth muscle relaxation to dilate blood vessels
  - Not with nitroglycerine—may cause hypotension
- Prostacyclins; orally, intravenous, subcutaneous, and inhaled routes
  - Dilate pulmonary and systemic vessels
  - Iloprost-inhaled
  - Epoprostenol-intravenous
  - May cause hypotension
- Bosentan; oral
  - Endothelin receptor antagonist
  - Decreases pulmonary artery pressure
  - Monitor liver function

Reinforcement of Priority Teaching

- Client and family reinforcement of teaching related to safe administration of medications and need to move/rise slowly after administration
- Portable oxygen to observe safety measures
- Ensure that clients and family understand the roles of diet, activity, and lifestyles in heart health and optimal respiratory function

Next Gen Clinical Judgment

A client undergoes a heart transplant secondary to severe pulmonary hypertension. What medications might be used to prevent organ rejection? What nursing care is indicated for clients on these medications?

Acute respiratory distress syndrome (ARDS)

Pathophysiology/Description

- Sudden and advanced progression of acute respiratory failure with large variability of impact and symptoms
- Characterized by hypoxemia, dyspnea, and decreased lung compliance despite increases in oxygen delivery
- Inflammatory response causing neutrophil collection, increased pulmonary capillary membrane permeability, vasoconstriction, decreased collagen, and microemboli
- Exists in 3 phases including injury/exudative (days 1-7, alveolar edema and atelectasis), reparative/proliferative (weeks 1-2, increased inflammation and fibrosis), and fibrotic (weeks 2-3, scarring, fibrosis, and decreased compliance)
- Related to systemic inflammatory response syndrome (SIRS), may be infectious or non-infectious and associated with multiorgan dysfunction syndrome (MODS)

Priority Data Collection or Cues

- Monitor for risk factors such as aspiration, viral /bacterial pneumonia, sepsis, trauma/injury, near-drowning, embolism
- Auscultate breath sounds which may be normal or include fine crackles to diffuse crackles and sonorous wheezes
- Observe for symptoms of phase 1 including dyspnea, tachypnea, cyanosis, pallor, cough, retractions, and increased work of breathing
- Watch for symptoms of phase 2 including the above and increasing hypoxemia, restlessness, and tachycardia
- Observe for symptoms of phase 3 including the above, marked hypoxia, and signs of pulmonary hypertension

Priority Laboratory Tests/Diagnostics

- ABGs show hypoxia, hypoxemia, and hypercarbia (indicate fatigue and respiratory failure), respiratory alkalosis due to tachypnea and exhalation of CO_2
- Chest X-ray showing scattered infiltrates, edema of alveoli and interstitial tissues
- Pulmonary function tests showing decreased tidal volume, compliance, and functional residual capacity
- Measured via PaO_2/FIO_2 ratio (normal PaO_2 is 85-100 mmHg at 0.21 % O_2-room air = >400). Acute lung injury ratio is 200-300. ARDS ratio is <200
- Pulmonary wedge pressure < 18 mmHg

Priority Interventions or Actions

- Identify and treat underlying cause
- Oxygen via mask, cannula, or endotracheal tube/positive pressure ventilation with positive end-expiratory pressure (PEEP)
- Check oxygen saturation frequently and keep oxygen at lowest concentration to maintain PaO_2 > 80 mmHg
- Nutrition and hydration, may include parenteral and enteral routes
- Continuous lateral rotation therapy/turning and prone positioning
- Sedation as indicated
- ECMO (extracorporeal membrane oxygenation)

Priority Potential & Actual Complications

- Sepsis/infections
- Stress ulcers
- Dysrhythmias and decreased cardiac output
- Pulmonary barotrauma
- Delirium
- Tracheomalacia or tracheal stenosis/ulceration
- MODS (multiple organ dysfunction syndrome)
- Ventilator-associated pneumonia (VAP)
- Oxygen toxicity
- May be fatal (50% mortality rate)

Priority Nursing Implications

- VAP prevention to include sterile technique with suctioning, handwashing, and oral care
- Ventilator bundle to include elevate HOB 30-45 degrees, sedation holidays to determine readiness for potential extubation, ulcer disease protocol, venous thrombosis prevention, and oral care daily with chlorhexidine
- Reduce barotrauma with lowest effective ventilator pressures

Priority Medications

- Dopamine/dobutamine/norepinephrine
  - Used to increase and maintain blood pressure/organ perfusion in critically ill clients
  - Carefully titrated via intravenous route and infusion pump
- Furosemide
  - To decrease pulmonary hypertension and edema
  - Given via intravenous when rapid effect needed. May also be given orally

Reinforcement of Priority Teaching

- Support client during this frightening experience, anxiety may increase oxygen hunger and physiological stress/ symptoms
- Family on the disease, associated stressors, course of illness, treatment, and equipment
- Refer to spiritual and emotional support systems

Chest trauma/pneumothorax

Pathophysiology/Description

- Chest trauma may be related to motor vehicle or other accidents, abuse/violence, falls, gun shot injuries, and other etiologies
- Blunt trauma (struck by an object-may include laceration of lung/cardiac tissues, compression of chest, or contralateral injuries) or penetrating trauma (open wound injuries)
- Issues include rib fracture, flail chest, pulmonary contusions, and pneumothorax; some clients may need ventilatory support related to respiratory failure
- Pneumothorax occurs when the negative pressure inside the pleural space is lost and the lung collapses
- Pneumothorax may be spontaneous (from the rupture of an emphysematous or other bleb), iatrogenic (puncture from a medical procedure or ventilator), open/traumatic (from an opening or wound in the chest wall), or tension (when there is too much positive pressure in the pleural space related to a chest injury or mechanical ventilation)
- Hemothorax is blood in pleural space. Chylothorax is lymph fluid in pleural space

Priority Data Collection or Cues

- Ask about for history of an injury, ventilator support, or other risk factors
- Monitor the respiratory status: Absent breath sounds on the affected side, cyanosis, decreased chest expansion on affected side, increased work of breathing, hypotension, tracheal deviation, tachycardia, tachypnea, sucking sound with a chest wound, subcutaneous emphysema
- Observe subjective findings: Severe chest pain, dyspnea, local pain
- Monitor for bruising, abrasions, open wound

Priority Laboratory Tests/Diagnostics

- Chest X-ray to confirm pneumothorax
- Arterial blood gases to monitor oxygenation/ventilation status
- Thoracentesis to confirm hemothorax

Priority Interventions or Actions

- Apply oxygen
- Sit client up and apply an occlusive dressing to open wound
- Prepare client and care for client with chest tube
- Stabilize flail chest with hand and then tape
- Tension pneumothorax may require needle decompression/ thoracentesis prior to or instead of chest tube drainage
- Intravenous access and fluid resuscitation/infusion of maintenance fluids
- Medicate for pain as indicated to enhance ventilation and comfort
- Monitor drainage from the chest tube and maintain the pleural drainage system

Priority Potential & Actual Complications

- Rib fractures are characterized by pain and impaired respirations
- Flail chest may be associated with blunt chest trauma, hemothorax, and fractured ribs-chest segment becomes paradoxical to rest of chest, leading to paradoxical respirations, dyspnea, cyanosis, severe pain, tachycardia, hypotension, and decreased breath sounds
- Acute respiratory failure and mechanical ventilation
- If open wound is covered, client may experience a tension pneumothorax
- Subcutaneous emphysema is air leaking into tissue around chest tube or wound site
- Cardiac tamponade is blood in pericardial sac compresses heart and prevents ventricular filling

Priority Nursing Implications

- Consider the fear, anxiety, and apprehension in a client suffering from chest trauma/pneumothorax and provide sensitive and caring support
- Chest tubes designed to drain and re-establish negative pressure in the pleural space
- During chest tube insertion, provide support and information as time will allow, assemble equipment, pre-medicate or sedate as able, position the client, and stay at the bedside to provide comfort and assistance as needed, along with monitoring client status
- Smaller wounds or those with less drainage may be relieved by a chest tube connected to a Heimlich/flutter valve and drainage system
- Pleural drainage systems include a drainage chamber, a water-seal chamber, and a suction chamber. The drainage chamber collects air and drainage. The water-seal fluctuates with respiration (tidaling), while the slow rolling bubbles in the suction chamber indicate suction is on. The amount of suction is regulated by the level of water-seal, not the amount of bubbling in the suction chamber
- Clamping of a chest tube is not recommended—if disconnected, place end of tube in water. Some practitioners clamp a chest tube before it is removed to determine client readiness, or clamp the tube intermittently during hospitalization, but practices differ

Priority Medications

- Comfort and sedation medications as indicated

Reinforcement of Priority Teaching

- Clients may go home on flutter valve systems. Reinforce teaching on home management
- Injury prevention and safety
- After a pneumothorax, educate clients about potential complications and respiratory symptoms that need to be reported to a health care provider

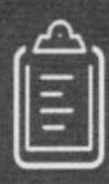

NurseThink® Quiz Questions

1. **What ultrasound finding indicates the need to add genetic testing for cystic fibrosis into a client's prenatal plan?**
   a. Ventral wall defect.
   b. Nuchal translucency.
   c. Hyperechoic bowel.
   d. Anencephaly.

2. **The nurse cares for a child with cystic fibrosis and discusses the treatment plan with the child's parents. What treatment does the nurse describe that will aid in lung health?**
   a. Administration of pancrelipase.
   b. Routine antibiotic therapy.
   c. Handwashing.
   d. Chest physical therapy.

3. **Based on the provider's note, what classification of chronic obstructive pulmonary disease severity does the nurse identify for this client?**

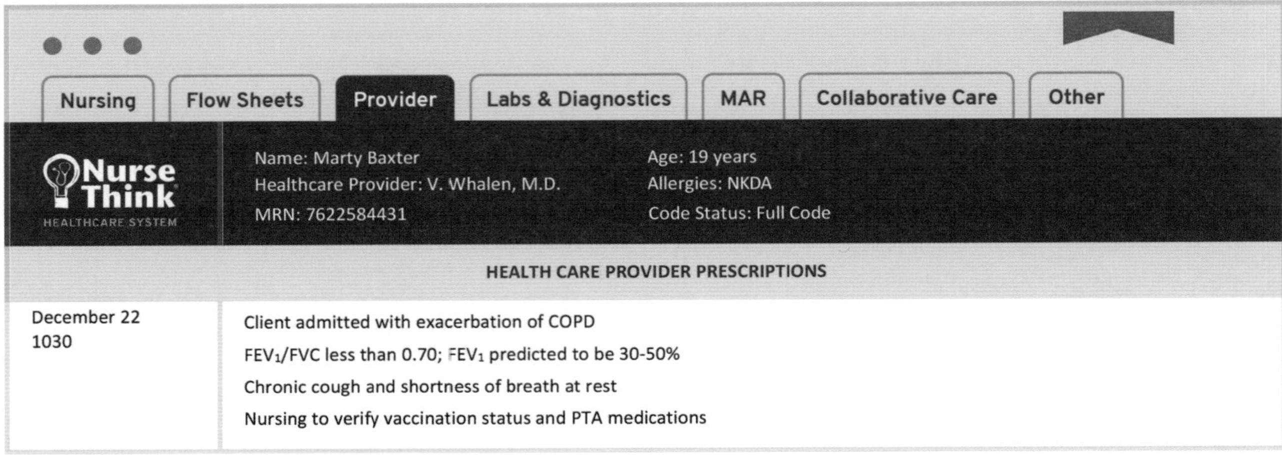

Nursing | Flow Sheets | Provider | Labs & Diagnostics | MAR | Collaborative Care | Other

Nurse Think HEALTHCARE SYSTEM

Name: Marty Baxter
Healthcare Provider: V. Whalen, M.D.
MRN: 7622584431

Age: 19 years
Allergies: NKDA
Code Status: Full Code

HEALTH CARE PROVIDER PRESCRIPTIONS	
December 22 1030	Client admitted with exacerbation of COPD FEV_1/FVC less than 0.70; FEV_1 predicted to be 30-50% Chronic cough and shortness of breath at rest Nursing to verify vaccination status and PTA medications

   a. Gold 1: Mild.
   b. Gold 2: Moderate.
   c. Gold 3: Severe.
   d. Gold 4: Very severe.

4. **The nurse provides care for a client with chronic obstructive pulmonary disease. What class of medications does the nurse expect the provider to prescribe when the client also has asthma?**
   a. Corticosteroids.
   b. Bronchodilators.
   c. NSAIDs.
   d. Methylxanthine.

5. **A client is brought to the emergency department with a spontaneous pneumothorax. What treatment does the nurse expect to assist with to help re-expand the lung?**
   a. Intubation and mechanical ventilation.
   b. Chest tube insertion.
   c. Bag-valve mask rescue breathing.
   d. Cardiopulmonary resuscitation.

6. **What findings does the nurse attribute to a client's asthma diagnosis? *Select all that apply.***
   a. Bradycardia.
   b. Tachypnea.
   c. Wheezing.
   d. Anxiety.
   e. Chest tightness.

7. **When planning care for an older adult with asthma, the nurse considers which common childhood cause a less likely trigger for adults?**
   a. Muscular weakness.
   b. Smoking.
   c. Allergies.
   d. Immune changes.

8. **The ICU nurse cares for a client with acute respiratory distress syndrome (ARDS). What finding does the nurse report as an indication of a complication from ventilator therapy?**
   a. Urine output of 50 milliliters in 2 hours.
   b. Oxygen saturation reading is greater than 90%.
   c. Asymmetrical chest rise on inspiration.
   d. Telemetry is showing sinus tachycardia.

9. **A client with Acute Respiratory Distress Syndrome (ARDS) receives BiPAP (bi-level positive airway pressure) treatment. Their respiratory rate is 35 breaths/minute, oxygen saturation is 80%, and their breathing is very labored. How does the nurse proceed?**
   a. Monitor the client closely as these findings are expected.
   b. Prepare for immediate intubation and ventilator support.
   c. Change the client to a continuous positive airway pressure system.
   d. Switch the client to 100% non-rebreather oxygen mask delivery.

10. **Which tuberculin skin test result requires treatment?**
   a. PPD 15 mm, first-time positive, no changes on chest x-ray, and asymptomatic.
   b. PPD 2 mm, has a cough for two weeks, and nausea.
   c. PPD 3 mm with an extensive area of redness surrounding the test site.
   d. PPD 7 mm, arrived from an endemic country.

11. **When evaluating a client with pneumonia, what findings does the nurse attribute to a potential complication? *Select all that apply.***
   a. Development of empyema.
   b. Pleuritis.
   c. Pleural effusion.
   d. Lung abscess.
   e. Pleuritic pain.

12. **What medication does the nurse expect to administer to a client with pneumonia whose sputum culture tested positive for Chlamydia pneumoniae?**
   a. Penicillin.
   b. Ceftriaxone.
   c. Erythromycin.
   d. Doxycycline.

13. **When reviewing a client's risks for bronchiolitis, what factor does the nurse note as a likely cause for the development of this disease?**
   a. Inhalation of sand in Iraq.
   b. History of pneumonia.
   c. Failure to receive the yearly influenza vaccine.
   d. Past pneumothorax.

14. **Place in order the stages in the infectious process. All steps may not be used.**
   a. Prodromal stage.
   b. Illness stage.
   c. Incubation stage.
   d. Convalescent stage.
   e. Acute symptomatic stage.

15. **What medications does the nurse expect to administer for almost all forms of upper respiratory infection?**
   a. Antibiotics.
   b. Corticosteroids.
   c. Bronchodilators.
   d. Diuretics.

16. **What finding causes the nurse to suspect the client has croup?**
   a. Cough improvement at night.
   b. Loud, barking cough.
   c. Hypothermia.
   d. Bradycardia.

17. **What findings does the nurse immediately report to the provider when caring for a client with croup?**
   a. Drooling and swallowing difficulty.
   b. Slow and deep breathing.
   c. Hoarseness.
   d. Fever.

18. **The nurse reinforces education for a client with pulmonary hypertension. What medication does the nurse discuss to emphasize prevention of its significant side effects?**
   a. Sildenafil.
   b. Salmeterol.
   c. Theophylline.
   d. Furosemide.

19. **What information does the nurse provide to the parent of a newborn diagnosed with sickle cell anemia? *Select all that apply.***
   a. Symptoms may not appear until 4-6 months of age.
   b. Stroke is a risk even in childhood.
   c. They should avoid low oxygen environments.
   d. Chest tightness and shortness of breath is an emergency.
   e. Side effects of hydroxyurea.

20. **Which statement by the client with sickle cell anemia illustrates the need for further reinforcement of teaching regarding their treatment plan?**
   a. "I need to be sure to stay current with vaccinations."
   b. "I should discuss family planning before becoming pregnant."
   c. "I should be careful to avoid low oxygen environments."
   d. "I need to restrict fluids in my diet to prevent fluid overload."

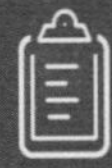

NurseThink® Quiz Answers

1. **What ultrasound finding indicates the need to add genetic testing for cystic fibrosis into a client's prenatal plan?**
   a. Ventral wall defect.
   b. Nuchal translucency.
   c. Hyperechoic bowel.
   d. Anencephaly.

   Topic/Concept: Respiration **Subtopic:** Cystic fibrosis (peds) **Bloom's Taxonomy:** Applying **Clinical Problem-Solving Process:** Planning **NCLEX-PN®:** Basic Care and Comfort **QSEN:** Patient-centered care **CJMM:** Analyze Cues

   Rationale: Hyperechoic bowel indicates potential cystic fibrosis prompting the need for genetic testing so appropriate medical planning can be done before the infant's birth. Ventral wall defects indicate a structural birth defect. Nuchal translucency is indicative of Down syndrome. Anencephaly is a defect on its own in which no brain has formed in the cranial cavity.

   THIN Thinking: *Top Three* – Prenatal testing can help parents prepare for childhood diseases like cystic fibrosis, where survival is not likely past a certain age.

2. **The nurse cares for a child with cystic fibrosis and discusses the treatment plan with the child's parents. What treatment does the nurse describe that will aid in lung health?**
   a. Administration of pancrelipase.
   b. Routine antibiotic therapy.
   c. Handwashing.
   d. Chest physical therapy.

   Topic/Concept: Respiration **Subtopic:** Cystic fibrosis (peds) **Bloom's Taxonomy:** Applying **Clinical Problem-Solving Process:** Planning **NCLEX-PN®:** Reduction of Risk Potential **QSEN:** Evidence-based Practice **CJMM:** Generate Solutions

   Rationale: Chest physical therapy helps to loosen mucus from the lungs, prevent consolidation, and allow it to be expelled, reducing the risk of lung infections. Pancrelipase aids in digestion issues. Antibiotic therapy is not given routinely as it can create superinfections. Handwashing is good to reinforce general infection control but does not directly target lung health.

   THIN Thinking: *Top Three* – Parents need to be educated on the proper care of their child that has a specific disease process to ensure quality of life and minimize complications. The child will likely be educated on their care by the parent, so the parent must understand the disease and treatment plan.

3. **Based on the provider's note, what classification of chronic obstructive pulmonary disease severity does the nurse identify for this client?**
   a. Gold 1: Mild.
   b. Gold 2: Moderate.
   c. Gold 3: Severe.
   d. Gold 4: Very severe.

   Topic/Concept: Respiration **Subtopic:** Chronic obstructive pulmonary disease **Bloom's Taxonomy:** Analyzing **Clinical Problem-Solving Process:** Data Collection **NCLEX-PN®:** Physiological Adaptation **QSEN:** Evidence-based Practice **CJMM:** Recognize Cues

   Rationale: According to the classification of COPD by severity, this measurement falls under Gold 3, severe.

   THIN Thinking: *Clinical Problem-Solving Process* – Understanding the severity of an illness helps the nurse identify expected data collection findings, treatment goals, treatment pathways, and potential prognosis.

4. **The nurse provides care for a client with chronic obstructive pulmonary disease. What class of medications does the nurse expect the provider to prescribe when the client also has asthma?**
   a. Corticosteroids.
   b. Bronchodilators.
   c. NSAIDs.
   d. Methylxanthine.

   Topic/Concept: Respiration **Subtopic:** Chronic obstructive pulmonary disease **Bloom's Taxonomy:** Applying **Clinical Problem-Solving Process:** Planning **NCLEX-PN®:** Pharmacological Therapies **QSEN:** Evidence-based Practice **CJMM:** Generate Solutions

   Rationale: All of these medications can be used in COPD, but corticosteroids are only added in the event of an asthma component in the disease.

   THIN Thinking: *Top Three* – The nurse needs to fully understand the purpose and actions of each medication used in order to evaluate effectiveness.

5. **A client is brought to the emergency department with a spontaneous pneumothorax. What treatment does the nurse expect to assist with to help re-expand the lung?**
   a. Intubation and mechanical ventilation.
   b. Chest tube insertion.
   c. Bag-valve mask rescue breathing.
   d. Cardiopulmonary resuscitation.

   Topic/Concept: Respiration **Subtopic:** Pneumothorax **Bloom's Taxonomy:** Applying **Clinical Problem-Solving Process:** Implementation **NCLEX-PN®:** Coordinated Care **QSEN:** Teamwork and Collaboration **CJMM:** Take Action

Rationale: CPR is not needed unless the client becomes pulseless. Bag-valve mask and intubation with mechanical ventilation will not re-expand the lungs. A chest tube will re-balance the pressure in the chest cavity and re-expand the lungs.

THIN Thinking: *Help Quick* – The nurse should evaluate respiratory effort and evenness when observing pneumothorax. They are responsible for positioning, pain management, monitoring, and maintaining sterility during chest tube insertion.

6. **What findings does the nurse attribute to a client's asthma diagnosis? *Select all that apply.***
   a. Bradycardia.
   b. Tachypnea.
   c. Wheezing.
   d. Anxiety.
   e. Chest tightness.

Topic/Concept: Respiration **Subtopic:** Asthma (peds) **Bloom's Taxonomy:** Analyzing **Clinical Problem-Solving Process:** Data Collection **NCLEX-PN®:** Physiological Adaptation **QSEN:** Patient-centered care **CJMM:** Recognize Cues

Rationale: Tachycardia, tachypnea, wheezing, anxiety, and chest tightness are all symptoms attributed to an asthma attack.

THIN Thinking: *Clinical Problem-Solving Process* – Understanding expected and unexpected findings will help the nurse distinguish between expected findings and potentially life-threatening complications of an illness.

7. **When planning care for an older adult with asthma, the nurse considers which common childhood cause a less likely trigger for adults?**
   a. Muscular weakness.
   b. Smoking.
   c. Allergies.
   d. Immune changes.

Topic/Concept: Respiration **Subtopic:** Asthma (adult) **Bloom's Taxonomy:** Applying **Clinical Problem-Solving Process:** Planning **NCLEX-PN®:** Coordinated Care **QSEN:** Teamwork and Collaboration **CJMM:** Prioritize Hypotheses

Rationale: Muscle weakness, immune changes, and smoking are more likely to develop and trigger asthma in adults. Allergies are the most likely trigger for children.

THIN Thinking: *Identify Risk to Safety* – Understanding the triggers for an asthma attack will help lessen the number of attacks a client experiences by learning how to avoid those triggers.

8. **The ICU nurse cares for a client with acute respiratory distress syndrome (ARDS). What finding does the nurse report as an indication of a complication from ventilator therapy?**
   a. Urine output of 50 milliliters in 2 hours.
   b. Oxygen saturation reading is greater than 90%.
   c. Asymmetrical chest rise on inspiration.
   d. Telemetry is showing sinus tachycardia.

Topic/Concept: Respiration **Subtopic:** Acute respiratory distress syndrome **Bloom's Taxonomy:** Applying **Clinical Problem-Solving Process:** Evaluation **NCLEX-PN®:** Reduction of Risk Potential **QSEN:** Evidence-based Practice **CJMM:** Evaluate Outcomes

Rationale: Although the urine output is beginning to show kidney dysfunction, this would not be specifically related to the ventilator. The pulse oximeter reading is at the low level of normal. Asymmetrical chest expansion and tracheal deviation indicate the client has had a pneumothorax, which is a complication of mechanical ventilation. An increased heart rate does not indicate a complication of the ventilator and has many likely causes.

THIN Thinking: *Identify Risk to Safety* – Ventilator care carries high risks for clients with ARDS. Higher pressures are needed to expand and fill the lungs, and higher pressures create a higher likelihood of complications.

9. **A client with Acute Respiratory Distress Syndrome (ARDS) receives BiPAP (bi-level positive airway pressure) treatment. Their respiratory rate is 35 breaths/minute, oxygen saturation is 80%, and their breathing is very labored. How does the nurse proceed?**
   a. Monitor the client closely as these findings are expected.
   b. Prepare for immediate intubation and ventilator support.
   c. Change the client to a continuous positive airway pressure system.
   d. Switch the client to 100% non-rebreather oxygen mask delivery.

Topic/Concept: Respiration **Subtopic:** Acute respiratory distress syndrome **Bloom's Taxonomy:** Analyzing **Clinical Problem-Solving Process:** Implementation **NCLEX-PN®:** Physiological Adaptation **QSEN:** Patient-centered care **CJMM:** Take Action

Rationale: BiPAP is the highest level of non-ventilator support, so if the client is experiencing difficulty breathing, intubation is the next step. All others listed are lesser oxygen support. Monitoring will not help as the client will crash quickly.

THIN Thinking: *Help Quick* – If the client is unstable on BiPAP, the only next step for oxygen support is to be on a mechanical ventilator. ARDS often requires mechanical ventilation as part of the treatment course and is an expected intervention.

10. Which tuberculin skin test result requires treatment?

a. PPD 15 mm, first-time positive, no changes on chest x-ray, and asymptomatic.
b. PPD 2 mm, has a cough for two weeks, and nausea.
c. PPD 3 mm with an extensive area of redness surrounding the test site.
d. PPD 7 mm, arrived from an endemic country.

Topic/Concept: Respiration **Subtopic:** Tuberculosis **Bloom's Taxonomy:** Analyzing **Clinical Problem-Solving Process:** Data Collection **NCLEX-PN®:** Safety and Infection Control **QSEN:** Safety **CJMM:** Recognize Cues

Rationale: Clients with latent TB infection need to be treated to avoid becoming an active case. PPD of 2 mm is not positive, redness around the test does not count as a positive, and 7mm is not positive for this patient.

THIN Thinking: *Identify Risk to Safety* – Clients with latent TB require treatment to prevent active disease. Active disease cases require treatment by law and can be charged as a danger to the public and placed in jail to complete treatment if they are non-compliant.

11. When evaluating a client with pneumonia, what findings does the nurse attribute to a potential complication? *Select all that apply.*

a. Development of empyema.
b. Pleuritis.
c. Pleural effusion.
d. Lung abscess.
e. Pleuritic pain.

Topic/Concept: Respiration **Subtopic:** Pneumonia (peds) **Bloom's Taxonomy:** Analyzing **Clinical Problem-Solving Process:** Evaluation **NCLEX-PN®:** Physiological Adaptation **QSEN:** Evidence-based Practice **CJMM:** Evaluate Outcomes

Rationale: Pleuritis and pleuritic pain are expected in pneumonia, but empyema, pleural effusion, and lung abscess are all complications of pneumonia.

THIN Thinking: Identify Risk to Safety: The nurse should monitor and treat pneumonia complications to prevent permanent lung tissue damage. To correct these issues quickly, the nurse must recognize them quickly.

12. What medication does the nurse expect to administer to a client with pneumonia whose sputum culture tested positive for Chlamydia pneumoniae?

a. Penicillin.
b. Ceftriaxone.
c. Erythromycin.
d. Doxycycline.

Topic/Concept: Respiration **Subtopic:** Pneumonia (adult) **Bloom's Taxonomy:** Applying **Clinical Problem-Solving Process:** Planning **NCLEX-PN®:** Pharmacological Therapies **QSEN:** Evidence-based Practice **CJMM:** Generate Solutions

Rationale: The drug of choice for this form of pneumonia is doxycycline; secondary options are macrolides and fluoroquinolones.

THIN Thinking: *Clinical Problem-Solving Process* – To treat pneumonia effectively, getting a proper sample for culture and sensitivity is essential to ensure the appropriate medication is administered.

13. When reviewing a client's risks for bronchiolitis, what factor does the nurse note as a likely cause for the development of this disease?

a. Inhalation of sand in Iraq.
b. History of pneumonia.
c. Failure to receive the yearly influenza vaccine.
d. Past pneumothorax.

Topic/Concept: Respiration **Subtopic:** Bronchitis **Bloom's Taxonomy:** Analyzing **Clinical Problem-Solving Process:** Data Collection **NCLEX-PN®:** Physiological Adaptation **QSEN:** Patient-centered care **CJMM:** Recognize Cues

Rationale: Inhalation of infectious and irritating organisms is a likely cause. Those that served in Iraq have a higher incidence, likely due to inhalation of sands.

THIN Thinking: *Clinical Problem-Solving Process* – Understanding increased risks is the only way to prevent exposure and screen for potentially affected people.

14. Place in order the stages in the infectious process. All steps may not be used.

a. Prodromal stage.
b. Illness stage.
c. Incubation stage.
d. Convalescent stage.
e. Acute symptomatic stage.

Answer: C, A, B, D–E is not used

Topic/Concept: Respiration **Subtopic:** Upper airway infections **Bloom's Taxonomy:** Applying **Clinical Problem-Solving Process:** Data Collection **NCLEX-PN®:** Safety and Infection Control **QSEN:** Safety **CJMM:** Recognize Cues

Rationale: The stages of the infectious process are Incubation Stage, Prodromal Stage, Illness Stage, and Convalescent Stage. Acute Symptomatic is not a stage.

THIN Thinking: *Clinical Problem-Solving Process* – Understanding the stages and the chain of infection will help prevent the spread of contagions.

15. What medications does the nurse expect to administer for almost all forms of upper respiratory infection?

a. Antibiotics.
b. Corticosteroids.
c. Bronchodilators.
d. Diuretics.

Topic/Concept: Respiration **Subtopic:** Upper airway infections **Bloom's Taxonomy:** Applying **Clinical Problem-Solving Process:** Planning **NCLEX-PN®:** Pharmacological Therapies **QSEN:** Patient-centered care **CJMM:** Prioritize Hypotheses

Rationale: Since most upper respiratory infections are bacterial, the nurse can expect to administer antibiotics. Not all cases will require bronchodilators. Very few will require diuretics. Corticosteroids may be needed but very sparingly, as they can allow infection to progress easily.

THIN Thinking: *Top Three* – When the nurse can recognize what medications are expected in a treatment course, they are better equipped to recognize errors or inconsistencies in treatment plans.

16. What finding causes the nurse to suspect the client has croup?

a. Cough improvement at night.
b. Loud, barking cough.
c. Hypothermia.
d. Bradycardia.

Topic/Concept: Respiration **Subtopic:** Croup (peds) **Bloom's Taxonomy:** Analyzing **Clinical Problem-Solving Process:** Data Collection **NCLEX-PN®:** Coordinated Care **QSEN:** Patient-centered Care **CJMM:** Analyze Cues

Rationale: Tachycardia, symptoms worsening at night, fever, and a loud, barking cough are all signs of croup.

THIN Thinking: *Top Three* – Even though the nurse does not diagnose, the nurse must recognize signs of particular diseases so things are not missed and treatment is not misguided.

17. What findings does the nurse immediately report to the provider when caring for a client with croup?

a. Drooling and swallowing difficulty.
b. Slow and deep breathing.
c. Hoarseness.
d. Fever.

Topic/Concept: Respiration **Subtopic:** Croup (peds) **Bloom's Taxonomy:** Applying **Clinical Problem-Solving Process:** Implementation **NCLEX-PN®:** Basic Care and Comfort **QSEN:** Evidence-based Practice **CJMM:** Take Action

Rationale: The nurse can expect a client with croup to have a fever and be hoarse. They will also be tachypneic. They should not be drooling or have difficulty swallowing.

THIN Thinking: *Help Quick* – Complications dealing with the respiratory center often have life-threatening consequences and need to be identified quickly.

18. The nurse reinforces education for a client with pulmonary hypertension. What medication does the nurse discuss to emphasize prevention of its significant side effects?

a. Sildenafil.
b. Salmeterol.
c. Theophylline.
d. Furosemide.

Topic/Concept: Respiration **Subtopic:** Pulmonary hypertension **Bloom's Taxonomy:** Applying **Clinical Problem-Solving Process:** Planning **NCLEX-PN®:** Physiological Adaption **QSEN:** Evidence-based Practice **CJMM:** Generate Solutions

Rationale: Sildenafil, a drug marketed primarily as an erectile dysfunction drug, was created to treat pulmonary hypertension through vasodilation of the lower body to release pressures in the upper body. The client needs to be well educated because if they use this in combination with nitroglycerin, they can cause severe and life-threatening hypotension. Salmeterol and theophylline are bronchodilators. While this affects the respiratory system, it impacts the blood flow to the lungs and not the airflow in the bronchus, so these are not useful. Furosemide is also not needed as clients do not routinely develop fluid in their lungs with this illness either.

THIN Thinking: *Identify Risk to Safety* – Many drugs have multiple uses that are not their primary use. The nurse must know what other uses a medication has and the major side effects to advise the client to decrease risks of injury.

19. **What information does the nurse provide to the parent of a newborn diagnosed with sickle cell anemia? *Select all that apply.***
    a. Symptoms may not appear until 4-6 months of age.
    b. Stroke is a risk even in childhood.
    c. They should avoid low oxygen environments.
    d. Chest tightness and shortness of breath is an emergency.
    e. Side effects of hydroxyurea.

Topic/Concept: Respiration **Subtopic:** Sickle cell anemia (peds) **Bloom's Taxonomy:** Applying **Clinical Problem-Solving Process:** Planning **NCLEX-PN®:** Reduction of Risk Potential **QSEN:** Safety **CJMM:** Prioritize Hypotheses

Rationale: All of these and many more things should be taught to the parents. They need to identify medical crises and emergencies, understand potential complications, and be aware of medication side effects for the best outcomes.

THIN Thinking: *Clinical Problem-Solving Process* – Proper treatment in pediatric clients relies heavily on the proper education of their parents. They set the tone for their early life and habits that children will have in caring for their disease throughout their lives. The better they care for their children as they grow, the less likely they will develop complications and disability.

20. **Which statement by the client with sickle cell anemia illustrates the need for further reinforcement of teaching regarding their treatment plan?**
    a. "I need to be sure to stay current with vaccinations."
    b. "I should discuss family planning before becoming pregnant."
    c. "I should be careful to avoid low oxygen environments."
    d. "I need to restrict fluids in my diet to prevent fluid overload."

Topic/Concept: Respiration **Subtopic:** Sickle cell anemia (adults) **Bloom's Taxonomy:** Analyzing **Clinical Problem-Solving Process:** Evaluation **NCLEX-PN®:** Basic Care and Comfort **QSEN:** Patient-centered care **CJMM:** Evaluate Outcomes

Rationale: Pregnancy is risky and complicated for mom and baby when mom has sickle cell anemia, so the client should discuss any plans of becoming pregnant with her provider. Low oxygen environments and dehydration will trigger a crisis, so these need to be avoided. They are at higher risk of infection, so infection prevention and proper vaccination are crucial in these clients.

THIN Thinking: *Help Quick* – Educating clients on prevention and health maintenance to prevent complications and injury will promote quality and length of life.

CHAPTER

10

Regulation

Cellular / Intracranial / Thermoregulation

This chapter addresses conditions that impact the body's regulation: Cellular, Intracranial and Thermoregulation. Cellular regulation allows the body to regulate the reproduction, proliferation and growth of cells. Intracranial regulation allows for homeostasis in the brain, thus maintaining important functions such as perfusion, and thermoregulation enables the body to maintain its core body temperature. There are conditions like cancer, hydrocephalus, and brain injuries that negatively impact the body's regulation.

Nurses play a critical role in caring for clients with impaired regulation. Nurses collect data on clients with body temperature changes, provide nursing interventions for clients with cancer, and reinforce teaching plans for clients with disorders associated with increased intracranial pressure.

Priority Exemplars:

- Skin cancers
- Hyperthermia
- Hypothermia
- Acute traumatic brain injury
- Blood-borne cancers
- Hydrocephalus
- Lymph cancers
- Other cancers
- Thrombocytopenia
- Polycythemia

Clinical Hint

The nursing care for clients with cancer, or disruptions in cellular regulation, is often focused on reducing or alleviating the side effects arising from the treatment. These side effects may be more distressing for clients than the cancerous processes.

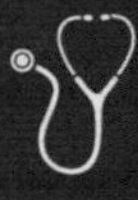

Go To Clinical

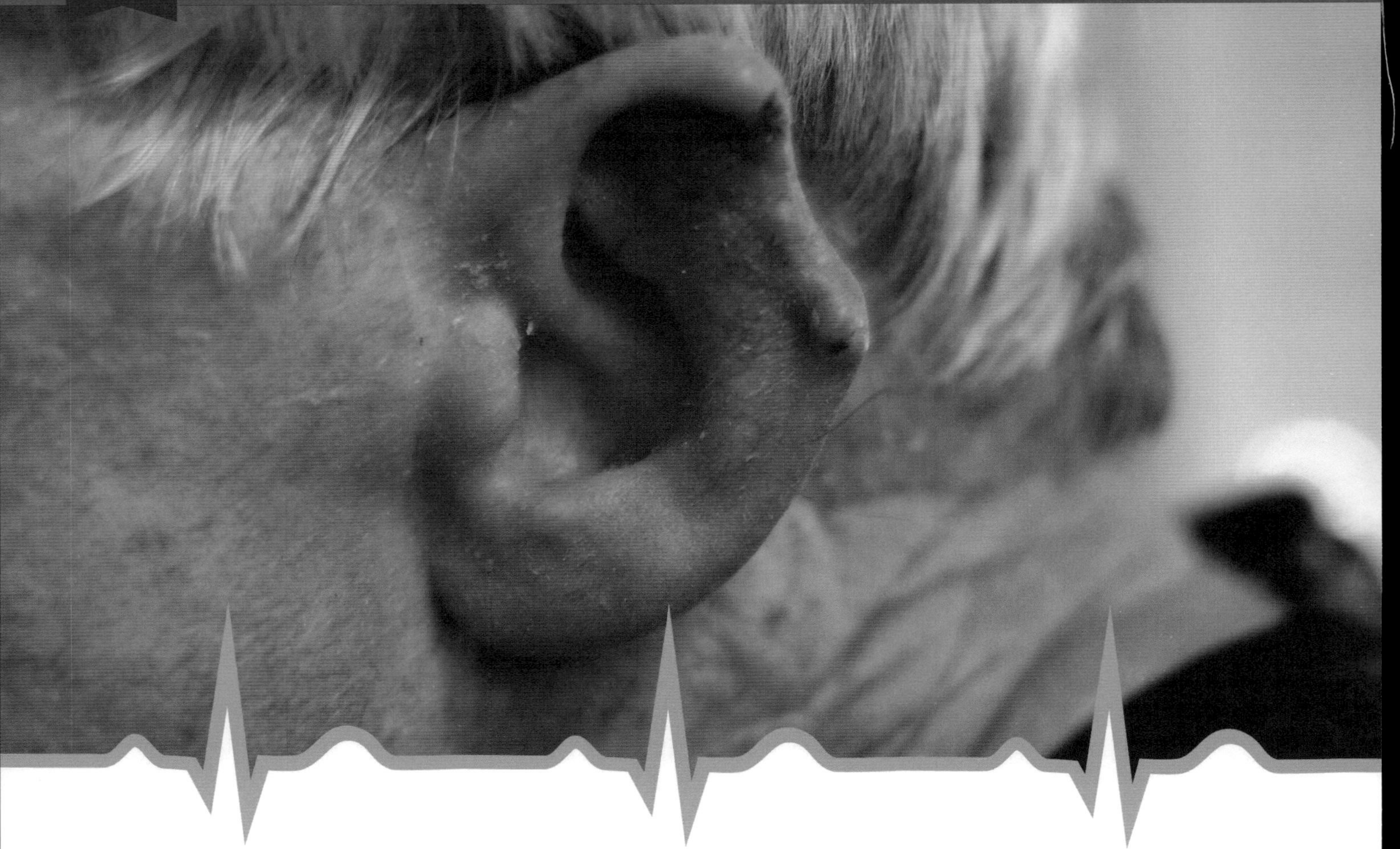

Go To Clinical Case 1

A 77-year-old Caucasian man presents to the community health clinic with a "sore on his ear that won't heal." His wife noted it a few weeks ago. His wife states "it is reddish-black and not healing. Sometimes it bleeds if he dries it too hard with a towel." The client denies itching but says "It hurts when my hat rubs on it. It's pretty tender when you touch it." The client currently takes losartan for hypertension. He had a left inguinal hernia repair at age 45 and a right inguinal hernia repair at age 62. The client is retired from the county where he worked in facilities and as a gardener. He reports he worked outside mowing lawns, gardening, and "keeping the public buildings looking nice." The nurse takes his vital signs, completes data collection, and prepares the client for an examination by the health care provider.

Vital signs: Vital signs: HR 76 beats/minute, RR 18 breaths/minute, BP 132/84 mmHg, and T 98.1°F (37°C).

NurseThink® Time

Using the NurseThink® system, complete the priorities. Check your answers designated by 💡 in the Skin cancers Priority Exemplar.

Next Gen Clinical Judgment

Nurses often provide health promotion counseling to clients who require significant lifestyle changes. This client was exposed to skin-damaging sunlight as part of his work responsibilities.

1. What might the nurse suggest?
2. What other lifestyle changes might be difficult for clients to change?
3. How can nurses assist clients to change habits to ensure optimal health?

NurseThink® Time

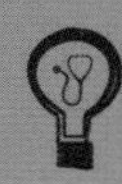

Priority Data Collection or Cues

1.

2.

3.

Priority Laboratory Tests/Diagnostics

1.

2.

3.

Priority Interventions or Actions

1.

2.

3.

Priority Potential & Actual Complications

1.

2.

3.

Priority Nursing Implications

1.

2.

3.

Priority Medications

1.

2.

3.

Reinforcement of Priority Teaching

1.

2.

3.

Skin cancers

Pathophysiology/Description

- Skin cancer is uncontrolled growth of abnormal skin cells
- Most common cancer in United States
- Three types of skin cancer
  - Basal cell carcinoma
  - Squamous cell carcinoma
  - Melanoma
- Melanoma is the least common, but the most lethal of the three
  - Occurs when melanocytes (cells that produce pigment) mutate and become cancerous
  - Peaks between ages 20 and 45
  - Risk factors are ethnicity (Caucasian most common), exposure to ultraviolet rays, fair-skinned in complexion and skin with large moles
  - Uses TNM (tumor, lymph nodes, metastasis) staging system and is staged based on the thickness of the tumor

Priority Data Collection or Cues

- Perform thorough skin inspection in good lighting. Palpate lymph nodes in area of lesions
- Use the ABCDEs to collect data on moles on the body:
  - **A**symmetry, which is an unbalanced lesion with irregular surface
  - **B**order is irregular and indistinct
  - **C**olor is variegated and not uniformly colored. A blue shade is bad (ominous)
  - **D**iameter, with moles larger than 6 mm being more suspicious
  - **E**levation or evolution (change over time)
- Ask about pain, pruritus, and tenderness of mole (These do not exist in a nevus that is benign). Ask about family history (melanoma occurs in families)

Priority Laboratory Tests/Diagnostics

- Biopsy confirms the disease; gives information on the thickness, type, and level of disease
- After diagnosis is made stage the extent of the disease by performing
  - Complete blood count
  - Liver function test
  - Computed tomography (CT) scan

Priority Interventions or Actions

- Prepare client for excision of lesion
- Administer and monitor chemotherapy and immunotherapy
- Observe client for pain related to surgical excision
- Monitor excision site for bleeding, healing and signs of infection
- Monitor graft site (if grafting of skin is done)
- Provide emotional and holistic support (surgery may cause disfiguring)
- Reinforce client education about course of treatment (To defray anxiety and doubt)
- Monitor symptoms to determine metastasis

Priority Potential & Actual Complications

- Surgical site infection
- Metastasis (Deeper and thicker melanoma tissue has higher risks of metastasis)
- Recurrence of melanoma

Type of Skin Cancer

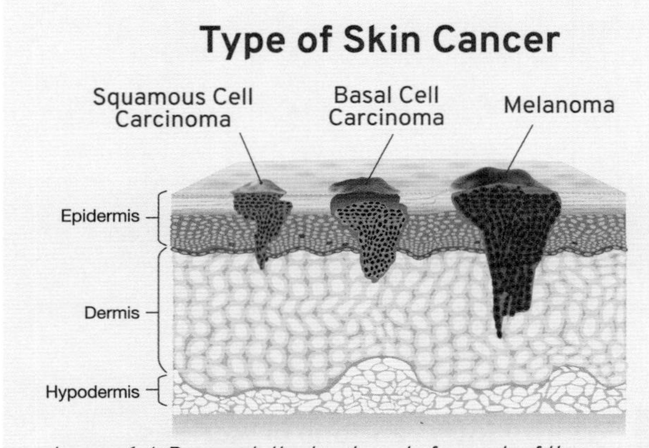

Image 6-1: Research the treatments for each of these cancer processes. How will the nursing care of each of these cancerous process be the same? How will they be different?

Clinical Hint

Annual skin assessments by a health care provider are recommended for all adult clients who may be at risk for skin lesions or cancers.

Priority Nursing Implications

- Know that client will need emotional support because surgery may cause disfigurement
- Awareness that melanoma is familial so provide client recommendations about the importance of follow-up with other close family members
- Understand complications of melanoma and reinforce client education

Priority Medications

- Radiotherapy
  - Uses a series of radiation over several days to kill cancer cells
  - Used alone or in combination with chemotherapy, immunotherapy or surgery
  - Blistering, redness, peeling, itching and weeping of the skin are side effects of radiation
- Dacarbazine, temozolomide, paclitaxel
  - Chemotherapy agents
  - Administered intravenously or orally
  - Collect data on bleeding, fatigue and infection. Monitor red and white blood cell counts and platelets
- Interferon-alpha, interleukin-2
  - Cytokines for immunotherapy
  - Administered intramuscularly, intravenously, subcutaneously or directly into the lesion
  - Injection site reaction, flu-like symptoms, dizziness, GI upset, and headaches are common side effects

Reinforcement of Priority Teaching

- How to do skin self-examination monthly (Will need a hand-held as well as full-length mirror, and good lighting)
- Ensure client understands the signs of melanoma and what findings to report to the physician
- Emphasize the side effects of treatment and complications of the condition
- Ensure client understands the importance of getting an annual skin health assessment
- Ensure client understands how to avoid sun exposure
  - Wear sunscreen (Must block ultraviolet A and B radiation)
  - Apply sunscreen about 15 minutes before exposure and every 2 hours while exposed
  - Avoid the sun on the hottest days
  - Avoid getting sunburned
  - Avoid tanning beds
  - Avoid sunbeds and sunlamps

Go To Clinical Answers

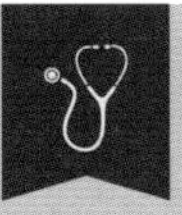

Text designated by 💡 are the top answers for the Go To Clinical related Skin cancers.

Clinical Hint

Rates of skin cancer are growing along with increased life expectancy, environmental changes, and other factors.

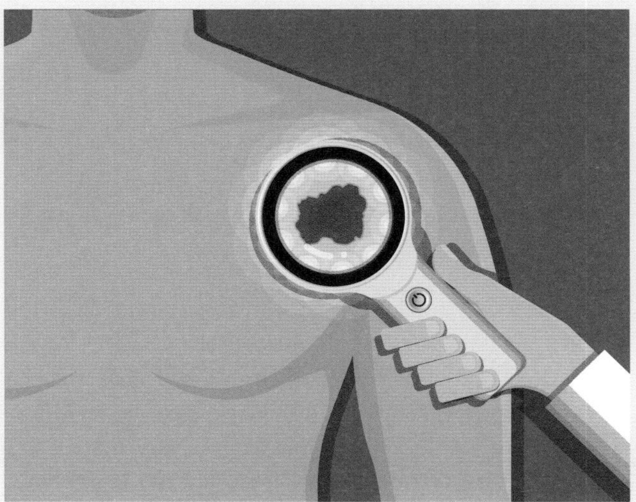

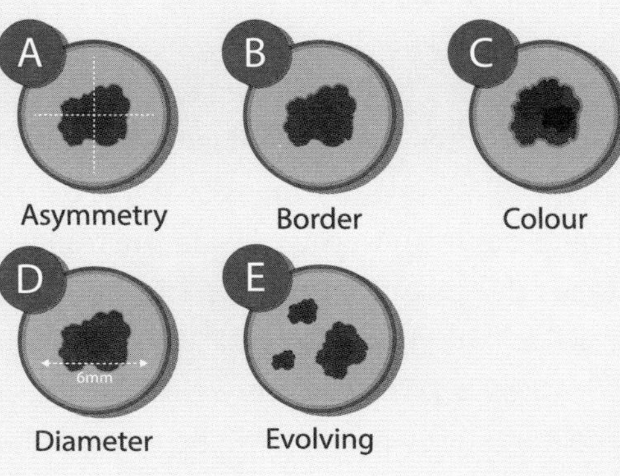

Image 10-2: How can the nurse use the ABCDE's of skin cancer to reinforce when a client should contact a health care provider?

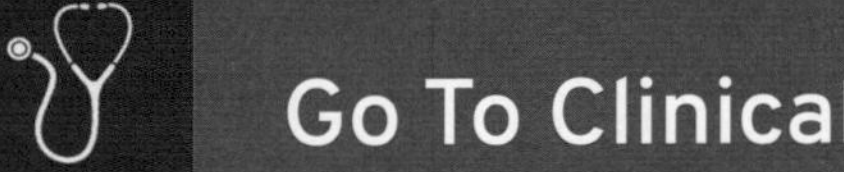

Go To Clinical

Go To Clinical Case 2

The nurse provides homecare for a 69-year-old woman with a history of fibromyalgia, osteoarthritis, and depression. The nurse's visits are focused on hygiene, ensuring medication administration, providing range of motion exercises, ensuring safe use of the walker, monitoring the client's eating and use of Meals on Wheels services, and determining the need for registered nurse or health care provider services. The client lives in a trailer with no air conditioning and the nurse notes that it is extremely hot inside the trailer. The nurse determines that it is over 104°F outside and it is even warmer inside the trailer. The nurse takes the client's vital signs: HR 132 beats/minute, RR 28 breath/minute, BP 100/68 mmHg, T 103.9°F (39.9°C). The pulse is weak and thready. While the nurse provides a bath, the nurse notes that the client feels very warm, the client appears very confused, and the client's skin is dry.

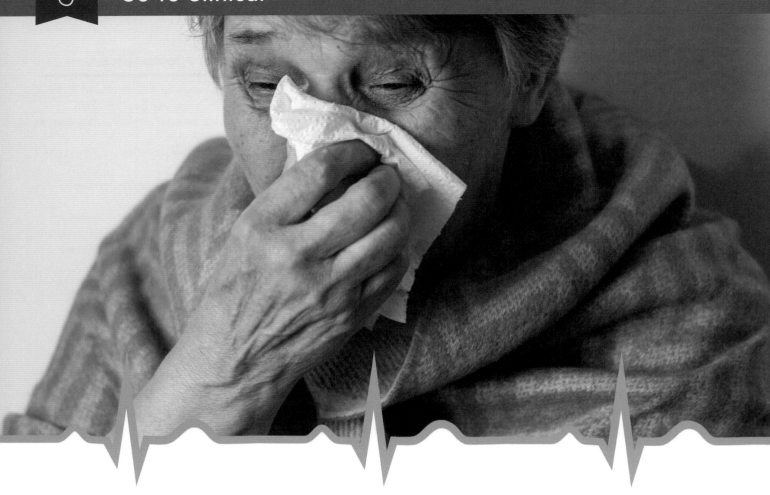

The nurse notes that the client has had very little urine output this morning. The client states "I just don't feel like eating or drinking anything!" The nurse conducts a comprehensive data collection in preparation for calling the homecare nursing supervisor.

NurseThink® Time

Using the NurseThink® system, complete the priorities. Check your answers designated by 💡 in the Hyperthermia Priority Exemplar.

Next Gen Clinical Judgment

Hyperthermia is a common condition requiring nursing care. What conditions may cause hyperthermia? What cues would indicate a client is experiencing hyperthermia? What nursing actions would be recommended to address hyperthermia?

NurseThink® Time

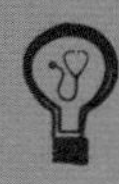

Priority Data Collection or Cues

1.

2.

3.

Priority Laboratory Tests/Diagnostics

1.

2.

3.

Priority Interventions or Actions

1.

2.

3.

Priority Potential & Actual Complications

1.

2.

3.

Priority Nursing Implications

1.

2.

3.

Priority Medications

1.

2.

3.

Reinforcement of Priority Teaching

1.

2.

3.

Hyperthermia

Pathophysiology/Description

- High body temperature-body no longer regulates heat from the environment; threatened body functioning
- Sustained body temperature that is usually greater than 102.2°F (39°C)
- Forms of hyperthermia
  - Heat stroke, heat cramps, heat exhaustion, heat fatigue and heat syncope
- There are many risk factors. The list below is not exhaustive
  - Lifestyle such as inadequate intake of fluids, lack of air conditioning, overcrowding, poor or lack of access to transportation, immobility issues and homelessness
  - Health-related factors such as cardiac or renal diseases, salt-restricted diets, reduced sweating, dehydration, over/under weight and intake of alcohol

Priority Data Collection or Cues

- Measure vital signs (pulse might be weak and thready with increased rate)
- Ask about what may have triggered the condition
- Observe for presenting symptoms to determine the form of hyperthermia
- Monitor neuro status as there can be confusion, especially with heat exhaustion
- Monitor urine output and hydration status
- Ask about living and health conditions

Priority Laboratory Tests/Diagnostics

- Electrolytes, primarily sodium. Sodium will be low because of profuse sweating

Priority Interventions or Actions

- Monitor temperature. Tympanic or rectal gives more accurate core body temperature
- Monitor heart rate and blood pressure
- Anticipate the need for oxygen therapy and have it ready. Metabolic demand for oxygen is increased with hyperthermia
- Remove excess clothing and covers from client
- Monitor environmental temperature and adjust as indicated
- Encourage and provide fluids by mouth if allowed
- Provide cooling mattress and cool packs
- Bathe client in tepid water
- Adjust cooling process based on the client's response
- Anticipate administration of normal saline (NS) so ensure a patent intravenous line. Normal saline restores fluid loss
- Administer and monitor internal cooling measures in severe cases with use of rectal and gastric ice water lavage

Priority Potential & Actual Complications

- Complications of hyperthermia occur when the condition is not treated
  - Sustained mental confusion
  - Coma
  - Death, occurring more commonly in older adults and the very young

Priority Nursing Implications

- Nurses may need to assist those alone or older adults to access alternate dwellings
- Nurses should be alert to heat waves and times when risk is highest

Priority Medications

- No specific medications to treat hyperthermia, medications may be used based on affected system
- Intravenous normal saline to replace fluid loss

Reinforcement of Priority Teaching

- Emphasize signs and symptoms, fluid intake, and remaining inside during a heatwave
- Adherence to air pollution alerts
- If no air conditioning in the home, recommend to go to places that have air conditioning like shopping malls, libraries, senior centers, religious sites, or health agencies
- Educate on seeking out cooling stations/centers that religious groups or health agencies set up in the community
- Alcohol intake may impair thermoregulation
- Encourage intake of 8 glasses of water daily, if not contraindicated
- Immediate treatment of suspected hyperthermia
  - Drink adequate fluids, water or fruit/vegetable juices
  - Take a shower or sponge bath with cool water
  - Place cold wet cloth to areas where blood passes close to the surface of the skin, like armpits, neck, groin and wrists. This helps to cool the blood

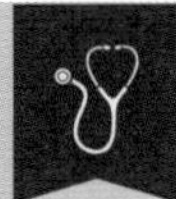

Go To Clinical Answers

Text designated by the bulb icon are the top answers in the Go to Clinical related to Hyperthermia.

Pathophysiology/Description

- Hypothermia occurs when the core body temperature decreases to below 95°F (35°C)
- Stages of hypothermia are based on severity
  - Mild (mental confusion, shivering, increased heart and respiratory rates). With these responses, the body is trying to maintain heat. Body temperature ranges from 93.2 to 96.8°F (34-36°C)
  - Moderate (Shivering is more pronounced, movements slowed, fingers/toes/lips/ears turn blue, paleness occurs, heart and respiratory rates slow, metabolic rate decreases). Body temperature ranges from 89.6 to 93.2°F (32-34°C)
  - Severe (gross confusion, heart/respiratory/blood pressure rates decrease, metabolism shuts down, behavior is irrational, skin appears blue, reflexes absent, pupils fixed). Body temperature is below 89.6°F (32°C)
- Causes include exposure to cold temperatures and any condition with more heat loss than production

Priority Data Collection or Cues

- Determine adequacy of airway, breathing and circulation
- Monitor vital signs (temperature must be taken with a low-temperature thermometer and esophageal measurement is the most accurate)
- Anticipate the results of electrocardiogram replace with hyphen or colon Osborn J wave which closely resembles the ST elevation that is evident in a myocardial infarction
- Ask about living conditions (homelessness is a risk factor), social history (substance abuse is a risk factor), and health conditions (some conditions, like hypothyroidism, are risk factors)
- Collect data on neurological status, blood glucose levels, or extremities for discoloration or damage due to exposure to cold

Priority Laboratory Tests/Diagnostics

- Other tests may be done depending on impact on body systems

Priority Interventions or Actions

- Mild hypothermia
  - Provide warm beverages
  - Put warm clothing on client
  - Encourage physical activity
  - Ongoing measurement of temperature
- Moderate hypothermia
  - Place heating blankets on client
  - Administer intravenous fluid that is warmed. Rewarming is ongoing with a goal of an increase in the body temperature to 90°F (32°C)
  - Ongoing measurement of temperature
- Moderate and severe hypothermia
  - May need to manage extracorporeal membrane oxygenation (ECMO)
  - Manage cardiopulmonary bypass
  - Ongoing measurement of temperature
  - If client has no pulse, then intervene with cardiopulmonary resuscitation (CPR)
- Treat any other systemic effects of hypothermia, like hypoglycemia

Priority Potential & Actual Complications

- Frostbite (freezing and crystallization of body tissue), coma and death

Priority Nursing Implications

- A low-temperature thermometer must be used. Temperature is measured in the esophagus, bladder or rectum
- Resources may be needed to return the client to safe living conditions and/or safe modified lifestyle
- Frostbite may cause loss of body parts; psychological and physical support may be needed

Reinforcement of Priority Teaching

- Proper dress, complications of hypothermia, and the impact of alcohol intake on hypothermia
- If homebound, recommend someone checks on the client frequently and ensure the home is kept at 64°F or above
- Assist clients who are homeless, poor, or elderly with resources such as shelters, clothing, and financial assistance
- The importance of taking medications for existing health conditions that may impact body temperature, like hypothyroidism

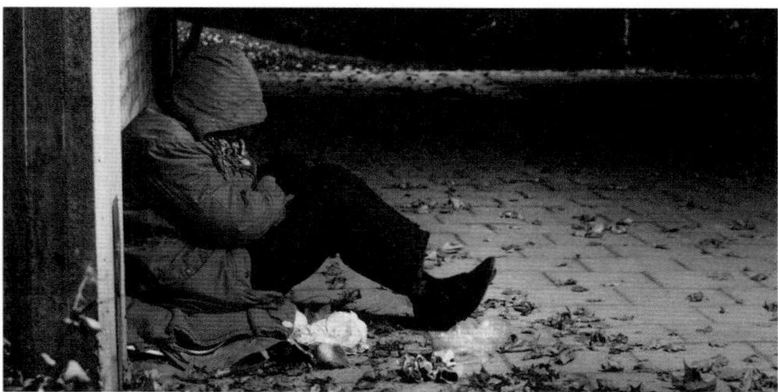

Image 10-3: Why are people who are homeless at risk for hypothermia? How can nurses assist to prevent exposure to environmental hazards? How can nurses advocate for those exposed to environmental hazards?

Acute traumatic brain injury

Pathophysiology/Description

- Defined as a disruption in the brain's normal function due to some type of trauma
  - Penetrating force to the head
  - Blow received to the head
  - Bumping the head
  - Jolt to the head
- A seemingly minor head injury can result in disrupted blood flow, poor tissue perfusion and major brain damage
- Signs and symptoms of traumatic brain injury (TBI) can occur immediately, or can be delayed
- Traumatic brain injury is considered mild or moderate-severe
  - Mild: neurological function loss is temporary and there is no visible structural damage (as in a concussion)
  - Moderate-severe: From minimal brain damage (bruising) to more widespread damage (damage to brain hemispheres, intracranial bleeding)
- Far-reaching physical and psychological effects can result from TBI

Priority Data Collection or Cues

- Initial Data Collection
  - Ask about the time, cause and source of the injury. If client unconscious, elicit information from family members or others who may have witnessed the injury
  - Determine if other injuries exist on any other part of body
  - Measure vital signs
- Initial and ongoing data
  - Glasgow Coma Scale
  - Determine neurological status
- Respiratory cues
  - Injury to brain can alter respiratory function
  - Can experience hypoxemia due to systemic changes from head injuries
- Cardiovascular cues
  - At risk for deep vein thrombosis because of immobility (if unconscious)
  - May develop cardiac dysrhythmias, hypo or hypertension
- Integumentary cues
  - Immobility due to unconsciousness causes risk of skin breakdown
- Consider age-related differences in manifestations of increased intracranial pressure (IICP). Infants may have sunsetting eyes, bulging fontanels, and changes in head circumference/sutures. Infants and children are more likely to vomit with IICP

Priority Laboratory Tests/Diagnostics

- Magnetic resonance imaging (MRI) shows extent of brain injury
- Computed tomography (CT) scans are done ongoing to monitor the injury
- Intracranial pressure monitoring determines pressure in the brain

Priority Interventions or Actions

- Anticipate client's needs as injury may prevent ability to make needs known
- Monitor level of consciousness and motor function, looking for changes in neurological status
- Level of consciousness is the best indicator of change in neurological function
- Manage the airway. An obstructed airway fosters CO_2 retention which can cause the vessels in the brain to dilate, creating an increase in intracranial pressure (ICP)
- Monitor for the signs of possible hematoma or brain hemorrhage
- If client is unconscious
  - Maintain head of bed at 30 degrees to decrease venous ICP
  - Suction effectively as secretions elicit coughing, which increases ICP
  - Monitor blood gasses because they need to be in normal range to support flow of blood to brain

Priority Potential & Actual Complications

- Cerebral edema and herniation, hematomas and hemorrhage, decreased cerebral perfusion, impaired ventilation and oxygenation, seizures, and headaches
- Long-term complications include disability and death

Priority Nursing Implications

- Baseline and ongoing neurologic monitoring is crucial so that subtle changes can be identified quickly
- Understand the association between vital signs and the client's ICP
  - Increasing systolic blood pressure, slowed/irregular respirations, slowed heart rate and widening pulse pressure are indicative of increasing ICP
- All body systems are potentially impacted by a brain injury so the nurse must ensure measures that support all body systems
- Client and family will need long-term community involvement to help with future client needs
- Monitor potassium when on furosemide because the drug is potassium-wasting

Priority Medications

- Mannitol, furosemide
  - Diuretics used to decrease fluid and reduce pressure in brain; monitor serum potassium levels
  - Administered via intravenous solution
  - Test dose of mannitol should be done in clients with renal impairment
- Nimodipine
  - Calcium channel blocker
  - Widens blood vessels and fosters improved blood flow to brain
  - Administered orally and can be given via gastric tube
- Phenytoin
  - Antiepileptic drug to prevent seizures
  - Administered intravenous and orally
  - A loading dose is usually given followed by a maintenance dose

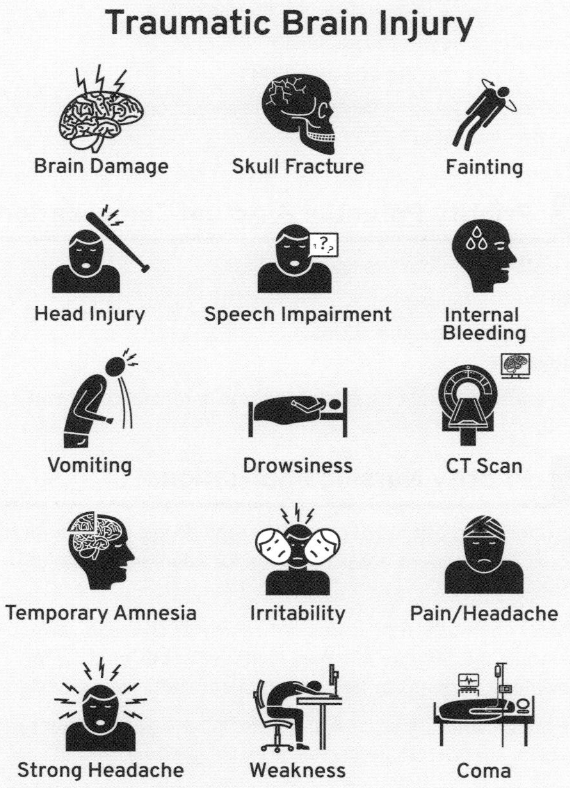

Traumatic Brain Injury

Brain Damage
Skull Fracture
Fainting
Head Injury
Speech Impairment
Internal Bleeding
Vomiting
Drowsiness
CT Scan
Temporary Amnesia
Irritability
Pain/Headache
Strong Headache
Weakness
Coma

Image 10-4: Consider these signs and symptoms associated with traumatic brain injury. What signs and symptoms would an adult manifest with increased intracranial pressure? How are these the same or different from the signs and symptoms manifested by an infant or child?

Reinforcement of Priority Teaching

- If client is being discharged to home
  - Reinforce client's prognosis with client and family
  - Ensure client's limitations are understood by client and family
  - Emphasize self-care management strategies
  - Reinforce safety for the client, such as fall prevention techniques
  - Emphasize about complications that require a call to the neurologist
  - If being discharged with seizure and other medications, reinforce teaching plan about the medication
  - Discuss home care environment modifications that are to be made to accommodate the client
- If client is being discharged to rehabilitation or long-term care
  - Assist family with locating rehabilitation or long-term care placement
  - Differentiate what to expect at these two levels of care (acute care versus rehabilitation)

BEHAVIOR	RESPONSE
Eye Opening 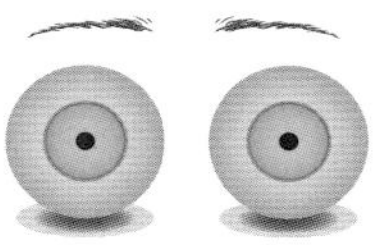	4. Spontaneously 3. To speech 2. To pain 1. No response
Verbal 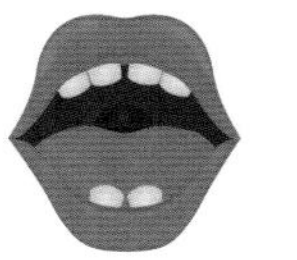	5. Oriented to time, person and place 4. Confused 3. Inappropriate words 2. Incomprehensible sounds 1. No response
Motor 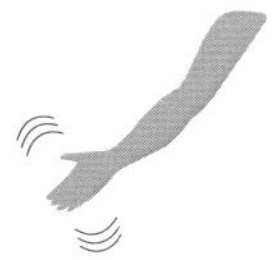	6. Obeys command 5. Moves to localized pain 4. Flex to withdraw from pain 3. Abnormal flexion 2. Abnormal extension 1. No response

Image 10-5: Glasgow Coma Scale (GCS): Consider how a client would appear with a GCS score of 15? 10? 5? What are the implications of these scores for client management and prognosis?

Pathophysiology/Description

- Acute lymphocytic leukemia (ALL) is an aggressive cancer of the blood and bone marrow caused by out of control growth of abnormal white blood cells
- The exact cause of ALL is unknown but possible risk factors are exposure to chemicals and radiation (higher incidence in Caucasians and among males)
- A bone marrow transplant (BMT) for ALL replaces the dysfunctional WBCs with healthy matched donor cells

Priority Data Collection or Cues

- Ask about influenza-like symptoms, which are fatigue, fever, anorexia, shortness of breath and pain/tenderness in the bones or joints
- Determine if there is bleeding, bruising, bone soreness, swollen lymph nodes, enlargement of spleen, and infection. Infection results from neutropenia
- Collect data on all body systems (respiratory, renal and cardiac are crucial)
- Monitor vital signs
- Determine client's understanding of treatment protocol
- Watch for graft-versus-host-disease (GVHD). This indicates a rejection of the host tissue by the implanted donor tissue

Priority Laboratory Tests/Diagnostics

- Complete blood count with differential. Likely to see low platelets causing bruising and bleeding, low red blood cells (RBC) causing tiredness and shortness of breath, and low-normal white blood cells, increasing risk of infection
- Blood chemistries and coagulation to determine kidney and liver dysfunction caused by the cancer spreading or by side effects of chemotherapy
- Bone marrow aspiration and biopsy. Results will identify leukemic blasts, which are immature cells in the bone marrow
- Lumbar puncture to determine presence of blasts in the cerebrospinal fluid
- Computed tomography (CT), magnetic resonance imaging (MRI), ultrasound. These determine any organ enlargement and/or metastasis of the cancer

Priority Interventions or Actions

- Prepare client for bone marrow biopsy and monitor for bleeding, pain and client's level of consciousness post procedure
- Maintain thorough hand washing, keeping environment clean and using strict aseptic technique for all procedures
- Ensure client is educated about the process of bone marrow transplant and side effects, and is prepared to start the conditioning phase
- Conditioning Phase is aimed at destroying damaged cells
  - Administer several regimens of high dose chemotherapy and monitor for side effects
  - Administer RBCs, platelets and antibiotics as ordered
  - Support through radiation if combined with chemotherapy
  - Monitor for hemorrhagic cystitis
  - Watch for low neutrophil count and place client in positive pressure isolation if required. An absolute neutrophil count of less than 500 cells/uL is considered severe neutropenia
- Infusion and engraftment phase
  - Administer and monitor infusion
  - Monitor for signs of bleeding and sepsis
  - Administer immunosuppressants (to prevent rejection), antiemetics and antibiotics as ordered
- Post-transplant
  - Assist with scheduling of follow-up visits
  - Determine psychosocial status
  - Observe for late effects of BMT
  - Prepare for long term use of immunosuppressant medications to deter rejection

Priority Potential & Actual Complications

- Graft-versus-host-disease (GVHD)
- Stem cell failure
- Viral and fungal infections
- Bleeding
- Sterility, cataracts, gastrointestinal and liver complications

Priority Nursing Implications

- Understand effects of chemotherapy drugs and radiation; conduct frequent data collection for adverse effects of therapy
- Most chemotherapy drugs are vesicants that can cause significant damage if leaked from veins; be watchful for swelling, redness or pain at the client's intravenous site
- Provide supportive care and determine needs of client for social support upon discharge
- Create an environment that decreases the risk of infection
- Epoetin alfa can cause life-threatening heart or circulatory problems
- Prednisone can cause corticosteroid withdrawal if stopped abruptly
- Methotrexate at high doses causes severe bone marrow suppression so must be given with a rescue antidote called leucovorin

Priority Medications

- Vincristine, daunorubicin, asparaginase, methotrexate
  - Chemotherapy protocols
  - Administered intravenously, intramuscularly in large muscle, or orally
  - Common side effects of chemotherapy drugs are myelosuppression, hair loss, nausea and vomiting, fatigue and infection
- Prednisone
  - Corticosteroid used to treat possible allergic reactions caused by chemotherapy drugs
  - Administered orally in liquid or tablet form. Given with food or milk to decrease stomach upset
  - Dosage is tapered to prevent prednisone withdrawal
- Epoetin alfa
  - Hemopoietic factor that promotes red blood cell growth
  - Administered via intravenous or subcutaneous routes and dosage is weight based
- Filgrastim (commonly known as G-CSF)
  - Colony-stimulating factor that treats neutropenia
  - Administered daily subcutaneous or intravenous. Stopped when absolute neutrophil is above 10,000 cells/mm^3

Reinforcement of Priority Teaching

- Signs and symptoms of GVHD, cell graft failure, infection and bleeding prevention
- Limiting exposure to other people, animals, some fresh fruits and vegetables, and plants/flowers
- Getting adequate rest
- Exposure to sun should be limited
- Cleanliness of environment
- Nutritional intake
- Using a toothbrush with soft bristles to brush teeth
- Contraception while on chemotherapy
- Driving and return to normal activities (Work, school, sexual activity, etc.)

Next Gen Clinical Judgment

What restrictions are included in neutropenic precautions? What client conditions would warrant the use of neutropenic precautions?

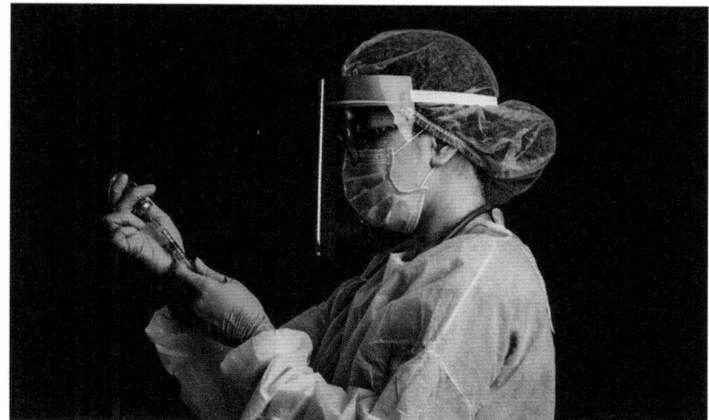

Image 10-7: How can a nurse provide comfort to a client in protective isolation? What precautions are warranted when a client is in protective isolation?

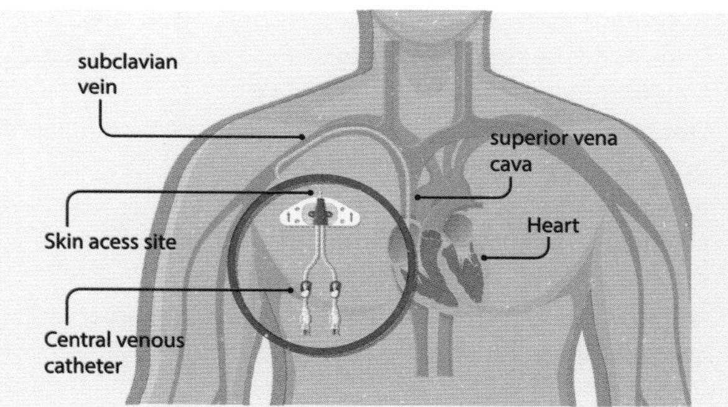

Image 10-8: Why is it preferable to use a central venous access device when administering chemotherapy? What are the potential negative effects of administering chemotherapy or vesicant medications through a peripheral intravenous access device?

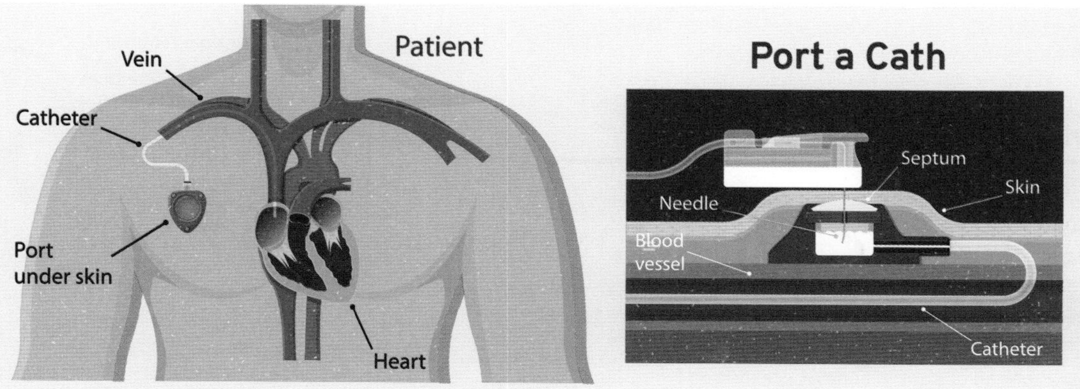

Image 10-6: For which clients is a port a cath preferable to a central venous access device?

Hydrocephalus

Pathophysiology/Description

- Cerebrospinal fluid brings nutrients to and removes waste from the brain, provides a cushioning effect for the brain and acts as a compensatory mechanism for changes in the amount of blood within the brain
- Conditions that impede the flow or absorption of CSF will result in excess accumulation and increased intracranial pressure, causing hydrocephalus
- Hydrocephalus can be defined as:
  - Congenital, present at birth and the cause might be genetic or an event that occurred in fetal development
  - Acquired, caused by conditions that develop after birth
- Treatment goal is to decrease pressure in the brain with a shunt or by performing a ventriculostomy (hole in the ventricle)

Priority Data Collection or Cues

- Complete neurological data collection to determine deficits
- Watch for change in infant's positioning. A change from flexion to extension is a sign of worsening neurological status
- Measure head circumference
- Determine if the infant's fontanel is bulging or pulsating. Determine the presence of McEwen's sign, a cracked-pot sound from percussion of the infant's head
- Observe eyes. With hydrocephalus, eyes can be bulging with downward deviation (called sunsetting)
- Ask caregivers(s) about poor feeding, irritability, vomiting, sleepiness, seizures, or high-pitched cry, all signs and symptoms of hydrocephalus
- Monitor vital signs for elevated systolic blood pressure, bradycardia, bradypnea

Priority Laboratory Tests/Diagnostics

- Ultrasound to determine the size of the ventricles in the brain
- Magnetic resonance imaging (MRI) to view cross-sectional images of the brain
- Computed tomography (CT) scan to view cross-sectional images of the brain (CT provides less detailed imaging than an MRI and is used mostly in an emergency)

Priority Interventions or Actions

- Prepare infant for surgery
- Post shunt Interventions
  - Elevate head of bed as prescribed to ensure stable intracranial pressure
  - Monitor for signs of increased intracranial pressure to determine if the shunt is functioning well
  - Measure head circumference at prescribed frequency
  - Check level of consciousness and pupillary reaction every 2-4 hours or as needed
  - Inspect dressing immediately postoperative, hourly for first 3-4 hours and then at least every 4 hours thereafter
  - Provide pain medication as needed
  - Observe for seizures, infection, or excessive irritability

Priority Potential & Actual Complications

- Untreated hydrocephalus causes brain damage
- Complications post-surgery
  - Blockage, disconnection and infection of shunt
- Seizures

Priority Nursing Implications

- Observe for proper functioning of the shunt, decreasing intracranial pressure and preventing infection
- Compare head circumference measurement and periodic measurements after surgery to determine effectiveness of the surgery
- Keep environment calm for the infant and caregivers(s) to decrease anxiety
- Understand the need for social interaction with the infant, incorporating talk and play as appropriate

Priority Medications

- Use of medication is controversial. Usually used to treat post hemorrhagic hydrocephalus in infants

Reinforcement of Priority Teaching

- Shunts may need revision or replacement as the child grows
- Wash incision daily with mild soap, rinse and dry by patting gently
- Monitor for complications and malfunctioning of shunt
- Provide family with a list of symptoms that require an immediate call to the health care provider (signs of infection or increased intracranial pressure)

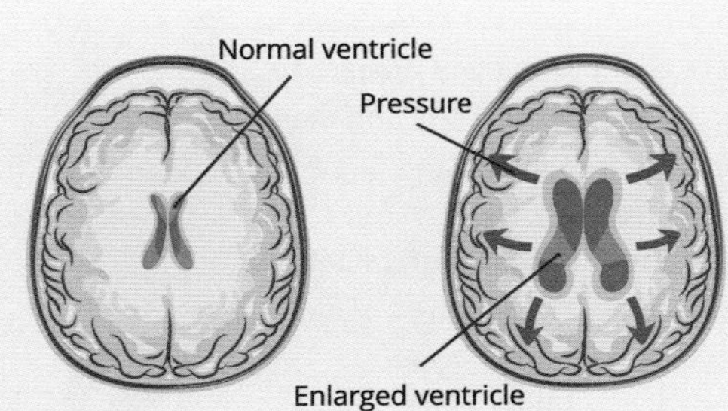

Image 10-9: An infant is suspected to have hydrocephalus with increased intracranial pressure (IICP). What are the specific and non-specific signs and symptoms of IICP in infants?

Pathophysiology/Description

- Lymphoma is a type of cancer that has its origin in lymphocytes. There are two types, Hodgkin's and non-Hodgkin's
- Hodgkin's lymphoma (HL)
  - Starts anywhere in the body where there is lymph tissue but is often found in a lymph node. The HL cells are called Reed-Sternberg cells
  - Peaks in early 20s and after age 50. Has familial tendency
  - Seen in military men who had Agent Orange exposure. Commonly seen in those receiving chronic immunosuppressive therapy
  - Linked to the Epstein-Barr virus. There are four stages to HL and Lugano classification is used to stage the disease

Priority Data Collection or Cues

- Collect data on enlarged painless lumps in the neck, under the arm, or in the groin
- Determine alcohol intake (Lumps may cause pain when alcohol is consumed)
- Determine signs and symptoms of invasion of HL to other organs, including: abdominal pain, cough, bone pain, and jaundice
- Ask the client about B symptoms which may predict how the cancer is likely to progress. These symptoms include drenching night sweats, fever and weight loss. Common in more rapidly growing lymphomas

Priority Laboratory Tests/Diagnostics

- Lymph node biopsy shows Reed-Sternberg cells
- X-ray and computed tomography (CT) scan of chest, abdomen and pelvis will help to define the clinical stage
- Positron emission tomography (PET) scan help to stage the disease as well as determine response to therapy
- Complete blood count (CBC), erythrocyte sedimentation rate (ESR) and platelet count do not diagnose the disease but help to determine involvement of other organs

Priority Interventions or Actions

- Prepare client for biopsy procedure
- Administer chemotherapy and monitor for adverse effects
- Administer prednisone and filgrastim and monitor for adverse effects
- Support the client through radiation
- Minimize risk of infections

Next Gen Clinical Judgment

List 10 side effects of chemotherapy. List 2 nursing actions to address or relieve each side effect.

Priority Potential & Actual Complications

- Complications are treatment related, including weakened immune system, herpes infections, cardiomyopathy, pericarditis, pneumococcal sepsis, development of secondary malignancies, and infertility

Priority Nursing Implications

- Understand that risk for infection is major for these clients
- Raynaud's phenomenon, which is discoloration of fingers and toes, is a consideration with therapy
- Vinblastine causes constipation
- Withhold etoposide for platelet count below 50,000 mm^3 or absolute neutrophil count below 500 mm^3
- Administer injections carefully to prevent leakage of drug into tissue; severe damage can occur with drug leakage
- Dexamethasone and prednisone can cause corticosteroid withdrawal if stopped abruptly

Priority Medications

- Adriamycin, bleomycin, vinblastine, dacarbazine (ABVD therapy)
  - Chemotherapy agents
  - Administered via intravenous infusion or injection, intramuscular or subcutaneous
  - Monitor for bleeding, fatigue and infection. Monitor red and white blood cell counts and platelets
- Mechlorethamine, doxorubicin, vinblastine, vincristine, bleomycin, etoposide, prednisone (Stanford V therapy)
  - Chemotherapy agents
  - Administered via oral and intravenous routes
  - Causes increased risk of infection, anemia and bleeding due to decreased platelets, red and white blood cells
- Prednisone
  - Corticosteroid used to treat possible allergic reactions caused by chemotherapy drugs
  - Administered orally in liquid or tablet form. Given with food or milk to decrease stomach upset
  - Dosage is tapered to prevent prednisone withdrawal
- Filgrastim (commonly known as G-CSF)
  - Colony-stimulating factor that treats neutropenia
  - Administered daily subcutaneous or intravenous. Stopped when absolute neutrophil is above 10,000 cells/mm^3

Reinforcement of Priority Teaching

- Education plan on the prevention of infection, long-term complications of the disease, not stopping prednisone abruptly, hair loss, and verbalization of feelings
- Discuss infertility and the need for men to consider sperm banking if they desire to have children
- Potential long term effects and monitoring for recurrence

Pathophysiology/Description

- Breast cancer
  - Rapidly growing malignant cells in the breast
  - Can invade surrounding tissue or metastasize to distant areas of the body
  - Can start anywhere in the breast but point of origin is quite often the ducts that carry milk to the nipple
  - Symptoms are hard, painless lump with irregular edges (but some lumps might also be soft and round), breast swelling, dimpling, irritation, pain, discharge, redness and retraction of nipple
  - There are no prevention strategies for breast cancer but risk factors are obesity, inactivity, birth control, having had no children, first child after age 30, post-menopause hormone therapy and alcohol intake
  - Staging is with the TNM (tumor, lymph node, metastasis) staging system is used (stages 0 -IV). Higher stage means greater spread of the cancer
- Brain cancer
  - Defined as primary (develop from cells in the brain) or secondary (travel from somewhere else in the body to the brain, called metastasis)
  - Metastatic brain cancer is much more common than primary cancer
  - Signs and symptoms are confusion, memory loss, seizures, headaches, vision problems, gait disturbances, paralysis, aphasia
  - Treatment of metastatic brain cancer is palliative. If no treatment then median survival is one month. With treatment, survival is 3-6 months
  - Treated with surgery, radiation and chemotherapy
  - Brain cancer is not staged but graded as I-IV, with higher grade indicating more rapid growth
- Bone cancer
  - Defined as with brain cancer (primary vs secondary)
  - Abnormal bone is formed, or bone is destroyed
  - Secondary (metastatic) bone cancer is the most common
  - Several types of bone cancer. The name is based on the cells that form the tumor or the part of the bone and tissue that is affected. Some types are multiple myeloma, osteosarcoma, chondrosarcoma, fibrosarcoma and Ewing sarcoma
  - Metastatic bone cancer primarily affects the femur, humerus, spine and skull
  - Treatment of metastatic bone cancer is palliative
  - Grading is as with brain cancer above (I- IV)
- Lung cancer
  - Defined as with bone cancer above (primary vs secondary)
  - Metastatic (secondary) lung cancer is the most common
  - Most lung cancer cases are related to inhalation of carcinogens, like cigarette smoke and asbestos
  - Lung cancer is classified as small-cell and non-small-cell. There is further classification for the non-small cell type
  - Non-small cell type is the most common lung cancer, 75-80% of all cases
  - Staged as I-IV, with stage I being the first stage of the condition and having the highest cure rate

Priority Data Collection or Cues

- Collect data related to breast, brain, bone and lung cancers
  - Complete a detailed health history
  - Review vital signs
  - Monitor for signs and symptoms of infection
  - Determine the impact of the client's illness on the family and work with others on the healthcare team to address these impacts
  - Determine baseline pain level and use it to inform changes in pain intervention
- Breast cancer
  - Determine the client's feelings about diagnosis, treatment and possible breast reconstruction
  - Ongoing observation of client's feelings about body image disturbance post-surgery
- Brain cancer
  - Conduct a thorough initial and ongoing focused neurological collection of data
  - Emaciation and muscle wasting are common in clients with brain cancer so it is critical to monitor the client's nutritional status
  - Consider the client's readiness to verbalize feelings about fear of dying, altered lifestyle or changed appearance
- Bone cancer
  - Determine the degree of disability because bone cancer often ends in amputation of limbs
  - Monitor for signs and symptoms of hypercalcemia (muscle weakness, vomiting, nausea, seizures). Hypercalcemia is a common and serious occurrence in bone cancer
  - Ask about fractures or related symptoms
  - Monitor for changes in the musculoskeletal system including numbness and tingling because cancer in the spine can elicit these symptoms
- Lung cancer
  - Monitor for persistent cough, shortness of breath, wheezing that has new onset, respiratory infections, hoarseness, chest pain worsened by laughing, breathing or coughing, blood in sputum
  - Ask about exposure to risk factors

Next Gen Clinical Judgment

What are the leading risk factors for breast, brain, bone, and lung cancer? How can risk factors assist the nurse to develop prevention strategies?

Priority Laboratory Tests/Diagnostics

- Breast cancer
  - Clinical breast exam
  - Screening mammograms, ultrasound, magnetic resonance imaging, breast tomosynthesis or 3D mammography are used to diagnose the disease
  - Breast biopsy is used to diagnose
- Brain Cancer
  - Computed tomography (CT) scan and magnetic resonance imaging (MRI). An MRI can find small tumors that a CT scan might miss
- Bone cancer
  - Computed tomography (CT) scan, magnetic resonance imaging (MRI), X-rays, bone scans and bone biopsy. These are used to diagnose the tumor
- Lung cancer
  - Chest X-ray, computed tomography (CT) scan, sputum cytology or fiberoptic bronchoscopy and lung biopsy. These are used to diagnose the tumor

Priority Interventions or Actions

- Interventions common to breast, brain, bone and lung cancers
  - Provide information related to before and after surgery
  - Monitor the surgical site for bleeding and signs of infection
  - Determine the client's readiness to view surgical site for first time
  - Discuss after surgery treatment including chemotherapy
  - Administer and monitor chemotherapy treatment
  - Provide medications to manage side effects of chemotherapy
  - Monitor for side effects of radiation therapy
  - Inspect the oral cavity daily (at risk for stomatitis)
  - Discuss hair loss and regrowth with client and family
  - Remove unpleasant odors and sights from environment during mealtime. They can stimulate anorexia and client already experiences increased. Nausea and vomiting
  - Encourage frequent rest periods to conserve energy (treatment depletes energy)
  - Manage pain
- Breast cancer
  - Initiate client's arm and shoulder exercise because restoration of arm function is priority
  - Manage surgical drains
  - Administer hematopoietic growth factor to help in reduction of chemotherapy-induced neutropenia
- Brain cancer
  - Frequent monitoring to detect subtle new changes that may impact outcome
- Bone cancer
  - Provide prompt treatment of hypercalcemia that can occur from bone breakdown
  - Prepare client for bone graft if applicable
  - Consider client's readiness to talk about loss of limb; discuss phantom pain
  - Discuss use of prosthesis
- Lung cancer
  - Prepare client for invasive testing procedures, like bronchoscopy and biopsy
  - Maintain proper airway clearance by performing suction, reinforcing client deep-breathing exercises and coughing
  - Administer oxygen
  - Monitor client's activity and ensure that energy conservation measures are used
  - Help client and family cope with the usual rapid progression of this disease
  - Consider readiness to discuss end-of-life treatment options

Priority Potential & Actual Complications

- Complications common to breast, brain, bone and lung cancers include, bleeding, infection, pain
- Breast cancer complications include hematoma or seroma, lymphedema, depression, loss of interest in sex, metastasis to brain, bone or lungs, and death
- Brain cancer complications include cerebral herniation, hydrocephalus, hemorrhage and stroke, coma and persistent vegetative state, and death
- Bone cancer complications include weakening of bones with susceptibility to fractures, hypercalcemia (dangerously high levels can occur), osteomyelitis, metastasis and death
- Lung cancer complications include respiratory failure with mechanical ventilation, pneumonitis, diminished cardiopulmonary function

Priority Nursing Implications

- Breast cancer
  - Need to also screen males for breast cancer
  - Not all breast cancer lumps are painless, with irregular edges. Some lumps have round edges and are painful so advise clients to see a healthcare professional for any new lumps observed in the breast. Reinforce teaching about self breast examination
  - Lower doses of epirubicin should be considered in clients with severe renal or liver impairment
  - With docetaxel, corticosteroid tablet is used to decrease the severity of allergic reaction and fluid retention caused by the drug
  - Dexamethasone and prednisone can cause corticosteroid withdrawal if stopped abruptly

- Brain cancer
  - Consider that this client is at high-risk for a deep vein thrombosis and pulmonary embolism, but anticoagulant is usually not prescribed because of the high-risk of brain hemorrhage
  - Consider the significant physical, psychosocial and financial burden that the complications of brain cancer have on the client and caregivers
  - Do not use bevacizumab within 28 days before or after a planned surgery as it interferes with wound healing
- Bone cancer
  - Bones can be weakened by cancer and fracture can occur
  - Disfigurement can occur, especially with amputations. Be sensitive to body image disturbances with client
  - Bones may become weakened and need structural support and stabilization to prevent pathological fractures. Bone cement, internal fixation or arthroplasty may be used to achieve stabilization
- Lung cancer
  - Lung cancer is a very subtle disease in that its growth is insidious

Priority Medications

- Doxorubicin, epirubicin, daunorubicin, paclitaxel, docetaxel, temozolomide, bevacizumab, vincristine, procarbazine, mitotane, cisplatin, etoposide
  - Chemotherapy drugs used in a variety of combinations and vary in duration
  - Administered via intravenous, injection or infusion
  - Monitor for bleeding, fatigue, and infection. Monitor red and white blood cell counts and platelets
- Filgrastim (commonly known as G-CSF)
  - Colony-stimulating factor that treats neutropenia
  - Administered daily subcutaneous or intravenous. Stopped when absolute neutrophil is above 10,000 cells/mm^3
- Dexamethasone, prednisone
  - Corticosteroids used to suppress immune response and reduce inflammation
  - Administered intravenous or orally, with food or milk to decrease stomach upset
  - Drugs must be tapered
- Epoetin alfa
  - Hemopoietic growth factor that promotes red blood cell growth
  - Administered via intravenous or subcutaneous routes and dosage is weight based
- Mannitol
  - Diuretic used to decrease fluid in brain
  - Administered via intravenous solution
  - Test dose should be administered in clients with renal impairment
- Phenytoin
  - Antiepileptic drug to prevent seizures in clients with brain cancer
  - Administered intravenous and oral but mostly given via the oral route
  - Gingival hyperplasia is a common adverse effect
- Calcitonin
  - Administered via subcutaneous or intramuscular routes
  - Used to decrease bone destruction
  - May cause increased bone pain in first few months of treatment

Reinforcement of Priority Teaching

- Breast, brain, bone and lung cancers
  - Inform clients of expectations of after surgery treatment, like chemotherapy
  - Ensure that client knows the side effects of chemotherapy, which are nausea, vomiting, hair loss, bad taste in mouth, mucositis and fatigue
  - Discuss management of complications such as antiemetics for nausea and bicarbonate solution for mucositis
  - Determine readiness to assume self-care and fill in any gaps in knowledge that may exist
  - Reinforce care of the incision site
  - Reinforce the importance of timely follow-up care
- Breast Cancer
  - Drain care and how to measure drainage. Advise client to call the health care provider with drainage greater than 30 mL or as instructed
  - Care of incision site, when to apply lotions and creams (when completely healed), range of motion exercises to affected arm, about phantom sensations, feeling like the breast is still present. Make the client aware that this feeling usually stays for a few months but will slowly go away
  - Client and partner may benefit from many community resources so assist with locating resources
- Brain cancer
  - There may be potential reoccurrence or worsening of brain cancer symptoms, that the client may require 24-hour long-term care, and about proper dental care due to gingival hyperplasia effects from phenytoin
  - Identify community resources
- Bone cancer
  - Discuss use of prosthesis and have client demonstrate donning and doffing
  - Ensure client knows how to secure assistive devices
- Lung cancer
  - Keeping the airway clear and means and importance of conserving energy
  - Assist client and family with pulmonary rehabilitation consultation if ordered

Pathophysiology/Description

- Thrombocytopenia is low platelet count. The normal range of platelets in the blood is 150,000 to 450,000 per microliter
- Has many causes including medications, other disease processes, and others
- Thrombocytopenia is increased destruction of platelets, decreased production of platelets or increased consumption of platelets

Priority Data Collection or Cues

- Review the result of the most recent complete blood count. The platelet count determines the severity of the client's symptoms
  - When count is less than 20,000/mcL, petechiae (tiny red spots on skin) and bleeding can occur
  - When count is less than 5,000/mcL, gastrointestinal and potentially lethal central nervous system hemorrhage can occur
- Determine the presence of petechiae and bruising, nosebleeds, oral bleeding, or bleeding from the rectum
- Ask about prolonged bleeding after a cut, surgery or dental procedure; blood in bowel movement or urine; medication history (heparin)
- Ask female about menstrual bleeding. Menstruation is excessive with thrombocytopenia
- If client is being administered heparin, consider heparin-induced thrombocytopenia (HIT)

Priority Laboratory Tests/Diagnostics

- Complete blood count: Less than 150,000 platelets/mcL of blood indicates thrombocytopenia

Priority Interventions or Actions

- Address intervention for underlying cause. If it is heparin-induced, stop the heparin
- Monitor platelet transfusion
- Administer corticosteroid and monitor for side effects as well as effectiveness of the drug

Priority Potential & Actual Complications

- Hemorrhage and significant blood loss
- Spontaneous bleeding when platelet count is less than 10,000
- Heparin-induced thrombocytopenia (HIT). With HIT, the client is at significant risk for developing a deep vein thrombosis or pulmonary embolism

Priority Nursing Implications

- Understand the impact of various platelet levels on the symptoms experienced by the client
- It is important to know the specific cause of the client's thrombocytopenia
- False Thrombocytopenia, called pseudo thrombocytopenia is common and occurs when platelets clump together on a complete blood count, causing a false low result. The blood must be redrawn if this is suspected
- Understand that bleeding is a major risk in a client so ensure daily observation for bleeding
- Dexamethasone and prednisone can cause corticosteroid withdrawal if stopped abruptly

Priority Medications

- Dexamethasone, prednisone
  - Corticosteroids used to suppress immune response and the antibodies for platelets
  - Administered orally with food or milk to decrease stomach upset
  - Must not be stopped abruptly
- Argatroban, bivalirudin and angiomax
  - Used for heparin-induced thrombocytopenia only
  - Administered via intravenous injection
  - Significant risk of hemorrhage

Reinforcement of Priority Teaching

- Delayed treatment might cause potentially fatal problems such as a heart attack or a pulmonary embolism
- Discuss avoiding any known agent that induced the condition, like heparin or alcohol
- Signs of disease exacerbation and how to contact the health care provider
- Information about observing skin for petechiae and bruising
- Bleeding prevention strategies including straining to have stools, constipation, using straight razors for shaving, using a toothbrush with hard bristles
- Recognize that if the platelet count is below 10,000/mcL, sexual intercourse should not be vigorous/rough due to risk of bleeding
- Discuss side effects of steroids. The most important is infections
- Caution when using over-the-counter medications that can impair platelet function, such as aspirin and ibuprofen. Tell client to speak with pharmacist before taking a new drug

Pathophysiology/Description

- Polycythemia: Bone marrow makes excess red blood cells. Platelets and white blood cells are usually in excess as well
- Blood becomes thickened, increasing potential for blood clots and subsequent stroke or heart attack
- More common in older adults
- With treatment, survival is over 10 years. Survival decreases to 6-18 months without treatment
- Two classifications of polycythemia
  - Primary (Polycythemia Vera): the result of genes that have mutated. Platelet, erythrocyte and leukocyte counts are elevated but the highest count is erythrocyte. Hematocrit may exceed 60%
  - Secondary: excessive erythropoietin production in response to situations where oxygen is reduced (i.e. high altitude). No treatment is necessary as it resolves when the cause is removed

Priority Data Collection or Cues

- Collect data for a complete health history
  - Ask about symptoms experienced
  - Ask about any previous associated illnesses like a stroke, blood clot or heart attack
  - Monitor for any abnormal bleeding and ask about risk factors
  - Determine social history, especially alcohol intake
- Ask about over-the-counter (OTC) supplements. Iron is in many vitamins and it can further stimulate the production of red blood cells
- Determine if the client has splenomegaly, gastric fullness or bloating, symptoms caused by an enlarged spleen, or itching, a common problem with the condition
- Measure vital signs

Priority Laboratory Tests/Diagnostics

- Complete blood count (CBC)
  - Erythrocytes, platelets, leukocytes, hemoglobin and hematocrit levels are elevated
- Erythropoietin test (EPO). Erythropoietin directs the production of red blood cells. The level in polycythemia is low because it is not directing RBC production

Priority Interventions or Actions

- Phlebotomy is important therapy—remove 500 mL blood weekly to decrease viscosity of blood and deplete iron stores
- Administer and monitor for adverse effects of medications and phlebotomy treatment
- Manage side effects of medications

Priority Potential & Actual Complications

- Tiredness from repeated phlebotomy
- Damaged veins from repeated phlebotomy
- Thrombosis, which can cause blood clots, stroke, heart attack and pulmonary embolism
- Enlarged spleen
- Long-term complications
  - Myelofibrosis where bone marrow no longer produces healthy functioning cells and scar tissue forms
  - Leukemia occurring over time. The longer the condition exists, the higher the risk of leukemia

Clinical Hint

Commercial multivitamins may contain iron. Request that clients bring their daily medications to a visit to be reviewed by a health care provider.

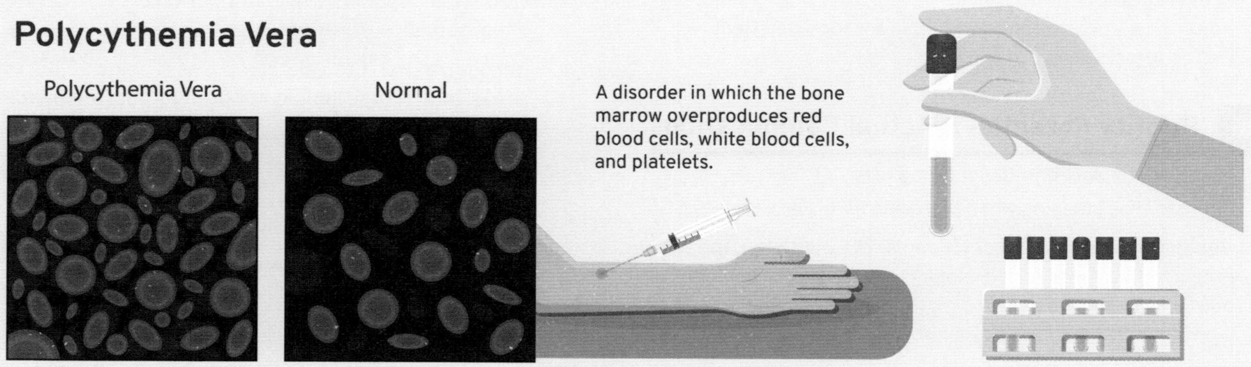

Polycythemia Vera

Polycythemia Vera

Normal

A disorder in which the bone marrow overproduces red blood cells, white blood cells, and platelets.

Image 10-10: Clients with polycythemia require ongoing follow-up. Which signs and symptoms should be reported immediately to the health care provider?

Priority Nursing Implications

- Consider the impact of treatment on the client and understand that tiredness will be evident
- Ensure that client understands the significant risk of blood clots

Priority Medications

- Hydroxyurea
  - An antimetabolite, chemotherapy agent
  - Administered orally as pill form. May be dissolved in water
  - Myelosuppression, edema, headache and drowsiness are the most common side effect
- Busulfan
  - Chemotherapy agent
  - Administered orally or intravenous; tablet form only available as brand name, Myleran
  - Infection, bleeding and anemia are common side effects
- Interferon-alpha
  - Cytokines for immunotherapy
  - Administered intramuscularly, intravenously, subcutaneously or directly in the lesion
  - Injection site reaction, flu-like symptoms, dizziness, GI upset, and headaches are common side effects
- Anagrelide
  - Platelet reducing agent
  - Decrease platelet count and reduce the risk of thrombotic events
  - Administered orally as capsules

Reinforcement of Priority Teaching

- Side effects of medications
- Long-term complications of the condition, like myelofibrosis
- Conditions that can exacerbate the condition, like smoking or high altitude
- How to reduce the risk of getting a blood clot (refrain from crossing the legs, do not wear clothing that is tight or restrictive, and stay active
- Decrease intake of alcohol to help reduce the risk of bleeding
- Do not take iron as it causes red blood cell production
- To help the itching
  - Use sodium bicarbonate in bath water
  - Apply cocoa butter to body
  - Use lotion and bath products that have oatmeal
  - Use cool or tepid bath water
  - Pat skin dry after bath; do not dry skin vigorously

Next Gen Clinical Judgment

Clients with polycythemia vera are at increased risk for clots.

1. What can a client do to avoid these clots?
2. Where may these clots form?
3. Which locations of clots cause the most severe health problems?

Diagnosis for Polycythemia Vera

Image 10-11: How should a nurse support a client during a bone marrow aspiration and biopsy?

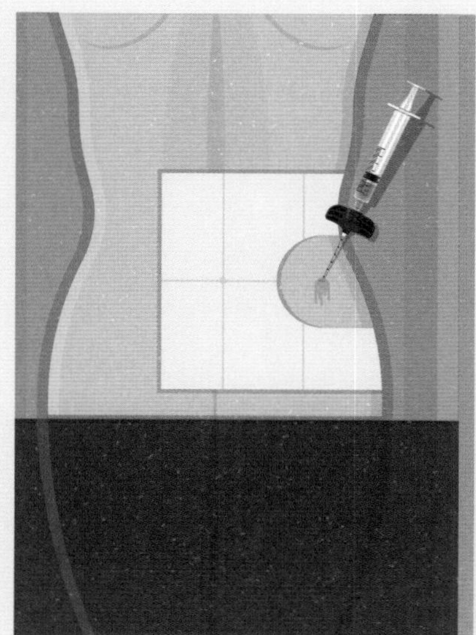

Bone Marrow Aspiration and Biopsy

Biopsy needle

Skin

Bone

Bone marrow

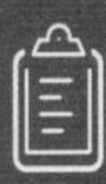

NurseThink® Quiz Questions

1. **The nurse cares for a pediatric client newly diagnosed with Wilms' tumor (nephroblastoma). Which information guides the nurse's evaluation of the client?**
   a. Auscultation of bowel sounds will reveal hyperactivity in the RLQ.
   b. Palpation and percussion of the abdomen should be avoided.
   c. Auscultation of lung sounds will reveal diminished sounds throughout.
   d. Percussion of the chest in the posterior lung fields is necessary.

2. **The nurse provides care for a client with leukemia receiving inpatient treatment of chemotherapy and radiation, resulting in myelosuppression. What intervention does the nurse implement first?**
   a. Administration of antiemetics.
   b. Initiate neutropenic precautions.
   c. Discuss hospice arrangements.
   d. Observe for excessive bruising.

3. **The nurse promotes skin cancer prevention in a community group. Which information does the nurse include about the appearance of malignant melanoma? *Select all that apply.***
   a. Asymmetric appearance.
   b. Rolled edges.
   c. Variations in color.
   d. Irregular borders.
   e. Visible telangiectasias ("spider veins").
   f. Evolving lesion.

4. **The school nurse reviews skin cancer prevention with a group of high school students. The nurse shares multiple images of normal and abnormal skin presentations and asks the students to identify them. When the nurse shares this image, which statement demonstrates accurate recognition of the image by the student?**

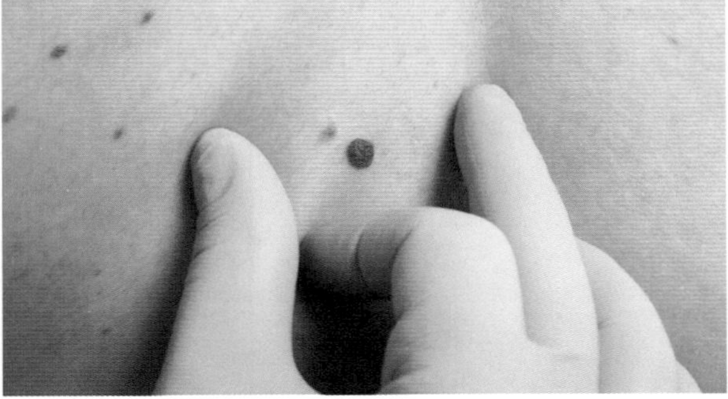

   a. "That is basal cell carcinoma because it's raised up."
   b. "That's big and irregular, so it's malignant melanoma."
   c. "There's no variation in color or shape. That's a mole."
   d. "That's squamous cell carcinoma because it's indurated."

5. **The nurse cares for a client receiving antineoplastic medications for the treatment of non-Hodgkin's lymphoma. What interventions does the nurse recommend for the discomfort associated with oral mucositis? *Select all that apply.***
   a. Using an oral saliva substitute PRN.
   b. Using a medium or firm toothbrush.
   c. Regular, gentle toothbrushing.
   d. Reducing the frequency of oral intake.
   e. Using 2% lidocaine mouth rinse.
   f. Oral rinsing every 2-4 hours.

6. **The nurse cares for a client receiving treatment for non-Hodgkin's lymphoma. The client begins experiencing symptoms related to superior vena cava syndrome, including edema of the neck and face. The nurse administers corticosteroids as prescribed. What signs that the condition is worsening does the nurse monitor for?**
   a. Dyspnea and tachypnea.
   b. Hypotension and tachycardia.
   c. Diminished breath sounds.
   d. Numbness to fingertips.

7. **The urgent care nurse reviews the initial presentation of a new client and is concerned that the client may have lung cancer. What initial diagnostic test is likely to provide this diagnosis?**

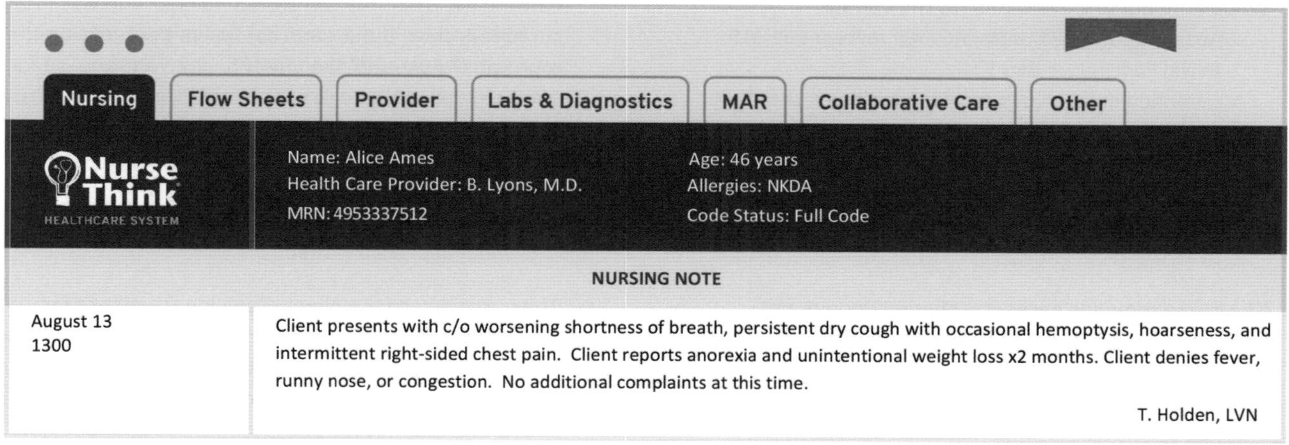

Nursing | Flow Sheets | Provider | Labs & Diagnostics | MAR | Collaborative Care | Other

Nurse Think HEALTHCARE SYSTEM

Name: Alice Ames
Health Care Provider: B. Lyons, M.D.
MRN: 4953337512

Age: 46 years
Allergies: NKDA
Code Status: Full Code

NURSING NOTE

August 13 1300	Client presents with c/o worsening shortness of breath, persistent dry cough with occasional hemoptysis, hoarseness, and intermittent right-sided chest pain. Client reports anorexia and unintentional weight loss x2 months. Client denies fever, runny nose, or congestion. No additional complaints at this time. T. Holden, LVN

a. CT scan.
b. Chest x-ray.
c. Complete blood count.
d. Thoracentesis.

8. **The nurse reviews the provider's prescriptions for a client diagnosed with a brain tumor. Which prescription does the nurse clarify before administration?**

a. Mannitol.
b. Carbamazepine.
c. Ondansetron.
d. Oxycodone.

9. **The nurse cares for a college student who suffered a head injury during an assault by a group of people outside a bar. Which of the client's lab values are most concerning to the nurse?**

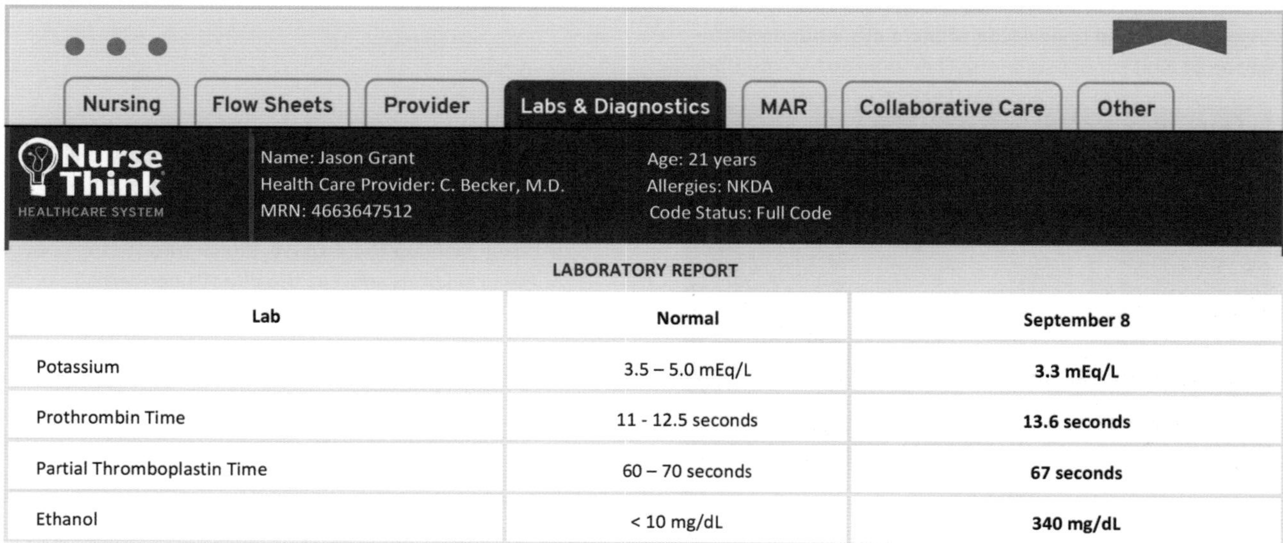

Nursing | Flow Sheets | Provider | Labs & Diagnostics | MAR | Collaborative Care | Other

Nurse Think HEALTHCARE SYSTEM

Name: Jason Grant
Health Care Provider: C. Becker, M.D.
MRN: 4663647512

Age: 21 years
Allergies: NKDA
Code Status: Full Code

LABORATORY REPORT

Lab	Normal	September 8
Potassium	3.5 – 5.0 mEq/L	**3.3 mEq/L**
Prothrombin Time	11 - 12.5 seconds	**13.6 seconds**
Partial Thromboplastin Time	60 – 70 seconds	**67 seconds**
Ethanol	< 10 mg/dL	**340 mg/dL**

a. Potassium.
b. Prothrombin Time.
c. Partial Thromboplastin Time.
d. Ethanol

10. The nurse cares for a client with a traumatic brain injury. To prioritize the client's plan of care, rank order each problem beginning with the most important.

a. Decreased level of consciousness, with potential for airway ineffectiveness.
b. Cerebral edema and reduced tissue perfusion.
c. Potential for impaired skin integrity related to immobility.
d. Hindrance of family coping related to uncertainty of outcome.
e. Brain injury, resulting in impaired thermoregulation.

11. The nurse supports a client with newly diagnosed polycythemia vera. What does the nurse discuss with the client to minimize symptoms?

a. Remind the client to lie supine while resting.
b. Encourage cold-weather exercise such as skiing.
c. Restrict fluid intake to less than 1.5 L/day.
d. Encourage elevation of the feet while at rest.

12. The nurse reviews the laboratory results of a client with polycythemia vera. What results are consistent with this diagnosis? *Select all that apply.*

a. Hemoglobin 20 g/dL.
b. Platelets 450,000 μL.
c. Iron 140 mcg/dL.
d. Hematocrit 42%.
e. Red Blood Cells 9.2 cells/L.

13. A child is brought to the school nurse during recess on a hot day. The child is alert and oriented but reports feeling dizzy, nauseous, and tired. Based on the nurse's immediate visual impression of the child, what does the nurse do first?

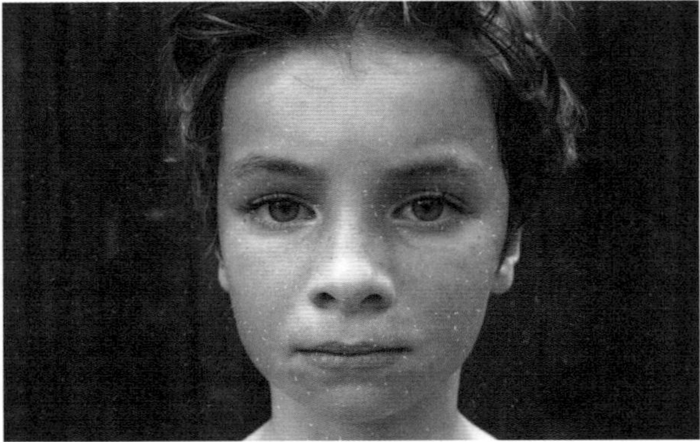

a. Move the child to lie down in a cool environment.
b. Move the child to sit in a chair and offer a cold soda.
c. Call 911 to transport the child to the ER.
d. Apply ice packs to the axilla and groin area.

14. A client was brought to the emergency room by a family member. The family member reports the client was push-mowing the grass for more than an hour and was found stumbling around the yard, confused. Upon sitting the client on the ground, the client began vomiting, so the family member called 911. Oral temperature is currently 104.8ºF. Which data supports the nurse's concern of heatstroke?

a. Client is sweating profusely.
b. Client is alert and oriented.
c. Client has red, dry skin.
d. Client reports leg cramps.

15. A client arrives at the emergency room after falling into a quarry after sunset. The outside temperature is 15ºF, and the client is pale, shivering, and soaking wet from head to toe. The client reports numbness to his fingers and toes, but no blistering or discoloration is noted. The nurse begins implementing which interventions for external warming? *Select all that apply.*

a. Administering warmed intravenous fluids.
b. Initiating bladder lavage with warmed fluids.
c. Removing all wet clothing.
d. Wrapping the client's head with a warm blanket.
e. Applying a forced warm air blanket.
f. Applying warmed, humidified oxygen.

16. The nurse cares for a client with a suspected diagnosis of osteosarcoma. What symptom does the nurse expect to see that will guide the plan of care?

a. Weight loss.
b. Malaise.
c. Localized pain.
d. Fever.

17. The nurse cares for a client with breast cancer who has recently undergone a bilateral mastectomy. The client explains that her mother and grandmother also had breast cancer, and she is concerned that her daughter will also develop the disease. Which information does the nurse provide to address the client's concerns?

a. "Your daughter may want to consider genetic testing for BRCA 1 and BRCA 2."
b. "Your daughter should consider a bilateral mastectomy immediately."
c. "Your daughter is not high-risk, so genetic testing is not likely to be performed."
d. "Your daughter may want to consider genetic testing for HER 2."

18. **The nurse cares for a client receiving chemotherapy for stage IIA breast cancer. What side effects of this treatment is the nurse likely to observe in the client? *Select all that apply.***
    a. Hair loss.
    b. Nausea.
    c. Desquamation.
    d. Dry cough.
    e. Mouth pain.
    f. Bowel changes.

19. **The nurse discusses treatments and likely side effects with a teenager with acute lymphocytic leukemia. Which statement by the client requires follow-up by the nurse?**
    a. "I should wash my hands often to prevent infection."
    b. "It is not a good idea to have plants and flowers in my room."
    c. "I should invite friends over to keep me company."
    d. "A soft toothbrush will reduce bleeding and pain."

20. **The nurse reviews the vital signs of a client with lung cancer receiving chemotherapy and radiation. What trend is most concerning to the nurse?**

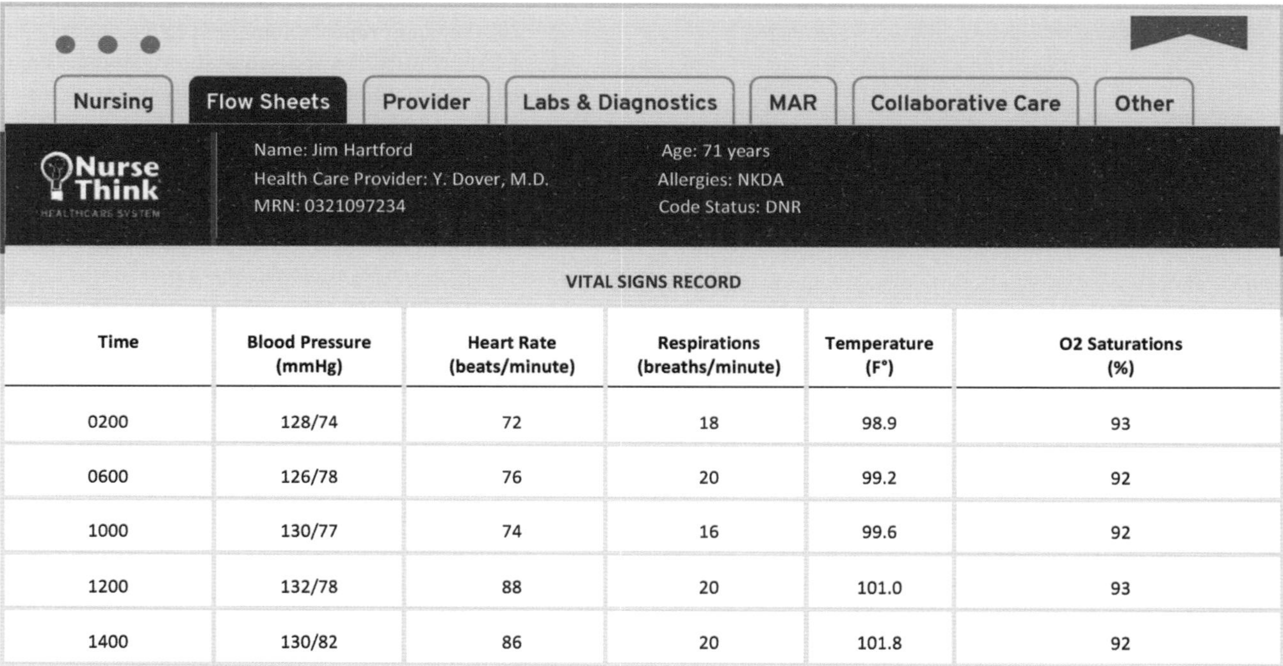

Nursing | Flow Sheets | Provider | Labs & Diagnostics | MAR | Collaborative Care | Other

Nurse Think HEALTHCARE SYSTEM

Name: Jim Hartford
Health Care Provider: Y. Dover, M.D.
MRN: 0321097234

Age: 71 years
Allergies: NKDA
Code Status: DNR

VITAL SIGNS RECORD

Time	Blood Pressure (mmHg)	Heart Rate (beats/minute)	Respirations (breaths/minute)	Temperature (F°)	O2 Saturations (%)
0200	128/74	72	18	98.9	93
0600	126/78	76	20	99.2	92
1000	130/77	74	16	99.6	92
1200	132/78	88	20	101.0	93
1400	130/82	86	20	101.8	92

a. The client's pulse is gradually increasing, indicating circulation concerns.
b. The client's blood pressure is labile, indicating an unstable cardiac output.
c. The client's O2 saturation is consistently <94%, indicating significant oxygenation issues.
d. The client's temperature is increasing, indicating a potential infection.

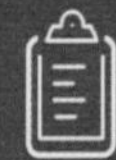

NurseThink® Quiz Answers

1. **The nurse cares for a pediatric client newly diagnosed with Wilms' tumor (nephroblastoma). Which information guides the nurse's evaluation of the client?**
   a. Auscultation of bowel sounds will reveal hyperactivity in the RLQ.
   b. Palpation and percussion of the abdomen should be avoided.
   c. Auscultation of lung sounds will reveal diminished sounds throughout.
   d. Percussion of the chest in the posterior lung fields is necessary.

   Topic/Concept: Regulation **Subtopic:** Bloodborne cancers (peds) **Bloom's Taxonomy:** Applying **Clinical Problem-Solving Process:** Data Collection **NCLEX-PN®:** Coordinated Care **QSEN:** Teamwork and Collaboration **CJMM:** Analyze Cues

   Rationale: Palpation of the abdomen is contraindicated as it may rupture the tumor and lead to the metastasis of cancer cells. Hyperactive bowel sounds and diminished bowel sounds are not specific data to be collected with Wilms' tumor. Wilms' tumor is in the abdomen, so percussion of the chest is irrelevant to this disease process.

   THIN Thinking: *Identify Risk to Safety* – Data Collection is an integral part of the nursing process, but the nurse must be aware of risks associated with certain techniques and avoid those approaches.

2. **The nurse provides care for a client with leukemia receiving inpatient treatment of chemotherapy and radiation, resulting in myelosuppression. What intervention does the nurse implement first?**
   a. Administration of antiemetics.
   b. Initiate neutropenic precautions.
   c. Discuss hospice arrangements.
   d. Observe for excessive bruising.

   Topic/Concept: Regulation **Subtopic:** Bloodborne cancers (adult) **Bloom's Taxonomy:** Applying **Clinical Problem-Solving Process:** Implementation **NCLEX-PN®:** Reduction of Risk Potential **QSEN:** Safety **CJMM:** Take Action

   Rationale: Myelosuppression is common after chemo/radiation and can have a significant impact on client safety. Neutropenia places the client at high risk for developing a potentially life-threatening infection that the body cannot fight. Initiation of neutropenic precautions is a priority. Continued observation of the client is important but is not the priority. Hospice arrangements can be addressed later and are not generally considered while the client is actively receiving chemo and radiation. Antiemetics may be administered, but this is not the priority.

   THIN Thinking: *Identify Risk to Safety* – The nurse should plan care based on priority. For the immunocompromised client, the priority is often prevention of infection. Exposure can be reduced with the implementation of neutropenic precautions.

3. **The nurse promotes skin cancer prevention in a community group. Which information does the nurse include about the appearance of malignant melanoma? *Select all that apply.***
   a. Asymmetric appearance.
   b. Rolled edges.
   c. Variations in color.
   d. Irregular borders.
   e. Visible telangiectasias ("spider veins").
   f. Evolving lesion.

   Topic/Concept: Protection **Subtopic:** Skin cancer **Bloom's Taxonomy:** Applying **Clinical Problem-Solving Process:** Planning **NCLEX-PN®:** Physiological Adaptation **QSEN:** Evidence-based Practice **CJMM:** Prioritize Hypotheses

   Rationale: Rolled edges and telangiectasias are consistent with basal cell carcinoma. All other listed signs indicate malignant melanoma.

   THIN Thinking: *Clinical Problem-Solving Process* – The nurse should instruct clients on evidence-based data collection and identification of cancer using terminology the client can understand.

4. **The school nurse reviews skin cancer prevention with a group of high school students. The nurse shares multiple images of normal and abnormal skin presentations and asks the students to identify them. When the nurse shares this image, which statement demonstrates accurate recognition of the image by the student?**
   a. "That is basal cell carcinoma because it's raised up."
   b. "That's big and irregular, so it's malignant melanoma."
   c. "There's no variation in color or shape. That's a mole."
   d. "That's squamous cell carcinoma because it's indurated."

   Topic/Concept: Protection **Subtopic:** Skin cancer **Bloom's Taxonomy:** Analyzing **Clinical Problem-Solving Process:** Evaluation **NCLEX-PN®:** Health promotion and maintenance **QSEN:** Patient-centered care **CJMM:** Evaluate Outcomes

   Rationale: This is an average mole. Color and shape are regular. There are no indurations, ulcerations, rolled edges, or telangiectasis. There is no scaling or flaking, and it's not large. The student who indicates this as a mole is correct.

   THIN Thinking: *Clinical Problem-Solving Process* – When giving a client information, the nurse must evaluate the client's understanding. One way to do this is to have the client provide feedback and repeat what is learned.

5. **The nurse cares for a client receiving antineoplastic medications for the treatment of non-Hodgkin's lymphoma. What interventions does the nurse recommend for the discomfort associated with oral mucositis? *Select all that apply.***

a. Using an oral saliva substitute PRN.
b. Using a medium or firm toothbrush.
c. Regular, gentle toothbrushing.
d. Reducing the frequency of oral intake.
e. Using 2% lidocaine mouth rinse.
f. Oral rinsing every 2-4 hours.

Topic/Concept: Regulation **Subtopic:** Lymph cancers **Bloom's Taxonomy:** Analyzing **Clinical Problem-Solving Process:** Implementation **NCLEX-PN®:** Reduction of Risk Potential **QSEN:** Evidence-based Practice **CJMM:** Generate Solutions

Rationale: Oral mucositis is common with antineoplastics and may result in pain and difficulty eating. These symptoms can be improved with gentle oral care. The client should use a soft toothbrush with gentle brushing, rinse the mouth frequently to keep it clean and moist, use an oral saliva substitute, and use lidocaine rinses as needed for discomfort. Poor oral intake may lead to dry mucosa, increasing discomfort, and painful swallowing.

THIN Thinking: *Clinical Problem-Solving Process* – The nurse should instruct the client on best practices for reducing risks associated with disease processes and treatment. In this case, the nurse should encourage frequent oral rinsing and gentle toothbrushing with a soft brush, oral saliva substitute, and 2% lidocaine mouth rinse.

6. **The nurse cares for a client receiving treatment for non-Hodgkin's lymphoma. The client begins experiencing symptoms related to superior vena cava syndrome, including edema of the neck and face. The nurse administers corticosteroids as prescribed. What signs that the condition is worsening does the nurse monitor for?**
   a. Dyspnea and tachypnea.
   b. Hypotension and tachycardia.
   c. Diminished breath sounds.
   d. Numbness to fingertips.

Topic/Concept: Regulation **Subtopic:** Lymph cancers **Bloom's Taxonomy:** Applying **Clinical Problem-Solving Process:** Evaluation **NCLEX-PN®:** Health promotion and maintenance **QSEN:** Patient-centered care **CJMM:** Evaluate Outcomes

Rationale: Superior vena cava (SVC) syndrome occurs with compression of the SVC, resulting in reduced venous return and venous congestion. Early signs are dyspnea and face/neck/eye edema. Later signs are more severe and include reduced cardiac output, resulting in a tachycardic response to hypotension.

THIN Thinking: *Top Three* – The nurse should plan to monitor the client closely for complications or worsening symptoms. Initial signs should be reported immediately to the provider.

7. **The urgent care nurse reviews the initial presentation of a new client and is concerned that the client may have lung cancer. What initial diagnostic test is likely to provide this diagnosis?**
   a. CT scan.
   b. Chest x-ray.
   c. Complete blood count.
   d. Thoracentesis.

Topic/Concept: Regulation **Subtopic:** Lung cancer **Bloom's Taxonomy:** Analyzing **Clinical Problem-Solving Process:** Data Collection **NCLEX-PN®:** Coordinated Care **QSEN:** Teamwork and Collaboration **CJMM:** Analyze Cues

Rationale: Based on the client's signs/symptoms, the client will likely undergo an initial chest x-ray. Most lung lesions are first found on chest x-ray, and additional testing will follow.

THIN Thinking: *Clinical Problem-Solving Process* – The nurse should be aware of expected diagnostic testing to efficiently prepare the client and implement the client's plan of care. A chest x-ray is often used as an initial diagnostic tool for conditions of the chest and abdomen.

8. **The nurse reviews the provider's prescriptions for a client diagnosed with a brain tumor. Which prescription does the nurse clarify before administration?**
   a. Mannitol.
   b. Carbamazepine.
   c. Ondansetron.
   d. Oxycodone.

Topic/Concept: Regulation **Subtopic:** Brain cancer **Bloom's Taxonomy:** Applying **Clinical Problem-Solving Process:** Implementation **NCLEX-PN®:** Physiological Adaptation **QSEN:** Evidence-based Practice **CJMM:** Take action

Rationale: Oxycodone is an opioid analgesic. Opioids are given cautiously in clients with brain injuries or tumors, as they may alter the client's LOC. Mannitol, carbamazepine, and ondansetron are commonly used in the treatment of brain tumors to reduce ICP, prevent/control seizures, and control nausea.

THIN Thinking: *Identify Risk to Safety* – The nurse should know side effects and potential complications associated with administered medications. The nurse should recognize a potential need for altered dosing of opioids in clients with brain disorders or injury to reduce the risk for complications related to physiologic alterations.

9. **The nurse cares for a college student who suffered a head injury during an assault by a group of people outside a bar. Which of the client's lab values are most concerning to the nurse?**
   a. Potassium.
   b. Prothrombin Time.
   c. Partial Thromboplastin Time.
   d. Ethanol

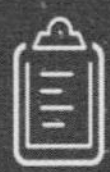

Topic/Concept: Regulation **Subtopic:** Acute traumatic brain injury **Bloom's Taxonomy:** Analyzing **Clinical Problem-Solving Process:** Data Collection **NCLEX-PN®:** Reduction of Risk Potential **QSEN:** Safety **CJMM:** Recognize Cues

Rationale: The client's ethanol level (blood alcohol content) is more than four times the legal limit for operating a motor vehicle. This is likely to significantly impact the client's level of consciousness (LOC), with or without a head injury, making a valid data collection difficult. Alcohol is also known to reduce clotting capability, placing the client at higher risk for a brain bleed. The other lab values are within or close to the normal range.

THIN Thinking: *Top Three* – The nurse should monitor laboratory values and recognize and report findings to the provider. Excessive ethanol levels increase the client's risk for bleeding and alter LOC, potentially impacting data collection and treatment.

10. The nurse cares for a client with a traumatic brain injury. To prioritize the client's plan of care, rank order each problem beginning with the most important.

a. Decreased level of consciousness, with potential for airway ineffectiveness.
b. Cerebral edema and reduced tissue perfusion.
c. Potential for impaired skin integrity related to immobility.
d. Hindrance of family coping related to uncertainty of outcome.
e. Brain injury, resulting in impaired thermoregulation.

Answer: A, B, E, D, C.

Topic/Concept: Regulation **Subtopic:** Acute traumatic brain injury **Bloom's Taxonomy:** Applying **Clinical Problem-Solving Process:** Planning **NCLEX-PN®:** Basic Care and Comfort **QSEN:** Patient-centered care **CJMM:** Prioritize Hypotheses

Rationale: Priorities for the client include maintaining a patent and effective airway, adequate circulation and tissue perfusion, and temperature regulation. Once life-threatening issues are addressed, the nurse can divert attention to caring for the client's family. Impaired skin integrity is a potential, not an immediate, concern and can be included in all elements of care for the client after emergent concerns are addressed.

THIN Thinking: *Identify Risk to Safety* – The nurse should implement care in the order of priority. Life-threatening issues should be addressed first, including patency and effectiveness of airway, breathing, and circulation.

11. The nurse supports a client with newly diagnosed polycythemia vera. What does the nurse discuss with the client to minimize symptoms?

a. Remind the client to lie supine while resting.
b. Encourage cold-weather exercise such as skiing.
c. Restrict fluid intake to less than 1.5 L/day.
d. Encourage elevation of the feet while at rest.

Topic/Concept: Regulation **Subtopic:** Polycythemia **Bloom's Taxonomy:** Applying **Clinical Problem-Solving Process:** Planning **NCLEX-PN®:** Reduction of Risk Potential **QSEN:** Patient-centered care **CJMM:** Generate Solutions.

Rationale: Symptom management with PV is to maintain quality of life. Elevation of the feet will allow for improved circulation and venous return. The nurse should instruct the client to engage in regular moderate exercise and avoid tight clothing and extreme temperatures. Lying flat may cause difficulty breathing, headache, and dizziness upon rising.

THIN Thinking: *Top Three* – The nurse should be aware of the progression and complications of PV and plan care that reduces risk factors. Circulation is a priority concern, and the nurse should instruct the client on strategies for improving venous return.

12. The nurse reviews the laboratory results of a client with polycythemia vera. What results are consistent with this diagnosis? *Select all that apply.*

a. Hemoglobin 20 g/dL.
b. Platelets 450,000 μL.
c. Iron 140 mcg/dL.
d. Hematocrit 42%.
e. Red Blood Cells 9.2 cells/L.

Topic/Concept: Regulation **Subtopic:** Polycythemia **Bloom's Taxonomy:** Applying **Clinical Problem-Solving Process:** Data Collection **NCLEX-PN®:** Physiological Adaptation **QSEN:** Evidence-based Practice **CJMM:** Analyze Cues

Rationale: Polycythemia vera is characterized by hyperviscosity of the blood. CBC results include increased RBCs > 6 cells/L, Hct > 60%, Hgb > 16.5 g/dL (men) and 16.0 g/dL (women), and increased platelets. The laboratory results for iron and Hct are within normal range.

THIN Thinking: *Top Three* – The nurse should monitor lab values closely and report unexpected or critical findings to the provider.

13. A child is brought to the school nurse during recess on a hot day. The child is alert and oriented but reports feeling dizzy, nauseous, and tired. Based on the nurse's immediate visual impression of the child, what does the nurse do first?

a. Move the child to lie down in a cool environment.
b. Move the child to sit in a chair and offer a cold soda.
c. Call 911 to transport the child to the ER.
d. Apply ice packs to the axilla and groin area.

Topic/Concept: Regulation **Subtopic:** Hyperthermia (peds) **Bloom's Taxonomy:** Applying **Clinical Problem-Solving Process:** Implementation **NCLEX-PN®:** Physiological Adaptation **QSEN:** Evidence-based Practice **CJMM:** Take Action

Rationale: Based on the child's complaints and visual appearance, the nurse should suspect that the child is overheated. Because the child is still sweating and alert, heatstroke is not indicated. The nurse's first action is to move the child to a cool environment and have them lie down due to the dizziness. The nurse should begin active cooling methods such as using fans and drinking cold water or sports drinks such as Gatorade if the child can tolerate it. 911 alert is not necessary, and soda should not be used for rehydration purposes. Until the child's temperature is evaluated and extremely elevated, ice packs are not indicated.

THIN Thinking: *Help Quick* – The nurse should prioritize care based on a rapid data collection in urgent situations. Because the child is still sweating and alert, heatstroke is not indicated. Thus, the nurse should begin by moving the client to an environment more suited for treating the client's condition.

14. A client was brought to the emergency room by a family member. The family member reports the client was push-mowing the grass for more than an hour and was found stumbling around the yard, confused. Upon sitting the client on the ground, the client began vomiting, so the family member called 911. Oral temperature is currently 104.8°F. Which data supports the nurse's concern of heatstroke?

a. Client is sweating profusely.
b. Client is alert and oriented.
c. Client has red, dry skin.
d. Client reports leg cramps.

Topic/Concept: Regulation **Subtopic:** Hyperthermia (adult) **Bloom's Taxonomy:** Analyzing **Clinical Problem-Solving Process:** Data Collection **NCLEX-PN®:** Reduction of Risk Potential **QSEN:** Patient-centered care **CJMM:** Analyze Cues

Rationale: Heatstroke manifests when the thermoregulatory mechanism fails, and the body temperature rises uncontrollably. Clients usually present with dry, red skin; confusion, delirium, seizures, or coma; core temperature greater than 104°F. The client's presentation, as well as red, dry skin, support hyperthermia and heatstroke. Sweating stops with heatstroke, and the client is generally disoriented and lethargic. Leg cramps are typically indicative of heat cramps, which occur much sooner than heatstroke.

THIN Thinking: *Clinical Problem-Solving Process* – The nurse should monitor the client closely and report findings to the provider. Heatstroke is a medical emergency that must be addressed immediately to prevent worsening complications.

15. A client arrives at the emergency room after falling into a quarry after sunset. The outside temperature is 15°F, and the client is pale, shivering, and soaking wet from head to toe. The client reports numbness to his fingers and toes, but no blistering or discoloration is noted. The nurse begins implementing which interventions for external warming? *Select all that apply.*

a. Administering warmed intravenous fluids.
b. Initiating bladder lavage with warmed fluids.
c. Removing all wet clothing.
d. Wrapping the client's head with a warm blanket.
e. Applying a forced warm air blanket.
f. Applying warmed, humidified oxygen.

Topic/Concept: Regulation **Subtopic:** Hypothermia **Bloom's Taxonomy:** Applying **Clinical Problem-Solving Process:** Implementation **NCLEX-PN®:** Safety and Infection Control **QSEN:** Safety **CJMM:** Take Action

Rationale: Passive external warming includes moving the client to a warmer environment, removing wet clothing and patting the client dry, covering the client with warm blankets, and wrapping the head to prevent heat loss. Active external warming includes external heat such as forced warm air (BAIR hugger) or heat lamps (kept carefully away from the skin). Warmed and humidified oxygen, warmed intravenous fluids, and bladder lavage are internal warming methods.

THIN Thinking: *Help Quick* – External warming is warming through external means. Invasive interventions, including administering warm oxygen, are internal strategies. In the early stages of hypothermia, external warming is usually adequate.

16. The nurse cares for a client with a suspected diagnosis of osteosarcoma. What symptom does the nurse expect to see that will guide the plan of care?

a. Weight loss.
b. Malaise.
c. Localized pain.
d. Fever.

Topic/Concept: Regulation **Subtopic:** Bone cancer **Bloom's Taxonomy:** Applying **Clinical Problem-Solving Process:** Planning **NCLEX-PN®:** Basic Care and Comfort **QSEN:** Patient-centered care **CJMM:** Prioritize Hypotheses

Rationale: Manifestations of osteosarcoma include localized pain lasting many months, intermittent pain as injury occurs, and large, tender masses. Fever, malaise, and weight loss are associated with metastasis.

THIN Thinking: *Top Three* – Care should be addressed in order of priority. The nurse must plan to address immediate needs first. For the client with osteosarcoma, pain is a common and priority concern. The nurse should treat pain when appropriate and notify the provider of an inability to achieve a tolerable pain level.

17. **The nurse cares for a client with breast cancer who has recently undergone a bilateral mastectomy. The client explains that her mother and grandmother also had breast cancer, and she is concerned that her daughter will also develop the disease. Which information does the nurse provide to address the client's concerns?**
    a. "Your daughter may want to consider genetic testing for BRCA 1 and BRCA 2."
    b. "Your daughter should consider a bilateral mastectomy immediately."
    c. "Your daughter is not high-risk, so genetic testing is not likely to be performed."
    d. "Your daughter may want to consider genetic testing for HER 2."

Topic/Concept: Regulation **Subtopic:** Breast cancer **Bloom's Taxonomy:** Applying **Clinical Problem-Solving Process:** Planning **NCLEX-PN®:** Psychosocial Integrity **QSEN:** Patient-centered care **CJMM:** Generate Solutions

Rationale: Genetic testing for BRCA 1 and 2 should be considered if two 1st degree relatives are diagnosed before age 50 or there is a family history. The other responses are not appropriate as they are not indicated or are incorrect.

THIN Thinking: *Clinical Problem-Solving Process* – The nurse should be honest and provide evidence-based information in educating the client and addressing psychosocial concerns.

18. **The nurse cares for a client receiving chemotherapy for stage IIA breast cancer. What side effects of this treatment is the nurse likely to observe in the client? *Select all that apply.***
    a. Hair loss.
    b. Nausea.
    c. Desquamation.
    d. Dry cough.
    e. Mouth pain.
    f. Bowel changes.

Topic/Concept: Regulation **Subtopic:** Breast cancer **Bloom's Taxonomy:** Analyzing **Clinical Problem-Solving Process:** Evaluation **NCLEX-PN®:** Pharmacological Therapies **QSEN:** Evidence-based Practice **CJMM:** Evaluate Outcomes

Rationale: Common side effects of chemotherapy include hair loss, nausea and vomiting, mouth pain, diarrhea or constipation, neuropathy, rashes, and nail changes. A nonproductive cough may be seen with pneumonitis associated with radiation therapy. Desquamation or shedding of outer skin layers may also be seen with radiation therapy.

THIN Thinking: *Clinical Problem-Solving Process* – The nurse should be aware of expected side effects and address them accordingly. The nurse should also be prepared to identify and address unexpected complications of treatment.

19. **The nurse discusses treatments and likely side effects with a teenager with acute lymphocytic leukemia. Which statement by the client requires follow-up by the nurse?**
    a. "I should wash my hands often to prevent infection."
    b. "It is not a good idea to have plants and flowers in my room."
    c. "I should invite friends over to keep me company."
    d. "A soft toothbrush will reduce bleeding and pain."

Topic/Concept: Regulation **Subtopic:** Brain cancer (peds) **Bloom's Taxonomy:** Analyzing **Clinical Problem-Solving Process:** Evaluation **NCLEX-PN®:** Physiological Adaptation **QSEN:** Evidence-based Practice **CJMM:** Evaluate Outcomes

Rationale: The nurse should follow up if the client is not clear on how to reduce the risks of infection injury. The client with ALL should be mindful of the risks of infection and avoid overexposure to people, plants and flowers, and fresh fruits. Frequent handwashing will reduce the risk for infection, and soft toothbrushing will reduce bleeding and pain.

THIN Thinking: *Identify Risk to Safety* – The nurse should evaluate client understanding and intervene when teaching has not been effective. The nurse should explain the risks of exposure to other individuals, especially groups, and encourage the client to find other ways to connect with friends that do not involve in-person interaction in groups.

20. **The nurse reviews the vital signs of a client with lung cancer receiving chemotherapy and radiation. What trend is most concerning to the nurse?**
    a. The client's pulse is gradually increasing, indicating circulation concerns.
    b. The client's blood pressure is labile, indicating an unstable cardiac output.
    c. The client's O2 saturation is consistently <94%, indicating significant oxygenation issues.
    d. The client's temperature is increasing, indicating a potential infection.

Topic/Concept: Regulation **Subtopic:** Lung cancer **Bloom's Taxonomy:** Applying **Clinical Problem-Solving Process:** Data Collection **NCLEX-PN®:** Health promotion and maintenance **QSEN:** Patient-centered care **CJMM:** Analyze Cues

Rationale: The nurse should be concerned about infection in a client with an increasing temperature and a compromised immune system. The other vital signs are relatively stable. Moderately low oxygen saturation is not uncommon in a client with lung cancer, but the nurse should observe the client for dyspnea or worsening respiratory status.

THIN Thinking: *Top Three* – The nurse should closely monitor the immunocompromised client for signs of infection and report concerning findings to the provider for further evaluation.

CHAPTER 11

Nutrition

Digestion / Elimination

As living beings, we cannot sustain life without proper nutrition and so we are reliant on our body's nutritional processes to function appropriately so that we might get the nutrients needed to continue life. To that end, digestion is a must. However, there are times when our otherwise seamless process of digestion and elimination becomes hindered because of disease conditions that afflict our bodies.

Illnesses impacting the gastrointestinal system are prevalent and as nurses, you will spend a significant part of your role managing these illnesses. It is therefore paramount that you have a firm understanding of the diseases that can impact digestion and elimination so that you might positively impact the care of clients with these health conditions.

Clinical Hint

Clients' daily intake and output totals are critical measures of nutrition, digestion, and elimination.

Priority Exemplars:

- Gastroesophageal reflux
- Constipation
- Celiac disease
- Acute kidney disease/injury
- Benign prostatic hypertrophy/prostate cancer
- Gastritis
- Cleft lip and palate
- Chronic kidney disease/end-stage renal disease
- Cirrhosis
- Colorectal cancer
- Diverticular disease
- Intestinal obstruction
- Gallbladder conditions
- Hepatitis
- Inflammatory bowel disease: Crohn's disease/ ulcerative colitis
- Obesity
- Peptic ulcer disease
- Pyloric stenosis

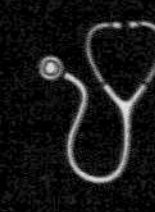

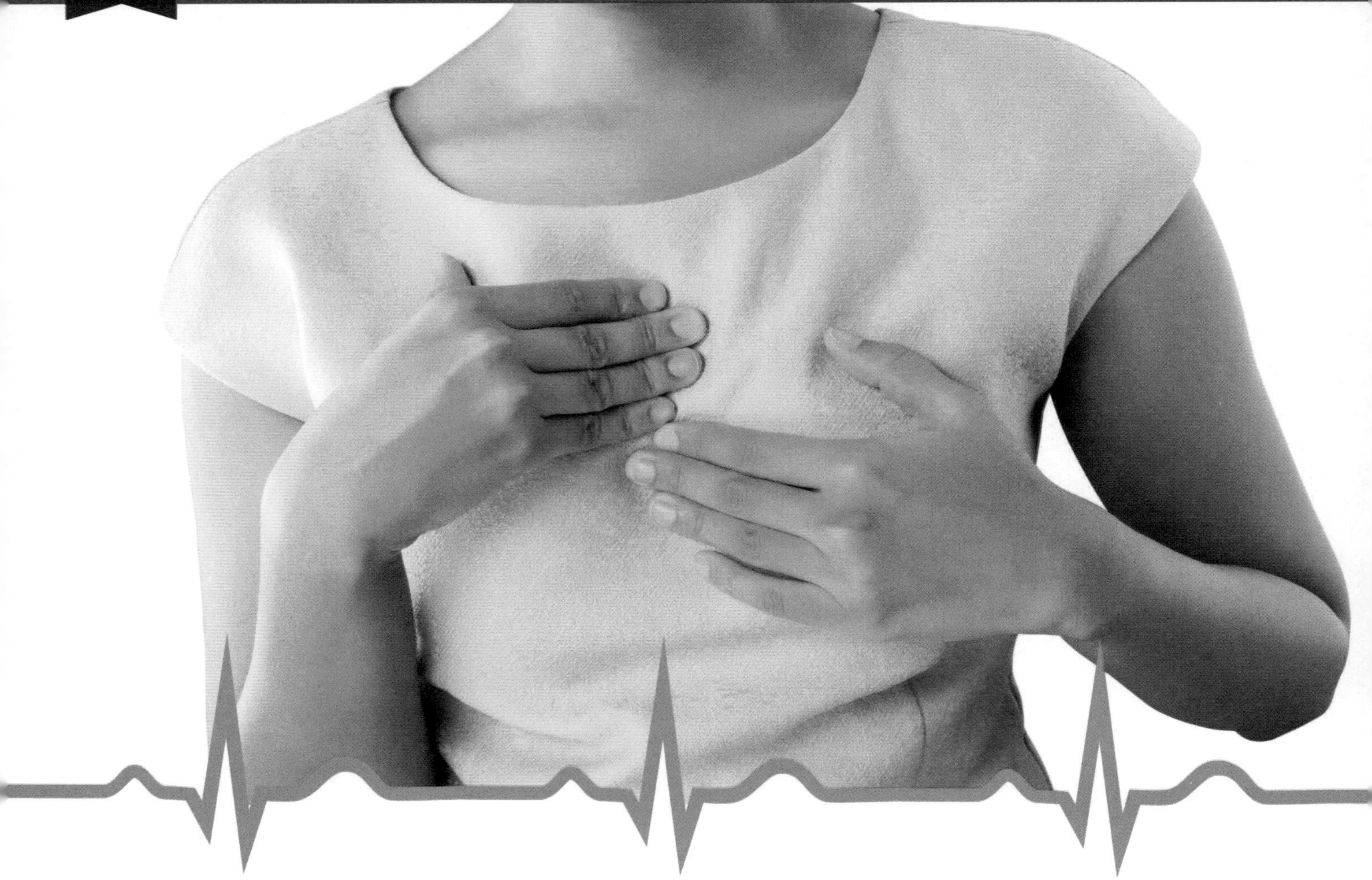

Go To Clinical

Go To Clinical Case 1

A young woman presents to the clinic complaining of epigastric pain. She states that the pain is worse when she eats spicy foods. She has tried some over-the-counter antacids and does have some relief when taking them. She states that she does occasionally smoke cigarettes but has been trying to stop. The client also states that she drinks alcohol on a weekly basis and drinks 3-4 cups of coffee a day. The client states the pain gets worse at night after eating dinner when laying in bed.

Upon arrival to the clinic, her vital signs were as follows: blood pressure 118/78 mmHg, pulse 87 beats per minute, respirations 18 breaths per minute, temperature 98.8°F. An ECG was performed after she complained of chest pain. The ECG showed normal sinus rhythm.

It is suspected that she is suffering from gastroesophageal reflux, or GER.

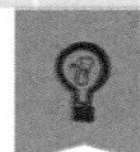

NurseThink® Time

Using the NurseThink® system, complete the priorities. Check your answers designated by in the Gastroesophageal reflux Priority Exemplar.

Next Gen Clinical Judgment

What diagnostic and laboratory tests are completed to differentiate a myocardial infarction from gastroesophageal reflux when a client presents with chest pain? How are the signs/symptoms the same? How are they different?

NurseThink® Time

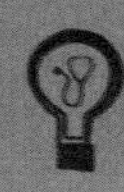

Priority Data Collection or Cues

1.

2.

3.

Priority Laboratory Tests/Diagnostics

1.

2.

3.

Priority Interventions or Actions

1.

2.

3.

Priority Potential & Actual Complications

1.

2.

3.

Priority Nursing Implications

1.

2.

3.

Priority Medications

1.

2.

3.

Reinforcement of Priority Teaching

1.

2.

3.

Gastroesophageal reflux

Pathophysiology/Description

- Gastroesophageal reflux (GER) is a common upper gastrointestinal (GI) problem that results from the backflow (reflux) of gastric contents into the esophagus. Pepsin and hydrochloric acid irritates the esophagus and produces inflammation
- Inflammation can be mild or severe depending on the contents that are refluxed
- Factors that predispose an individual to GER
  - A lower esophageal sphincter (LES) that does not function properly. This is the most common cause
  - Gastric emptying that is delayed
  - Motility from the esophagus that is impaired
  - Delayed stomach emptying
  - Hiatal hernia
  - Obesity
  - Cigarette smoking
- Normal function of the lower esophageal sphincter is to prevent food in the stomach from coming back up into the esophagus but with a non-functioning LES, food is allowed to backflow, especially when the individual is in a lying position
- It has been observed that the intake of certain foods, such as caffeinated beverages, fatty foods, peppermint, and alcohol cause the pressure of the LES to be decreased, while certain medications, such as metoclopramide causes increased pressure to the LES
- In extreme cases of where the individual has not responded to medical management, surgery may be indicated. The most common surgery for GER involves a fundoplication, where a portion of the gastric fundus around the esophageal sphincter is wrapped

Priority Data Collection or Cues

- Check for heartburn (pyrosis) and pain in the epigastric areas
- Check for pain in upper, center part of the abdomen, called dyspepsia
- Ask client about onset of heartburn, usually starts after eating foods that decrease LES pressure
- Ask client about meal intake, to determine the intake of foods that cause GER
- Ask about smoking habits, as smoking is a trigger for GER
- Ask about regurgitation of insipid tasting (described as sour or bitter) fluid in the mouth or throat
- Ask about difficulty swallowing, may occur from irritation and inflammation to the throat
- Check for wheezing and/or coughing
- Check for hoarseness
- Ask about a feeling of fullness in the throat due to presence of inflammation and soreness

Priority Laboratory Tests/Diagnostics

- Upper GI endoscopy will show status of LES. Expect to see scarring and inflammation with GER
- Esophageal biopsy to differentiate between esophageal cancer and Barrett's esophagus (change in esophageal cell type that is reversible but a precursor to esophageal cancer)
- Radionuclide test shows gastric content reflux and how fast the esophagus is clearing the reflux
- Manometric studies shows LES pressure and movement of the esophagus

Priority Interventions or Actions

- Elevate client's head by using 4 to 6-inch blocks, bricks or a long wedge pillow, to decrease likelihood of reflux
- Manage diet to ensure client's meal does not contain foods that induce reflux (aforementioned)
- Ensure client is not served anything to eat or drink 2 hours before bedtime so as not to cause reflux of food eaten into the esophagus
- Administer prescribed medications
- If client is having fundoplication surgery (in extreme cases), prepare client for surgery. Surgery is usually done laparoscopically
- Monitor vital signs

Priority Potential & Actual Complications

- Esophagitis
- Barrett's esophagus
- Several respiratory complications such as laryngospasms, bronchospasms, asthma, pneumonia
- Dental carries for prolonged exposure to stomach acid

Priority Nursing Implications

- Older adults with GER may have symptoms that are like angina pain. They may experience the pain as a squeezing in the chest area that radiates to the jaw and back. However, the pain will be relieved by using antacids
- The risk of fractures is increased when client takes a proton pump inhibitor (PPI) on a long-term basis

Priority Medications

- Proton pump inhibitors
  - Administered orally
  - Several drugs in this class are used. They decrease hydrochloric acid secretion and decrease gastric and esophageal mucosa irritation
  - This class of drug is among the most effective and common in treating GER
  - Available over-the-counter or by prescription
- Histamine receptor blockers
  - Administered orally
  - Several drugs in this class are used. They decrease hydrochloric acid secretion and decrease gastric and esophageal mucosa irritation
  - Like the proton pump inhibitors, this class of drugs is effective and commonly used
  - Available both as over-the-counter and prescription
- Cholinergic drug
  - Administered orally or subcutaneously
  - Urecholine is the only drug used in this class
  - Used to increase the pressure of LES and improve esophageal emptying
- Antacids
  - Administered orally
  - Several types of antacids in this class
  - Taken 1-3 hours after a meal and at bedtime, it neutralizes hydrochloric acid

Reinforcement of Priority Teaching

- Administration of prescribed medications
- Provide client with list of factors that cause decreased LES pressure and encourage avoidance
- Remind client not to eat 2 hours before bedtime, as this increases gastric acid secretion and likelihood of reflux
- Remind client that eating small meals at frequent intervals and drinking fluids in between meals
- Seek assistance of pharmacist before taking over-the-counter medications as some medications can increase likelihood of gastric acid reflux
- Smoking cessation for clients who smoke
- Encourage client who is obese to start a weight loss program

Go To Clinical Answers

Text designated by [icon] are the top answers for the Go To Clinical related to Gastroesophageal reflux.

Gastroesophageal Reflux Disease

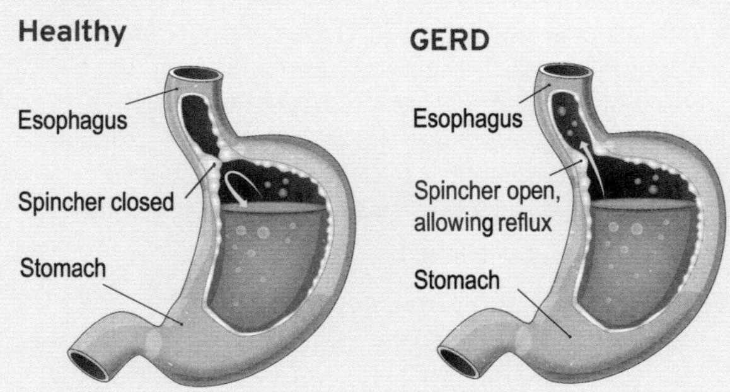

Image 11-1: How could the nurse use this image to reinforce the teaching plan for a client with GER?

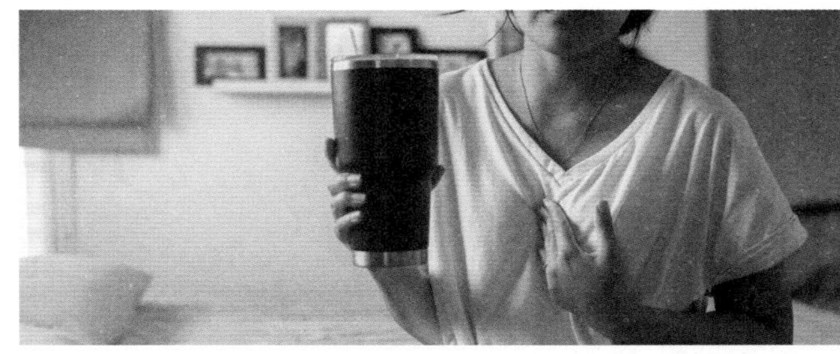

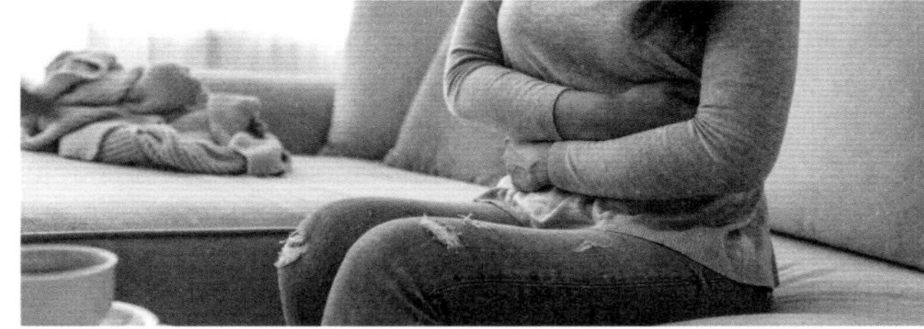

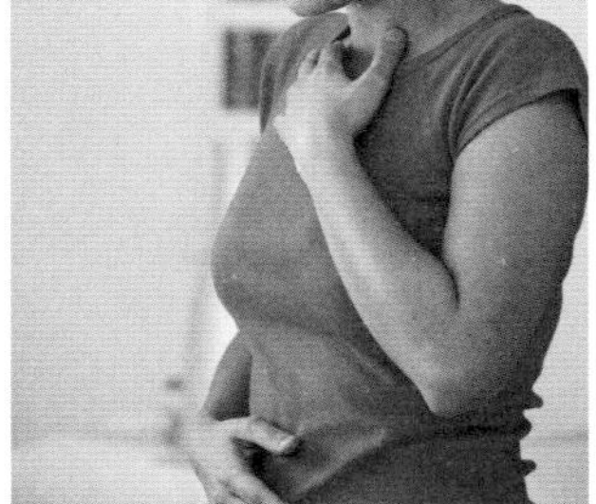

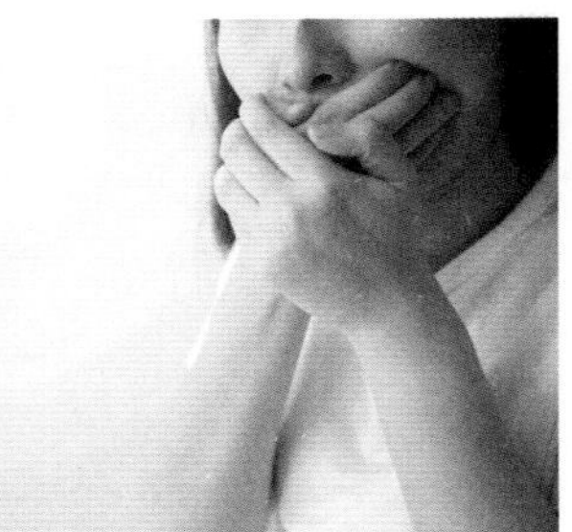

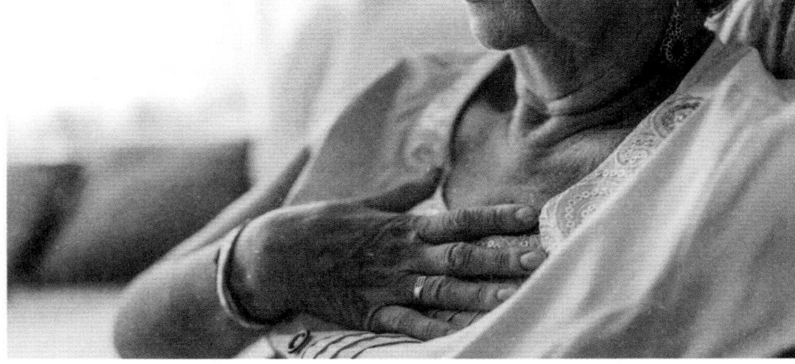

Image 11-2: What does each of these images portray? What words might clients use to describe their symptoms? What other signs would you anticipate? How might these conditions be managed?

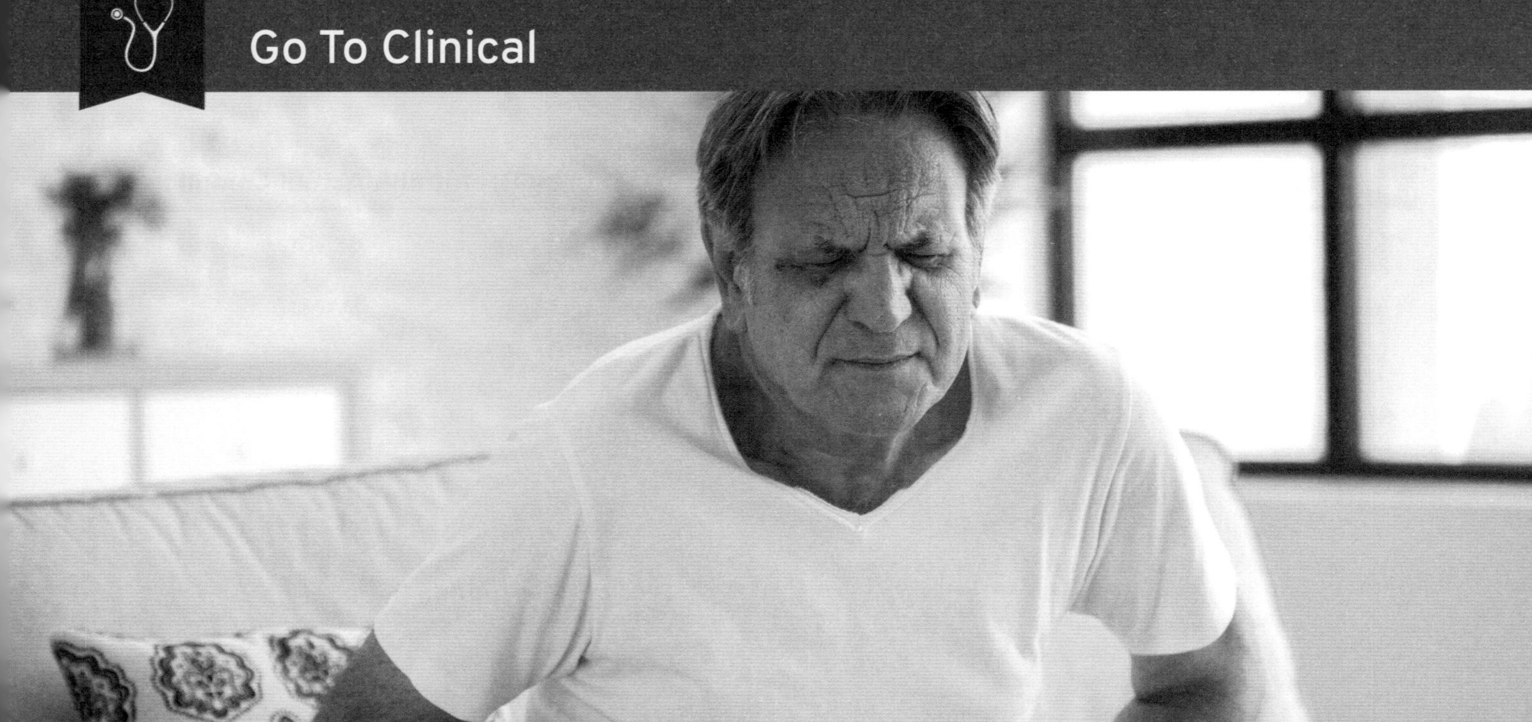

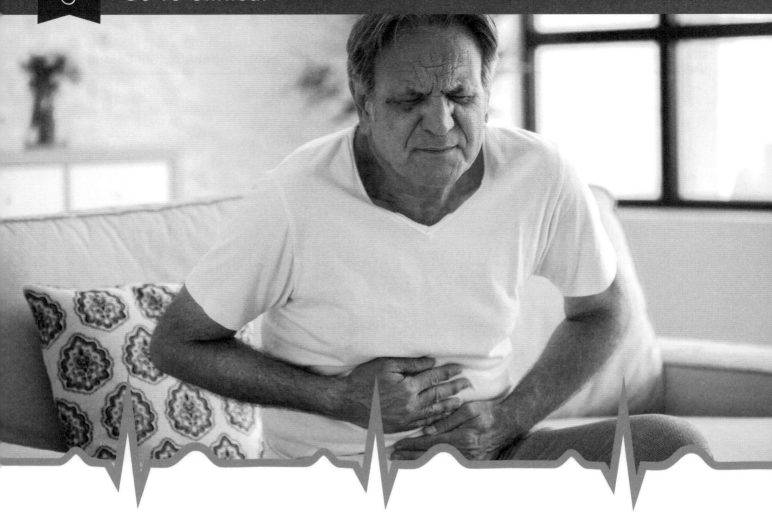

Go To Clinical Case 2

J. M. is a 68-year-old male who is at the clinic today complaining of abdominal pain. He rates his abdominal pain as a 6/10. He states that he has not had a bowel movement in a several days and is very uncomfortable. He is still passing gas. He states that he has not been moving around as much since he hurt his back. He is also been taking an opioid pain medication for pain due to the back injury. He states his back is not currently hurting. Upon further questioning, J. M. tells the nurse that he does not eat much fiber in his diet.

His current vital signs are: Temperature 97.9°F (36.6°C), Pulse 92 beats/minute, Respirations 18 breaths/minute, Blood pressure 128/80.

Clinical Hint

Every client receiving opioids should be monitored for constipation. Nurses should be vigilant to clients at risk for constipation and implement nursing actions early to prevent constipation before it evolves.

NurseThink® Time

Using the NurseThink® system, complete the priorities. Check your answers designated by 💡 in the Constipation Priority Exemplar.

NurseThink® Time

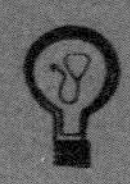

Priority Data Collection or Cues

1.

2.

3.

Priority Laboratory Tests/Diagnostics

1.

2.

3.

Priority Interventions or Actions

1.

2.

3.

Priority Potential & Actual Complications

1.

2.

3.

Priority Nursing Implications

1.

2.

3.

Priority Medications

1.

2.

3.

Reinforcement of Priority Teaching

1.

2.

3.

Pathophysiology/Description

- Constipation is the difficult and infrequent passage of stools that are hard and dry
    - Causes include: ignoring the urge to defecate, inadequate fluids, sedentary/decreased physical activity, decreased intake of fiber, drugs (opioids), and some diseases (Parkinson's, hypothyroid, others)
- Some individuals take laxatives regularly if they do not have a daily bowel movement. This results in a dependence on laxatives to have bowel movements

Priority Data Collection or Cues

- Check for abdominal distention and bloating
- Ask about abdominal pain
- Check for presence of rectal hemorrhoids, as these are common with chronic constipation
- Ask about quality of bowel movements. Stools are usually dry and hard
- Ask about difficulty passing stools. Straining is common because hard feces is difficult to pass
- Check for bowel perforation
- Check for fissures and ulcers to the rectal mucosa, caused by repeated straining and irritation from dry stools
- Ask client about bowel movement habits and patterns

Priority Laboratory Tests/Diagnostics

- Abdominal X-rays will likely show constipation
- Colonoscopy shows entire colon and can detect complications of constipation, such as polyps, and cancer
- Sigmoidoscopy, shows hemorrhoids, polyps and fissures
- Barium enema can see impacted fecal matter or can detect complications such as polyps
- Anorectal manometry and rectal balloon expulsion tests are used to measure muscle tone of the anal sphincter and coordination between the rectal and anal muscles
- Colonic transit test, used to determine how long it takes food to travel through the colon

Priority Interventions or Actions

- Prepare client for diagnostic tests, such as barium enema
- Provide diet high in fiber
- Provide adequate liquids
- Administer laxative and/or enema in acute constipation
- Check client's rectal vault for impaction, if indicated
- Provide adequate privacy for client to defecate
- Use a safe odor eliminator to minimize odor
- Keep client nothing by mouth (NPO) if nausea and vomiting then diet as tolerated

Priority Potential & Actual Complications

- Perforation of colon, diverticulosis, rectal ulcers, rectal hemorrhoids
- Surgery with use of fecal diversions (such as colostomy)

Priority Nursing Implications

- Important for client to know the risk of repeated straining to have a bowel movement, called Valsalva maneuvers. Can cause decreased heart rate, less return of blood to the heart, and less blood flow from the heart when straining. Can cause a fatal outcome. Clients with heart conditions and/or swelling in the brain are particularly at risk
- Surgery because of constipation is not common

Priority Medications

- Stool softeners
    - Given orally to soften feces by lubricating intestinal tract
    - Usually cause bowel movement in 72 hours
- Bulk-forming laxatives
    - Absorb water and cause increase bulk, thus stimulating peristalsis; administered orally
    - Usually cause bowel movement within 24 hours
- Stimulants
    - Work by irritating colon wall and increasing peristalsis
    - Usually cause bowel movement in 10 to 12 hours
- Saline and osmotic solutions
    - May be administered various routes
    - Work by retaining fluid in the intestines
    - Usually cause bowel movement in 20 minutes to 3 hours

Reinforcement of Priority Teaching

- Eat foods high in fiber
- Drinking 8 glasses of water daily, if not contraindicated
- Encourage daily exercise
- Inform client to defecate when the urge is felt
- Assist client to create a schedule for bowel movements (like every morning before breakfast) and keep to that schedule as best as possible
- Inform client that placing feet on a small footstool while defecating allows the thighs to be flexed

Go To Clinical Answers

Text designated by the icon are the top answers for the Go To Clinical related to Constipation.

Pathophysiology/Description

- Celiac disease is an autoimmune disease where there is damage to the small intestines from intake of rye, wheat and barley. The disease is also commonly known as gluten sensitive enteropathy or celiac sprue
- There are specific peptides in gluten that bind to the celiac disease human leukocyte antigen and initiate an inflammatory response. The inflammation causes destruction of the microvilli and brush border of the small intestine. This results in a decrease in surface area that is needed for nutrient absorption to occur
- Risk factors
    - European ancestry (common in this ethnic group)
    - First and second-degree relatives to someone with celiac disease
    - Ninety percent of persons with Celiac disease have the antigen for the disease
- Symptoms of celiac disease are most often seen in childhood, between the ages of 1 to 5 years

Priority Data Collection or Cues

- Check for flatulence and fatty stool (steatorrhea)
- Check for diarrhea and foul-smelling diarrhea, from malabsorption
- Check for abdominal distention from gas accumulation
- Check for muscle wasting and weight loss
- Ask about nausea and vomiting
- Check for folate and iron-deficiency. Check vitamin B12 levels
- Examine mouth, poor dentition is likely
- Ask about lactose intolerance, which is likely with celiac disease
- Examine skin for vesicular lesions on various parts of the body that are pruritic (itchy)
- Check for osteoporosis due to bone weakening from inadequate vitamin D absorption and poor calcium intake
- Check for celiac crisis: profuse watery diarrhea, nausea, vomiting
- Check for dehydration and electrolyte imbalances
- Check vital signs, may be tachycardic and hypotensive
- Perform meticulous skin care and apply skin barrier to prevent skin breakdown from profuse diarrhea

Priority Laboratory Tests/Diagnostics

- Tissue Transglutaminase Antibodies (tTG-IgA) test, will be positive in about 98% of patients with celiac disease who are on a gluten-containing diet
- Biopsy of small intestines will show loss of villi and flattened mucosa, damage that is consistent with celiac disease
- Genetic testing for the HLA-DQ2 and/or HLA-DQ8 antigens, will show an increased risk for celiac disease

Priority Interventions or Actions

- Refer client to have a dietary consult
- Ensure that client is served meals that are gluten-free
- Administer all necessary vitamins such as A, D, E, K, folic acid and iron. Malabsorption causes client to be deficient
- If client is in a celiac crisis, do not give oral food. Keep NPO until crisis is resolved and client can tolerate foods by mouth
- Provide intravenous fluids to prevent dehydration
- Administer electrolytes to compensate for electrolyte imbalance

Priority Potential & Actual Complications

- Increased risk of Hodgkin's lymphoma and gastrointestinal cancers

Priority Nursing Implications

- Ensure that the client and/or caregiver is provided with adequate discharge teaching and resources on how to live a gluten-free life. Provide information for community, local and national resources, such as the Celiac Disease Foundation and the Celiac Sprue Association

Priority Medications

- Corticosteroids (several in the class)
    - Several drugs in this category can be used. Choice of drug depends on severity. Routes may also vary, orally is most common
    - Used to manage refractory celiac disease (when a gluten-free diet doesn't work)

Reinforcement of Priority Teaching

- Encourage screening of close relatives for the disease
- A diet free from gluten, avoiding barley, oats, wheat and rye
- Assist with locating community resources
- Show client and/or caregiver how to read food labels
- Explain to client and/or caregiver that a gluten-free diet will need to be maintained for life
- Provide the celiac disease website to client as an excellent source for resources: www.celiac.org

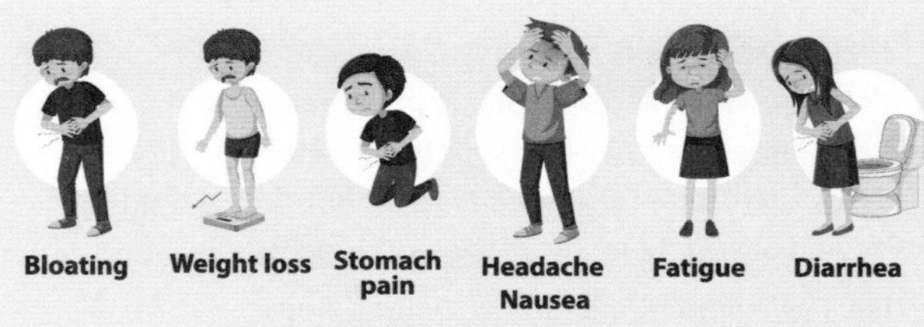

Image 11-3: What dietary restrictions are needed for a client with Celiac disease to avoid these symptoms?

Acute kidney disease/injury

Pathophysiology/Description

- Acute kidney disease (AKD) is defined as rapid loss of kidney function because of prerenal, intrarenal or postrenal damage to the kidneys. In AKD, the onset is sudden, but the condition is usually reversible once the cause is addressed
- Prerenal damage: caused by factors that occur outside of the kidneys that reduces or depletes intravascular volume such as, hemorrhage, decreased cardiac output and dehydration, among others
- Intrarenal: caused by factors that cause direct damage to the renal parenchyma, such as acute glomerulonephritis, acute tubular necrosis and effects of drugs on the kidneys, among others
- Postrenal: caused by factors that impede the flow of urine between the kidney and the urethra, such as benign prostate hyperplasia, calculi and bladder cancer, among others
- Phases associated with AKD
  - Oliguric: reduction in urine output to less than 400 mL/24 hours, occurring within 1-7 days of kidney injury is usually first sign of AKD. This phase can have a 10 to 14 days duration, but longer oliguric phase represents poorer prognosis for kidney recovery. Some clients will not experience oliguria
  - Diuretic: daily urine output starts to increase and can get as high as 5 L/day. The kidneys have not recovered but this urine output indicates that the kidneys are able to eliminate wastes from the body. The diuretic phase may last for up to 3 weeks
  - Recovery: glomerular filtration rate increases, and urine volume normalizes. Full kidney function occurs slowly, and it may take up to 1 year for kidney function to fully stabilize
- Continuous renal replacement therapy (CRRT) is sometimes done for clients with AKD
  - Double lumen catheter placed in the clients femoral or jugular vein and connected to a hemofilter where solutes are removed, and the client's blood is filtered of toxins until AKD is resolved
- Many clients with AKD recover well but if recovery does not proceed well through the phases, then the client may progress to end-stage kidney disease

Priority Data Collection or Cues

- Check for sudden decrease in urine output
- Check for anorexia, nausea and vomiting
- Check for signs of neurological impairment
- Check neck veins, which may be distended
- Check lungs for crackles, indicating fluid in the lungs
- Check for pericarditis, manifested by friction rub, and chest pain upon inspiration
- Check for signs of fluid overload
- Check respirations, may find Kussmaul respirations because of metabolic acidosis, caused by depletion of sodium bicarbonate
- Check for increased urine volume
- Check for hypovolemia and hypotension, tachycardia
- Check for normalized urine output (recovery phase)
- Check for manifestations of infection
- If client getting CRRT monitor vital signs, intake and output, and hemodynamic status hourly. Monitor the vascular access site for infection, and maintain patency of the CRRT system

Priority Laboratory Tests/Diagnostics

- Electrolytes: in oliguric phase, serum sodium and bicarbonate levels are decreased while potassium, blood urea nitrogen (BUN) and creatinine levels are increased
- Urinalysis showing elevated white blood cell count, casts, hematuria, pyuria and protein, indicate an intrarenal cause for AKD
- Kidney ultrasound to look for obstructions and/or other abnormalities of the urinary system
- Computed tomography (CT) scan to look for complications of the condition, such as renal masses and vascular abnormalities
- Renal scan to look at renal tubular function and kidney blood flow
- Renal biopsy is used to determine cause of the kidney injury and is considered the most definitive way to diagnose AKD caused by intrarenal factors
- EKG: widening of QRS complex and ST segment depression may indicate hyperkalemia

Priority Interventions or Actions

- Measure intake and output
- Administer diuretics as prescribed, to treat fluid overload
- Weigh client daily using the same scale and at the same time
- Use aseptic technique where needed
- Provide prescribed diet
- Provide measures to prevent blood clots from immobility
- Provide measures to prevent skin breaks
- Prepare client for renal replacement therapy, if prescribed
- Administer enteral feeding if cannot tolerate oral
- Administer treatment for hyperkalemia as prescribed

Priority Potential & Actual Complications

- Infection
- Hyperkalemia
- Chronic kidney disease
- Dialysis
- Renal transplantation

Priority Nursing Implications

- When caring for clients who are older adults, it is important to know that they may not recover from AKD as do younger clients. They may not regain full function of their kidneys after AKD
- Clients on dialysis who are in AKD, their response to fever is blunted so they may not respond to an infection with a fever
- Contrast media must not be used in tests for clients with AKD

Priority Medications

- Furosemide
    - Most commonly given orally, but may be given intravenous
    - Loop diuretic to treat fluid overload in oliguric phase
    - Potassium-wasting drug so monitor potassium
- Several drugs are used to treat hyperkalemia associated with AKD. Below are a few of these drugs
    - Sodium bicarbonate
    - Patiromer
    - Calcium gluconate

Reinforcement of Priority Teaching

- Importance of monitoring urinary status
- The impact of diet on the kidneys
- Importance of medications
- Importance of regular follow-up with health care provider to assess kidney function
- Remind client the indicators of recurrent kidney disease and when to contact health care provider
- Remind client that full recovery after AKD may take several months
- Discuss with client possibilities if kidneys do not fully recover, such as dialysis or kidney transplantation
- Assist client with seeking appropriate resources for counseling, if needed
- Discuss that certain drugs worsen kidney function

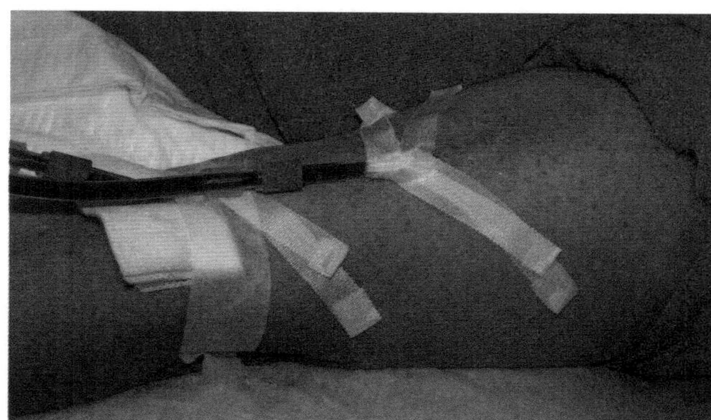

Image 11-4: How can a nurse determine that a fistula for hemodialysis is patent?

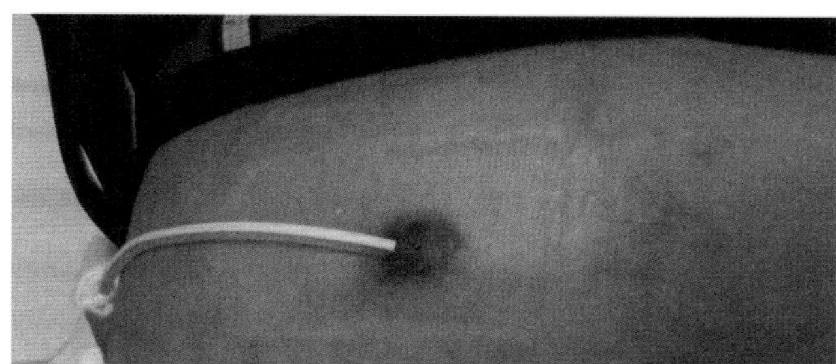

Image 11-5: What is the significance of a distended or hard abdomen in clients receiving peritoneal dialysis?

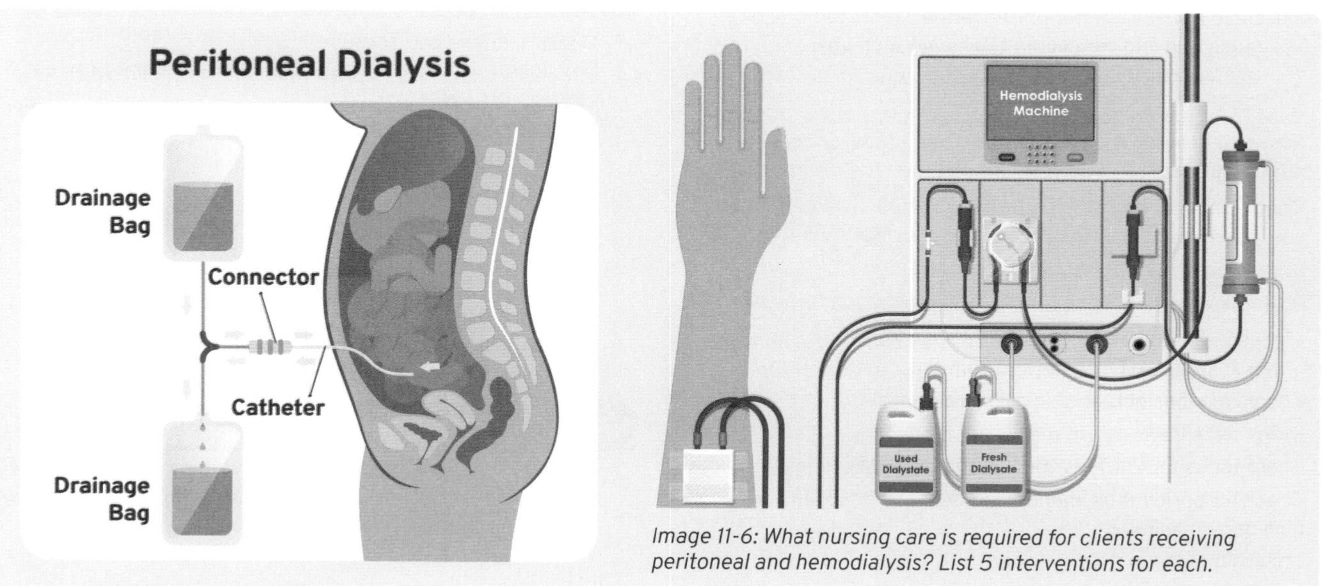

Image 11-6: What nursing care is required for clients receiving peritoneal and hemodialysis? List 5 interventions for each.

Pathophysiology/Description

- Benign prostatic hypertrophy (BPH) is the increase of the prostate gland causing disruption in the outflow of urine. Conversely, prostate cancer is a slow-growing, malignant growth of the prostate gland that can spread to various parts of the body
- Decrease in testosterone as men age, coupled with an excess dihydrotestosterone, and higher proportion of estrogen may account for increase cell growth, causing BPH
- The urethra is compressed as the prostate grows causing partial obstruction and urinary difficulty
- Risk factors for BPH
    - Genetic predisposition with family history of first-degree relative having BPH
    - Erectile dysfunction, diabetes
    - Alcohol intake, smoking, obesity, physical inactivity
- Risk factors for prostate cancer
    - Age 50 and older
    - Ethnicity, as higher incidence seen in African American men
    - Diet low in vegetables and fruits but high in fats, red and processed meats
    - Interactions with chemicals such as pesticides in farming
- Both prostate cancer and BPH are slow growing and the client may not see manifestations until prostate is large and/or cancer has progressed beyond the early stage
- Prostate cancer is staged using the commonly used Tumor, Node Metastasis (TNM) staging system. Stages are from I to V, with V being the most poorly differentiated cells

Priority Data Collection or Cues

- Ask about nocturia, as this is usually one of the first symptoms
- Ask about urinary frequency and urgency, dysuria
- Ask client to describe the urine stream
- Ask about the time it takes to start a urine stream
- Ask about dribbling at the end of the stream
- Use the American Urological Association symptom index for BPH tool to guide data collection of symptoms of voiding related to BPH
- Check bladder, may find that it is distended. Check for painless, gross hematuria, indicating prostate cancer
- Check client's understanding of surgery
- Postoperative monitoring for BPH and prostate cancer surgery
    - Check for symptoms of transurethral resection syndrome (TUR), manifested by nausea, vomiting, hypertension, bradycardia, increased intracranial pressure, disorientation
    - Check for bladder spasms. Check for infection and bleeding
    - Examine color of irrigation drainage to determine effectiveness of irrigation. It should be light pink in color and with no clots
    - Monitor vital signs

Priority Laboratory Tests/Diagnostics

- Digital rectal examination tells the size and consistency of the prostate
- Urinalysis shows elevated white blood cell count or hematuria, indicating inflammation or infection
- Prostate-specific antigen (PSA) will be elevated in BPH and prostate cancer
- Transrectal ultrasound to differentiate between BPH and prostate cancer and to do a biopsy of the tumor
- Magnetic resonance imaging (MRI) ultrasound fusion biopsy, a new biopsy technique that examines cancer tumor
- Serum creatinine to rule out insufficiency of renal system
- Uroflowmetry determines volume of urine that is coming from the bladder, which can then determine degree of urethral blockage
- Cystoscopy to look at inside of urethra and bladder and view the prostate enlargement
- Postvoid residual urine shows the extent of the urine flow obstruction
- Serum alkaline phosphatase will be increased if prostate cancer has metastasized to the bone

Priority Interventions or Actions

- Administer antibiotics preoperatively as prescribed
- Administer antiemetics for nausea
- Insert urinary drainage preoperatively, may need to use a catheter with a special tip
- Provide opportunity for client and partner to discuss the effect of surgery on sexual function
- Initiate administration of drugs for androgen deprivation therapy, if used
- Assist with procedure to remove testes(orchiectomy) to augment androgen deprivation therapy
- Prepare client for radiation, used with or without surgery
- Postoperative specific interventions for BPH and prostate cancer
    - Irrigate bladder either manually or continuously after TURP, as prescribed to prevent clots
    - Administer analgesics for pain. Administer antispasmodics for bladder spasms as prescribed
    - Have client practice Kegel exercises to strengthen pelvic floor several times while awake
    - Clean perineal area well after each bowel movement, especially if client had a radical prostatectomy, to prevent infection
    - Change dressings using sterile technique. Empty and document drainage from surgical drains
    - Dressing from a suprapubic prostatectomy procedure will drain urine at the surgical site, change dressing often and perform good site care
    - Remove suprapubic catheter when residual urine volume is less than 75 mL and client is consistently emptying the bladder

- Monitor hematocrit and hemoglobin levels
- Administer stool softeners to prevent client from straining at stools postoperatively
- Assist client to ambulate early postoperatively to minimize complications of post-surgical immobility, such a blood clot

Priority Potential & Actual Complications

- TUR, hemorrhage, urinary retention, deep vein thrombosis, wound dehiscence, sexual dysfunction, sterility

Priority Nursing Implications

- It is important to recognize a potentially serious complication of the TURP procedure, called transurethral resection syndrome (TUR), manifested by nausea, vomiting, hypertension, bradycardia, disorientation. The syndrome occurs as a result of bladder irrigation that is prolonged in surgery, and hyponatremia
- When the client has a perineal prostatectomy, rectal probes, tubes, thermometers must not be used as they increase the risk of trauma, which can cause infection and/or bleeding
- Consider health and cultural beliefs of the client. Prostate cancer and BPH affect a man's sensitive part of his body and in some cultures, surgery on that part of the body is viewed as a significant onslaught on his manhood and how he is perceived as a "man." At some point pre or post treatment, this issue should be broached and discussed

Priority Medications

- Finasteride
    - 5a-Reductase Inhibitor, a common oral drug, used to reduce the size of the prostate
    - Must not be handled by pregnant women as it may cause anomalies with a male fetus
- Dutasteride/Tamsulosin
    - 5a-Reductase Inhibitor, a common oral drug, used to reduce the size of the prostate
    - This is a combination therapy so both drugs are taken together
- Dutasteride
    - 5a-Reductase Inhibitor, a common oral drug, used to reduce the size of the prostate
    - May also lower the risk of prostate cancer
- Alfuzosin
    - An orally administered adrenergic receptor blocker relaxes smooth muscles making urination better in BPH
    - Causes hypostatic hypotension, and is worsened if taking antihypertensive drugs
- Silodosin
    - A-Adrenergic receptor blocker relaxes smooth muscles making urination better in BPH
    - If difficulty swallowing, open capsule and sprinkle on applesauce
- Prazosin
    - An orally administered adrenergic receptor blocker relaxes smooth muscles making urination better in BPH
- Tadalafil
    - Erectogenic drug that decreases the symptoms of BPH
    - Has added benefit of helping erectile dysfunction that is sometimes associated with BPH
- Oxybutynin
    - Antimuscarinic, given orally, used to treat bladder spasms in BPH and prostate cancer
- Several drugs from various classes are used for androgen deprivation therapy in prostate cancer. Below are a few common ones
    - Leuprolide
    - Triptorelin
    - Degarelix
    - Bicalutamide
- The use of chemotherapy in prostate cancer is palliative and not curative and administered by a RN
    - Cabazitaxel
    - Docetaxel and prednisone
    - Estramustine

Reinforcement of Priority Teaching

- For active surveillance (for BPH) or androgen suppression therapy (for prostate cancer)
    - Decrease intake of caffeine, spicy foods and artificial sweeteners
    - Fluid intake of up to 2000 to 3000 mL daily, if not contraindicated. Restrict fluids at night before bed
    - Take medications as prescribed
    - Monitor symptoms carefully
    - Contact health care provider for worsening symptoms
    - Have annual PSA and digital rectal examination
    - Avoid alcohol intake
    - Speak with pharmacist before taking over-the-counter medications and herbal remedies
    - Do not suppress the urge to urinate as it causes stasis of urine
    - Proper administration and side effects of drugs used for androgen suppression
- After surgery for BPH and prostate cancer
    - Proper handling of surgical site, to prevent infection
    - Monitoring site for bleeding and infection
    - The possibility of retrograde ejaculation and erectile dysfunction
    - Return of sexual function may be 1 to 2 years
    - Take medications prescribed to help sexual function
    - Be aware of incontinence and that it should resolve
    - Drink water and urinate 2 to 3 times daily
    - Signs and symptoms to report immediately and who to call

Pathophysiology/Description

- Gastritis is inflammation of the gastric mucosa
- Acute gastritis usually has a duration of hours to a few days. The mucosa is usually completely healed after the episode
- Chronic gastritis occurs over extended periods. Atrophy of stomach mucosa occurs causing loss of parietal cells. This results in loss of intrinsic factor needed for absorption of vitamin B_{12}, which is essential in red blood cell maturation
- The etiology of gastritis relates to a breakdown in the normal mucosal barrier. This mucosal barrier breakdown allows hydrochloric acid to damage the mucosa causing irritation, erosion, edema and inflammation
- There are several risk factors for gastritis such as
    - Dietary eating spicy foods, large amounts of food or intaking alcohol
    - Pathogens, such as Helicobacter pylori (H. pylori)
    - Drugs, such as non-steroidal anti-inflammatory drugs (NSAIDs)
    - Environmental, such as smoking
    - Disease processes, such as burns
    - Autoimmune atrophic gastritis, where immune response damages stomach cells. This is an inherited condition seen in women of northern European descent

Priority Data Collection or Cues

- Check for nausea, vomiting, feeling of fullness, anorexia and epigastric tenderness
- Check client for gastric hemorrhage, which indicates alcohol associated gastritis
- Ask about excessive belching
- Check for anemia, caused by lack of vitamin B12 with chronic gastritis
- Ask client about intake of foods that cause gastritis
- Check vital signs, hypotension and tachycardia may indicate bleeding
- Ask client about exposure to environmental factors that cause gastritis
- Check for sour taste in mouth, occurring more with chronic gastritis
- Check for vitamin B 12 deficiency, occurring with chronic gastritis

Priority Laboratory Tests/Diagnostics

- Test for H. Pylori via breath, blood and stool, will be positive
- Stool tested for occult blood, may be positive
- Endoscopy stomach examination and biopsy will show H. Pylori and biopsy can rule out gastric cancer
- Complete blood count may indicate anemia because of lack of B12

Priority Interventions or Actions

- Acute gastritis
    - Maintain nothing by mouth (NPO)
    - Administer intravenous fluids to prevent dehydration
    - Monitor intake and output
    - Monitor nasogastric (NG) tube for bleeding
    - If no NG, check vomitus for signs of gastric bleeding
    - Administer antiemetics as prescribed
    - Re-introduce a clear liquid diet when symptoms have subsided
    - Administer medications to manage gastritis symptoms
    - Administer antibiotics to treat H. Pylori

Priority Potential & Actual Complications

- Peptic ulcer
- Pernicious anemia
- Cancer called gastric mucosa-associated lymphoid tissue (MALT) lymphoma because of chronic H. pylori gastritis

Priority Nursing Implications

- Clients with pernicious anemia from chronic gastritis must be educated on the fact that they will need to take B12 injections for life

Priority Medications

- Proton pump inhibitors
    - Administered via the oral route
    - Several drugs in this class are used. They decrease hydrochloric acid secretion and decrease gastric mucosa irritation
    - Available over-the-counter or by prescription
- Histamine receptor blockers
    - Several drugs in this class are used. They decrease hydrochloric acid secretion and decrease gastric and esophageal mucosa irritation
    - Like the proton pump inhibitors, this class of drugs is effective and commonly used orally
    - Available both as over-the-counter and prescription

Reinforcement of Priority Teaching

- Assist with administration of prescribed medications
- Avoid spicy and well-seasoned foods
- Prevention of alcohol intake
- Client to stop smoking
- Remind client to take all of the prescribed antibiotics for H. pylori, even if symptoms have subsided
- Increase diet back to normal, as tolerated, after an acute episode
- The intake of 6 small meals instead of large meals
- Remind client to monitor for signs and symptoms of gastric bleeding and contact health care provider immediately

Cleft lip and palate

Pathophysiology/Description

- Cleft lip and palate are congenital anomalies that cause abnormalities in closure of the lip and palate. Tissue that makes up the palate and lip normally fuse together in the second and third months in pregnancy
- Cleft lip and palate can occur bilaterally or unilaterally
- Causes include: Genetics, with high incidence in children with family history of cleft lip/palate defects, chromosomal abnormality syndrome, exposure to teratogens while pregnant, the mother having diabetes before pregnancy, or obesity during pregnancy
- Surgery is the only means of fixing a cleft lip and palate. A cleft lip is usually repaired first at around the third month of life
- Cleft palate is repaired in several surgeries. The first surgery occurs between 6 to 12 months. Focus of the first surgery is on the creation of a palate that is functional and that minimizes the likelihood of fluid accumulating in the middle ear. This first surgery also helps the child develop facial bones and teeth

Priority Data Collection or Cues

- Check for difficulty feeding. Examine baby's lip and palate, will observe abnormal openings in lip and palate. Ask caregiver about regurgitation of fluids through the baby's mouth and nose
- Ask caregiver about ear infections as chronic ear infections are common with cleft lip and palate
- Examine baby's teeth (if there are teeth yet), expect misalignment of teeth
- Check baby's ability to breathe without having difficulty
- Check baby's voice, usually sounds nasal with cleft lip and palate
- Check for nutritional and fluid intake, may be poorly nourished because of difficulty eating

Priority Laboratory Tests/Diagnostics

- Cleft lip and palate can be diagnosed 16 weeks into a woman's pregnancy. The physical appearance of the newborn after birth confirms the diagnosis

Priority Interventions or Actions

- Feed baby using a special nipple. Hold baby in a semi-upright seated position and stabilize the baby's head with one hand while feeding with the other. Keep a bulb suction to suction feeding from the nasal passage if needed
- Feed using the ESSR method of feeding: Enlarge the nipple, Stimulate the reflex for sucking, allow baby to Swallow and Rest to give the baby time to swallow what is in its mouth. Feed baby small amounts and burp baby often
- Allow caregiver(s) to verbalize feelings about the baby's appearance
- Postoperative interventions
  - Check surgery site for bleeding and signs of infection. A metal bar may be used on the face to protect the cleft lip surgery incision. Adhesive strips (Steri Strips) may also be used
  - Keep restraint on baby's hands and arms, unless a guardian or nurse is in the room with the baby
  - Place baby to sleep on side and back and not stomach, to prevent pressure on incision
  - Change dressings using sterile technique to minimize risk of infection. Antibiotic ointment may be prescribed
  - Administer pain medication to manage baby's pain
  - Monitor surgical packing that is secured to the child's palate, if used. Check for bleeding
  - Do not brush teeth, if present
  - Do not place objects in child's mouth while collecting data on the palate incision as objects may damage the incision
  - Initiate appropriate consults such as to dietitian, dentist and speech therapist

Priority Potential & Actual Complications

- Speech difficulties and dental problems
- Impaired sucking ability and decreased nutrition, ear infections and hearing loss
- Parental psychological distress

Priority Nursing Implications

- The child born with a cleft lip and palate can be very distressing for the parents as they may see their child as being disfigured. Be sensitive and allow parents to verbalize their feelings

Priority Medications

- Analgesics: Used for managing child's pain after surgery. The choice and dose of medication will vary

Reinforcement of Priority Teaching

- Use the ESSR method to feed baby
- Provide information on support groups
- Do not place anything hard, like a spoon, in baby's mouth after surgery. Give baby a small amount of water after feeding to cleanse the mouth of food that might cause buildup of bacteria in mouth, causing infection
- The use of a cradle hold to prevent injury to the surgical site
- Baby will wear a restraint for a few weeks to prevent from rubbing or touching the incision
- Remind caregiver not to use aspirin for baby's pain

Pathophysiology/Description

- Chronic kidney disease (CKD) is progressive, irreversible loss of kidney function. End-stage renal disease with the need for dialysis or kidney transplantation is the result of CKD
- Unlike acute kidney injury that is sudden, CKD has a slow onset, often progressing over several years and is characterized by significantly decreased glomerular filtration rate (less than 60 mL/min for more than 3 months) and kidney damage (for more than 3 months)
- There are 5 stages of CKD. Stage 1 manifests kidney damage with glomerular filtration rate (GFR) of 90 mL/min or greater. As the stages progress and CKD worsens, GFR decreases until the 5th stage, kidney failure, is reached with a GFR of less than 15 mL/min. At this stage the client requires dialysis or kidney transplantation to sustain life
- All body systems are negatively impacted
- Diabetes and hypertension are the predominant causes of CKD. African Americans, Hispanics and Native Americans have much higher rates
- With end-stage renal disease, the client will need dialysis or kidney transplantation. There are several types of dialysis
- Peritoneal dialysis
    - The peritoneum is used as a semipermeable membrane to perform dialysis treatment via a catheter that is inserted through the client's abdomen. Dialysate is instilled in client's abdomen and dwells there for a few hours, pulling toxins via the peritoneum's semipermeable membrane. It is then drained from the abdomen
- Hemodialysis
    - Removal of waste from a client's body by use of a hemodialyzer (artificial kidney). A fistula or graft is created in a client's body, usually in the lower or upper arm and these are accessed and connected to the dialyzer. One lumen takes blood from the client to the dialyzer and the other brings blood back from the dialyzer to the client
- Continuous renal replacement therapy
    - Double lumen catheter placed in the client's femoral or jugular vein and connected to a hemofilter where solutes are removed, and the client's blood is filtered of toxins

Priority Data Collection or Cues

- Check for anorexia, nausea and vomiting, lethargy and fatigue, indicative of very high BUN level
- Check for metallic taste to mouth and uremic fetor (urine like smell) from ammonia buildup
- Check for signs of neurological impairment due to accumulation of ammonia from nitrogenous waste
- Check for peripheral neuropathy and asterixis
- Check for fractures of small bones, caused by associated mineral and bone disorder
- Check skin for itching caused by uremic frost, crystallization of uremia on skin due to elevated BUN
- Ask client about use of prescription and over-the-counter medications as many drugs are toxic to the kidneys
- Check for signs of fluid overload
- Check blood glucose, may find hyperglycemia
- Check for symptoms of metabolic acidosis
- Check respirations, may find Kussmaul respirations
- Check for bleeding due to decreased coagulopathy
- Check for infections as CKD places client at high risk
- Check client's long-term support system, since CKD and end-stage renal disease are life-altering conditions
- For client on hemodialysis
    - Monitor for hypotension
    - Check for nausea, vomiting, chest pain, and visual changes due to rapid fluid removal
    - Check for muscle cramps associated with low sodium dialysis solution
    - Check post dialysis bleeding from factors such as poor rinsing of blood for the dialyzer
    - Check the fistula by feeling the thrill (purring at the fistula site) and listening to the bruit (sound of rushing water, like a washing machine) with a stethoscope
    - Check client for steal syndrome (shunting of blood from distal extremity in dialysis), manifested by pain distal to the access site, poor capillary refill and numbness that worsens with dialysis
    - Check insertion site for bleeding, hematoma or infection
- Additionally for client on peritoneal dialysis (PD)
    - Check the catheter insertion site for infection
    - Check for peritonitis
    - Check for hernias and back pain, due to weight of the dialysate causing increased pressure in the abdomen
    - Check respiratory status for complications such as pneumonia, and atelectasis

Priority Laboratory Tests/Diagnostics

- Urine will show elevated albumin, white blood cell count, protein, casts and glucose
- Glomerular filtration rate (GFR) shows degree of kidney damage
- Elevated potassium, blood urea nitrogen (BUN) and creatinine levels are expected
- Kidney ultrasound to look for obstructions and/or other abnormalities of the urinary system
- Computed tomography (CT) scan to look for complications of the condition
- Renal scan to look at renal tubular function and kidney blood flow
- Renal biopsy is used to determine cause of the kidney disease and is considered the most definitive

Priority Interventions or Actions

- Administer diuretics as ordered, to treat fluid overload
- Weigh client daily
- Administer medications as prescribed
- Refer client to dietitian for nutritional counseling
- Monitor client taking nephrotoxic drugs
- Allow client adequate rest
- Maintain client on sodium and phosphate restricted diet
- Provide information to client on all types of dialysis procedures
- Maintain prescribed diet and fluid restrictions
- Provide measures to prevent blood clots from immobility
- Provide measures to prevent skin breaks
- Provide comfort measures as needed
- Administer enteral feeding if client cannot tolerate oral intake
- Interventions for client on hemodialysis
  - Monitor vital signs pre-during and post dialysis
  - Weigh client before and after dialysis
  - Monitor client for bleeding as heparin is used in dialysis
  - Monitor for fluid status
  - Ensure client with femoral vein catheter sits up at less than a 45-degree angle and does not lean forward due to risk of catheter occlusion or kinking
  - Monitor graft/shunt for clotting, manifested by inability to feel a thrill and hear a bruit, and by client's complaint of tingling and discomfort in arm
- Interventions for client on peritoneal dialysis
  - Administer antibiotics for infection
  - Apply orthopedic binders for complaint of back pain
  - Monitor dialysis fluid outflow to ensure consistency in flow. Maintain drainage bag below client's abdomen. Check outflow for color, odor, presence of blood
  - Ongoing monitoring of protein loss to prevent loss that is too high, placing client at risk for malnutrition

Priority Potential & Actual Complications

- Cardiovascular complications, dyslipidemia, bone disease
- End-stage renal disease and dialysis, catheter site infection and peritonitis with PD
- Renal transplantation

Priority Nursing Implications

- Chronic kidney disease impacts every system in the body. Cardiovascular disease is the most common cause of death in clients with CKD, so meticulous monitoring of the cardiovascular system must be made when caring for clients with CKD
- Nurses must remember that blood pressure and venous access must never be performed in the client's arm that has a vascular access because of the risk of clotting of the vascular access
- A temporary access can be used for dialysis until a fistula or graft matures and can be used. The temporary access is made via the femoral or jugular veins. These should not be mistaken for regular intravenous lines

Priority Medications

- Several drugs are used to treat hyperkalemia associated with CKD such as, Sodium bicarbonate, Sodium polystyrene sulfonate, Patiromer, and Calcium gluconate
- Calcium acetate
  - Used orally as a phosphate binder to bind phosphate and excrete it in stool
- Calcitriol
  - Given orally or intravenous to treat secondary hyperparathyroidism in end-stage renal disease
  - Measure serum calcium at least twice weekly during start of drug therapy
- Erythropoietin
  - May be given intravenous or subcutaneously
  - Treat anemia associated with chronic kidney disease
  - Monitor iron stores and administer iron if serum ferritin is below 100 ng/mL
  - Monitor hemoglobin to prevent cardiovascular complications
- Atorvastatin
  - Given orally to treat dyslipidemia in CKD

Reinforcement of Priority Teaching

- Follow the prescribed diet restrictions. Demonstrate how to read food labels
- Discuss barriers to dialysis with client
- Assist with information regarding resources
- How to measure blood pressure and blood glucose. Have client do return demonstration
- Remind client to examine PD catheter insertion site for infection
- Remind client to avoid intravenous catheters or blood pressure measurements in the arm with a graft or shunt for dialysis
- Remind client to avoid submerging the shunt in water
- Signs of shunt infection and when to contact the health care provider
- Importance of regular follow-up with health care provider
- Remind the client to take prescribed medications
- Remind client to ask the pharmacist before taking any over-the-counter drugs or herbal preparations
- Remind client on dialysis that they may or may not produce urine

Cirrhosis

Pathophysiology/Description

- Cirrhosis is chronic end-stage liver disease characterized by irreversible destruction and degeneration of liver cells
- Due to repeated injury of the cells, scar tissue forms. The new cells are abnormal leading to the lobes of liver having a irregular size and shape. Normal blood flow is inhibited. This leads to poor liver function
- Causes of cirrhosis include: chronic hepatitis, excessive alcohol intake, nonalcoholic steatohepatitis (caused by accumulation of fat in liver), extreme dieting, biliary conditions and hepatic encephalopathy

Priority Data Collection or Cues

- Check for anorexia, nausea and vomiting. Check for ascites, measure abdominal girth
- Check for muscle wasting from poor nutritional status
- Check color of urine, color is dark brown in presence of jaundice
- Check stools, color is tan or gray in presence of jaundice
- Check respiratory status, dyspnea and hyperventilation
- Check for presence of jaundice
- Ask client about itching, common in liver failure
- Check for melena or hematemesis from bleeding varices
- Check for bleeding esophageal and gastric varices (a medical emergency)
- Check for symptoms of hepatorenal syndrome
- Check for symptoms of hepatic encephalopathy
- Check for a sweet, musty odor on client's breath (called fetor hepaticus), because of accumulated liver byproducts

Priority Laboratory Tests/Diagnostics

- Esophagogastroduodenoscopy (EGD), will show esophageal and stomach varices
- Liver biopsy used to make definitive diagnosis of cirrhosis
- Liver function test, enzymes will be elevated at first because they are released from inflamed cells but may be normal in end-stage cirrhosis due to damage of hepatocytes
- Increased bilirubin and decreased serum protein and albumin are expected
- Ultrasound elastography, shows liver fibrosis. Liver with cirrhosis will be stiffer than healthy one
- Complete blood cell (CBC), may show increased white blood cell count due to inflammation

Priority Interventions or Actions

- Provide oral hygiene before meals
- Administer medications as prescribed
- Monitor intake and output
- Weigh client daily. Manage nutritional deficits
- Monitor for orthostatic hypotension with bleeding varices
- Administer intravenous fluids if blood loss from varices
- Administer supplemental vitamins
- Elevate head of bed to help client breathe better
- Measure abdominal girth throughout treatment to determine effectiveness of treatment for ascites
- Allow client to remain on bedrest. Provide range of motion exercises
- Assist client with deep breathing and coughing exercises
- Monitor and document fluid and electrolyte imbalances
- Provide good skin care. Ensure client is turned every two hours or more frequent if needed. Elevate extremities that are edematous
- Prepare client for procedure to remove fluid from the abdominal cavity (paracentesis)
- Allow client to verbalize feelings regarding disease

Priority Potential & Actual Complications

- Portal hypertension, ascites, jaundice, hepatorenal syndrome
- Bleeding esophageal varices, defects in coagulation, encephalopathy, and may be fatal

Priority Nursing Implications

- When a balloon tamponade is used for bleeding varices, it is important that each tube is labeled so they are easily identified. The tube must be secured to prevent accidental occlusion of airway and balloons deflated per the hospital's policy

Priority Medications

- Albumin
    - Administered intravenously
    - Used to help maintain intravascular volume and adequate urine output in ascites
    - Administer additional albumin within 15 to 30 minutes if response to initial dose was inadequate

- Spironolactone
  - Several diuretics used to treat ascites, spironolactone is a commonly used oral drug in the class
  - Used to treat ascites and does not cause potassium to be depleted
- Tolvaptan
  - Given orally to treat hyponatremia that is common in cirrhosis
- Nadolol
  - Administered orally
  - Used to treat clients with esophageal or gastric varices. Reduce portal pressure and decrease risk of varices rupturing and hemorrhage
- Octreotide acetate
  - May be given subcutaneously or intravenously
  - Used to stop the bleeding in varices so additional intervention can be started
  - Causes vasoconstriction and decreases portal blood flow, thus decreasing portal hypertension
- Lactulose
  - Administered orally or as an enema
  - Used to treat hepatic encephalopathy
- Rifaximin
  - Administered orally
  - Used to reduce risk of hepatic encephalopathy
  - May cause dizziness
- Cholestyramine
  - Administered orally
  - Used to treat pruritus (itching)

Reinforcement of Priority Teaching

- Encourage client experiencing pruritus to use knuckles to rub itchy area, instead of using nails
- Remind client the importance of not drinking alcohol
- Avoid straining such as during a bowel movement
- Assist client with information on help with quitting alcohol
- Remind client to follow the sodium restricted diet carefully
- Demonstrate how to read food labels for sodium content
- Follow prescribed diet and oral nutritional supplement
- Potential symptoms and when to contact their health care provider
- Remind client to keep follow-up medical appointments as cirrhosis requires ongoing medical care
- Encourage client to speak with pharmacist before taking any over-the-counter medications

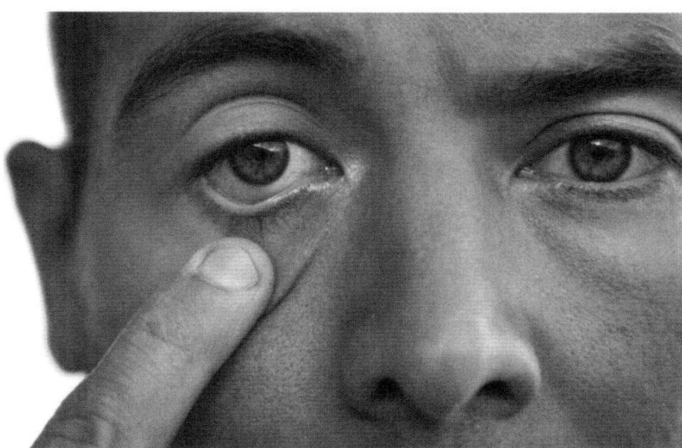

Image 11-7: The nurse observes the above client. What additional information would the nurse want to gather from the client?

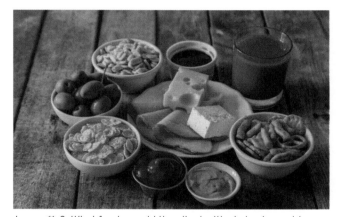

Image 11-8: What foods would the client with cirrhosis want to limit? Provide specific examples.

Clinical Hint

Pruritis is a common issue with cirrhosis. Effective interventions may include using warm (not hot) water, providing moisturizing lotions, keeping environmental temperatures moderate, maintaining adequate hydration, and using medications as needed.

Colorectal cancer

Pathophysiology/Description

- Colorectal cancer is a malignant growth that occurs in the rectum and/or colon. It is the third most common cancer in the United States and ranks as the second leading cause of death from all cancers
- Risk factor
  - First-degree family or personal history of colorectal polyps
  - Family history of colorectal cancer
  - Personal history of inflammatory bowel disease
  - Personal history of diabetes mellitus
  - Age, usually seen in older than 50 years
  - Smoking
  - Obesity
  - Excessive alcohol intake, usually more than 4 to 5 drinks weekly
  - Consumption of large amounts of red meat, usually greater than 6-7 servings weekly
- Metastasis is a major concern with colorectal cancer because as it spreads to the liver (a common site of metastasis), it can then move from the liver to several other parts of the body
- Colorectal cancer is staged using the commonly used Tumor Node Metastasis (TNM) staging system. Stages are from 0 to IV and as the stages increase, prognosis worsens
- There are several types of surgical ostomies that can be done with colorectal cancer. The choice of ostomy is dependent on the location of the tumor and the severity of the cancer

Priority Data Collection or Cues

- Check for blood in stool
- Ask client about change in bowel habits, diarrhea or constipation. This can indicate the location of the tumor
- Ask about size of stools, as in a decrease from large stools to pencil-sized. This change can indicate partial obstruction
- Check for nausea, vomiting, anorexia and weight loss
- Check for presence of an abdominal mass
- Check appearance of abdomen, may appear distended
- Check for ascites, which indicates liver involvement
- Check for muscle wasting (cachexia)
- Check for bowel perforation and signs of peritonitis
- Check client's understanding of surgery
- Check client's psychological status and intervene accordingly

Priority Laboratory Tests/Diagnostics

- Colonoscopy shows entire colon, polyps visualized can be removed and tissue biopsy done
- Fecal occult and fecal immunochemical tests show blood in stool. Since bleeding from tumor does not occur continuously, these tests must be done frequently
- Stool DNA test (New test called Cologuard) can show DNA markers that can indicate colorectal cancer
- Computed tomography (CT) scan, magnetic resonance imaging (MRI) and abdominal ultrasound to look for metastasis of the cancer
- Barium enema to look for structural abnormalities
- Complete blood count
- Liver function tests, to determine involvement of the liver
- Blood culture may show infection in blood
- Carcinoembryonic antigen (CEA) level may be elevated

Priority Interventions or Actions

- Keep client nothing by mouth in acute phase
- Monitor intravenous fluids to prevent dehydration
- Administer medications as prescribed
- Monitor intake and output
- Monitor for bowel perforation
- Prepare client for radiation to decrease tumor size, if indicated
- Allow client time to verbalize feelings
- Surgical interventions (polypectomy during colonoscopy, abdominal-perineal resection, colectomy with ostomy)
  - Perform preoperative preparation and care
  - Insert nasogastric tube to suction
  - Manage post-surgical devices such as ostomy pouch
  - Perform colostomy irrigations
  - Manage surgical drains, empty and document drainage
  - Check surgical site for infection
  - Check viability of stoma and report any negative findings, such as a brown-black stoma color, which indicates necrosis. Healthy stoma is pink in color
  - Initiate consult with the hospital's wound, ostomy and continence nurse (WOCN)
  - Initiate consult with dietitian to discuss, modifications in diet
  - Give close attention to surgical site in the immediate postoperative period. Reinforce dressings as needed and monitor for excessive bleeding. Perform ongoing sterile dressing changes

- Provide clear liquids after the acute phase and progress diet as tolerated
    - Allow client to participate in self-care of surgical site, in preparation for home care
    - Allow early mobility to prevent post-surgery complications, such as pneumonia and blood clots

Priority Potential & Actual Complications

- Bowel obstruction and perforation
- Hemorrhage and peritonitis
- Fistula
- Permanent bowel diversion device (like colostomy)
- Sepsis
- May be fatal

Priority Nursing Implications

- Colorectal cancer usually does not manifest until the disease has progressed to an advanced stage. Therefore, clients must be provided with information on the importance of getting a screening colonoscopy at scheduled intervals
- Having a bowel diversion device on the body and dealing with everything that comes with that device and the diagnosis of cancer, can be challenging and distressing for clients. It is important that clients get presurgical psychological preparation as this will increase the likelihood of better coping after the surgery

Priority Medications

- 5-fluorouracil, oxaliplatin, irinotecan, bevacizumab, panitumumab, trifluridine/tipiracil, aflibercept, regorafenib
    - Chemotherapy drugs used in a variety of combinations most likely to be administered by the RN
    - Monitor for bleeding fatigue, and infection. Monitor red and white blood cell counts and platelets

Reinforcement of Priority Teaching

- Show client how to properly care for surgical site at home, such as empty device, change device, check stoma, irrigate colostomy, check for signs of infection, protect skin, reduce odor
- Have WOCN provide detailed client teaching on care of ostomy. Reinforce education provided by WOCN
- Assist the client to contact the WOCN with concerns or questions
- Assist the client on where to get ostomy supplies
- Phantom rectal pain and the need to have a bowel movement. Let client know that this is normal and will subside over time
- Explain to client that excessive gas for the first two weeks after surgery is normal
- Eat balanced meals and take vitamins to prevent deficits in nutrition
- Drink adequate fluids, if not contraindicated, at least 2000 to 3000 mL daily to prevent dehydration
- Encourage the client to avoid foods that produce excessive gas and odor, such as broccoli, eggs and cheese, among others
- Client with an ileostomy to expect that stools will be liquid and to provide meticulous skin care around the stoma to prevent skin breaks
- Ensure client has psychological support to cope with diagnosis and change in lifestyle due to new bowel diversion device
- Verbalize future care needs on topics such as palliative and end-of-life care
- Assist client and family with securing hospice or palliative care if needed
- Importance of keeping all follow-up medical appointments
- Importance of educating family members on timely colorectal screens, since there is a genetic predisposition to the condition. Provide client with list of when screenings must be done based on risk factors

Colon Cancer Risk Factors

Being older than 50 years of age

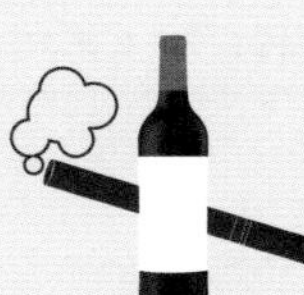

Use of alcohol and tobacco

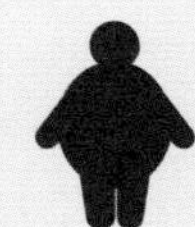

Lack of physical exercise

Low-fiber diet

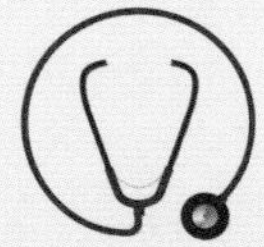

Personal history of inflammatory intestinal conditions

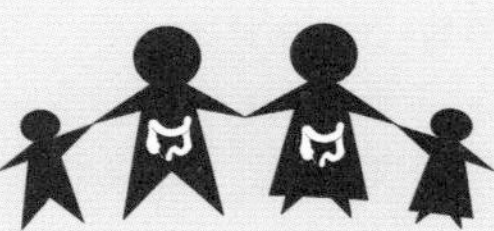

Family history of colon cancer

Image 11-9: What suggestions can the nurse provide to lower the risk of colorectal cancer? Which are modifiable or non-modifiable risk factors?

Diverticular disease

Pathophysiology/Description

- Diverticular disease encompasses two conditions, diverticulosis and diverticulitis. Diverticula are herniation or saccular dilations of the intestinal mucosa. When there are many of these diverticula present, it is called diverticulosis. When one or more diverticula become inflamed, diverticulitis occurs
- Diverticula occur mostly at points in the intestines where the wall is weak, and they can be formed anywhere in the gastrointestinal tract. However, they are most commonly located in the descending, sigmoid colon
- Causes include low intake of fiber, constipation, obesity, excessive alcohol intake, western populations, and smoking
- Diverticular disease is often asymptomatic, diagnosed only when an individual has a screening colonoscopy

Priority Data Collection or Cues

- Ask about nausea and vomiting
- Check for abdominal pain in the left lower quadrant that usually worsens when client lifts, strains or coughs
- Check for a palpable abdominal mass
- Ask client about flatulence, which is common with diverticulitis
- Check for blood in the stool
- Check for bowel perforation and signs of peritonitis
- Check client's understanding of surgery, if surgery indicated

Priority Laboratory Tests/Diagnostics

- Colonoscopy and sigmoidoscopy show entire colon and diverticular disease will be visualized
- Chest and abdominal X-rays determine if there are other associated diseases for the abdominal pain
- Computed tomography (CT) scan with contrast shows inflamed diverticula
- Complete blood cells show elevated white blood cell count
- Blood cultures may show infection in blood

Priority Interventions or Actions

- Keep client nothing by mouth in acute phase, to let the colon rest and heal
- Maintain intravenous fluids to prevent dehydration
- Provide clear liquids after the acute phase and progress diet as tolerated
- Administer medications as prescribed
- Monitor intake and output
- Monitor for bowel perforation which may include tachycardia, restlessness, abdominal distention, increased temperature
- If surgery is indicated (resection of diseased part of colon, temporary colostomy)
    - Check post-surgical devices such as ostomy pouch
    - Nasogastric (NG) tube to suction
    - Check for bleeding, infection and viability of stoma
    - Allow client to participate in self-care of surgical site, in preparation for home care
    - Allow early mobility to prevent post-surgery complications, such as pneumonia and blood clots

Priority Potential & Actual Complications

- Bowel perforation, Peritonitis, Permanent bowel diversion device, Sepsis, May be fatal

Priority Nursing Implications

- Most clients in an acute attack, can be managed outside of the acute care setting. However, severe cases may require hospitalization

Priority Medications

- Stool softeners
    - Soften feces by lubricating intestinal tract
    - Taken orally usually cause bowel movement in 72 hours
- Bulk-forming laxatives
    - Absorb water and cause increase bulk, thus stimulating peristalsis causing a bowel movement within 24 hours
    - Usually administered orally
- Stimulants
    - Administered orally
    - Work by irritating colon wall and increasing peristalsis
    - Usually cause bowel movement in 10 to 12 hours
- Saline and osmotic solutions
    - Work by retaining fluid in the intestines
    - Usually cause bowel movement in 20 minutes to 3 hours
- Several different types of antibiotics used to treat acute diverticulitis

Reinforcement of Priority Teaching

- Consume a high fiber diet
- Remind client to avoid excessive fat and meat intake
- Adequate fluid intake to prevent constipation, if not contraindicated, at least 2000 mL daily
- Remind the client to defecate when the urge occurs
- Remind client to avoid activities that increase intraabdominal pressure, such as heavy lifting, straining or bending as they can cause an attack of diverticulitis
- Explain when to contact the health care provider
- Smoking cessation for clients who smoke, as smoking is a risk factor for diverticular disease
- Weight reduction if client is obese as obesity is a risk factor for diverticulitis

Intestinal obstruction

Pathophysiology/Description

- Intestinal obstruction results when passage of intestinal content through the gastrointestinal (GI) tract is impaired
- Bowel obstruction, in the presence of poor blood flow can cause major problems. Tissues can become edematous and cyanotic leading to gangrene and intestinal infarction. This is a medical emergency requiring quick attention to prevent the possibility of septic shock and death
- Obstruction can be described as partial or complete and strangulated (no blood supply) or simple
- Mechanical bowel obstruction (physical obstruction of intestinal lumen)
- One part of intestines folds into another (Intussusception): Bowel twisting on itself (volvulus), Colorectal cancer, Crohn's disease, Diverticular disease, or no obvious cause
- Nonmechanical bowel obstruction (obstruction due to altered neuromuscular transmission or bowel innervation). Causes: Paralytic ileus, Inflammatory responses, Electrolyte imbalances, or Interruption to blood supply to the intestines
- Types of surgery, if required, include: Ileostomy, Colectomy, or Colostomy

Priority Data Collection or Cues

- Ask about recent surgeries
- Check bowel sounds
- Ask about abdominal pain that client may describe as colicky
- Ask about quality of vomiting as it can indicate the area of obstruction. For example, with distal obstruction vomiting is gradual and has a foul, fecal smell
- Ask about last bowel movement, client is usually constipated
- Check vital signs. If strangulation, expect elevated temperature, indicating inflammation and infection
- Check abdomen for distention and visible masses
- If client had surgery, perform ongoing monitoring of surgical site to ensure no infection and bleeding
- Check urine and drainage from surgical drains (if used) for proper functioning

Priority Laboratory Tests/Diagnostics

- Abdominal X-rays and computed tomography (CT) scans will likely show obstruction
- Colonoscopy and sigmoidoscopy show entire colon obstruction of colon will be visualized
- Sigmoidoscopy, shows hemorrhoids, polyps and fissures
- Complete blood count will show elevated white blood cell count if perforation or strangulating has occurred. Decreased hematocrit and hemoglobin may indicate bleeding
- Metabolic profile may show electrolyte imbalances due to dehydration

Priority Interventions or Actions

- Administer pain medications as prescribed
- Maintain client nothing by mouth (NPO) until obstruction is resolved; may have a nasogastric tube
- Administer intravenous fluids using lactated ringers or normal saline to prevent dehydration
- Monitor intake and output. Empty drains and urinary catheter
- Start client on clear liquid diet when able to eat, increase diet as tolerated. Perform oral care regularly
- Additional interventions if surgery is indicated
  - Manage post-surgical devices such as ileal pouch
  - Check for bleeding, infection and viability of stoma
  - Allow client to participate in self-care of surgical site, in preparation for home care

Priority Potential & Actual Complications

- Perforation of bowel, strangulated and necrotic bowel, septic shock, surgery with permanent use of fecal diversions, may be fatal

Priority Nursing Implications

- If client has surgery and will need to wear an ileal pouch, body image disturbances may occur so be sensitive and allow client to deal with this emotional issue

Priority Medications

- There are a myriad of different classes of pain medications that can be used to treat the client's abdominal pain, if medication is needed. The health care provider decides the best choice

Reinforcement of Priority Teaching

- Remind client to defecate when the urge is felt and to create a schedule for bowel movements
- Symptoms of bowel obstruction and when to contact health care provider
- Risk factors for bowel obstruction
- Remind client how to minimize the risk of a paralytic ileus, especially after a surgery
- For clients with ostomies, demonstrate how to care for the stoma and ostomy device, and how to check for infection
- Resume normal activities slowly
- Importance of follow-up appointments

Pathophysiology/Description

- Diseases of the gallbladder are very common in the United States. These include gallstones (cholelithiasis) and gallbladder inflammation (cholecystitis)
- Cholelithiasis occurs more in women than men and is more commonly seen in women over 40 years. Because cholesterol production is impacted by oral contraceptives and causes saturation of cholesterol in the gallbladder, younger women who take contraceptives have a high-risk of getting gallbladder disease. The same is true for women who are postmenopausal and take hormone replacement
- Obesity is also known to increase the likelihood of getting gallbladder disease
- There is also a noted tendency for gallbladder disease to be in families
- Cholelithiasis
    - Supersaturation of bile with cholesterol occurs causing cholesterol to precipitate into stones
    - Protein, bile salts and calcium also precipitate into stones in the gallbladder
    - Conditions such as pregnancy, obstructive lesions or inflammation of the biliary system and immobility, decrease flow and/or stasis of bile and increase the risk of gallstones formation
    - Gallstones frequently stay in the gallbladder but may move to the ducts, causing obstruction and pain. If bile is unable to flow out from the ducts, this can precipitate an inflammation (cholecystitis)
- Cholecystitis
    - Can occur as acute or chronic. Acute gallbladder inflammation occurs as a result of obstruction that is caused by biliary sludge or gallstones
    - Chronic disease is caused when the wall of the gallbladder becomes scarred and tissue becomes fibrotic, causing a shrunken gallbladder and decreased function
    - In acute cholecystitis, the gallbladder becomes swollen, and usually contains pus
    - Cholecystitis can occur in the absence of gallstones, called acalculous cholecystitis. This predisposes the client to infections

Priority Data Collection or Cues

- Check for pain that client may describe as severe, steady and colicky. Pain that usually goes away after an hour, leaving a feeling of tenderness in the right upper quadrant, usually indicate cholelithiasis
- Check for pain in the epigastric region that client might describe as radiating to the right scapula shoulder area, indicating cholecystitis
- Ask client what factors precipitate the pain. Pain with cholelithiasis/cholecystitis is usually precipitated by intake of a meal high in fat
- Check for nausea and vomiting
- Watch for belching, flatulence and indigestion, primarily with cholecystitis
- Additional data to be collected if bile flow is obstructed
    - Monitor client for signs of infection, such as fever
    - Monitor for jaundice, indicating obstruction. Bile is not flowing into the duodenum and bilirubin is accumulating in the blood
    - Examine urine, will be dark brown in color and foamy, indicating bilirubin is being excreted by the kidneys and not going to the small intestines for conversion as is the norm
    - Check stools, will show fat (steatorrhea) and clay color due to lack of fat digestion in the absence of bile
    - Ask client about itching skin (pruritus), due to bile salts being deposited on skin
    - Check for bleeding. Vitamin K is not being absorbed which causes a decrease in the production of clotting factor, prothrombin
    - Monitor vital signs, temperature may be elevated due to obstruction causing reflux of bacteria into systemic circulation from biliary tract
    - Check for bleeding due to decreased production of prothrombin by the liver

Priority Laboratory Tests/Diagnostics

- Abdominal ultrasound shows gallstones
- Endoscopic retrograde cholangiopancreatography (ERCP) to examine the biliary structures and remove bile for culture, if infection suspected
- Percutaneous transhepatic cholangiography, done as a follow-up test if a blockage of the bile duct is shown on ultrasound. May show poor filling of biliary and hepatic ducts
- Liver enzymes may be elevated. Bilirubin level may be elevated
- Complete blood cell (CBC), may show increased white blood cell count due to inflammation

Priority Interventions or Actions

- Administer pain medications and antiemetics as prescribed
- Maintain nothing by mouth (NPO) status
- Monitor the nasogastric (NG) tube
- Administer intravenous fluids
- Provide a low-fat diet when intake by mouth is started
- Administer fat-soluble vitamins
- Monitor intake and output
- Provide client with frequent mouth care when vomiting
- Explain to client the process of removal of stones via papillotomy or lithotripsy
- Administer anti-pruritic medication as prescribed

- Postoperative interventions (cholecystectomy)
  - Monitor punctures to abdomen for signs of infection and bleeding
  - Manage T-tube if an open cholecystectomy was performed. Monitor and measure drainage
  - Administer pain medications as needed
  - Prevent respiratory problems. Ensure adequate ventilation
  - Encourage coughing and deep breathing to prevent respiratory compromise
  - Position client on left side with right knee flexed to minimize the common complaint of pain to the shoulder caused by the CO_2 used in surgery
  - Assist client to ambulate to prevent complications of immobility

Priority Potential & Actual Complications

- Acalculous cholecystitis with perforation and infection
- Bleeding from decreased production of prothrombin
- Injury to common bile duct during laparoscopic cholecystectomy

Priority Nursing Implications

- Acalculous cholecystitis occurs more commonly in clients who are critically ill due to increased viscosity of bile from various pathological processes related to the critical illness, such as dehydration and fever

Priority Medications

- Non-steroidal anti-inflammatory drugs (NSAIDs)
  - Most commonly administered orally
  - Used to treat mild pain
  - There are several NSAIDs that can be used
  - Most significant adverse effect of NSAIDs is gastrointestinal bleeding
- Morphine
  - Various routes such as orally, intravenous or IM
  - Used initially in acute phase to manage pain and NSAIDs used after
  - Causes depressed respirations so monitor client's respiratory rate
- Anticholinergic and antispasmodic drugs
  - Most common route is oral
  - Used to decrease biliary ductal tone and relax the smooth muscles
  - Several drugs in the two classes
- Ursodeoxycholic acid
  - Administered orally
  - Dissolve gallbladder stones
  - Not widely used because of the risk of gallstones returning
- Cholestyramine
  - Administered orally
  - Used to treat pruritus (itching)

Reinforcement of Priority Teaching

- Proper medication administration such as vitamin replacement and medications for pain and spasms
- Inform client that discharge after a laparoscopic cholecystectomy is usually the day of or the day after surgery
- Show client how to care for surgical puncture or open incisional site after a cholecystectomy
- Remind the client of signs and symptoms of infection
- If client has a transhepatic biliary catheter placement to drain bile, demonstrate on cleaning skin at the insertion site with antiseptic daily to maintain cleanliness. Encourage client to observe for and report any signs of catheter obstruction manifested as fever, nausea and sudden pain in abdomen
- Drink beverages that contain electrolytes to replace fluid lost in the biliary drainage
- Importance of avoiding foods that are high in saturated fats
- Eat small meals
- Encourage client who had cholecystectomy to increase diet gradually, from liquid to regular as tolerated
- Avoid heavy lifting for 4-6 weeks after surgery
- Lose weight, if obese
- Remind client to keep follow-up medical appointments

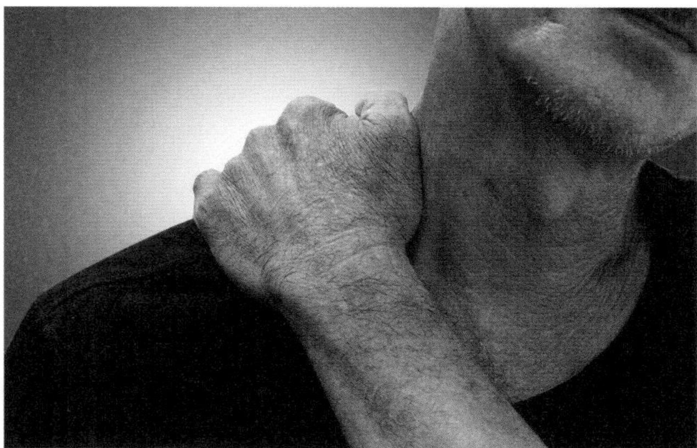

Image 11-10: The client who has been admitted for cholecystitis asks the nurse if the pain in this area could be related to the current condition. What is the best response by the nurse?

Hepatitis

Pathophysiology/Description

- Hepatitis is inflammation of the liver caused by viruses, or other substances such as alcohol or medications. With hepatitis, the virus causes many liver cells to be killed, which triggers a myriad of impaired functions in the body
- There are five different types of viral hepatitis: Hepatitis A virus (HAV), Hepatitis B virus (HBV), Hepatitis C virus (HCV), Hepatitis D virus (HDV), Hepatitis E virus (HEV)
- Even though there are commonalities among all types of viral hepatitis in terms of clinical manifestations, each has its own specific mode of transmission
- Hepatitis A virus
  - Transmission: primarily via fecal-oral route
  - At risk: crowded conditions, poor hygiene of food handlers, poor sanitation
  - Incubation: 15 to 50 days
  - Prevention: Good handwashing, HAV vaccine (need 2 doses at least 6 months apart)
- Hepatitis B virus
  - Transmission: via blood or body fluids
  - At risk: Healthcare workers, intravenous drug abusers, individuals who reside with persons who have HBV, Individuals who undergo dialysis
  - Incubation: 45 to 160 days
  - Prevention: Good handwashing, HBV vaccine, needle precautions, avoiding unprotected contact with body fluids of infected persons, blood donor screening, testing of women who are pregnant
- Hepatitis C virus
  - Transmission: via blood or body fluids
  - At risk: Healthcare workers, intravenous drug users, high-risk sexual practices, blood transfusions prior to 1992
  - Incubation: 14 to 180 days
  - Prevention: Good handwashing, blood donor screening, needle precautions, avoid unprotected sex with infected persons. No vaccine available
- Hepatitis D
  - HDV must have HBV in order to replicate and causes infection only when there is active HBV infection. Not common in the United States. No vaccine available
- Hepatitis E
  - Not very common in the United States. No worldwide vaccine available

Priority Data Collection or Cues

- Acute hepatitis
  - Check for nausea and vomiting
  - Ask about bowel habits, constipation or diarrhea
  - Ask client about meal intake
  - Check for flu-like symptoms, fatigue, or malaise
  - Ask about aches and pains, myalgias and arthralgias
  - Ask client about living conditions
  - Ask about risky sexual behaviors and intravenous drug abuse as these are risk factors for HBV, HCV and HDV
  - Ask about meal preparation and food and water sources
  - Ask about recent travels
  - Ask about the client's work
  - Check liver and spleen, both are likely to be enlarged
  - Check client's sense of taste and smell
  - Check color of urine, dark brown indicates jaundice
  - Check stools, expect clay-colored stools
  - Check for presence of jaundice
  - Ask client about itching of skin
  - Check vital signs, likely to find elevated temperature
- Additional collection of data for chronic hepatitis
  - Determine type of hepatitis infection
  - Check integumentary system, likely to find red palms (palmar erythema) and small branching arteries showing on the surface of the skin (spider angiomas)
  - Check for edema, likely to see edema of lower extremities and ascites
  - Check for swollen lymph nodes (lymphadenopathy)
  - Check neurologic system. Confusion may be seen due to encephalopathy
  - Check for bruising and bleeding
  - Check client for asterixis (rapid flexion and extension of hands when the arm/hands are stretched out), which is common in liver encephalopathy

Priority Laboratory Tests/Diagnostics

- There is a myriad of tests to distinguish between the various viral hepatitis to determine the specific one the client has. For example, there is Anti-HAV immune globulin M (IgM) for hepatitis A and Anti-HCV (antibody to HCV) for hepatitis C, among many others
- Aspartate aminotransferase (AST) alanine aminotransferase (ALT) will be elevated at first because they are released from inflamed cells but will decrease as hepatitis is resolved and jaundice disappears
- Serum and urine bilirubin increased due to liver damage
- Alkaline phosphatase and γ-Glutamyl transpeptidase increased due to liver damage
- Prothrombin time is prolonged due to decreased production in the liver
- Liver biopsy for chronic hepatitis, will show the degree of chronic injury to the liver

- Ultrasound elastography, shows liver fibrosis. Liver with cirrhosis will be stiffer than healthy one
- FibroSure is a biomarker serum test that determines the extent of liver fibrosis

Priority Interventions or Actions

- Allow client to rest in acute hepatitis as it helps with regeneration of liver cells
- Administer medications as prescribed
- Administer direct-acting antivirals as prescribed
- Provide client with a balanced nutritional diet as tolerated
- Encourage small, frequent meals instead of large meals, to help with nausea and vomiting, may need intravenous nutrition
- Provide adequate fluids. 2500 to 3000 mL daily
- Monitor intake and output. Monitor fluid and electrolyte
- Place patient in a private room for HAV if possible
- Provide range of motion exercises to minimize risk of blood clots while client is on bedrest

Priority Potential & Actual Complications

- Chronic liver disease, Fulminant hepatitis, Cirrhosis, Encephalitis, Liver cancer, Liver failure, May be fatal

Priority Nursing Implications

- Clients with hepatitis must be made aware of fulminant hepatitis, a serious complication of acute hepatitis. It causes liver failure which then triggers a myriad of other serious malfunctions in the body, including the possibility of death. Fulminant hepatitis is manifested as gastrointestinal bleeding, encephalopathy, renal failure, respiratory failure, disseminated intravascular coagulopathy and hypoglycemia, among a myriad of other severe imbalances. Prognosis is poor, and a liver transplant is the cure
- Understand that there are risk factors for acute viral hepatitis to progress to a chronic stage. These include fatty liver disease, metabolic syndrome, co-infection with HIV, alcohol intake and being male
- When a food handler contracts HAV, all food handlers at the client's place of work should be vaccinated with hepatitis A immune globulin (IG)

Priority Medications

- Direct-acting antivirals
  - Administer orally once a day
  - Drug: simeprevir, administered with another drug called sofosbuvir
  - Works by preventing HCV replication
- Sofosbuvir
  - Administered orally
  - Works by preventing HCV replication
  - Administered with simeprevir
- Antiemetics
  - Promethazine
  - Used to treat nausea and administered via several routes
- Nucleoside and nucleotide analogs
  - Administered orally
  - Lamivudine
  - Works by inhibiting viral replication in chronic HBV and liver inflammation

Reinforcement of Priority Teaching

- Provide client information on vaccines for hepatitis
- Explain the importance of rest to client
- Demonstrate the method of proper hand washing
- Encourage preventative measure
- Maintaining good personal hygiene
- Maintain good environmental hygiene
- Avoid drinking alcohol
- Complications of hepatitis and how to recognize symptoms of complications
- Remind client that HBV and HCV can relapse
- Avoid donating blood if infected with HBV or HCV
- Remind client to keep follow-up medical appointments

Compare and Contrast Hepatitis A, B, & C:

	A	B	C
Causes jaundice			
Vaccine available			
Spread via blood			
Spread via body fluids			
Spread via feces from infected person			
May cause chronic infection			

Table 11-1: Compare and contrast the three types of hepatitis.

Inflammatory bowel disease: Crohn's disease/ulcerative colitis

Pathophysiology/Description

- Inflammatory bowel disease (IBD) describes an incurable, chronic condition that is marked by inflammation of the gastrointestinal tract. The condition is not continuous but presents with periods of exacerbations and remissions. Crohn's disease and ulcerative colitis are the 2 conditions that are classified as IBD
- Factors associated with IBD
  - Genetics: it is seen that there are frequent occurrences of IBD in family members of individuals with IBD
  - Environmental: smoking, stress, air pollutants, among others, cause increase susceptibility to IBD
  - Dietary: intake of foods high in polyunsaturated fats, and meat increase the risk of getting IBD
- Crohn's disease usually affects any part of the GI system, from the mouth to the anus, but it quite commonly occurs in the proximal colon and the terminal ileum
- Ulcerative colitis is more localized and involves the rectum, spreading up toward the cecum
- It is common for both conditions to affect teenagers, adults in their third decade of life and those after 60-years-old
- The GI inflammation seen with ulcerative colitis is continuous while with Crohn's, inflammation is seen in a skipped pattern (commonly termed skipped lesions), meaning that there can be areas of normal bowel between portions that are diseased. All layers of the bowel are involved with Crohn's causing deep ulcerations and the classic "cobblestone" look. However, with ulcerative colitis, only the mucosal layer is involved
- Abscess and peritonitis are likely in Crohn's because of bowel perforation, causing bowel contents to leak into the peritoneal cavity. Narrowed lumen, ulcerations, scarring and fistulas are common in Crohn's disease
- With ulcerative colitis, inflamed mucosa prevents the absorption of electrolytes and water and the lack of absorption causes the client to have diarrhea with electrolyte loss. Finger-like projections (called pseudopolyps) may be formed because of the inflamed mucosa. These are not common to Crohn's disease
- Certain dietary measures can be taken to decrease the risk of both diseases. Eating a high intake of vegetables is known to decrease the risk of ulcerative colitis, while the risk of Crohn's can be decreased with high fruit and fiber consumption

Priority Data Collection or Cues

- Check for fever, cramping abdominal pain, diarrhea with pus, rectal bleeding and weight loss with Crohn's disease. Weight loss occurs as a result of malabsorption from inflammation
- Check for mild to severe constant abdominal pain, bloody diarrheal stools and tenesmus (painful and constant need to empty bowel), indicative of ulcerative colitis. Check number of bowel movements daily, expect 4-20 with ulcerative colitis
- Check stools for infection
- Ask about client's health history
- Check for anemia, as blood loss in stools can cause anemia. Bleeding occurs more in ulcerative colitis than Crohn's
- Check for nutritional deficiency due to malabsorption. Monitor for dehydration and electrolyte imbalance due to fluid and electrolytes loss in liquid stools
- Check vital signs, hypotension, tachycardia and fever, likely due to fluid issues and inflammation
- Check for malnutrition, expect that it may be more pronounced in Crohn's disease due to malabsorption issues
- Check for signs and symptoms of peritonitis, occurring from bowel perforation, more likely with Crohn's disease
- Check client's understanding of surgery, if indicated
- Determine client's readiness to look at surgical site and learn self-care, if surgery was indicated

Priority Laboratory Tests/Diagnostics

- C-reactive protein and white blood cell count elevated due to inflammation. Stool test shows mucus, blood and pus. Stool culture shows infection
- Metabolic profile shows decreased potassium, sodium, bicarbonate, chloride due to diarrhea and vomiting and low Albumin because of inadequate nutrition
- Imaging such as computed tomography, magnetic resonance imaging (MRI), barium enema, small bowel follow through, help in the diagnosis. Colonoscopy and endoscopy are used to look for diseased areas in various parts of the gastrointestinal tract
- Complete blood count shows anemia because of blood loss in stools

Priority Interventions or Actions

- Prepare client for imaging tests
- Collect stool samples and send to lab
- Weigh client daily, numerous diarrhea and fluid loss causes weight loss. Monitor intake and output
- Maintain client nothing by mouth (NPO) in acute phase. Administer intravenous fluids and electrolytes to replace loss from diarrhea. Restrict activity to decrease intestinal motility. Provide diet high in proteins, vitamins and caloric value to compensate for malabsorption and malnutrition
- Dietary consults for client's nutritional needs
- Monitor stools noting consistency and amount. Note presence of blood
- Monitor for bowel perforation, which may include tachycardia, restlessness, abdominal distention, increased temperature
- Monitor bowel sounds, abdominal tenderness and pain
- Clean client's perineal area with plain water and apply barrier cream to prevent skin breaks from frequent diarrhea
- If surgery is indicated
  - Perform preoperative care
  - Insert nasogastric tube if prescribed

- Perform post-surgical care as prescribed
- Manage post-surgical devices such as ileal pouch
- Manage care of surgical site. Monitor for bleeding, infection and viability of stoma
- Allow client to participate in self-care of surgical site, in preparation for home care
- Monitor for initial ileostomy output, which may be up to 1800 mL/24 hours

* Administer medications as prescribed

Priority Potential & Actual Complications

- Fistulas and abscess of the perineal area, strictures, perforation causing peritonitis with hemorrhage
- Toxic megacolon requiring colectomy, colorectal cancer (primarily with ulcerative), small intestinal cancer (primarily with Crohn's)
- May be fatal

Priority Nursing Implications

- If client has surgery and will need to wear an ileal pouch, body image disturbances may occur
- Long-term therapy with sulfasalazine may result in abnormal production of sperm, which can cause infertility
- Clients with ulcerative colitis can be significantly fatigued. Rest periods must be considered when performing care to the client with this condition in the acute setting
- A yellow-orange discoloration of the skin may be caused by taking sulfasalazine, so client must be made aware
- 6-mercaptopurine and azathioprine can cause suppression of bone marrow so complete blood count must be monitored when these drugs are being taken
- Methotrexate has serious side effect of hepatoxicity and bone marrow suppression, so CBC must be monitored frequently. Remind female clients taking the drug not to become pregnant
- Natalizumab, one of the biologic and targeted therapies, has a risk of progressive multifocal leukoencephalopathy. Therefore, its use is restricted

Priority Medications

- Sulfasalazine
  - Administered orally with full glass of water
  - Main drug to maintain remission and prevent exacerbations (flare-ups)
- Olsalazine
  - Administered orally
  - Main drug to maintain remission and prevent exacerbations (flare-ups)
- Mesalamine
  - Administered orally
  - Main drug to maintain remission and prevent exacerbations (flare-ups)
- Corticosteroids
  - Different ones in the class are used and dosages depend on the drug and severity of the condition
  - Intravenous corticosteroids may be used for short duration with severe inflammation
- Chemotherapy medications may also be used. These medications are typically administered by the RN. Two common medications are 6-mercaptopurine and Methotrexate
- Azathioprine
  - Immunosuppressant
  - Dose for ulcerative colitis is administered intravenously using various variations of dosages
- Biological and targeted therapy
  - Several medications in this class of drugs used to treat Crohn's disease
  - Used mostly to induce and maintain remission in clients who have had no success with other treatments

Reinforcement of Priority Teaching

- Perform frequent and proper perineal care due to multiple bowel movements. Avoid harsh soaps. A skin barrier cream may be used to preserve skin integrity
- A diet high in protein, calories and vitamins to maintain nutritional status
- Importance of stress reduction
- Remind the client to get adequate rest
- Assist client to schedule psychotherapy to deal with the emotional toll of a chronic condition and/or issues surrounding body image disturbances from ostomy device
- Review the symptoms of the disease and when to contact the health care provider
- Explain the importance of smoking cessation for clients who smoke, as smoking can worsen both Crohn's disease and ulcerative colitis
- If surgery was done, reinforce education:
  - How to empty and change ostomy device
  - How to care for, and check the stoma
  - Have client do return demonstration of ostomy care
  - Signs of infection and to check stoma site for infection
  - That a second surgery may be needed
  - On Kegel exercises that serve to strengthen the sphincter muscles and pelvic floor
- Remind the client it may take several weeks before client feels well enough to resume normal activities
- Review how to administer medications and about adverse effects for which the health care provider must be notified
- Importance of keeping follow-up appointments

Pathophysiology/Description

- Obesity, a major disease globally, is characterized by excessive amounts of body fat that is beyond the individual's physical body requirements
- Cause of primary obesity includes excessive calorie intake and not enough expenditure of energy
- Causes of secondary obesity include: lesions in the central nervous system, metabolic imbalances, congenital anomalies, drugs
- Classifications of obesity
  - Body mass index: obese is 30 kg/m^2 and greater
  - Waist-to-hip ratio: greater than 0.8 increases the risk of health problems
  - Waist circumference: increased health risk if greater than 30 inches in men and greater than 35 inches in women
  - Body shape: apple and pear-shaped bodies have greater risks of health conditions
- Genetics, environmental and psychological contributory factors
  - Genes recently identified as having linkage to obesity
  - Greater access to fast and unhealthy foods
  - Increased tendency to eat outside the home
  - Reliance on use of technology and less physical activity
  - Increased portion sizes of meals. Use of food for comfort and reward
  - Lack of areas for recreational activities in poorer neighborhoods. Lower socioeconomic status
  - Use of food for comfort and reward
- Obesity can be managed with diet and exercise but there are times when an individual chooses to have a bariatric surgery to help with weight loss
- Bariatric surgery procedures
  - Sleeve gastrectomy: portion of stomach removed, and remainder has a sleeved shape
  - Adjustable gastric banding: inflatable band placed around the stomach to decrease the size. Stomach size can be manipulated by injecting fluid in an inflatable/deflectable port
  - Intragastric balloons: balloon placed in stomach and is filled with saline, gives sense of fullness in the stomach so client eats less
  - Roux-en-Y gastric bypass: this is the gold standard for bariatric surgeries. A small gastric pouch is created and attached directly to the small intestines. Dumping syndrome is an issue with this procedure because of contents emptying too rapidly in the small intestines
  - Implantable gastric stimulation: Device implanted in abdomen that allows client to send signal of stomach fullness to the brain

Priority Data Collection or Cues

- Check for cause of obesity
- Check weight and height. Check motivation to lose weight and barriers to weight loss
- Ask about current diet
- Pre and postoperative for bariatric surgery
  - Check for use of assistive devices
  - Preoperatively, reinforce how to cough and deep breathe, use incentive spirometry and reposition in bed postoperatively
  - Check vital signs pre and postoperatively
  - Check client's knowledge of the surgical procedure
  - Check skin to ensure no skin breaks from immobility
  - Check surgical dressing for bleeding
  - Check surgical site for wound dehiscence, evisceration or infection
  - Check respiratory status to ensure no compromise

Priority Laboratory Tests/Diagnostics

- There are no specific labs for obesity. Labs and diagnostics are done based on symptoms from complications of obesity

Priority Interventions or Actions

- Restrict dietary meal intake to below energy requirement
- Initiate dietary consult
- Discuss weight loss goals with client and assist client with initiating weight loss plans
- Offer praise when weight goals are met
- Preoperative interventions for bariatric surgery
  - Coordinate care across specialties if client has other comorbidities
  - Gather all appropriately sized equipment that will be used pre and postoperative
  - Perform preoperative care
- Postoperative interventions
  - Administer pain medications as prescribed
  - Keep the client's head positioned at 35 to 40 degree angle to foster lung expansion and reduce pressure on the abdomen
  - Assist client to ambulate as prescribed
  - Empty urinary catheter and measure output
  - Assist client to use incentive spirometry
  - Monitor intravenous fluid and insertion site. Document intake and output
  - Provide water and sugar-free clear liquids in the immediate postoperative period

Priority Potential & Actual Complications

- Cancer, obesity is a risk factor for several cancers
- Musculoskeletal problems due to stress on joints
- Cardiovascular problems such as hypertension
- Gastrointestinal problems such as gallstones
- Endocrine problems such as diabetes
- Respiratory problems such as sleep apnea
- Psychological problems mainly from having to manage the stigma of obesity

Priority Nursing Implications

- In caring for clients with obesity, it is important to remember cultural considerations

Priority Medications

- Bupropion/Naltrexone (a combination drug)
  - Administered orally
  - Antidepressant/opioid antagonist
- Orlistat
  - Administered orally
  - Blocks the breakdown of fat and its absorption in the intestines
  - Has unpleasant side effect of flatulence and leakage of stool
- Lorcaserin
  - Administered orally
  - Suppress appetite causes sense of fullness
  - Selective serotine agonist
- Liraglutide
  - Administered subcutaneously once daily
  - Glucagon-like peptide that induces fullness
- Phentermine/topiramate
  - Administered orally
  - Sympathomimetic anorectic/antiseizure drug that works to increase satiety

Reinforcement of Priority Teaching

- Eat a balanced meal
- Drink adequate water
- Explain the risk of fad diets
- Drugs must be combined with diet and exercise to be effective in losing weight
- Set realistic weight loss goals
- Assist client with locating community social support
- Explain the importance of starting an exercise program
- Post bariatric surgery
  - Explain to client that vomiting usually occurs in the early postoperative phase. Remind client to eat small meals
  - Eat slowly and do not eat past fullness
  - Do not eat and drink at the same time
  - Eat the prescribed diet (high protein)
  - Follow fluid restrictions
  - Signs and symptoms of wound infection
  - Explain the importance of walking daily
  - Alert client to the fact that weight loss will be significant in first few months and to not be alarmed with loose skin
  - Let client know that complications can occur late in recovery, keep follow-up medical appointments

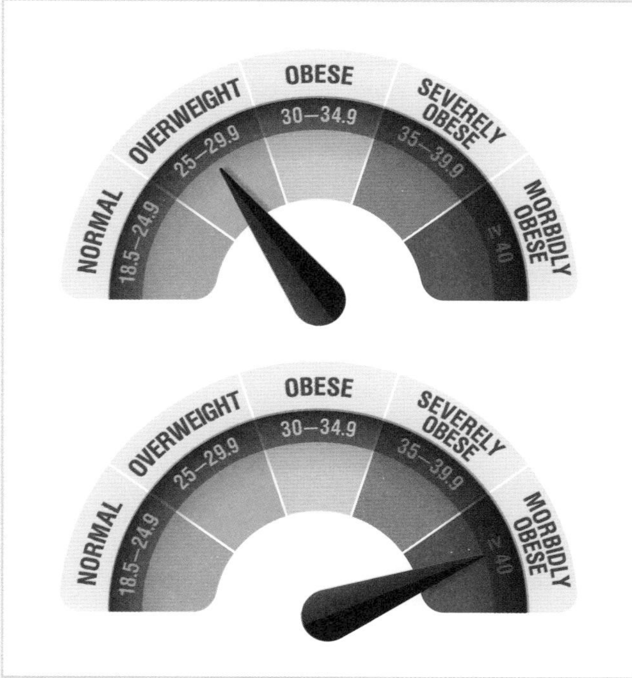

Image 11-11: As BMI increases, the risks for other diseases also increase. What diseases and disorders should the nurse be aware of for these clients?

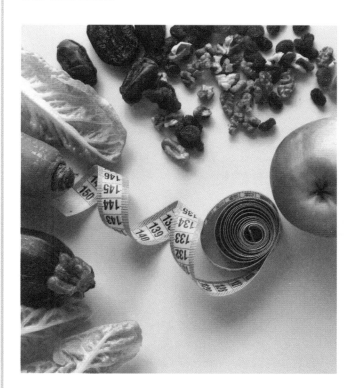

Image 11-12: A client has begun medication to lose weight. What specific education should the nurse reinforce regarding diet and exercise for this client?

Peptic ulcer disease

Pathophysiology/Description

- A peptic ulcer is an ulceration in the gastric mucosa. It can occur in several locations in the gastrointestinal (GI) system, esophagus, stomach, pylorus and duodenum. Peptic ulcers thrive in an acid environment and so any situation that causes excess acid production in the GI system contributes to peptic ulcer formation
- Classification of peptic ulcers
    - Acute vs chronic
    - Esophageal, gastric or duodenal
- Acute ulcers are short in duration, superficial, heal quickly, and cause minimal inflammation
- Chronic ulcers last months to years, are deep, and are more common
- Gastric ulcers
    - Adults over 50 years and women have the highest incidence of gastric ulcers
    - Higher risk of causing obstruction and mortality rate higher due to age
- Duodenal ulcers
    - Most peptic ulcers are duodenal ulcers
    - Age of highest incidence is 35-45 years
    - H. pylori is the most common cause of duodenal ulcers
- Factors that predispose to peptic ulcers
    - Dietary–spicy foods, large amounts, and alcohol
    - Helicobacter pylori (H. pylori)
    - Certain drugs, such as non-steroidal anti-inflammatory drugs (NSAIDs) and corticosteroids
    - Caffeine and alcohol stimulate gastric acid secretion and smoking which delay gastric ulcer healing
    - Certain diseases predispose an individual to peptic ulcers, especially duodenal ulcers. These include liver cirrhosis, chronic pancreatitis, chronic kidney disease, among others
    - Stress is known to impact peptic ulcer disease

Priority Data Collection or Cues

- Ask about conditions that are risk factors for peptic ulcer disease
- Check for pain occurring in the mid-epigastric region or toward the back. Clients usually describe it as a burning pain that occurs about 1½ to 3 hours after a meal, indicating a duodenal ulcer
- Ask about sleep pattern
- Check for pain occurring in the high epigastric region. Clients usually describe it as a gnawing pain that worsens 30 to 60 minutes after a meal, indicating a gastric ulcer
- Ask client about pain relieving strategies used. Eating a meal aggravates a gastric ulcer while eating relieves pain caused by a duodenal ulcer
- Ask about duration of symptoms. Duodenal ulcers may occur for a long duration, like a few months, disappear for a long while and then recur
- Ask about nausea, vomiting and bloating, experienced by some clients
- Check for active bleeding

Priority Laboratory Tests/Diagnostics

- Test for H. Pylori via breath, blood and stool, will be positive
- Stool tested for occult blood, may be positive
- Endoscopy stomach examination and biopsy will show H. Pylori and biopsy can rule out gastric cancer
- Rapid urease testing is done for H. pylori using a biopsy sample. H. pylori secretes the urease enzyme and test will be positive for the bacteria
- Barium contrast study to detect gastric ulcers if a client cannot do an endoscopy. It also diagnoses gastric outlet obstruction
- Complete blood count may indicate anemia due to bleeding

Priority Interventions or Actions

- Acute Care
    - Maintain nothing by mouth (NPO)
    - Administer intravenous fluids to prevent dehydration
    - Monitor intake and output
    - Monitor nasogastric (NG) tube and suction
    - If no NG tube, check vomitus and stools for active bleeding
    - Administer medications as prescribed
    - If actively bleeding, monitor for hypovolemic shock
    - Watch for perforation
    - Provide client with a quiet, calm and restful environment
    - Monitor blood transfusion, if prescribed
    - Monitor intake and output
    - Re-introduce a clear liquid diet when symptoms have subsided
- Additional interventions if surgical procedure (partial gastrectomy, vagotomy, pyloroplasty or closure of perforation)
    - Ongoing monitoring of vital signs
    - Maintain NPO until peristalsis returns and oral intake is tolerated
    - Monitor for postoperative complications
    - Ongoing bowel collection of data, looking for signs of bowel obstruction

Priority Potential & Actual Complications

- Hemorrhage
- Perforation
- Gastric outlet obstruction
- Postoperative complications:
    - Hemorrhage at surgery site, dumping syndrome, bile reflux, hypoglycemia (postprandial) vitamin B12 deficiency

Priority Nursing Implications

- The client who has a gastrectomy must understand the symptoms of dumping syndrome and how to control it
  - Cause of dumping syndrome: Stomach no longer has control over the amount of chyme that enters the small intestines so large amounts of hypertonic fluid enter the intestine pulling fluid with it into the bowel. This causes distention of the lumen and rapid movement so that within a few minutes after eating the client gets the strong urge to have a bowel movement, associated with sweating, palpations and dizziness
  - Managing dumping syndrome: Eat six small meals instead of a few large meals and chew food properly. Do not eat concentrated sweets as they can cause diarrhea. Increase protein and complex carbohydrate intake instead of fatty foods. Do not drink fluids with, or within 30 minutes after a meal, and refrain from eating dairy products
- The risk of fractures is increased when client takes a proton pump inhibitor on a long-term basis
- It is important to note that some over-the-counter drugs contain aspirin. Clients must understand that they must seek advice from health care providers and pharmacists before taking OTC drugs and herbal remedies to ensure they are not increasing their risk of bleeding
- Clients with renal failure should not take antacids containing magnesium due to a potential risk of magnesium toxicity. Use antacids that contain sodium cautiously in older adults with conditions such as heart failure and hypertension as it may cause fluid retention

Priority Medications

- Proton pump inhibitors (PPI)
  - Several oral drugs in this class are used. They decrease hydrochloric acid secretion and decrease gastric mucosa irritation
  - This class of drug is among the most effective and common in treating peptic ulcers. Often used in combination with antibiotics to treat ulcers when the cause is H. pylori
  - Available over-the-counter or by prescription
- Histamine receptor blockers
  - Several oral drugs in this class are used. They decrease hydrochloric acid secretion and promote healing of ulcer
  - Like the proton pump inhibitors, this class of drugs is effective and commonly used
  - Available both as over-the-counter and prescription
- Antacids
  - Work by neutralizing hydrochloric acid
  - Several oral drugs in this class, available over-the-counter or with prescription
  - Best taken after meals for a longer effect
- Antiulcer protectant
  - Only one used is sucralfate, taken orally
  - Taken on an empty stomach for maximum effect
- Amoxicillin
  - Antibiotic, administered orally
  - Used in triple-drug therapy with a PPI, and clarithromycin to treat H. pylori infection
- Clarithromycin
  - Antibiotic, administered orally
  - Used in triple-drug therapy with a PPI, and amoxicillin to treat H. pylori infection
- Tetracycline
  - Antibiotic, administered orally
  - Used in quadruple drug therapy with a PPI, bismuth, and metronidazole to treat H. pylori infection
- Metronidazole
  - Antibiotic, administered orally
  - Used with a PPI, bismuth, and tetracycline to treat H. pylori infection
- Bismuth
  - Administered orally
  - Antacid and antidiarrheal
  - Used with a PPI, metronidazole and tetracycline to treat H. pylori infection

Reinforcement of Priority Teaching

- Strict administration of prescribed medications to ensure full healing of ulcer
- Take all of the prescribed antibiotics for H. pylori, even if symptoms have subsided
- Remind client that an endoscopic follow-up examination will be done about 3-6 months after treatment to evaluate the ulcer
- Avoid foods that are irritating to the ulcer, such as pepper, hot and spicy foods, caffeinated and carbonated beverages
- Remind client that aspirin and NSAID's must not be taken for 4-6 weeks
- Encourage client not to interchange brands of medications without first speaking with the health care provider
- If client had surgery, reinforce signs and symptoms of postoperative complications and when to contact the health care provider
- Avoid alcohol
- Stop smoking
- Advance diet back to normal, as tolerated, after an acute episode
- Intake of 6 small meals instead of large meals
- Signs and symptoms of gastric bleeding or perforation and to contact health care provider immediately
- Demonstrate administration of B12 injections and have client do a return demonstration
- Maintain adequate rest
- Limit stress

Pathophysiology/Description

- Narrowing of the pyloric canal between the stomach and duodenum as a result of hypertrophy of the muscles of the pylorus. The result of this is a blockage of food from entering the small intestines causing forceful vomiting and constant hunger. Pyloric stenosis is not present at birth but develops after
- A definitive cause of a baby having pyloric stenosis is not known but possible risk factors have been identified
- Risk factors
  - More common in Northern European ancestry
  - Familial tendency. Higher rates of the condition found in babies born to mothers who had the condition
  - Mothers who were treated with antibiotics in late pregnancy
  - Babies who were treated with antibiotics in the first weeks after birth
  - Occurs more in male babies than females
  - Bottle feeding
  - Babies born prematurely
  - Smoking in pregnancy
- Treatment for pyloric stenosis is always surgical. Surgery is a Laparoscopic pyloromyotomy which opens a wider channel in the pylorus to allow food to pass through. The surgery is almost always done laparoscopically unless there are complications in surgery that cause a change to the open surgical procedure

Priority Data Collection or Cues

- Check for vomiting after feeding. Vomiting may be projectile. Ask about belching
- Ask caregiver about the baby's bowel movements. With food not getting to the intestines, baby may be constipated
- Check skin for an olive-shaped lump by the baby's umbilicus, in the epigastric area
- Inspect baby's abdomen, wave-like contractions may be seen across baby's stomach caused by the muscles if the stomach trying to push food through the pylorus that is narrowed
- Weigh the baby. Compare baby's weight now to birthweight
- Check baby's hydration status
- Check baby's feeding habits
- Ask about irritability
- Check baby's activity, usually less active with pyloric stenosis

Priority Laboratory Tests/Diagnostics

- Ultrasound to look at the pylorus, confirms the diagnosis
- Blood tests to look for electrolyte imbalance or dehydration

Priority Interventions or Actions

- Monitor intake and output
- Obtain daily weights
- Prepare baby for surgery (laparoscopic pyloromyotomy)
- Place nasogastric tube preoperatively to decompress stomach
- Postoperative interventions
  - Maintain the baby nothing by mouth (NPO) until able to tolerate oral feeding
  - Monitor nasogastric tube
  - Monitor intake and output
  - Monitor for abdominal distention
  - Monitor surgical wound for bleeding, and infection
  - Change dressing using aseptic technique
  - Initiate small feedings
  - Administer pain medication as prescribed

Priority Potential & Actual Complications

- Failure to thrive
- Jaundice
- Dehydration
- Electrolyte imbalances
- Erosion and bleeding of the stomach/aspiration

Priority Nursing Implications

- A child with pyloric stenosis will likely show signs of poor hydration and will be hungry all the time because of excessive vomiting and food not getting to the small intestines

Priority Medications

- Analgesics: Used for managing child's pain after surgery. The choice and dose of medication is at the discretion of the physician

Reinforcement of Priority Teaching

- Remind caregiver to report the following to the health care provider
  - The baby has pain and pain medication is not helping
  - The baby is not able to have a bowel movement
  - Fever greater than 101.3°F by oral or rectal thermometer
  - Vomiting even after drinking only clear liquids
  - Redness, bleeding or pus at the surgical incision site
- Importance of keeping follow-up medical appointments

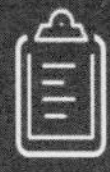

NurseThink® Quiz Questions

1. **The nurse cares for a child, post-op cleft lip repair using z-plasty. When demonstrating appropriate care to the child's parent, where does the nurse introduce the nipple for feeding?**

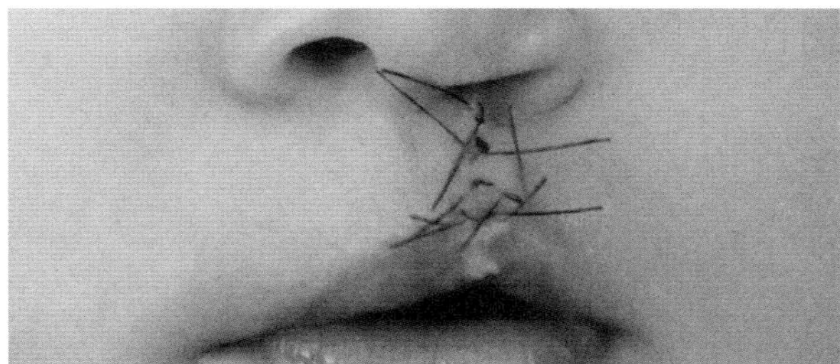

   a. From the bottom lip, with the nipple slanting upward.
   b. From the side of the mouth, to the left or right of the suture line.
   c. From the upper lip, with the nipple slanting downward.
   d. The nurse should use a syringe, not a nipple, for feeding.

2. **The nurse cares for a client with gastroesophageal reflux disease (GERD). The client complains of persistent bloating, "heartburn," and nausea, as well as frequent regurgitation. Which question does the nurse prioritize when speaking with the client?**
   a. "Do you take over-the-counter antacids or acid-blockers?"
   b. "Are you experiencing any difficulty swallowing?"
   c. "Do you see your dentist every six months?"
   d. "How often and how much per day are you eating?"

3. **The nurse reviews the laboratory results of a male client with chronic gastritis. Which lab value best indicates the client is at risk for the development of pernicious anemia?**

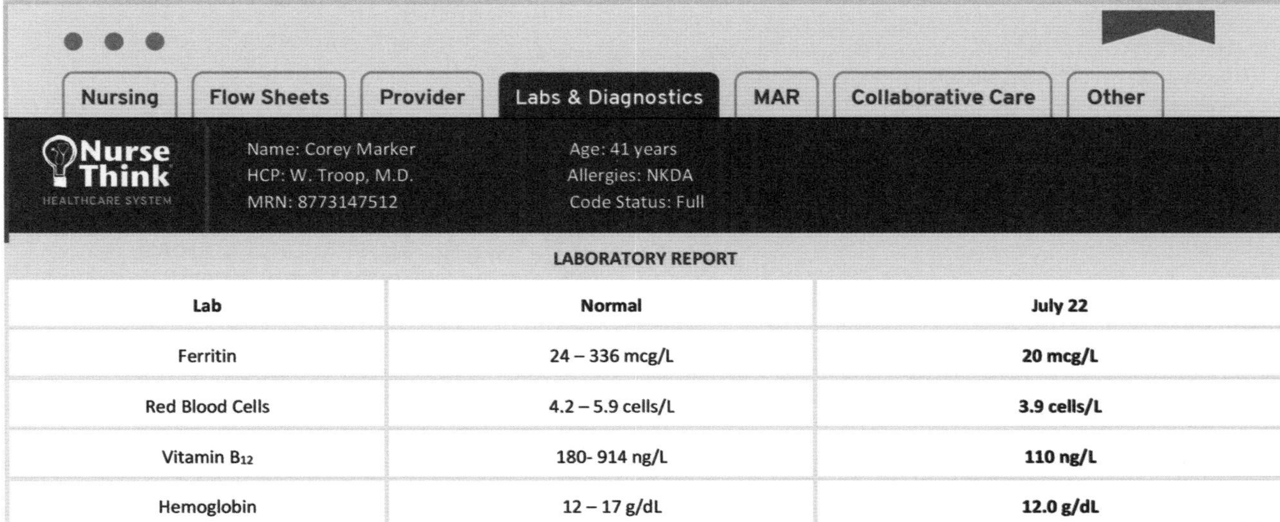

LABORATORY REPORT

Lab	Normal	July 22
Ferritin	24 – 336 mcg/L	**20 mcg/L**
Red Blood Cells	4.2 – 5.9 cells/L	**3.9 cells/L**
Vitamin B_{12}	180- 914 ng/L	**110 ng/L**
Hemoglobin	12 – 17 g/dL	**12.0 g/dL**

   a. Ferritin.
   b. Red blood cells.
   c. Vitamin B12.
   d. Hemoglobin.

4. **A client with peptic ulcer disease is going home later today. What instructions does the nurse give the client prior to discharge? *Select all that apply.***
   a. Stop taking PPIs when symptoms subside.
   b. Avoid nonsteroidal anti-inflammatory medications.
   c. Limit coffee, tea, alcohol, and carbonated beverages.
   d. Cigarette smoking will help reduce stress levels.
   e. Contact provider if blood is seen in the stool.
   f. Avoid the use of flavored antacids.

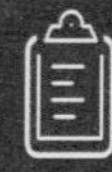

NurseThink® Quiz Questions

5. **The nurse develops a plan of care for a client diagnosed with celiac disease. Which type of diet does the nurse include in the referral to the dietitian?**
   a. Low-carbohydrate.
   b. Low-sodium, high-calcium.
   c. Fat-free, low-calorie.
   d. Gluten-free.

6. **The nurse evaluates a client who presents with persistent nausea after eating pizza and vomiting. Suspecting cholecystitis, what client data is most important for the nurse to collect? *Select all that apply.***
   a. The client's response to RUQ palpation while taking a deep breath.
   b. The presence of jaundice in the client's skin and sclera.
   c. The presence of left flank tenderness and bruising.
   d. The client's temperature.
   e. The presence of periumbilical bruising.
   f. The type and severity of the client's pain.

7. **The nurse plans home care for a client post-op after an open cholecystectomy. What discharge information does the nurse provide?**
   a. "You may resume a regular diet as soon as you are hungry."
   b. "You may experience constipation as a result of the procedure."
   c. "You should avoid heavy lifting for four to six weeks after surgery."
   d. "You should bathe, not shower, until the drainage tube is removed."

8. **The nurse cares for an older adult experiencing chronic constipation. Which statement by the client requires follow-up from the nurse?**
   a. "I go for a walk around the neighborhood almost every day."
   b. "I only use a laxative once in a while."
   c. "I stop drinking water before dinner, so I don't have to wake up to urinate."
   d. "Every morning, I eat oatmeal with blueberries."

9. **The nurse cares for a pediatric client with constipation. What information does the nurse report to the health care provider as evidence of a complication?**
   a. Vomiting with dark, foul-smelling emesis.
   b. Leaking of stool between bowel movements.
   c. Hiding while having bowel movements.
   d. Presence of an anal wink.

10. **A client verbalizes an urge to defecate but has been unable to pass stool or flatus for more than 12 hours. Which additional data best supports the nurse's suspicion of small bowel obstruction?**
   a. Presence of borborygmi.
   b. Intermittent abdominal cramping.
   c. Ribbon-like stools around impaction.
   d. Projectile vomiting with fecal odor.

11. **The nurse and a client are reviewing information about diverticulitis. The nurse asks the client to point to the area of the abdomen where pain most commonly occurs with exacerbation of the disease. Which location, as indicated by the client, indicates understanding?**

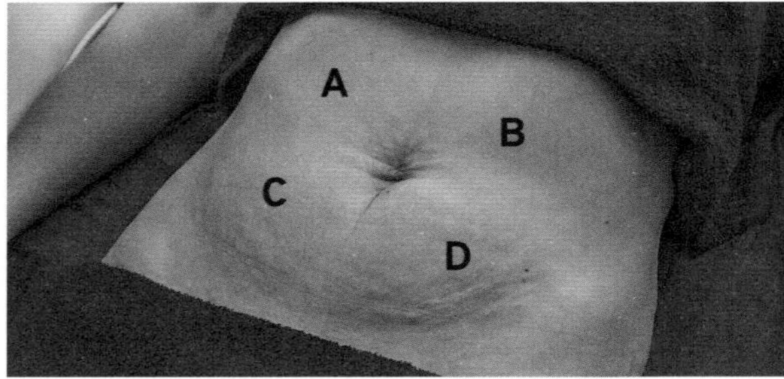

   a. Right upper quadrant.
   b. Left upper quadrant.
   c. Right lower quadrant.
   d. Left lower quadrant.

12. **The nurse prepares a client for a wireless capsule endoscopy to rule out the presence of colorectal cancer. What information does the nurse give the client to prepare them for the procedure?**
   a. "Sedation is necessary for this type of endoscopic procedure."
   b. "You will be asked to change positions repeatedly to distribute the barium."
   c. "It will take about eight hours for the camera to pass through the GI tract."
   d. "After you expel the barium, your intestine will be inflated with air."

13. **The nurse is planning a community health class at a senior citizens' center. The nurse will be promoting risk reduction of colon cancer. What information does the nurse present? *Select all that apply.***
   a. Consume a low-fat, low-carbohydrate diet
   b. Have regular, age-specific colorectal screenings
   c. Consume a calcium-rich, high-fiber diet
   d. Engage in regular physical exercise
   e. Reduce or eliminate alcohol intake.

14. **The nurse provides care for an unconscious client with a history of Hepatitis C. The nurse concerned about exposure to Hepatitis C through what routes of transmission? *Select all that apply.***
   a. Feces.
   b. Mucosal blood.
   c. Urine.
   d. Percutaneous blood.
   e. Emesis.

15. The nurse cares for a pediatric client with pyloric stenosis. Due to extensive vomiting and dehydration, the nurse plans to monitor the client's lab values for which physiologic response?

a. Metabolic acidosis.
b. Metabolic alkalosis.
c. Respiratory acidosis.
d. Respiratory alkalosis.

16. The nurse collects information about risk factors contributing to a client's diagnosis of class 1 obesity. What environmental factors does the nurse expect to find? *Select all that apply.*

a. Availability and access to unhealthy foods.
b. Automation of food preparation.
c. Leptin and melanocortin-4 receptor mutation.
d. Stress and binge eating.
e. Increase in average portion size.
f. Physical inactivity or sedentary lifestyle.

17. The nurse discusses the plan of care for a pediatric client with obesity with the client's parents. Which recommendations does the nurse provide for the parents in managing their child's health? *Select all that apply.*

a. Encourage the child to eat quickly to fill up faster.
b. Restrict eating in front of the television or computer.
c. Discourage the child from skipping meals.
d. Promote an increase and change in physical activity.
e. Set daily screen time at 4-8 hours per day.
f. Provide some choices in meals and snacks.

18. The nurse is planning home care for a client who has undergone brachytherapy for prostate cancer. Which instructions does the nurse reinforce to the client regarding sexual activity?

a. Abstain from sexual intercourse for four weeks after treatment.
b. Always urinate before and after sexual intercourse.
c. Abstain from sex for two weeks, then resume with condom use.
d. Sex with a condom may resume as soon as you feel you are able.

19. The nurse reviews the prescriptions of a client with end-stage renal disease. Which medication does the nurse clarify with the provider?

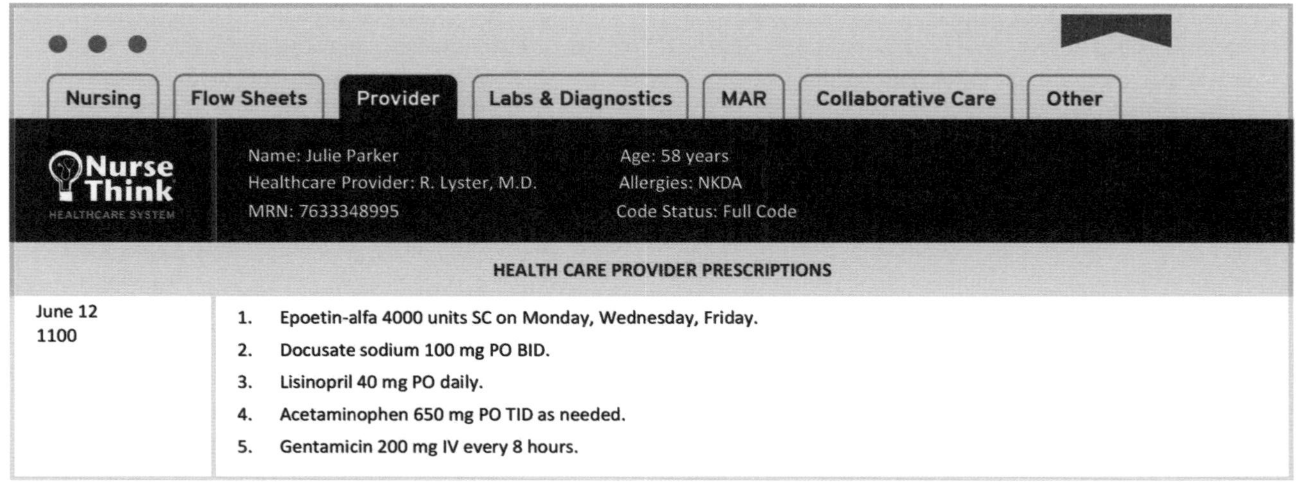

HEALTH CARE PROVIDER PRESCRIPTIONS	
June 12 1100	1. Epoetin-alfa 4000 units SC on Monday, Wednesday, Friday. 2. Docusate sodium 100 mg PO BID. 3. Lisinopril 40 mg PO daily. 4. Acetaminophen 650 mg PO TID as needed. 5. Gentamicin 200 mg IV every 8 hours.

a. Epoetin-alfa.
b. Lisinopril.
c. Gentamicin.
d. Acetaminophen.

20. The nurse cares for a client with a renal injury due to kidney trauma. The nurse carefully monitors the client's laboratory findings for which manifestation of renal injury?

a. Impaired excretion of potassium resulting in hyperkalemia.
b. Conservation of sodium resulting in hypernatremia.
c. Increased excretion of chloride resulting in hypochloremia.
d. Shift of magnesium resulting in hypomagnesemia.

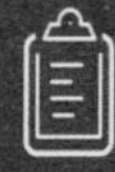

NurseThink® Quiz Answers

1. **The nurse cares for a child, post-op cleft lip repair using z-plasty. When demonstrating appropriate care to the child's parent, where does the nurse introduce the nipple for feeding?**
   a. From the bottom lip, with the nipple slanting upward.
   b. ● From the side of the mouth, to the left or right of the suture line.
   c. From the upper lip, with the nipple slanting downward.
   d. The nurse should use a syringe, not a nipple, for feeding.

   Topic/Concept: Nutrition **Subtopic:** Cleft lip **Bloom's Taxonomy:** Applying **Clinical Problem-Solving Process:** Implementation **NCLEX-PN®:** Basic Care and Comfort **QSEN:** Patient-centered care **CJMM:** Take Action

   Rationale: The nurse should plan to introduce the nipple for feeding on either side of the suture line to protect the surgical wound from infection and prevent damage to the sutures and incision.

   THIN Thinking: *Clinical Problem-Solving Process* –The nurse should plan to introduce the nipple for feeding on either side of the suture line to protect the surgical wound from infection and prevent damage to the sutures and incision.

2. **The nurse cares for a client with gastroesophageal reflux disease (GERD). The client complains of persistent bloating, "heartburn," and nausea, as well as frequent regurgitation. Which question does the nurse prioritize when speaking with the client?**
   a. "Do you take over-the-counter antacids or acid-blockers?"
   b. ● "Are you experiencing any difficulty swallowing?"
   c. "Do you see your dentist every six months?"
   d. "How often and how much per day are you eating?"

   Topic/Concept: Nutrition **Subtopic:** Gastroesophageal Reflux **Bloom's Taxonomy:** Applying **Clinical Problem-Solving Process:** Data Collection **NCLEX-PN®:** Physiological Adaptation **QSEN:** Evidence-based Practice **CJMM:** Analyze Cues

   Rationale: The nurse should check for dysphagia or odynophagia, indicating esophagitis or esophageal stenosis. The nurse needs to review the client's typical intake and use of antacids, but it is not the priority question. Acid reflux can cause damage to the teeth, and dental care is also important but is not the priority.

   THIN Thinking: *Identify Risk to Safety* – It's important that the nurse checks for significant damage to the oral cavity and esophagus. Dysphagia may indicate the presence of esophagitis or esophageal stenosis, which may impair swallowing and place the client at risk for aspiration.

3. **The nurse reviews the laboratory results of a male client with chronic gastritis. Which lab value best indicates the client is at risk for the development of pernicious anemia?**
   a. Ferritin.
   b. Red blood cells.
   c. ● Vitamin B12.
   d. Hemoglobin.

   Topic/Concept: Nutrition **Subtopic:** Gastritis **Bloom's Taxonomy:** Analyzing **Clinical Problem-Solving Process:** Data Collection **NCLEX-PN®:** Reduction of Risk Potential **QSEN:** Evidence-based Practice **CJMM:** Analyze Cues

   Rationale: Chronic gastritis damages the stomach's parietal cells, including intrinsic factor, resulting in decreased absorption of vitamin B12. Without B12, Hgb cannot be synthesized, leading to pernicious anemia. Low RBCs and a reduced Hgb may be present with other types of anemia, and low iron is expected with iron-deficiency anemia.

   THIN Thinking: *Identify Risk to Safety* – The nurse should recognize the client's risk for pernicious anemia related to chronic gastritis and monitor labs closely. The nurse should report abnormal laboratory values to the provider and implement new orders as received.

4. **A client with peptic ulcer disease is going home later today. What instructions does the nurse give the client prior to discharge? *Select all that apply.***
   a. Stop taking PPIs when symptoms subside.
   b. ● Avoid nonsteroidal anti-inflammatory medications.
   c. ● Limit coffee, tea, alcohol, and carbonated beverages.
   d. Cigarette smoking will help reduce stress levels.
   e. ● Contact provider if blood is seen in the stool.
   f. ● Avoid the use of flavored antacids.

   Topic/Concept: Nutrition **Subtopic:** Peptic ulcer disease **Bloom's Taxonomy:** Applying **Clinical Problem-Solving Process:** Planning **NCLEX-PN®:** Basic Care and Comfort **QSEN:** Patient-centered care **CJMM:** Generate Solutions

   Rationale: The nurse should instruct the client to avoid anything that may irritate the stomach lining, including smoking, carbonated beverages, coffee, tea, alcohol, NSAIDs, and stress. Flavored antacids delay stomach emptying and should also be avoided. PPI regimens should be completed as prescribed.

   THIN Thinking: *Clinical Problem-Solving Process* –When planning care, the nurse must include reinforcing client teaching about lifestyle practices that may potentiate or worsen the client's condition. It's also important for the nurse to advise the client signs and symptoms to report to the provider.

5. **The nurse develops a plan of care for a client diagnosed with celiac disease. Which type of diet does the nurse include in the referral to the dietitian?**
   a. Low-carbohydrate.
   b. Low-sodium, high-calcium.
   c. Fat-free, low-calorie.
   d. Gluten-free.

Topic/Concept: Nutrition **Subtopic:** Celiac Disease **Bloom's Taxonomy:** Applying **Clinical Problem-Solving Process:** Planning **NCLEX-PN®:** Coordinated Care **QSEN:** Teamwork and Collaboration **CJMM:** Generate Solutions

Rationale: The client with celiac disease should avoid gluten. Foods containing gluten are often higher in carbohydrates, but gluten is the ingredient that needs to be avoided. Neither low-sodium, high-calcium nor fat-free, low-calorie diets are indicated with Celiac disease.

THIN Thinking: *Clinical Problem-Solving Process* –When managing care, the nurse should communicate needs and expected outcomes to those involved in treatment. The nurse should make the referral request as ordered and communicate the client's needs.

6. **The nurse evaluates a client who presents with persistent nausea after eating pizza and vomiting. Suspecting cholecystitis, what client data is most important for the nurse to collect? *Select all that apply.***
   a. The client's response to RUQ palpation while taking a deep breath.
   b. The presence of jaundice in the client's skin and sclera.
   c. The presence of left flank tenderness and bruising.
   d. The client's temperature.
   e. The presence of periumbilical bruising.
   f. The type and severity of the client's pain.

Topic/Concept: Nutrition **Subtopic:** Gallbladder conditions **Bloom's Taxonomy:** Analyzing **Clinical Problem-Solving Process:** Data Collection **NCLEX-PN®:** Physiological Adaptation **QSEN:** Evidence-based Practice **CJMM:** Recognize Cues

Rationale: The nurse should check the client for the presence of Murphy's sign (RUQ palpation during deep inspiration), jaundice (in the case of a blocked bile duct), fever, and colicky or radiating pain. Cholecystitis can be difficult to identify as symptoms may vary, and pain can be general. The nurse needs to document a comprehensive review of findings. Periumbilical bruising (Cullen's Sign) and flank bruising (Turner's Sign) are rare but indicate retroperitoneal hemorrhage associated with pancreatitis.

THIN Thinking: *Top Three* – The nurse should check the client thoroughly and document findings. The nurse needs to identify abnormal findings and report those to the provider.

7. **The nurse plans home care for a client post-op after an open cholecystectomy. What discharge information does the nurse provide?**
   a. "You may resume a regular diet as soon as you are hungry."
   b. "You may experience constipation as a result of the procedure."
   c. "You should avoid heavy lifting for four to six weeks after surgery."
   d. "You should bathe, not shower, until the drainage tube is removed."

Topic/Concept: Nutrition **Subtopic:** Gallbladder conditions **Bloom's Taxonomy:** Applying **Clinical Problem-Solving Process:** Planning **NCLEX-PN®:** Coordinated Care **QSEN:** Teamwork and Collaboration **CJMM:** Generate Solutions

Rationale: After an open cholecystectomy, the nurse should instruct the client to avoid heavy lifting and baths and to advance to solid foods gradually. The nurse should also instruct the client that diarrhea, not constipation, is common and that stools will return to brown within a week.

THIN Thinking: *Identify Risk to Safety* – When caring for post-operative clients, the nurse must know expected outcomes, potential complications, and client needs for progression and discharge. Post-operatively, the nurse should focus on reducing client risk and promoting safety and healing.

8. **The nurse cares for an older adult experiencing chronic constipation. Which statement by the client requires follow-up from the nurse?**
   a. "I go for a walk around the neighborhood almost every day."
   b. "I only use a laxative once in a while."
   c. "I stop drinking water before dinner, so I don't have to wake up to urinate."
   d. "Every morning, I eat oatmeal with blueberries."

Topic/Concept: Nutrition **Subtopic:** Constipation **Bloom's Taxonomy:** Analyzing **Clinical Problem-Solving Process:** Evaluation **NCLEX-PN®:** Reduction of Risk Potential **QSEN:** Evidence-based Practice **CJMM:** Evaluate Outcomes

Rationale: Adequate hydration is vital in managing constipation, so the nurse needs to ensure the client gets enough fluid throughout the day. A low-fat, high-fiber diet is recommended for constipation. Inactivity and prolonged use of laxatives can contribute to constipation.

THIN Thinking: *Identify Risk to Safety* – The nurse should prepare to implement orders to reduce constipation and improve elimination which should improve the client's appetite and oral intake overall, improving nutritional status.

9. The nurse cares for a pediatric client with constipation. What information does the nurse report to the health care provider as evidence of a complication?

a. Vomiting with dark, foul-smelling emesis.
b. Leaking of stool between bowel movements.
c. Hiding while having bowel movements.
d. Presence of an anal wink.

Topic/Concept: Nutrition **Subtopic:** Constipation (peds) **Bloom's Taxonomy:** Applying **Clinical Problem-Solving Process:** Implementation **NCLEX-PN®:** Basic Care and Comfort **QSEN:** Patient-centered care **CJMM:** Take Action

Rationale: Manifestations of constipation in children include hard, infrequent, and painful stools, leaking stool between bowel movements, holding behaviors, nausea, and reduced appetite. The presence of an anal wink is a positive and normal data collection finding. With or without noted impaction, vomiting may indicate bowel obstruction and should be reported to the provider.

THIN Thinking: *Help Quick* – The nurse should recognize abnormalities during data collection. The presence of vomiting with dark, foul-smelling emesis may indicate an intestinal obstruction that warrants immediate notification of the provider.

10. A client verbalizes an urge to defecate but has been unable to pass stool or flatus for more than 12 hours. Which additional data best supports the nurse's suspicion of small bowel obstruction?

a. Presence of borborygmi.
b. Intermittent abdominal cramping.
c. Ribbon-like stools around impaction.
d. Projectile vomiting with fecal odor.

Topic/Concept: Nutrition **Subtopic:** Intestinal obstruction **Bloom's Taxonomy:** Analyzing **Clinical Problem-Solving Process:** Data Collection **NCLEX-PN®:** Physiological Adaptation **QSEN:** Patient-centered care **CJMM:** Analyze Cues

Rationale: Borborygmi may be present with small and large bowel obstructions. Small bowel obstructions are also associated with visible peristaltic waves, epigastric or upper abdominal pain and distention, and metabolic alkalosis, as well as projectile vomiting. Ribbon-like stools around impaction and intermittent abdominal cramping are indicative of large bowel obstructions.

THIN Thinking: *Clinical Problem-Solving Process* –The nurse should be aware of normal and abnormal findings during data collection. Projectile vomiting of emesis with a fecal odor may indicate an intestinal obstruction, a medical emergency that should be reported to the provider.

11. The nurse and a client are reviewing information about diverticulitis. The nurse asks the client to point to the area of the abdomen where pain most commonly occurs with exacerbation of the disease. Which location, as indicated by the client, indicates understanding?

a. Right upper quadrant.
b. Left upper quadrant.
c. Right lower quadrant.
d. Left lower quadrant.

Topic/Concept: Nutrition **Subtopic:** Diverticular disease **Bloom's Taxonomy:** Analyzing **Clinical Problem-Solving Process:** Data Collection **NCLEX-PN®:** Health promotion and maintenance **QSEN:** Evidence-based Practice **CJMM:** Analyze Cues

Rationale: Diverticulitis typically occurs over the sigmoid colon, located in the LLQ of the abdomen. Pain in other quadrants is typically associated with other conditions.

THIN Thinking: *Clinical Problem-Solving Process* –The nurse should evaluate the client's understanding by asking the client to report back or demonstrate evidence of learning. The nurse should intervene and provide additional information if the client indicates a lack of understanding.

12. The nurse prepares a client for a wireless capsule endoscopy to rule out the presence of colorectal cancer. What information does the nurse give the client to prepare them for the procedure?

a. "Sedation is necessary for this type of endoscopic procedure."
b. "You will be asked to change positions repeatedly to distribute the barium."
c. "It will take about eight hours for the camera to pass through the GI tract."
d. "After you expel the barium, your intestine will be inflated with air."

Topic/Concept: Nutrition **Subtopic:** Colorectal cancer **Bloom's Taxonomy:** Applying **Clinical Problem-Solving Process:** Planning **NCLEX-PN®:** Basic Care and Comfort **QSEN:** Evidence-based Practice **CJMM:** Generate Solutions

Rationale: Wireless capsule endoscopy is known as the pill camera. The client swallows the pill containing the camera, and the camera captures video throughout the GI tract over approximately 8 hours, at which time the camera is then expelled. No sedation, barium, or invasive procedure is required.

THIN Thinking: *Clinical Problem-Solving Process* –The nurse should ensure that the client understands the procedure and expected outcomes. The nurse should notify the provider if the client indicates misunderstanding to ensure the client has provided informed consent for the procedure.

13. **The nurse plans a community health class at a senior citizens' center. The nurse will be promoting risk reduction of colon cancer. What information does the nurse present? *Select all that apply.***
    a. Consume a low-fat, low-carbohydrate diet
    b. Have regular, age-specific colorectal screenings
    c. Consume a calcium-rich, high-fiber diet
    d. Engage in regular physical exercise
    e. Reduce or eliminate alcohol intake.

Topic/Concept: Nutrition **Subtopic:** Colorectal cancer **Bloom's Taxonomy:** Applying **Clinical Problem-Solving Process:** Planning **NCLEX-PN®:** Reduction of Risk Potential **QSEN:** Patient-centered care **CJMM:** Generate Solutions

Rationale: Regular screenings are important to reducing the risk of colorectal cancer. Clients should also be instructed to consume low-fat, low-carb, calcium-rich, high-fiber foods, engage in physical activity, and avoid smoking and excessive alcohol intake.

THIN Thinking: *Clinical Problem-Solving Process* –The nurse should plan to provide information on risk factors and screening to the community in layman's terms.

14. **The nurse provides care for an unconscious client with a history of Hepatitis C. The nurse concerned about exposure to Hepatitis C through what routes of transmission? *Select all that apply.***
    a. Feces.
    b. Mucosal blood.
    c. Urine.
    d. Percutaneous blood.
    e. Emesis.

Topic/Concept: Nutrition **Subtopic:** Hepatitis **Bloom's Taxonomy:** Applying **Clinical Problem-Solving Process:** Data Collection **NCLEX-PN®:** Safety and Infection Control **QSEN:** Safety **CJMM:** Recognize Cues

Rationale: Hepatitis B and C are transmitted via percutaneous and mucosal blood, body fluids, and sharp instrument and needle sticks. Hepatitis A may be spread through feces.

THIN Thinking: *Top Three* – When caring for any client, universal precautions should be implemented. However, the nurse needs to be aware of additional risks and take precautions to limit exposure or transmission.

15. **The nurse cares for a pediatric client with pyloric stenosis. Due to extensive vomiting and dehydration, the nurse plans to monitor the client's lab values for which physiologic response?**
    a. Metabolic acidosis.
    b. Metabolic alkalosis.
    c. Respiratory acidosis.
    d. Respiratory alkalosis.

Topic/Concept: Nutrition **Subtopic:** Pyloric Stenosis **Bloom's Taxonomy:** Applying **Clinical Problem-Solving Process:** Planning **NCLEX-PN®:** Health promotion and maintenance **QSEN:** Patient-centered care **CJMM:** Prioritize Hypotheses

Rationale: The client is at risk for metabolic alkalosis due to the loss of chloride from vomiting. The other conditions are not typically present as a result of vomiting and dehydration.

THIN Thinking: *Identify Risk to Safety* – The nurse should monitor the client and laboratory values. Evidence of metabolic alkalosis should be reported to the provider for further evaluation and treatment.

16. **The nurse collects information about risk factors contributing to a client's diagnosis of class 1 obesity. What environmental factors does the nurse expect to find? *Select all that apply.***
    a. Availability and access to unhealthy foods.
    b. Automation of food preparation.
    c. Leptin and melanocortin-4 receptor mutation.
    d. Stress and binge eating.
    e. Increase in average portion size.
    f. Physical inactivity or sedentary lifestyle.

Topic/Concept: Nutrition **Subtopic:** Obesity (adult) **Bloom's Taxonomy:** Applying **Clinical Problem-Solving Process:** Data Collection **NCLEX-PN®:** Coordinated Care **QSEN:** Teamwork and Collaboration **CJMM:** Recognize Cues

Rationale: Environmental factors contributing to obesity include availability and access to high-fat, high-calorie, convenience foods with large portions. Other factors may be genetic or behavioral.

THIN Thinking: *Identify Risk to Safety* – The nurse can provide more detailed information on reducing risk and promoting wellness with a better understanding of risk factors for specific conditions.

17. **The nurse discusses the plan of care for a pediatric client with obesity with the client's parents. Which recommendations does the nurse provide for the parents in managing their child's health? *Select all that apply.***
    a. Encourage the child to eat quickly to fill up faster.
    b. Restrict eating in front of the television or computer.
    c. Discourage the child from skipping meals.
    d. Promote an increase and change in physical activity.
    e. Set daily screen time at 4-8 hours per day.
    f. Provide some choices in meals and snacks.

Topic/Concept: Nutrition **Subtopic:** Obesity (peds) **Bloom's Taxonomy:** Applying **Clinical Problem-Solving Process:** Implementation **NCLEX-PN®:** Psychosocial Integrity **QSEN:** Evidence-based Practice **CJMM:** Take Action

Rationale: Management of the child with obesity requires lifestyle changes and an individualized weight loss plan. This includes giving the child choices of healthy meals and snacks, encouraging regular meals and physical activity, and discouraging distracted eating. The child should be encouraged to eat slowly to allow the brain to recognize fullness. Screen time should be limited to 2-3 hours/day to limit sedentary behaviors.

THIN Thinking: *Clinical Problem-Solving Process* –The nurse should identify the client's developmental level and recommend age-appropriate strategies for making positive lifestyle changes.

18. The nurse plans home care for a client who has undergone brachytherapy for prostate cancer. Which instructions does the nurse reinforce to the client regarding sexual activity?

a. Abstain from sexual intercourse for four weeks after treatment.
b. Always urinate before and after sexual intercourse.
c. Abstain from sex for two weeks, then resume with condom use.
d. Sex with a condom may resume as soon as you feel you are able.

Topic/Concept: Nutrition **Subtopic:** Prostate Cancer **Bloom's Taxonomy:** Applying **Clinical Problem-Solving Process:** Planning **NCLEX-PN®:** Physiological Adaption **QSEN:** Patient-centered care **CJMM:** Generate Solutions

Rationale: Brachytherapy is a procedure in which permanent radioactive seeds are placed in the prostate to target a precise location, losing radioactivity over time. The client should abstain from sex initially and return to sexual activity with a plan to reduce the risk of radiation exposure to the partner. Abstaining for more than two weeks and urinating before and after intercourse are not indicated. Sexual intercourse before two weeks is not safe and is not recommended.

THIN Thinking: *Identify Risk to Safety* – The nurse should plan care around reducing risk to the client, as well as those at risk for exposure. The client should be instructed to abstain from sex for two weeks after the procedure and then wear a condom to protect his partner from radiation exposure.

19. The nurse reviews the prescriptions of a client with end-stage renal disease. Which medication does the nurse clarify with the provider?

a. Epoetin-alfa.
b. Lisinopril.
c. Gentamicin.
d. Acetaminophen.

Topic/Concept: Nutrition **Subtopic:** ESRD **Bloom's Taxonomy:** Applying **Clinical Problem-Solving Process:** Implementation **NCLEX-PN®:** Reduction of Risk Potential **QSEN:** Safety **CJMM:** Take Action

Rationale: The nurse would want to clarify the order for Gentamicin in the client with ESRD as aminoglycosides may be nephrotoxic and may require an alternative medication or a dose adjustment. The other medications are not contraindicated with ESRD.

THIN Thinking: *Identify Risk to Safety* – The nurse should review medication orders closely and contact the provider with prescriptions that may pose a risk to the client.

20. The nurse cares for a client with a renal injury due to kidney trauma. The nurse carefully monitors the client's laboratory findings for which manifestation of renal injury?

a. Impaired excretion of potassium resulting in hyperkalemia.
b. Conservation of sodium resulting in hypernatremia.
c. Increased excretion of chloride resulting in hypochloremia.
d. Shift of magnesium resulting in hypomagnesemia.

Topic/Concept: Nutrition **Subtopic:** Kidney injury **Bloom's Taxonomy:** Analyzing **Clinical Problem-Solving Process:** Data Collection **NCLEX-PN®:** Basic Care and Comfort **QSEN:** Patient-centered care **CJMM:** Analyze Cues

Rationale: The nurse should monitor laboratory values in the client with renal injury, paying close attention to impaired excretion of potassium (resulting in hyperkalemia) and an inability to conserve sodium (hyponatremia). Conservation of sodium, excretion of chloride, and hypomagnesemia are not generally seen with renal injury.

THIN Thinking: *Identify Risk to Safety* – The nurse should plan care that includes close monitoring of the client's status. Significant changes in laboratory values may indicate progression of the client's condition, and the provider should be informed.

CHAPTER

12

Hormonal

Neuroendocrine / Glucose Regulation

This chapter addresses conditions that impact the body's hormonal processes. The neuroendocrine system is an intricate design of interwoven processes that involve the nervous and endocrine systems. The nervous and endocrine systems often function perfectly in a process called neuroendocrine integration to ensure that the body's physiological processes regulate effectively. The interaction between the endocrine system and the nervous system is made possible because of the hypothalamus and the significant role it plays in controlling endocrine glands such as the pituitary gland.

The functions regulated by the various glands in the body manage life and so when there is impairment in any aspect of neuroendocrine function, the threat to life is significant. Therefore, nurses must understand the pathophysiological processes that affect the effective functioning of each gland in the system but more importantly, they must be knowledgeable and prepared to provide quality care to clients who present to their facilities with neuroendocrine disorders.

Priority Exemplars:

- Gestational diabetes
- Addison's disease
- Hypothyroidism
- Cushing's syndrome
- Diabetic ketoacidosis
- Diabetes insipidus
- Diabetes mellitus–type 2
- Diabetes mellitus–type 1
- Hyperglycemic hyperosmolar syndrome
- Hypoparathyroidism
- Hyperparathyroidism
- Hyperthyroidism
- Metabolic syndrome
- Syndrome of inappropriate antidiuretic hormone (SIADH)
- Wilms tumor

Clinical Hint

Disorders of regulation are common co-morbidities with other diagnoses and illnesses.

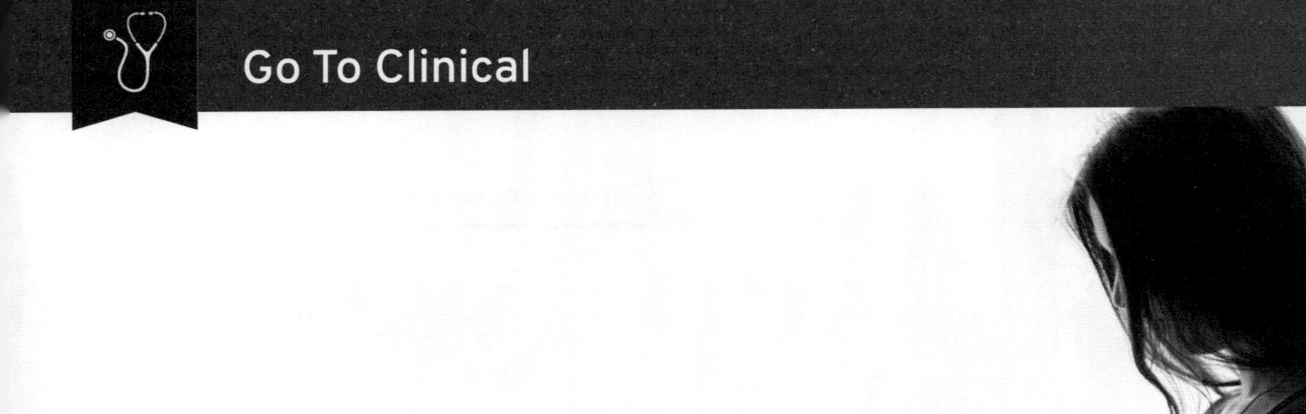

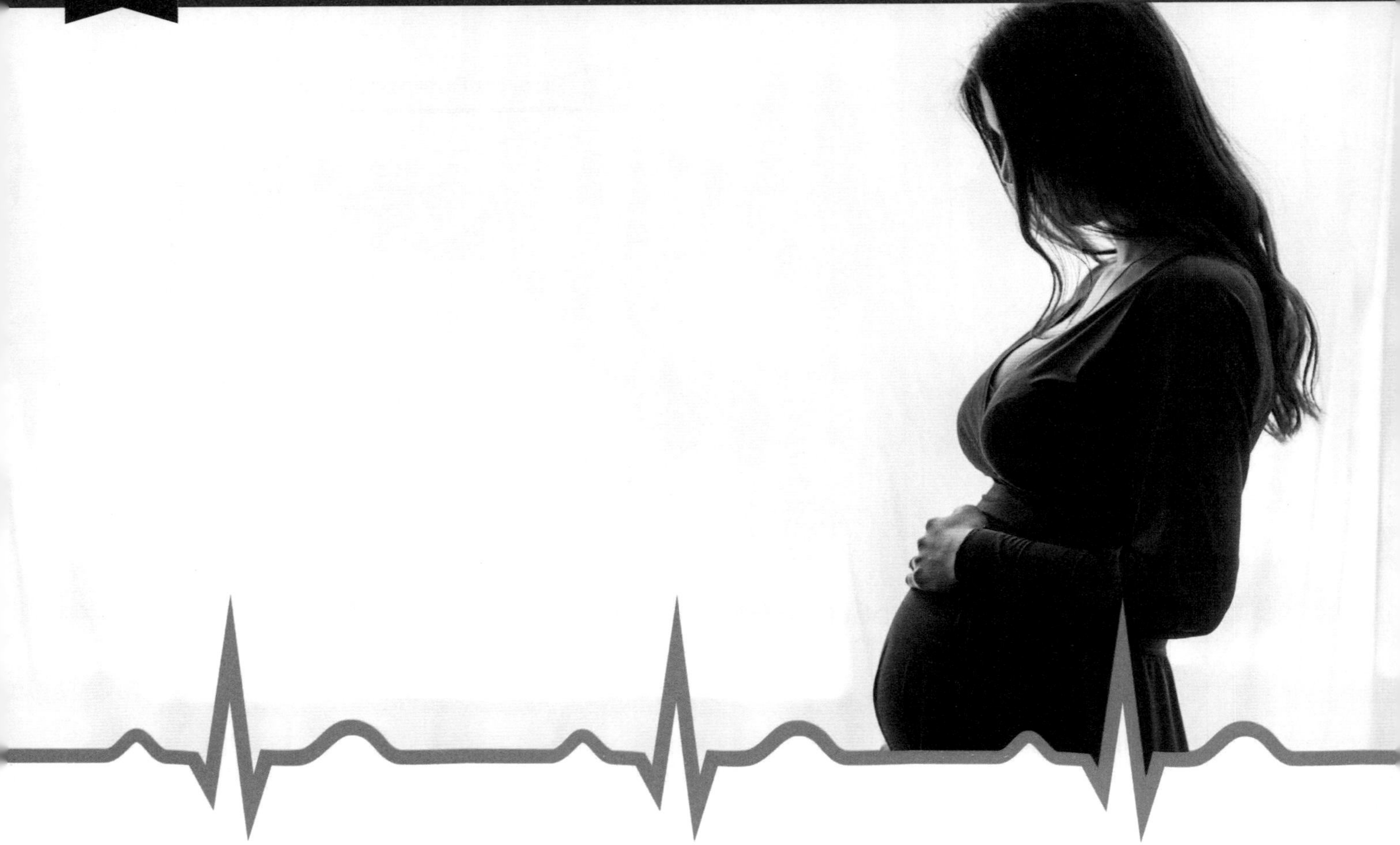

Go To Clinical Case 1

The client K.H. is 36 years old. She is a 25-week pregnant female who presents to the clinic for a second gestational diabetes screening. The results of her first oral glucose tolerance test were 165 mg/dL. This is her first pregnancy, and she has no significant past medical or surgical history. There is a family history of type 2 diabetes. Her spouse is with her and they both have questions regarding the health of the unborn child if the diagnosis is confirmed.

She confirms that she is fasting and has not had anything to eat or drink in the past eight hours. She states that she has been more thirsty than usual and urinating more, but she thinks that is just part of the pregnancy. Her vital signs are as follows: Blood pressure 120/78 mm Hg, heart rate 89 bpm, temperature 98.8°F, and respirations 22 bpm.

The client was at the clinic for a total of 3 hours for the test. The results from this oral glucose tolerance test are: Fasting–148 mg/dL; 1 hour–184 mg/dL; 2 hours–175 mg/dL; 3 hours–170 mg/ dL. The client was instructed to return tomorrow for her scheduled appointment to discuss the findings with her health care provider.

Next Gen Clinical Judgment

How does the care of a client with gestational diabetes differ from the care of a client with type 1 or type 2 diabetes who is pregnant? How is the care similar?

NurseThink® Time

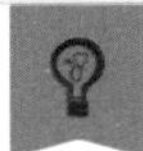

Using the NurseThink® system, complete the priorities. Check your answers designated by 💡 in the Gestational diabetes Priority Exemplar.

NurseThink® Time

Priority Data Collection or Cues

1.

2.

3.

Priority Laboratory Tests/Diagnostics

1.

2.

3.

Priority Interventions or Actions

1.

2.

3.

Priority Potential & Actual Complications

1.

2.

3.

Priority Nursing Implications

1.

2.

3.

Priority Medications

1.

2.

3.

Reinforcement of Priority Teaching

1.

2.

3.

Gestational diabetes

Pathophysiology/Description

- Diabetes that develops during pregnancy and resolves after pregnancy
- In pregnancy, the placenta makes hormones that make it more difficult for insulin to work
- Women at high risk include: family history of diabetes, advanced maternal age, obesity, and given birth to a large baby previously
- Impact of gestational diabetes include: birth injury or death to the infant
- Women are usually screened at 24-28 weeks using the oral glucose tolerance test (OGTT)
- Gestational diabetes is mostly controlled with diet, but some women may require insulin

Priority Data Collection or Cues

- Ask about the status of the fetus in utero
- Ask about symptoms such as polydipsia, polyuria, polyphagia. Determine blood glucose level
- Ask about diet and exercise habits
- Check knowledge of insulin preparation and administration
- Check ability to manage diabetes at home
- Measure vital signs
- Evaluate client's understanding of disease management and physical ability to prepare and administer insulin injections

Priority Laboratory Tests/Diagnostics

- Glucose challenge test. One hour after drinking a glucose solution, blood sample is taken to measure glucose level. If result is greater than 140 mg/dL, a second test called an oral glucose tolerance test (OGTT) is done. The OGTT is a fasting test
- Oral glucose tolerance test (OGTT). Performed as a follow-up to glucose challenge test. Blood glucose is tested every hour for three hours. The diagnosis of gestational diabetes is made if two of the three blood glucose levels are higher than normal

Priority Interventions or Actions

- Monitor blood glucose with expectation of the following results
  - Before a meal (preprandial) should be 95 mg/dL or less
  - 1-hour after a meal (postprandial) should be 140 mg/dL or less
  - 2-hours after a meal (postprandial) should be 120 mg/dL or less
- Administer insulin and monitor for adverse effects
- Monitor meal intake
- Schedule meeting with dietitian to talk with client about nutrition planning and ensure client's knowledge needs are met

Priority Potential & Actual Complications

- Complications in the infant include: birth defects, high birth weight, and hypoglycemia
- Complications in the mother include: cesarean section and developing type 2 diabetes
- Hypoglycemia, if on insulin
- Atrophy or hypertrophy of tissue at injection site

Priority Nursing Implications

- There is a 63% likelihood of developing type 2 diabetes within 16 years for women with a history of gestational diabetes
- Family members may be included in the education, as family roles may change

Priority Medications

- Rapid-acting insulin
  - Lispro, aspart; given subcutaneously
  - Onset 10-30 minutes, peak 30 minutes-3 hours, duration 3-5 hours
- Short-acting insulin
  - Regular; usually administered subcutaneously
  - Onset 30 minutes- 1 hour, peak 2-5 hours, duration 5-8 hours
  - Administered via subcutaneous route
- Intermediate-acting insulin
  - NPH; administered subcutaneously
  - Onset 1.5-4 hours, peak 4-12 hours, duration 12-18 hours
- Combination therapy
  - Several combinations of premixed insulins (2 insulins combined)

Reinforcement of Priority Teaching

- Prescribed diet and importance of eating with insulin
- If controlled with insulin, discuss storage, preparation, administration, injection, and side effects of insulin
- Have client demonstrate insulin administration and blood glucose checks. Discuss frequency and proper technique
- Remind client about signs and symptoms of hypo and hyperglycemia
- Likelihood of developing type 2 diabetes in the future

Go To Clinical Answers

Text designated by are the top answers for the Go To Clinical related to Gestational diabetes.

Addison's disease

Pathophysiology/Description

- Addison's disease results when there is hypofunction of the adrenal glands causing corticosteroids (mineralocorticoids, glucocorticoids, and androgens) to be insufficient. This is primary adrenal insufficiency. Adrenal insufficiency may also occur from insufficient pituitary adrenocorticotropic hormone as a secondary cause
- Majority of Addison's disease in the United States result from an autoimmune response that causes destruction to the adrenal cortex by antibodies
- Common clinical manifestations include: bronzed hyperpigmentation of skin, hypotension, lethargy, hypovolemia, decreased cardiac output, anorexia, weight loss, abdominal cramping, depression, confusion, delusions, hyperkalemia, sodium loss, salt craving, decreased libido, and decreased muscle size and tone
- Occurs most often in adults younger than age 60 and is not gender-specific

Priority Data Collection or Cues

- Check for the clinical manifestations of Addison's disease
- Check for Addisonian crisis, a life-threatening condition, which has added manifestations of severe abdominal and lower back pain, severe headache, severe hypotension, tachycardia, generalized weakness and shock

Priority Laboratory Tests/Diagnostics

- Adrenocorticotropic(ACTH) stimulation test
  - Baseline cortisol and ACTH are measured. Intravenous Addison's disease is indicated if cortisol level is increased minimally or not increased at all
- Corticotropin-releasing hormone (CRH) stimulation test (measured when ACTH test is abnormal)
  - Addison's disease is indicated if ACTH level is high, but cortisol level is absent
- Blood tests will show increased potassium and decreased blood glucose, sodium and chloride
- Electrocardiogram will show peaked T waves from hyperkalemia
- Computed tomography (CT) scan and magnetic resonance imaging (MRI) will show other non-autoimmune causes

Priority Interventions or Actions

- Assist with labs and diagnostic tests
- In acute Addisonian crisis, assist with medications and labs as needed
- Monitor weight, as unexplained, weight loss is an issue
- Administer medications replacement hormones as prescribed
- Allow client time to verbalize feelings about the disease

Priority Potential & Actual Complications

- Addisonian crisis
- Depression

Priority Nursing Implications

- It is crucial for individuals with Addison's disease to know how hormone replacement will be managed during times of added stress
- Understand the importance of carrying medications at all times in the event an emergency occurs. Clients must teach someone else how to administer hydrocortisone injections

Priority Medications

- Hydrocortisone
  - Used in Addisonian crisis to replace hormone
  - Used as maintenance hormone replacement
  - Hydrocortisone (has both mineralocorticoid and glucocorticoid properties)
  - Can be administered via various routes including orally or intravenous
- Fludrocortisone (most commonly prescribed mineralocorticoid)
  - Used as partial replacement therapy for Addison's disease
  - Adverse effects include fluid retention, hypertension and potential heart failure
  - Administered orally
- Dehydroepiandrosterone (DHEA)
  - Given to women as androgen replacement
  - Alert to the fact that DHEA can cause acne and unwanted, male-pattern hair growth in women (hirsutism)
  - Administered various routes including orally and IM

Reinforcement of Priority Teaching

- Signs and symptoms of Addisonian crisis
- Encourage wearing MedicAlert identification
- Remind client on the proper time of day to take prescribed glucocorticoids and mineralocorticoids
- Remind the importance of carrying a kit at all times to include, 100 mg of hydrocortisone with a syringe and clear instructions for use
- Importance of following up with health care provider visits
- Importance of lifelong hormone drug therapy
- In times of stress, such as illness, corticosteroid dosage will need to be increased
- Discuss the side effects of medication therapy and signs and symptoms of corticosteroid deficiency
- Avoid the stress of strenuous exercise
- Encourage adhering to a prescribed diet

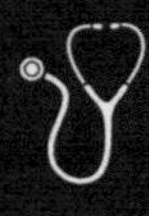

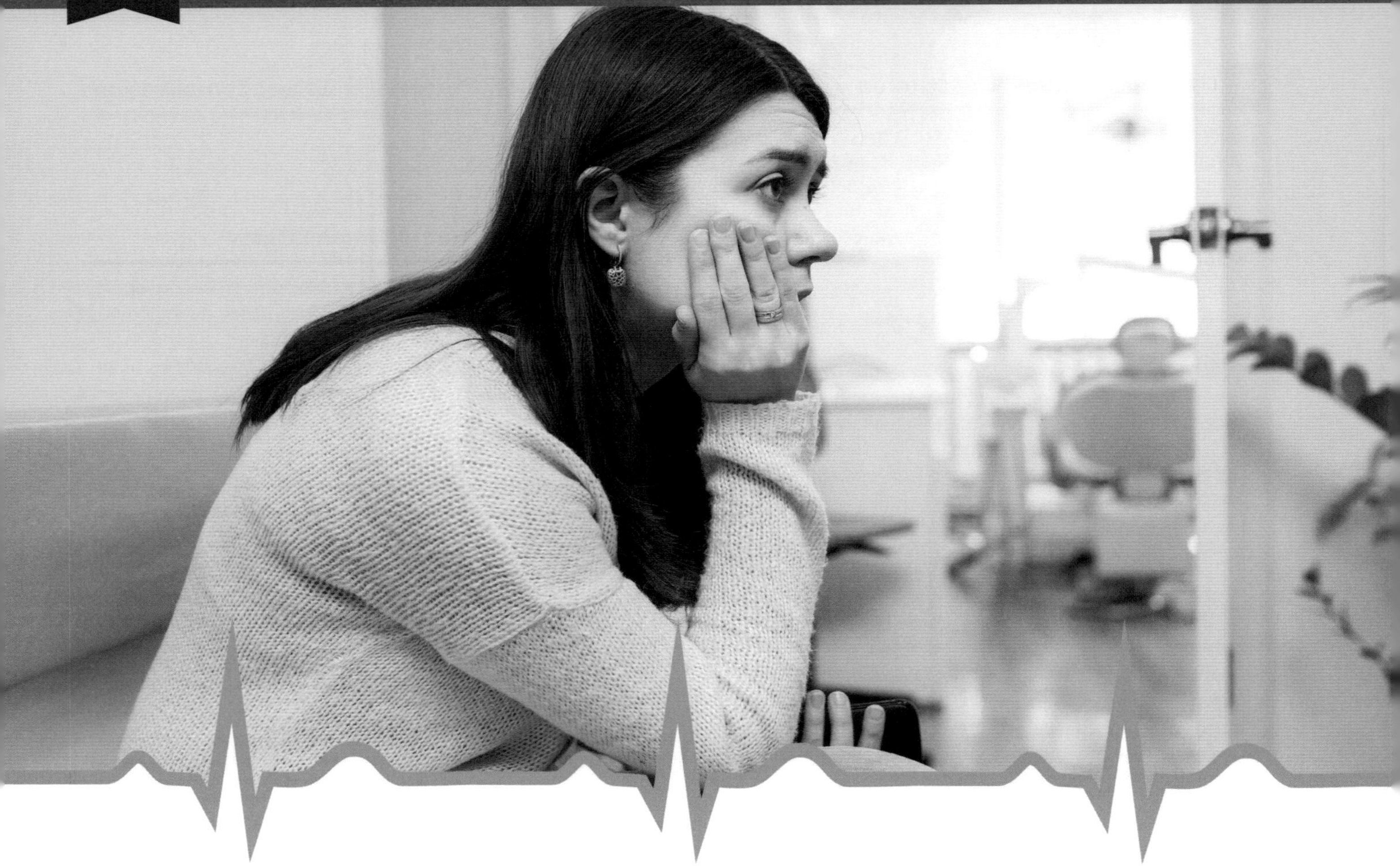

Go To Clinical

Go To Clinical Case 2

A 26-year-old white, female presents to the clinic with a chief complaint of fatigue and difficulty breathing. She also states that she has noticed being hoarse, having muscle aches, and gaining weight. Her current vital signs are as follows: Blood pressure 136/88 mm Hg, pulse 58 bpm, respirations 18 breaths per minute, and temperature is 98.9°F. Her oxygen saturation is 98% on room air.

She states that she is always cold and it is hard to stay warm, especially with it being cold outside. Additionally, she states that she experiences constipation but has used over-the-counter laxatives as needed. Lately, she has noticed a change in her hair and nails. She feels like they are becoming drier and brittle but is not sure if that is related to the other signs and symptoms she is experiencing.

She has not changed anything recently in her diet or routine. She has no medical conditions but reports her father has type 2 diabetes and has hypothyroidism. Her lab work reveals an increased TSH (Thyroid stimulating hormone) and low free T4. Other labs were unremarkable.

NurseThink® Time

Using the NurseThink® system, complete the priorities. Check your answers designated by 💡 in the Hypothyroidism Priority Exemplar.

Next Gen Clinical Judgment

Many of the endocrine disorders reflect inverse relationships. For example, clients with hypothyroid often feel cold; whereas, clients with hyperthyroid often feel warm or hot.

NurseThink® Time

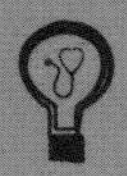

Priority Data Collection or Cues

1.

2.

3.

Priority Laboratory Tests/Diagnostics

1.

2.

3.

Priority Interventions or Actions

1.

2.

3.

Priority Potential & Actual Complications

1.

2.

3.

Priority Nursing Implications

1.

2.

3.

Priority Medications

1.

2.

3.

Reinforcement of Priority Teaching

1.

2.

3.

Hypothyroidism

Pathophysiology/Description

- Hypothyroidism occurs when there is not enough thyroid hormone (deficiency), causing a slowing of the body's metabolic rate. The condition is more commonly seen in women than men
- There are two classifications to the condition, primary and secondary
  - In primary hypothyroidism the thyroid tissue is destroyed, or synthesis of the hormone is defective. Atrophy of the thyroid gland is the most common cause. This is as a result of Graves' disease or Hashimoto's disease
  - Secondary hypothyroidism results when there is a disease of the pituitary gland
- Risk factors for hypothyroidism are family history, female and white, type 1 diabetes, Down syndrome, previous hyperthyroidism, radiation to neck and head, and goiter
- A thyroidectomy or iodine, used to destroy the thyroid gland in treating hyperthyroidism, can cause hypothyroidism. Certain drugs that contain iodine can also cause hypothyroidism. Hypothyroidism can also develop at birth (called cretinism). Screening for the condition in all infants occurs in the United States
- Hypothyroidism causes functions of the body to slow down. Clinical manifestations impact all body systems
- Myxedema occurs with longstanding hypothyroidism. Causes puffiness to skin, edema around the eyes (periorbital edema), facial edema, and a flat or masklike effect
- Myxedema coma results if myxedema is not treated early. Symptoms include: hypotension, subnormal body temperature, hypoventilation, and collapse of the cardiovascular system

Priority Data Collection or Cues

- Ask about past treatment for hyperthyroidism, antithyroid or iodine intake
- Check for known signs and symptoms including, but not limited to: bradycardia, dyspnea, lethargy, constipation, weakness, dry hair, decreased libido
- Check for myxedema
- Check vital signs, including oxygen saturation level
- Check response to treatment
- Ask about depression and body image disturbances

Priority Laboratory Tests/Diagnostics

- Thyroid stimulating hormone (TSH) will be low in secondary hypothyroidism and high in primary hypothyroidism. Thyroxine (T4) will be low in both primary and secondary hypothyroidism. Thyroid antibodies will be positive in Hashimoto's disease

Priority Interventions or Actions

- In acute situation
  - Ensure intravenous line, medications may be given intravenous
  - Provide cardiac monitoring and respiratory support
  - Monitor body temperature
  - Position client frequently to minimize risk of skin breakdown. Use pressure relief mattress
- Encourage exercise but space activities to conserve energy
- Administer medications to treat symptoms as indicated
- Administer thyroid hormone
- Monitor environmental temperature
- Orient to environment, since mental processing is slowed

Priority Potential & Actual Complications

- Loss of consciousness, mental sluggishness, myxedema coma, collapse of cardiovascular system

Priority Nursing Implications

- Altered self-image is a significant problem. Devise strategies to assist client with coping skills
- Understand that if a client has diabetes mellitus, blood glucose must be checked daily as return to a euthyroid state often causes an increase in insulin requirement

Priority Medications

- Thyroid hormone
  - Levothyroxine
  - Administered orally as long-term therapy

Reinforcement of Priority Teaching

- Remind client and family members about the signs and symptoms of hypothyroidism
- Remind client to avoid extreme cold temperatures
- Weight reduction measures
- A high-fiber diet and fluid intake
- Assist with referral to dietitian
- Assist with psychological referral if needed to manage depression and body image disturbance
- Remind the client of the importance of follow up visits
- Lifelong drug therapy
- Discuss the side effects of medication therapy
- Remind client not to switch brands of hypothyroid medication as it may alter the body's response to the drug

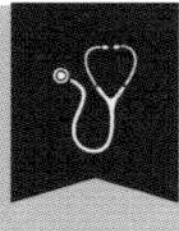

Go To Clinical Answers

Text designated by ⓥ are the top answers for the Go To Clinical related to Hypothyroidism.

Cushing's syndrome

Pathophysiology/Description

- Cushing's syndrome results when an individual experiences chronic exposure to corticosteroids
- Common causes include: use of corticosteroids or pituitary tumor
- Common clinical manifestations include lower extremities edema, hypertension, fatigue, muscle wasting in extremities, weakness, osteoporosis resulting in compression fractures, inhibition of immune and allergic responses, petechial hemorrhage, thin and fragile skin, bruises, purplish striae, problems with wound healing

Priority Data Collection or Cues

- Check for muscle wasting and weakness
- Check for classic appearance of hump, called buffalo hump and face for moon shaped appearance from fatty deposits
- Check for classic obesity to trunk with thin extremities and fatty deposits to supraclavicular area
- Check skin for reddish-purple stretch marks (called striae) on abdomen and thighs, resulting from inflamed and ruptured dermal tissue because of the weight gain associated with Cushing's syndrome
- Check for facial hair in women (called hirsutism) and gynecomastia in men
- Monitor blood pressure, blood glucose and sodium levels
- Monitor potassium and calcium levels
- Ask about depression and body image disturbances

Priority Laboratory Tests/Diagnostics

- Late night salivary cortisol is expected to be elevated above the normal range of 0.10-0.15 ug/dL with Cushing's syndrome. Normally, cortisol secretion is very low at late night
- Low dose dexamethasone suppression test. A serum cortisol level >1.7 µg/dL after the single dose dexamethasone is a positive test
- Urine free cortisol, levels higher than 80 -120 mcg/24 hour is positive for Cushing's syndrome
- ACH test to determine cause with results that may be normal, elevated or low depending on the cause of the condition
- Computed tomography (CT) scan and magnetic resonance imaging (MRI) to examine pituitary and adrenal glands for tumors

Priority Interventions or Actions

- Ensure intravenous line, assist with administration of fluid and medications
- Prepare client for surgery, radiation, or chemotherapy based on the cause
- Provide expectations regarding postoperative care
- Discontinue corticosteroid medications if cause of Cushing's syndrome is from exogenous intake of corticosteroids
- Postoperative interventions
  - Monitor urinary catheter and nasogastric tube (often used) postoperatively
  - Ensure placement of sequential leg compression device to minimize risk of blood clot formation
  - Monitor vital signs and for hemorrhage
  - Monitor subtle signs of infection (important as the inflammatory response is decreased)
  - During first 24-48 hours postoperative, constant monitoring for corticosteroid imbalance

Priority Potential & Actual Complications

- Osteoporosis resulting in fractures, hypertension, type 2 diabetes and infections, hemorrhage from surgery

Priority Nursing Implications

- If client is having surgery, ensure hypertension, hyperglycemia, and hypokalemia are controlled before surgery
- Surgery presents a significant risk of bleeding
- Taper slowly to avoid adrenal insufficiency manifested by increased weakness, vomiting, hypotension dehydration, peeling skin, joint pain, and pruritus

Priority Medications

- Ketoconazole
  - Used to control cortisol production by decreasing steroid hormone production in the adrenal gland
  - Causes liver toxicity at high doses
  - Administered orally
- Mifepristone
  - Used to treat high blood glucose associated with Cushing's syndrome in clients with type 2 diabetes (not used to treat diabetes outside of Cushing's syndrome)
  - Given orally to block the effect of excess cortisol
- Corticosteroids (hydrocortisone most common drug in class)
  - Various routes of administration

Reinforcement of Priority Teaching

- Signs and symptoms of corticosteroid therapy
- Assist client to schedule a home health nurse for ongoing teaching and evaluation
- Proper administration and side effects of drug therapy
- Assist with psychological referral if needed
- Importance of following up with health care provider visits
- Importance of lifelong drug therapy
- Encourage stress reduction strategies
- Encourage client to wear a MedicAlert identification

Diabetic ketoacidosis

Pathophysiology/Description

- Diabetic ketoacidosis (DKA) results when cells of the body cannot get the insulin they need for energy because there is profound insulin deficiency
- Usually occurs when the pancreas is unable to adjust to the extra need for insulin brought on by conditions such as significant stress or severe illness
- DKA is more common in type 1 diabetes, but may rarely occur in type 2
- Contributing factors to DKA include: Type 1 diabetes not diagnosed, illness, infection, poor management of diabetes, dosage of insulin inadequate, insulin pump malfunction
- How diabetic ketoacidosis occurs
  - Glucose gets to a very high level because there is no insulin to break it down to usable energy
  - The body needs energy, breaks down fats to use as fuel
  - When fats breakdown, ketone acids are produced
  - If the process is sustained, then ketones accumulate in the blood causing major problems on systems of the body
- Diabetic ketoacidosis progresses rapidly and is life-threatening if the individual does not get treatment readily. Fluid imbalance is a major factor in this disease

Priority Data Collection or Cues

- Check for patent airway and determine oxygen level. Check level of consciousness and cardiac status. Confusion and cardiac dysrhythmias can occur with DKA
- Check glucose levels. Expect blood glucose levels of 250 mg/dL or higher
- Determine urine output and signs and symptoms of dehydration. Watch for fluid overload as fluid resuscitation is initiated
- Ask about time of last food intake and insulin administration as well as overall self-management of diabetes
- Check all body systems as DKA impacts functions in all systems
- Check vital signs frequently

Priority Laboratory Tests/Diagnostics

- Blood glucose level, expected greater than 250 mg/dL
- Urinalysis positive for ketones
- Blood pH shows acidity.
- Electrolytes levels expected to be low because of the changing pH, acidosis and dehydration
  - Hyponatremia, hypokalemia, hypomagnesemia, hypocalcemia, hypophosphatemia
- Bicarbonate (HCO_3) expected to be low, less than 15 mEq/L
- Blood urea nitrogen (BUN) level expected to be high, greater than 20 mg/dL due to dehydration
- Creatinine expected to be high, greater than 1.5 mg/dL due to dehydration

Priority Interventions or Actions

- Ensure airway is patent
- Intravenous fluid with 0.9% NaCL at 1 L per hour. Once glucose is less than 250 mg/dL, 5%-10% dextrose may be added
- The client may need regular insulin intravenous. Monitor fluid balance and potassium levels
- If acidosis is severe, with pH less than 7.0, sodium bicarbonate may be used
- Potassium to correct issue of hypokalemia

Priority Potential & Actual Complications

- Cerebral edema from rapid lowering of the glucose, rapid administering intravenous fluids or administering the wrong intravenous fluid
- Coma
- May be fatal

Priority Nursing Implications

- Administration of insulin causes potassium to decrease. A potassium supplement may be needed
- Involve the family in the care as indicated

Priority Medications

- Regular insulin
  - Watch for hypoglycemia
  - Most commonly given subcutaneously
- Sodium bicarbonate
  - May be administered intravenous or PO
  - Reverses metabolic acidosis. Dosage dependent on the client's weight, age, health condition and lab data
- Potassium
  - Administered PO or intravenous for potassium loss

Reinforcement of Priority Teaching

- Insulin therapy
  - Storage and expiration date
  - Preparation
  - Administration and site rotation
  - Meal requirement with administration
- Measure blood glucose regularly
- Adhere to exercise and meal plan
- Signs and symptoms of hypo and hyperglycemia
- Managing insulin when sick
- Wear diabetes identification

Diabetes insipidus

Pathophysiology/Description

- Diabetes insipidus (DI) occurs when there is hyposecretion of antidiuretic hormone (ADH). This is caused by a deficit in secretion or production of ADH or the kidney's inability to respond appropriately to ADH, in the presence of adequate production of the hormone. There are three types of DI
  - Central DI, occurring when there is a problem with the production of ADH. This is the most common type of DI
  - Nephrogenic DI, occurring when there is inadequate response of renal system to ADH
  - Primary DI, occurring from excessive intake of water
- Clinical manifestations
  - Polyuria and polydipsia, excretion of significantly large amounts of urine, up to 20 L/day
  - Fatigue and exertional dyspnea, headache, muscle cramping
  - Nausea, vomiting and loss of appetite
  - When the sodium level decreases drastically (below 120 mEq/L), manifestations are more severe and include muscle twitching, cerebral edema, seizures and coma

Priority Data Collection or Cues

- Check urine output, expect large amounts of dilute urine
- Check skin and mucous membranes for dehydration
- Ask about fatigue, muscle weakness and headache
- Check for postural hypotension related to fluid loss
- Check the cardiovascular and neurological systems as several manifestations relate to these systems
- Check vital signs, likely to see tachycardia, and hypotension
- Check for neurologic impairment

Priority Laboratory Tests/Diagnostics

- Urine specific gravity expected to be less than 1.005
- Water deprivation test (if identified as central DI): Urine osmolality, volume, body weight and urine specific gravity are measured pretest then water deprivation occurs for 8- 12 hours. Desmopressin is then administered via subcutaneous or nasal routes. With central DI a dramatic increase in urine osmolality, to 600 mOsm/kg, will be seen along with decrease in volume of urine. If neurogenic DI, urine osmolality will not be greater than 300 mOsm/kg
- Test with ADH analog (if identified as central DI): Desmopressin is given. If cause is central DI, urine will be concentrated by the kidneys

Priority Interventions or Actions

- Administer fluids as the client tolerates
- Monitor blood glucose as glycosuria and hyperglycemia can cause osmotic diuresis
- Monitor intake and output carefully
- Monitor urine specific gravity as treatment starts
- Monitor neurologic status to determine resolution of neurologic symptoms
- Ensure accurate documentation of daily weights
- Administer medications to relieve thirst
- Administer thiazide diuretics as presecribed for nephrogenic DI

Priority Potential & Actual Complications

- Severe dehydration
- Seizures
- Brain damage

Priority Nursing Implications

- Chlorpropamide can cause significant hypoglycemia so blood glucose must be checked when taking this drug

Priority Medications

- Carbamazepine and chlorpropamide
  - Administered orally
  - Used to help control thirst that results from central DI
- Desmopressin
  - Can be administered via various routes
  - Used with severe ADH deficiency
  - Water intoxication is a serious adverse effect
- Thiazide diuretics
  - Most commonly administered orally
  - Reduce volume of urine in central DI and nephrogenic DI. Reduced volume results from reduction in extracellular volume and proximal tubule reabsorption.
- Indomethacin
  - Administered orally, but may also be given intravenous
  - Prostaglandin inhibitor that helps to increase responsiveness of renal system to ADH

Reinforcement of Priority Teaching

- Proper administration of medications
- Limiting of sodium intake
- Avoidance of foods that produce diuresis
- Encourage wearing of a MedicAlert bracelet and carrying a MedicAlert card
- Discuss signs and symptoms of DI and reinforce the importance of following up with health care provider visit

Diabetes mellitus – type 2

Pathophysiology/Description

- Diabetes is a multisystem disease of glucose metabolism that is marked by hyperglycemia
- Two most common types of diabetes mellitus are types 1 and 2. Type 2 diabetes is the most prevalent
- Type 2 is marked by insulin resistance, inadequate insulin secretion or a combination of both
  - Insulin resistance: Body tissues do not respond to insulin's action due to unresponsive or insufficient numbers of insulin receptors
  - Inadequate insulin secretion: Cells of the pancreas become fatigued and so insulin production is decreased
- Risk factors
  - Family history. More likely to get the condition if there are first degree relatives with it
  - Obesity or overweight. Fat cells are resistant to insulin
  - Certain ethnicities. It is more prevalent in Asian Americans, African Americans, Hispanics, Pacific Islanders and Native Americans
  - Age. Older than 40 years of age
- Type 2 diabetes has a gradual onset. Many persons do not know they have the condition until it is detected on routine lab testing
- Diabetes is a life-altering condition

Priority Data Collection or Cues

- Ask about symptoms such as polydipsia, polyuria, polyphagia, fatigue, recurrent infections, visual changes and poor wound healing. Determine blood glucose level
- Ask about management of the condition such as meal planning and medication administration
- Measure vital signs
- Check skin, focusing on feet. Diabetes causes neuropathy and individuals can have wounds on their soles without knowing it. Untreated wounds can lead to amputations
- Ask about recent eye exams. Blindness is a major complication of diabetes
- Review labs, including kidney function tests. Nephropathy is a major complication of diabetes
- Determine social support
- Check client's understanding of disease management

Priority Laboratory Tests/Diagnostics

- Diagnosis made with one of the following
  - Fasting blood glucose 126 mg/dL or higher
  - A1C of 6.5% or higher
  - Using a glucose load of 75 g during an oral glucose tolerance test, a two-hour plasma level that is equal to or greater than 200 mg/dL
  - Random blood glucose greater than or equal to 200 mg/dL in a client who has the classic symptoms of hyperglycemia or is in a hyperglycemic crisis
  - The first 3 items above must be repeated to confirm the diagnosis. However, the fourth does not need to be repeated

Priority Interventions or Actions

- Administer medications and monitor blood glucose for effectiveness of dosage
- Monitor meal intake
- Schedule meeting with dietitian to discuss nutrition planning
- Schedule meeting with diabetic educator to ensure client's knowledge needs are met

Priority Potential & Actual Complications

- Nephropathy, leading to kidney failure, neuropathy, leading to sores and amputations and retinopathy, leading to blindness
- Hyperglycemic hyperosmolar syndrome, hypoglycemia
- Conditions related to the heart, brain and blood vessels
- Gastroparesis
- Fungal infections

Priority Nursing Implications

- The need for lifestyle changes, including medication
- Persons with type 2 diabetes who take oral medications can require insulin in times of stress, as in acute illness

Priority Medications

- Biguanides
  - Metformin, the most effective first line treatment for type 2 diabetes
  - Decrease production of glucose in liver and enhances transport of glucose into cells
  - Must not be used if kidney or liver disease, or heart failure. Major side effect is lactic acidosis, stopped for surgery or if having a procedure that uses a contrast medium to avoid the risk of lactic acidosis
- Sulfonylureas
  - Administered orally
  - Glipizide, glyburide, glimepiride
  - Increase production of insulin by the pancreas
  - Major side effect is hypoglycemia
- Thiazolidinediones
  - Administered orally
  - Pioglitazone, rosiglitazone
  - Increase uptake of glucose in muscle and decrease endogenous production of glucose
  - Major side effect is adverse cardiovascular events
- A-Glucosidase inhibitors
  - Administered orally

- Acarbose, miglitol
- Cause absorption of starches from the gastrointestinal tract to be delayed
- Must be taken with the first bite of food, most effective in lowering postprandial blood glucose

- Dipeptidyl peptidase-4
  - Administered via the oral route
  - linagliptin, saxagliptin, sitagliptin, alogliptin
  - Increase the activity of incretin. Stimulate insulin release from pancreatic B-cells and decrease the liver's production of glucose
- Sodium-Glucose Co-Transporter 2
  - Administered via the oral route
  - Canagliflozin, dapagliflozin
  - Decrease reabsorption of glucose in the kidneys and increase its excretion through urine
  - Causes urinary tract and genital infections
- Glucagon-like Peptide-1 Receptor Agonists
  - Administered via the subcutaneous route
  - Exenatide, exenatide extended-release, dulaglutide, albiglutide, lixisenatide, liraglutide
  - Decrease secretion of glucagon, stimulate release of insulin and slow gastric emptying, thus causing a feeling of fullness and satiety
  - Exenatide causes acute pancreatitis and kidney problems liraglutide should not be used in clients with family or personal history of medullary thyroid cancer
- Combination oral therapy
  - Combination of two different classes of medications into one pill
  - Advantageous, as only 1 pill is taken instead of two different pills, thus increasing medication compliance

Reinforcement of Priority Teaching

- Measure blood glucose regularly
- Adhere to exercise and meal plan
- Signs and symptoms of hypo and hyperglycemia
- Ensure proper administration as well as understanding of adverse effects of medications
- Meal consumption in relationship to insulin administration
- Wear diabetes identification
- Remind the client on the importance of having A1C measured regularly to determine effectiveness of treatment protocol
- Remind client of proper foot care
- Remind client of the importance of getting eye exams
- Get annual physical, ensuring kidney function is checked

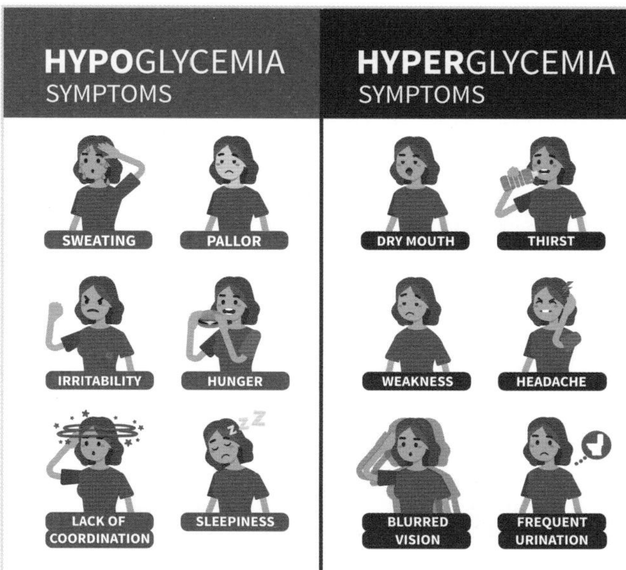

Image 12-1: What additional signs and symptoms would the nurse include when educating the client regarding hypo and hyperglycemia?

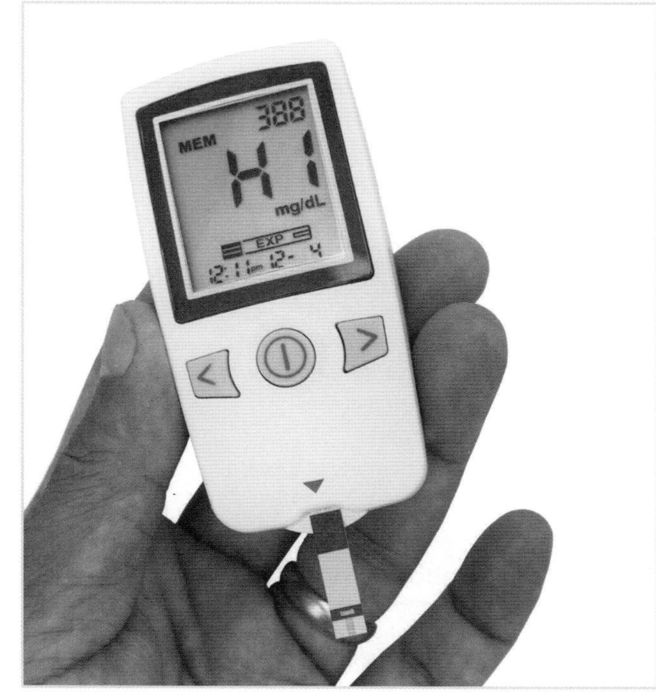

Image 12-2: Upon taking the blood glucose of a client, the nurse sees this image.

1. *What action should the nurse take next?*
2. *What could have led to this reading?*
3. *What client signs and symptoms should the nurse anticipate?*
4. *How could this be prevented in the future?*

Diabetes mellitus - type 1

Pathophysiology/Description

- Diabetes is a multisystem disease of glucose metabolism that is marked by hyperglycemia
- Type 1 is an autoimmune disorder where antibodies are developed against the pancreas B-cells or against insulin.
- Has a genetic link
- Has a sudden onset once the pancreas can no longer produce insulin. Some individuals are diagnosed initially when they are in diabetic ketoacidosis
- Classic symptoms, known as the 3 Ps
  - Polyuria (frequent voiding), because of the osmotic effect of glucose
  - Polydipsia (excessive thirst), because of the osmotic effect of glucose
  - Polyphagia (excessive hunger), because of lack of glucose usage for energy
- Exogenous insulin is required for life

Priority Data Collection or Cues

- Ask about symptoms such as polydipsia, polyuria, polyphagia, fatigue, weight loss. Determine blood glucose level
- Ask about management of the condition such as meal planning and medication administration
- Check knowledge of insulin preparation and administration
- Check for ability to manage diabetes at home
- Measure vital signs
- Check skin, focusing on feet
  - Diabetes leads to neuropathy, causing unknown wounds. Without treatment this can lead to amputations
- Check eyes; diabetes causes blindness
- Review labs, including kidney function tests. Nephropathy is a major complication of diabetes
- Determine social support
- Check client's understanding of disease management and physical ability to prepare and administer insulin injections

Priority Laboratory Tests/Diagnostics

- Diagnosis made with one of the following
  - Fasting blood glucose 126 mg/dL or higher
  - A1C of 6.5% or higher
  - Using a glucose load of 75 g during an oral glucose tolerance test, a two-hour plasma level that is equal to or greater than 200 mg/dL
  - Random blood glucose greater than or equal to 200 mg/dL in a client who has the classic symptoms of hyperglycemia or is in a hyperglycemic crisis
  - The first 3 items above must be repeated to confirm the diagnosis. However, the fourth does not need to be repeated

Priority Interventions or Actions

- Administer insulin and monitor blood glucose for effectiveness of dosage
- Monitor meal intake
- Schedule meeting with dietitian to talk with client about nutrition planning
- Schedule meeting with diabetic educator
- Have newly diagnosed client demonstrate blood glucose checks and insulin preparation and injection

Priority Potential & Actual Complications

- Nephropathy, leading to kidney failure. Neuropathy, leading to sores and amputations. Retinopathy, leading to blindness
- Hypoglycemia
- Somogyi Effect, caused by high dose of insulin that causes some counter regulatory hormones to be released, which then causes rebound hyperglycemia in the morning
- Dawn phenomenon occurs similar to the Somogyi effect but the treatment for both is different
- Diabetic ketoacidosis, hypoglycemia
- Atrophy or hypertrophy of tissue at injection site
- Conditions related to the heart, brain, and blood vessels
- Gastroparesis

Priority Nursing Implications

- Meal consumption must be timed with insulin administration
- Involve the family in the care as appropriate as diabetes is a life-altering disease
- Type 1 diabetes require exogenous insulin for life
- Premix insulin formulas are better for individuals who lack the ability to prepare insulin for themselves
- Insulin pumps may be used

Priority Medications

- Rapid-acting insulin
  - Lispro, aspart, glulisine
  - Onset 10-30 minutes, peak 30 minutes - 3 hours, duration 3-5 hours
  - Administered via subcutaneous route but can be given intravenous in a monitored setting
- Short-acting insulin
  - Regular
  - Onset 30 minutes- 1 hour, peak 2-5 hours, duration 5-8 hours
  - Administered via subcutaneous route
- Intermediate-acting insulin
  - NPH
  - Onset 1.5-4 hours, peak 4-12 hours, duration 12-18 hours
  - Administered via subcutaneous route

- Long-acting insulin
  - Glargine, detemir, degludec
  - Onset 0.8-4 hours, peak no identified/pronounced peak, duration 16-24 hours
  - Administered via subcutaneous route
- Inhaled insulin
  - Administered via an inhaler
  - Onset 12-15 minutes, peak 60 minutes, duration 2.5-3 hours
- Combination therapy
  - Several combinations of premixed insulins (2 insulins combined)
- More concentrated insulin
  - Humulin R U-500, toujeo U-300

Reinforcement of Priority Teaching

- Measure blood glucose regularly
- Insulin
  - Storage
  - Care of insulin container
  - Preparation and administration
  - Appropriate injection sites and injection site rotation
  - Side effects
- Demonstrate proper insulin administration and blood glucose checks
- Signs and symptoms of hypo and hyperglycemia
- Proper administration as well as adverse effects of medications
- Meal consumption in relationship to insulin administration
- Complications of insulin therapy
- Encourage the client to wear diabetes identification
- A1C measured regularly to determine effectiveness of treatment protocol
- Encourage proper foot care
- Importance of getting eye exams
- Encourage annual physicals, ensuring kidney function is assessed
- Options for insulin administration, like insulin pen and insulin pump

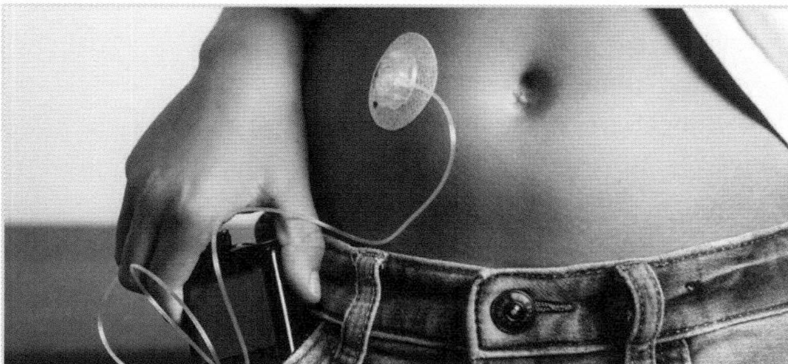

Image 12-3: What is the nursing care of a client with an insulin pump?

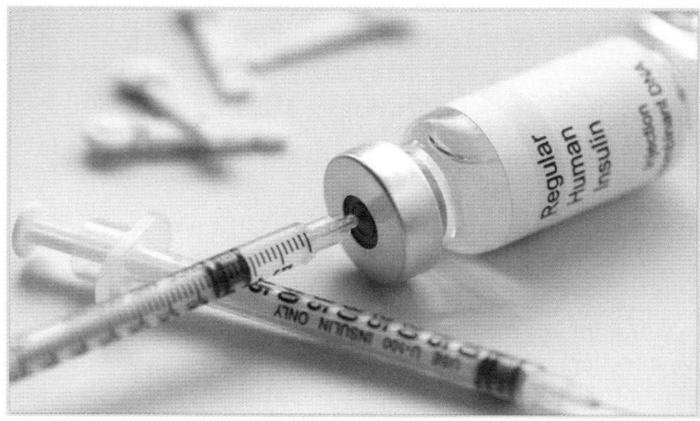

Image 12-4: What are the proper steps to withdrawing and administering 10 units of insulin as shown here?

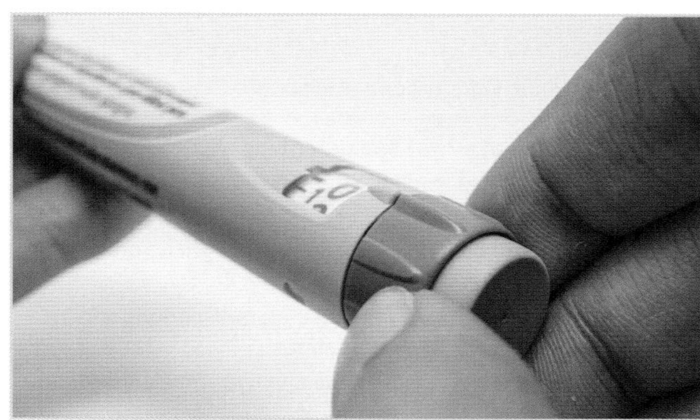

Image 12-5: An adolescent is self-administering insulin using an insulin pen. What steps should be followed when using an insulin pen?

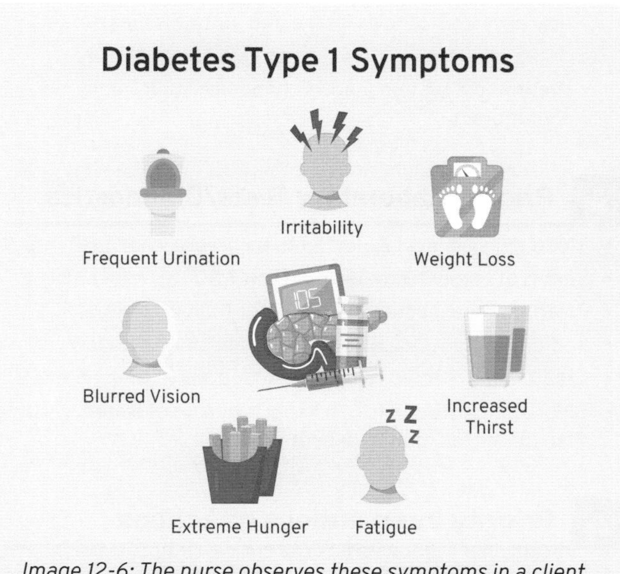

Image 12-6: The nurse observes these symptoms in a client previously diagnosed with type 1 diabetes. What action should the nurse take first?

Hyperglycemic hyperosmolar syndrome

Pathophysiology/Description

- The syndrome of hyperglycemic hyperosmolar syndrome (HHS) results when clients with diabetes whose pancreas still make some insulin, have severely high blood glucose levels
- Enough insulin is produced to prevent the breakdown of fats for energy that would result in DKA, but insulin is not produced in enough quantity to prevent hyperglycemia
- Contributing factors to HHS include: Sepsis, urinary tract infection, type 2 diabetes that is newly diagnosed or poorly controlled, pneumonia, acute illness, impaired sensation of thirst, not being able to replace fluids
- Results of severely high glucose levels in HHS include: Increase in serum osmolality, lethargy, sleepiness, seizures, aphasia, hemiparesis, coma

Priority Data Collection or Cues

- Check for patent airway and determine oxygen level
- Determine glucose level and dehydration. Profound dehydration is classic of HHS
- Check neurological status. Neurological deficits are prominent in HHS
- Review health history to include diet, medications and overall self-management of diabetes
- Measure vital signs (tachycardia and hypotension seen due to dehydration and fluid depletion)
- Determine efficacy of therapy by performing ongoing monitoring of the following
  - Lab values (show electrolytes and dehydration status)
  - Cardiac and respiratory systems
  - Renal system (shows intake and output issues)
  - Integumentary system (shows skin turgor status)
  - Neurologic system (shows changes in neurologic symptoms)

Priority Laboratory Tests/Diagnostics

- Blood glucose level expected to be greater than 600 mg/dL
- Serum pH expected to be less than 7.30
- Bicarbonate expected to be greater than 20 mEq/L
- Sodium and potassium expected to be normal to low
- Creatinine expected to be elevated (greater than 1.5 mg/dL)
- Blood urea nitrogen (BUN) expected to be elevated, greater than 20 mg/dL, due to dehydration

Priority Interventions or Actions

- Ensure airway is patent and a large bore intravenous access
- Intravenous fluid 0.9% or 0.45% NaCL
  - Large volumes of fluid are required but must be administered slowly due to increased risk of cardiac events from fluid overload
  - 5% to 10% dextrose may be added when the glucose is less than 250 mg/dL to prevent a quick drop in blood glucose levels
- Intravenous insulin may be used if not corrected with fluids
- Monitor electrolyte levels and correct as needed
- Monitor intake and output carefully. Have client drink fluids when safe to do so
- The underlying cause must be treated

Priority Medications

- Regular insulin
  - Monitor for decrease in blood glucose level
- Electrolyte replacement only if indicated

Priority Potential & Actual Complications

- Shock
- Seizures
- Stroke
- Coma
- May be fatal

Priority Nursing Implications

- The outstanding difference between DKA and HHS is that with HHS, the individual has some insulin production to prevent the breakdown of fats, so ketoacidosis does not become a factor
- Blood glucose can progress to very high levels before the issue is recognized. This is because fewer symptoms are seen in the early stages of the condition
- Symptoms of HHS may mimic other medical conditions, so proper diagnosis is imperative
- With HHS, the role of insulin is less important because ketoacidosis does not occur. Rehydration may be all that is needed to correct the problem
- Understand that HHS is a medical emergency that must be treated immediately. It has a high mortality rate

Reinforcement of Priority Teaching

- Insulin therapy
  - Storage/care of insulin
  - Preparation and administration
  - Appropriate injection sites and injection site rotation
  - Side effects
- Measure blood glucose regularly
- Adhere to exercise and meal plan
- Discuss signs/symptoms of hypo/hyperglycemia
- Discuss social/community support to assist in preventing recurrence of HHS
- Wear diabetes identification
- Encourage to seek medical care when needed
- Discuss adequate daily fluid intake

Hypoparathyroidism

Pathophysiology/Description

- Hypoparathyroidism occurs when circulating parathyroid hormone (PTH) is inadequate
- Parathyroid hormone (PTH) is needed to regulate phosphate and calcium levels
- Lack of PTH causes hypocalcemia because serum calcium levels cannot be maintained
- Common causes of hypoparathyroidism
  - Thyroidectomy, where the parathyroid gland is damaged accidentally
  - Autoimmune where the immune system develops antibodies against the parathyroid gland
- Treatment is focused on addressing the acute condition, such as managing tetany and normalizing calcium levels

Priority Data Collection or Cues

- Check airway, breathing and circulation. Acute condition with sudden decrease in calcium level can cause painful spasms to smooth and skeletal muscles, including laryngospasms and respiratory compromise
- Obtain a health history
- Monitor neurological status as anxiety and lethargy can occur with hypoparathyroidism
- Check for tetany, which occurs when there is sudden decrease in calcium levels
  - Mild tetany includes tingling around the mouth and hands
  - Severe tetany includes muscular spasms
- Check for Chvostek' sign
- Check for Trousseau's sign

Priority Laboratory Tests/Diagnostics

- Serum calcium expected to be low
- Serum phosphorus, expected to be high
- Parathyroid level expected to be low
- Serum magnesium expected to be low

Priority Interventions or Actions

- Administer calcium and monitor serum calcium levels
- Ensure electrocardiogram monitoring during acute intravenous calcium administration as cardiac dysrhythmias or arrest are adverse effects of high calcium levels
- Place oxygen, tracheostomy set and suction supplies at the bedside in the event of a cardiac event
- Ensure a patent intravenous line before starting calcium therapy
- Ensure intake of high calcium low phosphorus diet
- Ensure ordered labs are drawn and review results to determine efficacy of treatment
- Administer medications and monitor side effects

Priority Potential & Actual Complications

- Long-term low calcium levels, necessitating the intake of calcium and vitamin D supplements
- Paresthesia
- Tetany
- Heart arrhythmias
- Heart failure
- Slowed mental development
- Stunted growth
- Calcium deposits in brain

Priority Nursing Implications

- Calcium chloride is irritating to veins and can cause inflammation. Extravasation can result in tissue necrosis, so the intravenous line must be monitored to ensure patency

Priority Medications

- Calcium (for acute use)
  - Administered slowly via intravenous route
  - Electrocardiogram monitoring must occur
  - Administered in the acute phase only. Client will be discharged with oral calcium as calcium carbonate supplements
- Vitamin D
  - Administered orally
  - Calcitriol
  - Regulates serum calcium levels
- Parathyroid hormone
  - Given once daily via subcutaneous injection
  - Natpara
  - Restricted use due to potential risk of getting bone cancer

Reinforcement of Priority Teaching

- Side effects of medication and symptoms of hypo/hypercalcemia
- Administration of calcium and vitamin D supplements as prescribed
- Encourage foods that are low in phosphorus and rich in calcium. May need to consult dietary
- Keep all physician and lab appointments

Hyperparathyroidism

Pathophysiology/Description

- Hyperparathyroidism occurs when secretion of the parathyroid hormone is increased
- Parathyroid hormone (PTH) is needed to regulate phosphate and calcium levels
- Three classifications of hyperparathyroidism, primary, secondary and tertiary
  - Primary hyperparathyroidism is increased secretion of PTH resulting in conditions related to phosphate, calcium and bone metabolism. A benign tumor in the parathyroid gland is the most common cause
  - Secondary hyperparathyroidism occurs when there is a response that compensates for conditions that cause or induce hypocalcemia, since hypocalcemia is the primary stimulus for the secretion of PTH. A few of these conditions are chronic kidney disease, vitamin D deficiency, hypophosphatemia, malabsorption
  - Tertiary hyperparathyroidism is due to the parathyroid glands experiencing hyperplasia. Tertiary hyperparathyroidism is usually seen in kidney transplant clients who have had long duration of dialysis
- Most effective treatment for primary and secondary disease is surgery to partially or completely remove the parathyroid gland. Surgery has a high cure rate

Priority Data Collection or Cues

- Obtain a complete health history
- Check for hypophosphatemia and hypercalcemia
- Ask about fatigue, skeletal pain, and muscle weakness
- Check for cardiac and renal issues. Measure vital signs, particularly blood pressure, as high serum calcium levels can cause hypotension
- Determine the client's knowledge of surgery and follow-up care. Check for hemorrhage after surgery
- Examine post-surgery electrolytes levels and check for electrolyte disturbances
- Check for tetany, a sign of decreased calcium levels
  - Mild tetany includes tingling around the mouth and hands and resolves over time
  - Severe tetany includes muscular spasms and is treated with medications
- Check for Chvostek's sign, seen when the facial nerve is trapped in front of the ear. The muscle will contract
- Check for Trousseau's sign, seen as spasm of the muscles in the hand and forearm when a blood pressure cuff is inflated on the arm for 3 minutes and the brachial artery is occluded. The fingers adduct, wrist flex and joints extend. These result from hypocalcemia and neuromuscular irritability

Priority Laboratory Tests/Diagnostics

- Serum calcium expected to exceed 10 mg/dL
- Serum phosphorus, expected to be less than 3 mg/dL
- A 24-hour urine test
- Bone mineral density test, using dual energy X-ray absorptiometry (DXA) scan
- Magnetic resonance imaging (MRI) and computed tomography (CT) scan to look for an adenoma
- X-rays or other imaging tests of the abdomen to detect kidney abnormalities
- Serum potassium and magnesium levels

Priority Interventions or Actions

- Prepare client for parathyroidectomy and autotransplantation (if indicated)
- Monitor intake and output
- Monitor for dysrhythmias
- Ensure ordered labs are drawn and review results
- Encourage mobility as it fosters calcification of bone
- Ongoing care if no surgical intervention
  - Regular physical exams
  - Labs: calcium, PTH, phosphorua, phosphatase, blood urea nitrogen (BUN), and creatinine
  - Ongoing measurement of urinary excretion of calcium
  - Annual dual energy X-ray absorptiometry (DXA) scan
- Encourage moderate dietary intake of calcium and high fluid
- Administer medications and monitor side effects
- Monitor intravenous fluids for hydration

Priority Potential & Actual Complications

- Sustained low calcium levels, necessitating the intake of calcium and vitamin D supplements
- Impairment in speech due to damage to nerves controlling the vocal cords

Priority Nursing Implications

- Understand that surgery is indicated with the following criteria
  - Hypercalciuria above 400 mg/day, Calcium levels greater than 1 mg/dL above the upper limit of normal, Bone mineral density that is significantly reduced, Obvious symptoms such as kidney stones
- Client may opt to autotransplant normal parathyroid tissue in the arm close to the sternocleidomastoid muscle so that secretion of PTH can continue. If no autotransplant, or if the transplant fails, calcium will be needed for life
- Monitor potassium with furosemide, as it is potassium-wasting

Priority Medications

- Calcium gluconate
  - Administered intravenous
  - Must be readily available after parathyroidectomy surgery
- Loop diuretic
  - Most commonly given orally, but may be administered intravenous
  - Furosemide (common drug used)
  - Increase calcium excretion in urine
  - Inhibit calcium reabsorption in the renal tubule
- Bisphosphonates
  - Administered orally. Must remain upright for 30 minutes after administration
  - Administer with plain water only
  - Alendronate, most common drug in class
  - Inhibit resorption of osteoblastic bone, brings normalcy to serum calcium levels, improve mineral density of bone
- Calcimimetic agents
  - Administered orally
  - Cinacalcet
  - Cause sensitivity of calcium receptors on parathyroid gland to be magnified. It tricks the parathyroid gland into the release of less parathyroid hormone fostering lowered calcium levels and PTH
- Calcitonin
  - Most commonly administered IM or subcutaneously
  - Inhibits osteoclast activity of bones
  - Should not be taken if allergic to salmon (it is a salmon-based drug)

Reinforcement of Priority Teaching

- Remind client about side effects of medications
- Discuss symptoms of hypo and hypercalcemia
- Discuss expectations of parathyroid surgery
- Refrain from sedentary lifestyle, walk frequently
- Assist with adaption to meal plan (may need Dietitian)
- Encourage an exercise program as immobility can worsen bone loss
- Keep all physician appointments
- If taking alendronate—must be taken alone on an empty stomach, with a full glass of water, and remain in a upright position for 30 minutes (as it has a risk of causing ulcers in the esophagus)

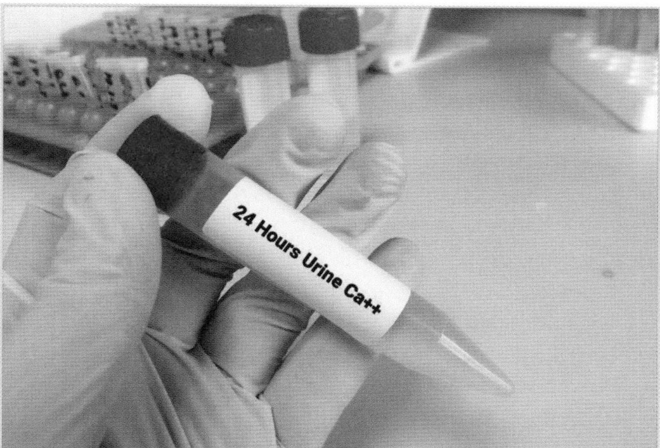

Image 12-7: The client has been instructed to collect a 24 hour urine specimen. What instructions should the nurse include?

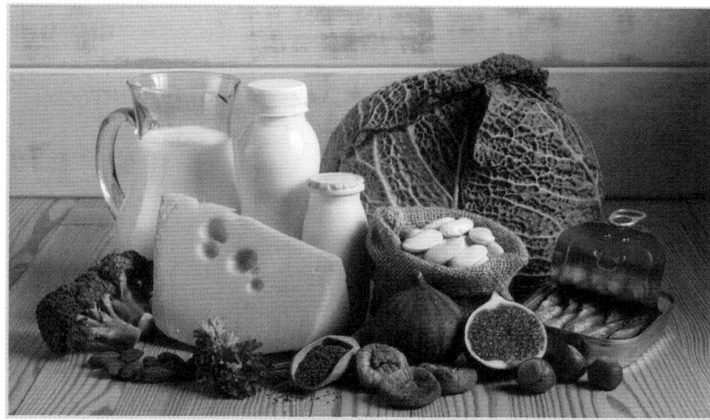

Image 12-8: Which foods would be recommended for a client who has been diagnosed with hyperparathyroidism?

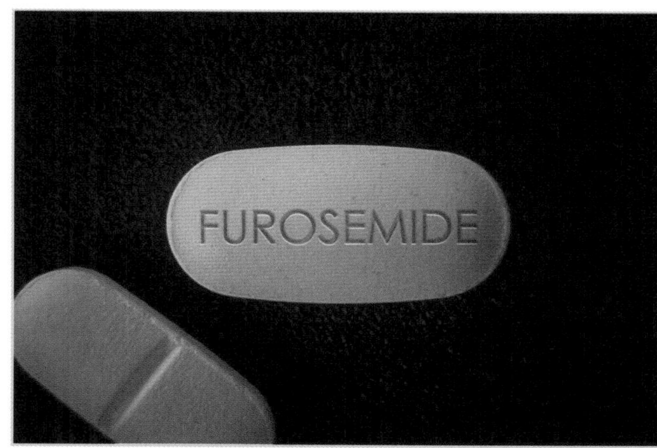

Image 12-9: A client has been prescribed furosemide. What should the nurse reinforce in the teaching plan for this client?

Hyperthyroidism

Pathophysiology/Description

- Hyperthyroidism occurs when the thyroid gland is hyperactive, causing continuous increase in the production and release of thyroid hormones (T3 and T4)
- Commonly seen in the 20 to 40 age range and occurs more often in women than men
- Common causes of hyperthyroidism
  - Graves' disease, thyroiditis, excess iodine intake, thyroid cancer, toxic nodular goiter, and pituitary tumor
- The clinical manifestations of hyperthyroidism are termed thyrotoxicosis
- Hyperthyroidism causes functions of the body to speed up
- The goal of hyperthyroidism management is to prevent complications, suppress over production of thyroid hormone and prevent adverse effects

Priority Data Collection or Cues

- Check for symptoms of acute thyrotoxicosis
- Check vital signs (heart rate likely to be greater than 100 beats per minute, hypertension)
- Check the cardiac system (arrhythmias, palpations, angina and systolic murmurs are common)
- Ask about appetite and meal consumption (causes increased appetite)
- Ask about sudden weight loss pattern (weight loss is likely)
- Ask about heat tolerance (increased heat sensitivity is likely)
- Determine sleep pattern (difficulty sleeping is an expectation)
- Check the integumentary system (likely to find thinning skin and hair that is fine and brittle)
- Examine the neck (a swelling at the base of the neck, called a goiter, is common)
- Check for bulging eyes, called exophthalmos (common with the disease)
- Ask about bowel elimination (likely to have increased number of bowel movements)
- Check the neurologic system (irritability, fine tremors of the hands and fingers, anxiety, depression and nervousness are common)
- Ask about menstrual changes, decreased libido and impotence (common occurrences)
- Ask about activity intolerance due to fatigue
- After thyroidectomy
  - Check respiratory status as breathing may be affected by neck swelling
  - Check client for tracheal compression and damage, frequent swallowing, choking, hemorrhage, sensation of fullness at insertion site
  - Check for tetany which can occur if the pituitary gland is damaged in surgery

Priority Laboratory Tests/Diagnostics

- Thyroid stimulating hormone (TSH) will be low or not detectable, free thyroxine (free T4) will be elevated
- Radioactive iodine uptake (RAIU) test
- Electrocardiogram, showing tachycardia and atrial fibrillation

Priority Interventions or Actions

- Provide oxygenation in thyrotoxicosis crisis
- Assist with process of radioactive iodine uptake test and iodine therapy
- Encourage adequate rest in a quiet, calm and cool environment
- Place light covering on client and change frequently if diaphoretic
- Administer antithyroid medications as prescribed
- Administer medications as prescribed, to treat the symptoms
- Apply artificial tears to moisten conjunctiva and prevent corneal injury and eye discomfort, if exophthalmos is present
- Monitor daily weights
- Monitor nutritional status due to increased rate of metabolism
- Help client with coping strategies for altered body image
- Interventions after thyroidectomy
  - Maintain patent airway
  - Position client in the semi-Fowler's position
  - Use pillows to support client's head
  - Administer pain medications

Priority Potential & Actual Complications

- Cardiac problems, thyrotoxicosis, thyroid storm, eye problems, brittle bones, accidental removal of thyroid gland, hemorrhage and injury to laryngeal nerve resulting in vocal cord paralysis

Priority Nursing Implications

- Individuals at risk for hyperthyroidism must be closely monitored if they have a procedure that involves the use of iodinated contrast medium, since iodine is a causative factor for the condition
- Understand that thyrotoxicosis is a medical emergency that must be treated quickly
- Client may be distressed looking at the scar after surgery, Encourage the wearing of a scarf and let client know that the scar will fade over time
- Check for thyroid storm when using methimazole and propylthiouracil
- Black box warning with beta blockers, used to treat the cardiac symptoms, indicate that they must be tapered over 1-2 weeks and not withdrawn abruptly

Priority Medications

- Antithyroid medication
  - Methimazole or propylthiouracil (PTU)
  - Propylthiouracil 100-150 mg/day administered orally
  - Both medications impede formation of thyroid hormone
- Beta Blockers
  - Propranolol, atenolol and metoprolol. Dose ranges vary for each
  - Used to treat the cardiac symptoms associated with hyperthyroidism
  - A common adverse effect is bradycardia

Reinforcement of Priority Teaching

- Discuss the signs and symptoms of hyperthyroidism
- Provide nutritional information, which may involve a dietitian
- Encourage the avoidance of caffeinated beverages
- Importance of following up with physician's visits
- Taking lifelong thyroid hormone if surgery was complete thyroidectomy
- Monitor heart rate when taking beta blockers

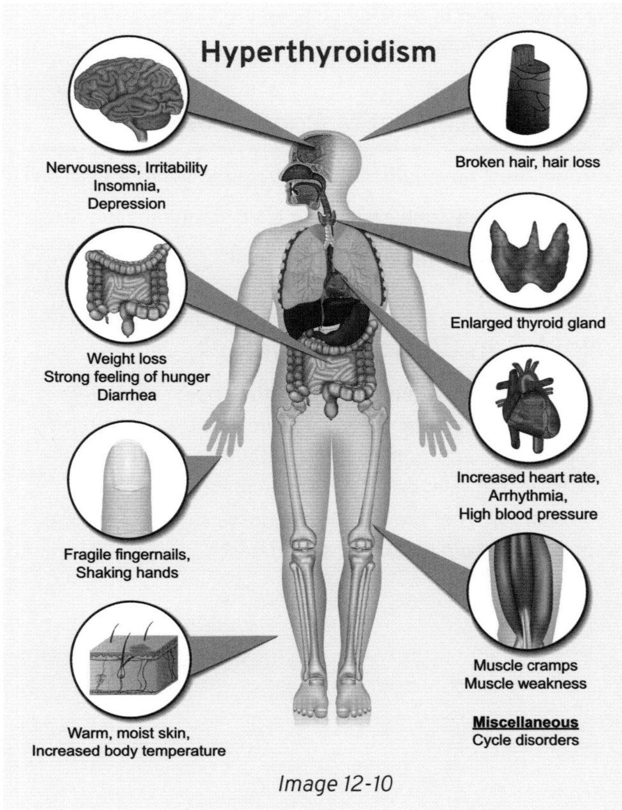

Image 12-10

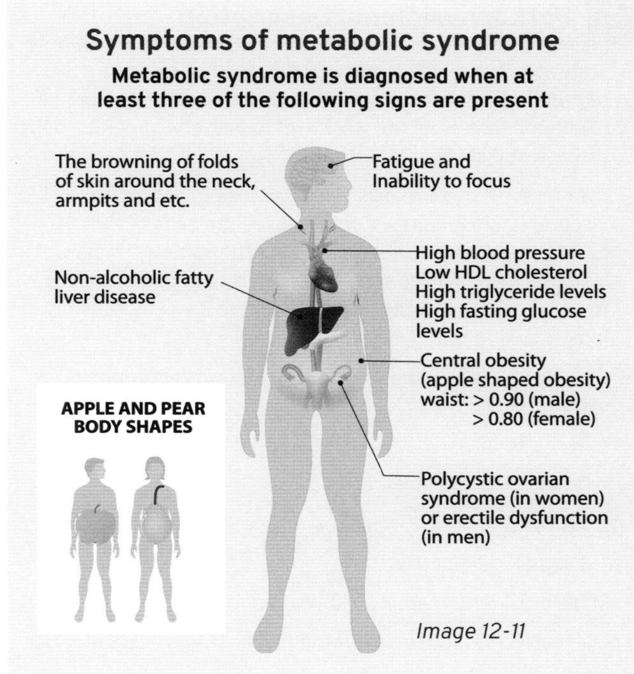

Image 12-11

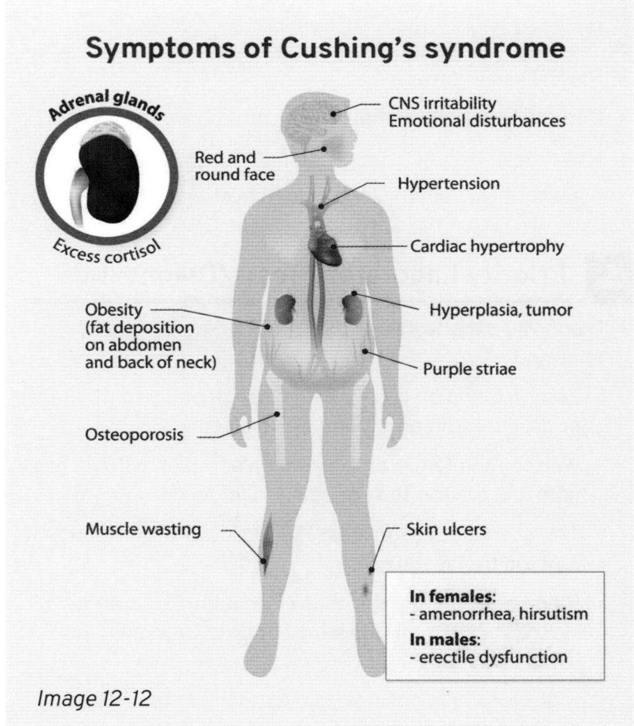

Image 12-12

Review the signs and symptoms of the disorders in the three images on this page. List three top nursing interventions for a client with each of these disorders. Is there a disorder that represents the opposite of the disorder? If so, list the three top nursing interventions for a client with these disorders that represent the opposite of the disorder.

Pathophysiology/Description

- Metabolic syndrome is not one disease but a group of metabolic risk factors that cause an increase in the likelihood that a person will develop diabetes mellitus, heart disease and stroke
- Risk factor is insulin resistance because of too much visceral fat. Insulin resistance causes the cells of the body to have decreased ability to respond to the action of insulin. The pancreas secretes more insulin in an attempt to compensate and this compounds the issue by causing hyperinsulinemia
- Cluster of health conditions associated with metabolic syndrome
  - Hypertension
  - Abnormal lipid levels
  - Obesity
  - High blood glucose
- More prevalent in adults, 60 years and older
- Untreated metabolic syndrome places the individual at risk for a multitude of conditions

Priority Data Collection or Cues

- Review health history
- Determine presence of diagnostic measures
- Measure vital signs
- Ask about barriers to lifestyle modification

Priority Laboratory Tests/Diagnostics

- Diagnosis is made if individual has 3 or more of the following
  - Fasting blood glucose greater than or equal to 110 mg/dL or drug treatment for high blood glucose
  - Waist circumference greater than or equal to 40 inches in men and greater than or equal to 35 inches in women
  - Triglycerides greater than 150 mg/dL or drug treatment for high triglycerides
  - Blood pressure greater than or equal to 130 mmHg systolic or 85 mmHg diastolic or drug treatment for hypertension
  - High-density lipoprotein cholesterol less than 40 mg/dL in men and less than 50 mg/dL in women or drug treatment for high cholesterol

Priority Nursing Implications

- Individuals who have metabolic syndrome and smoke are at a much higher risk of getting serious complications

Priority Interventions or Actions

- Schedule dietary consult
- Treat symptoms
- Treat conditions that predispose to metabolic syndrome, like high blood pressure and high cholesterol
- Provide resources for community support to reduce risk factors

Priority Potential & Actual Complications

- If metabolic syndrome is not addressed
  - Cardiovascular events
  - Diabetes
  - Stroke
  - Polycystic ovary syndrome
  - Renal disease

Priority Medications

- Drugs are not usually used to treat metabolic syndrome but if the individual is unable to lower risks with using lifestyle modification, or if there is a high-risk for diabetes mellitus or cardiac events, then blood pressure, cholesterol and diabetes medications may be given

Reinforcement of Priority Teaching

- Proper lifestyle modification. This is first line intervention
- Physical activity and assist with plans to engage in exercise
- Strategies to maintain a healthy weight

Next Gen Clinical Judgment

What are three unique aspects of the appearance of a client with metabolic syndrome? How do these aspects lead to signs and symptoms? What nursing actions are indicated to alleviate or reduce these signs and symptoms? What prevention measures should the nurse suggest to avoid metabolic syndrome?

Syndrome of inappropriate antidiuretic hormone (SIADH)

Pathophysiology/Description

- Occurs when ADH (Antidiuretic hormone) is released without a need for it
- Pathophysiology
  - Renal tubules and collecting ducts suffer increased permeability which causes fluid to be reabsorbed into the body's circulation. There is expansion of extracellular fluid volume. The overall result is increased glomerular filtration rate, expansion of extracellular fluid volume, decrease of plasma osmolality and decrease in sodium levels
- The pathophysiology results in: Fluid retention, Dilutional hyponatremia, Concentrated Urine, Low serum osmolality, and Hypochloremia
- Clinical manifestations
  - Increased body weight, decreased urine output and signs of fluid overload
  - Fatigue and exertional dyspnea, headache, muscle cramping
  - Nausea, vomiting and loss of appetite
  - When the sodium level decreases drastically (below 120 mEq/L), manifestations are more severe and include muscle twitching, cerebral edema, seizures and coma

Priority Data Collection or Cues

- Check for low urine output coupled with a high urine specific gravity
- Check electrolyte levels, be alert for low sodium level
- Check for weight gain in the absence of edema
- Check for signs of low sodium
- Check for neurologic impairment

Priority Laboratory Tests/Diagnostics

- Serum sodium, less than 134 mEq/L, serum osmolality less than 280 mOsm/kg and urine specific gravity that is greater than 1.025, indicate dilutional hyponatremia

Priority Interventions or Actions

- Monitor intake and output carefully
- Obtain weights daily to monitor gain or loss
- Treat underlying cause
- Monitor for signs of increased intracranial pressure
- Elevate head of bed no higher than 10 degrees
- Implement seizure precautions
- Conduct ongoing monitoring of electrolyte levels, serum and urine osmolality
- Monitor fluid restriction

Priority Potential & Actual Complications

- Seizures
- Cerebral edema
- Pulmonary edema

Priority Nursing Implications

- Understand that with severe hyponatremia, fluid must be managed carefully. Usually no more than 500 mL/day is given
- Monitor potassium, as a supplement may be needed if on a potassium wasting diuretic

Priority Medications

- Loop diuretic
  - Typically given orally, but may be administered intravenous
  - Furosemide (most commonly used) to promote diuresis
  - Carefully monitor blood pressure, electrolyte levels (especially sodium and potassium), and urine output
- Vasopressin antagonist
  - Conivaptan (administered intravenous) and tolvaptan (administered orally) (both used in acute setting)
  - Administer vasopressin antagonists with caution in liver disease, may worsen liver function

Reinforcement of Priority Teaching

- Remind client and family members about the signs and symptoms of SIADH
- Avoiding common medications that stimulate the release of antidiuretic hormone such as thiazide diuretics, some chemotherapy drugs and opioids, to name just a few
- Remind about importance of fluid restriction in chronic SIADH. Drink no more than 800-1000 mL/day
- Alternative to fluids to minimize thirst, such as sugarless gum and ice chips
- Assist with referral to dietitian
- Weigh daily
- Foods that contain potassium if taking furosemide
- Signs and symptoms of electrolyte imbalance and reinforce the importance of following up with health care provider visit

Next Gen Clinical Judgment

Compare and contrast the lab values of a client with SIADH and DI.

Wilms tumor

Pathophysiology/Description

- Wilms tumor is a rare solid malignant tumor that affects children. It occurs in the abdomen and kidney and is initiated from immature cells in the kidney
- It usually occurs unilaterally but can be bilateral
- The tumor may spread to the blood vessels that immediately surround the kidney in the form of a clot. Another common site of metastasis is the lungs
- Wilms tumor has a genetic predisposition, but certain congenital conditions are also associated with the disease. The incidence of Wilms tumor peaks at age 3
- Treatment is surgery, chemotherapy and/or radiation
- Clinical manifestations include: abdominal swelling, fever hypertension, hematuria, anemia, lethargy, anorexia, and dyspnea
- Treatment is based on the stage of the disease and the condition

Priority Data Collection or Cues

- Check abdomen for a firm mass, usually to one side but can be on both sides; avoid palpation of abdomen
- Measure vital signs, blood pressure and temperature are expected to be elevated due to fever and renin excess
- Check urine for presence of blood. Measure urine output
- Ask caregiver about meal intake and appetite
- Monitor neurologic system as lethargy is an issue
- Check respiratory system to determine lung involvement, evidenced by dyspnea and chest pain
- Check response to treatment
- Determine caregiver's knowledge about treatment plan
- Check surgical site for signs and symptoms of hemorrhage and infection

Priority Laboratory Tests/Diagnostics

- Ultrasound, computed tomography (CT) scan, magnetic resonance imaging (MRI) used to identify the tumor and determine its exact location
- Chest X-ray looks for metastasis to the lungs (a common organ of metastasis for this tumor)
- Lab tests (blood count and metabolic profile) to examine blood levels such as anemia, white blood cells and certain electrolytes that might be abnormal with cancerous processes in the body
- Kidney biopsy, looking at a piece of tumor tissue under a microscope, should show cancer cells

Priority Interventions or Actions

- Prepare client for treatment, as prescribed
- Ensure intravenous line
- Place sign at head of client's bed indicating that abdomen is not to be palpated
- Measure client's abdominal girth daily
- Monitor for hemorrhage and infection at surgery site
- Monitor gastrointestinal system
- Monitor intake and output
- Treat side effects of chemotherapy
- Allow caregiver time to verbalize feelings about child's disease

Priority Potential & Actual Complications

- Hemorrhage, intestinal injury bowel obstruction
- If both kidneys are affected, there will be complication of kidney function
- Spread of tumor to lungs, bone, liver or brain
- High blood pressure may occur due to the tumor or treatment

Priority Nursing Implications

- Never palpate the abdomen as it might cause the encapsulated tumor cells to spread in the abdomen and move into bloodstream and lymph system. The child must be moved and positioned with care
- Allow caregiver the opportunity to be involved in care of child

Priority Medications

- Dactinomycin, doxorubicin, vincristine, etoposide, cyclophosphamide, irinotecan
  - Chemotherapy drugs are most often given by a RN with specialized training
  - Increased risk of infection, anemia and bleeding due to decreased platelets red and white blood cells

Reinforcement of Priority Teaching

- Remind client and family members about the signs and symptoms of postoperative infection. Report fever to provider immediately
- Reinforce the importance of following up with health care provider visits
- Reinforce how to care for surgery site at home and how to check for hemorrhage
- Reinforce education about side effects of chemotherapy and ensure caregiver understand how to manage side effects
- Reinforce education regarding when to call health care provider

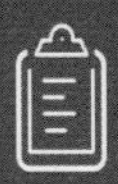

NurseThink® Quiz Questions

1. **The nurse cares for a client recently diagnosed with type 1 diabetes. The nurse expects the client to report which clinical manifestations of this form of diabetes? *Select all that apply.***
   a. Polydipsia.
   b. Oliguria.
   c. Polyphagia.
   d. Anuria.
   e. Weight loss.

2. **The nurse takes over the care of a pediatric client with Type I DM and reviews the medication administration record. Based on the administration time for Humulin R, when does the nurse expect the medication to be at its peak effectiveness?**

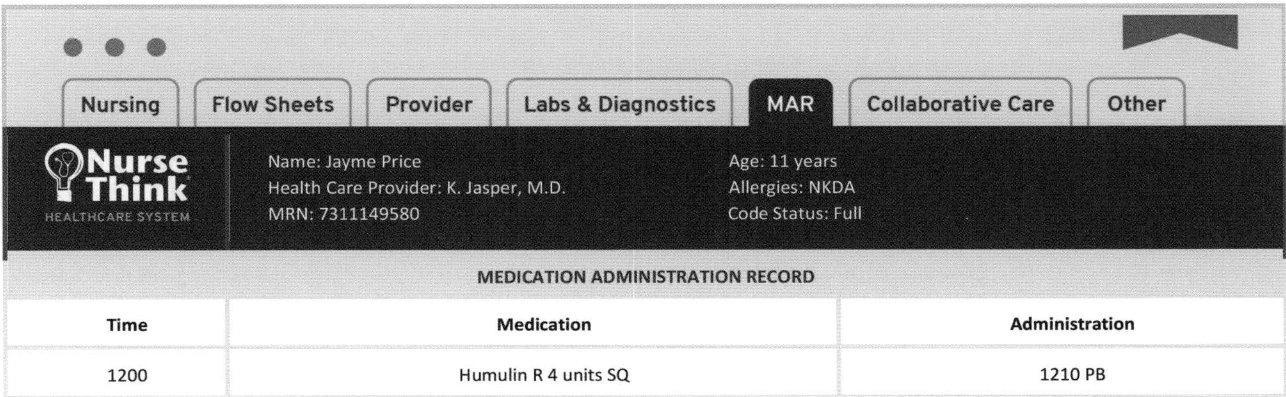

MEDICATION ADMINISTRATION RECORD

Time	Medication	Administration
1200	Humulin R 4 units SQ	1210 PB

   a. Between 1240 and 1330.
   b. Between 1400 and 1600.
   c. Between 1600 and 2000.
   d. Between 1215 and 1230.

3. **The nurse prepares a client to self-administer insulin at home. The provider has prescribed subcutaneous Humulin R before meals and at bedtime. What does the nurse emphasize to the client?**
   a. Avoid wearing a medical ID as it may impact emergency medical response.
   b. When eating high carbohydrate meals, double the prescribed dosage.
   c. Administer with an intradermal syringe when an insulin syringe is not available.
   d. Carry oral glucose with you at all times in case of hypoglycemia.

4. **The nurse supports a group of women with gestational diabetes. To manage the challenges of diabetes while pregnant, what behaviors does the nurse encourage the women to implement? *Select all that apply.***
   a. Eat small meals at regular intervals.
   b. Monitor blood glucose 4-5 times/day.
   c. Count carbohydrates and document intake.
   d. Minimize physical activity and exercise.
   e. Eat three large meals per day.

5. **The nurse cares for a client experiencing a hyperglycemic hyperosmolar state. The client has received 2 liters of 0.9% sodium chloride via rapid infusion. The client is responding well, and their current blood glucose is 362 mg/dL. Based on the client's current glucose level, what intravenous fluid does the nurse prepare to infuse?**
   a. The nurse continues rapid infusion of 0.9% sodium chloride.
   b. The nurse prepares to administer 0.45% sodium chloride.
   c. The nurse prepares to administer D5 0.45% sodium chloride.
   d. The nurse stops infusing all intravenous fluids at this time.

6. **The nurse cares for a client with hyperparathyroidism. The nurse instructs the client to avoid which foods in their diet? *Select all that apply.***
   a. Orange juice.
   b. Collard greens.
   c. Whole milk.
   d. Kiwi fruit.
   e. Lima beans.

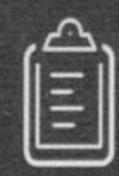

NurseThink® Quiz Questions

7. **The nurse cares for a client with hypoparathyroidism who is receiving intravenous calcium gluconate. Which findings alert the nurse that the client is now hypercalcemic?**
   a. Muscle cramps or spasms.
   b. Prolonged PR interval.
   c. Paresthesia of the hands.
   d. Hypotension.

8. **The nurse suspects the client is experiencing a thyroid storm. What priority items does the nurse ensure are in place at the bedside?**

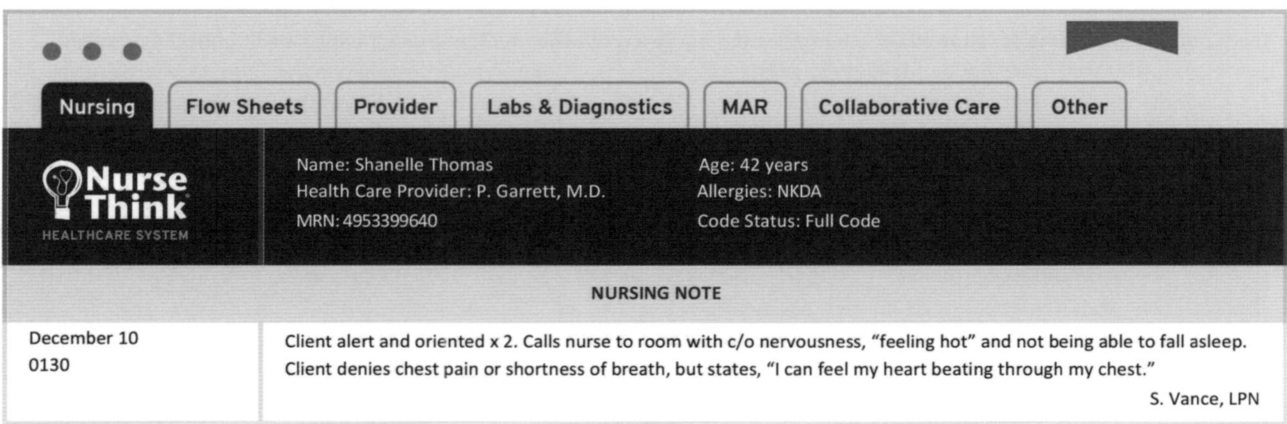

Nursing | Flow Sheets | Provider | Labs & Diagnostics | MAR | Collaborative Care | Other

Nurse Think
HEALTHCARE SYSTEM

Name: Shanelle Thomas
Health Care Provider: P. Garrett, M.D.
MRN: 4953399640

Age: 42 years
Allergies: NKDA
Code Status: Full Code

NURSING NOTE	
December 10 0130	Client alert and oriented x 2. Calls nurse to room with c/o nervousness, "feeling hot" and not being able to fall asleep. Client denies chest pain or shortness of breath, but states, "I can feel my heart beating through my chest." S. Vance, LPN

   a. Beta-adrenergic blockers.
   b. Supplies for suction and intubation.
   c. Nasal cannula and portable oxygen.
   d. Levothyroxine and lactated ringers.

9. **The nurse cares for a client with hypothyroidism who is one day post-op hip repair. The client is complaining of significant pain at the surgical site, and the nurse administers an opioid analgesic as prescribed. At this time, what follow-up does the nurse prioritize?**
   a. Monitoring changes in the client's cardiac rhythm.
   b. Observing the client for respiratory depression.
   c. Evaluating the client for signs of constipation.
   d. Observing the client for changes in skin turgor.

10. **The nurse reviews education with a client diagnosed with Cushing's syndrome. The nurse asks the client to indicate the area on the body, anteriorly, where fat is most likely to be distributed with this disease. Which location indicates the instruction was effective?**

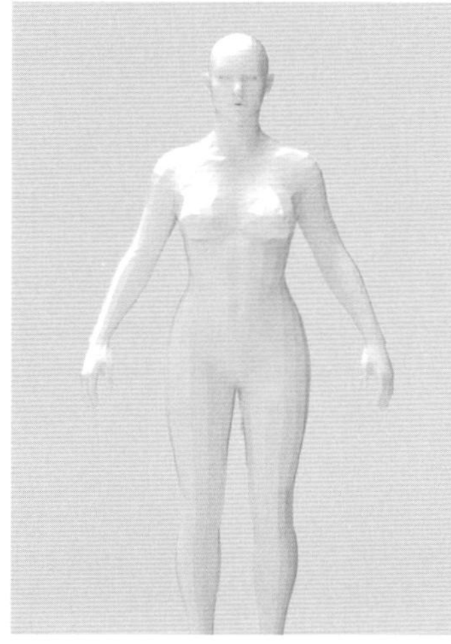

11. **The nurse cares for a client experiencing an Addisonian crisis. The client reports nausea and vomiting, abdominal pain, and dizziness. What intervention does the nurse initiate first?**
   a. Place the client on their left side.
   b. Apply oxygen via nasal cannula.
   c. Call for an electrocardiogram.
   d. Establish a peripheral intravenous and initiate infusion.

12. **The nurse cares for a client experiencing syndrome of inappropriate antidiuretic hormone (SIADH). What does the nurse include in the client's plan of care? *Select all that apply.***
   a. Strict monitoring of intake and output.
   b. Encourage 1000-2000 mL of water daily.
   c. Initiate a low-sodium diet.
   d. Daily weights at the same time each day.
   e. Closely monitor serum sodium levels.

13. **A client with diabetes insipidus (DI) is experiencing polyuria and polydipsia. What does the nurse plan to implement to maintain fluid balance?**
   a. Intravenous administration of isotonic fluids to correct hypovolemia.
   b. Restriction of oral fluids to < 1000 mL/day.
   c. Intravenous administration of hypotonic fluid to correct hypovolemia.
   d. Intravenous administration of hypertonic fluids to correct hypervolemia.

14. **The nurse cares for a child with a suspected Wilms' tumor. What physical finding does the nurse contribute to this diagnosis?**
    a. Hard, painless lump in the axillary.
    b. Soft, reducible lump at neck base.
    c. Lump at the waistband area.
    d. Soft, painful lump behind the ear.

15. **The nurse reviews information with a client at high risk for metabolic syndrome. If followed, which instruction by the nurse is most likely to reduce the client's overall risk?**
    a. Implement diet changes to manage diabetes.
    b. Consume foods to increase LDL levels.
    c. Walk 15 minutes a day, three times a week.
    d. Maintain fasting glucose >110 mg/dL.

16. **The new nurse plans care for a client with Type II Diabetes. What statement by the new nurse indicates a lack of understanding of risk reduction in diabetes?**
    a. "It's important that the client closely monitor blood glucose levels."
    b. "The client should exercise 30 minutes a day at least five days a week."
    c. "Snacks should contain less than 45 grams of carbohydrates."
    d. "The client should always avoid walking around barefoot."

17. **The nurse is reinforcing education to a client newly diagnosed with Cushing's disease. Which statement by the client indicates the need for follow-up by the nurse?**
    a. "I may notice swelling in my legs if I don't keep them elevated."
    b. "It's important that I urinate about the same amount that I drink."
    c. "I need to weigh myself at least once a week."
    d. "I should take my medications exactly as they are prescribed."

18. **The home health nurse visits a client with Addison's disease. What instructions does the nurse review with the client for optimal disease management? *Select all that apply.***
    a. Avoid becoming overheated.
    b. Maintain a low-sodium diet.
    c. Always carry emergency hydrocortisone.
    d. Do not discontinue glucocorticoids abruptly.
    e. Monitor and record weight accurately.

19. **The nurse implements an oral glucose tolerance test for a client who is pregnant. Rank order the steps of implementation from first to last.**
    a. Have the client drink the oral glucose.
    b. Obtain baseline fasting blood glucose.
    c. Monitor blood glucose at 30-minute intervals.
    d. Maintain NPO status 8-12 hours before the test.
    e. Obtain blood glucose 2 hours after initiation.

20. **The nurse cares for a client with newly diagnosed hypothyroidism who has been prescribed the medication in the image. What does the nurse ensure the client knows about this medication?**

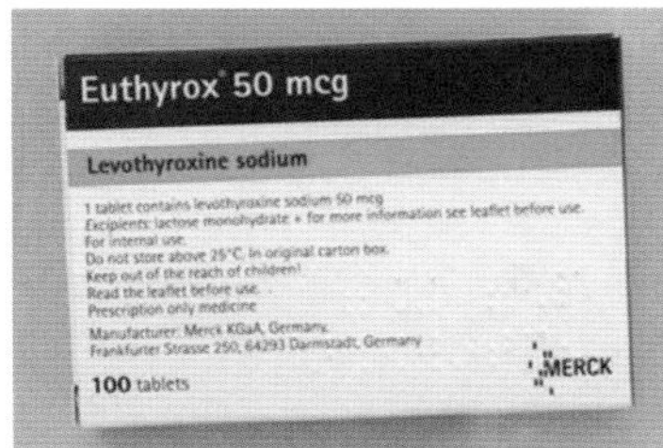

    a. This medication should be held 36-48 hours prior to surgery.
    b. This medication may be discontinued after the disease has resolved.
    c. This medication must be taken at the same time each morning.
    d. This medication should be taken in the evening, with food or milk.

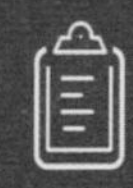

NurseThink® Quiz Answers

1. **The nurse cares for a client recently diagnosed with type 1 diabetes. The nurse expects the client to report which clinical manifestations of this form of diabetes? *Select all that apply.***
   a. Polydipsia.
   b. Oliguria.
   c. Polyphagia.
   d. Anuria.
   e. Weight loss.

   Topic/Concept: Hormonal **Subtopic:** Diabetes-Type I **Bloom's Taxonomy:** Applying **Clinical Problem-Solving Process:** Data Collection **NCLEX-PN®:** Physiological Adaptation **QSEN:** Evidence-based Practice **CJMM:** Analyze Cues

   Rationale: T1DM clinical manifestations include polyuria (excessive urine output), polydipsia (excessive thirst), polyphagia (increased appetite), fatigue, and weight loss. Oliguria (reduced urine output) or anuria (no urine output) may indicate renal failure.

   THIN Thinking: *Top Three* – The nurse should collect subjective and objective data to provide appropriate documentation. The nurse must be aware of common signs/ symptoms to ask appropriate questions.

2. **The nurse takes over the care of a pediatric client with Type I DM and reviews the medication administration record. Based on the administration time for Humulin R, when does the nurse expect the medication to be at its peak effectiveness?**
   a. Between 1240 and 1330.
   b. Between 1400 and 1600.
   c. Between 1600 and 2000.
   d. Between 1215 and 1230.

   Topic/Concept: Hormonal **Subtopic:** Diabetes-Type I (peds) **Bloom's Taxonomy:** Analyzing **Clinical Problem-Solving Process:** Evaluation **NCLEX-PN®:** Pharmacological Therapies **QSEN:** Safety **CJMM:** Evaluate Outcomes

   Rationale: Humulin R is short-acting, with onset in 30-60 minutes and a peak at 2-4 hours. The medication was administered at 1210, placing the peak at around 1400-1600. The nurse needs to understand the onset and peak times for the various types of insulin to manage care.

   THIN Thinking: *Clinical Problem-Solving Process* – The nurse should use the client's medication administration record to determine the expected outcomes of treatment. Being aware of peak times for insulin will help the client in recognizing signs of hypoglycemia.

3. **The nurse prepares a client to self-administer insulin at home. The provider has prescribed subcutaneous Humulin R before meals and at bedtime. What does the nurse emphasize to the client?**
   a. Avoid wearing a medical ID as it may impact emergency medical response.
   b. When eating high carbohydrate meals, double the prescribed dosage.
   c. Administer with an intradermal syringe when an insulin syringe is not available.
   d. Carry oral glucose with you at all times in case of hypoglycemia.

   Topic/Concept: Hormonal **Subtopic:** Diabetes-Type II **Bloom's Taxonomy:** Applying **Clinical Problem-Solving Process:** Planning **NCLEX-PN®:** Pharmacological Therapies **QSEN:** Evidence-based Practice **CJMM:** Generate Solution

   Rationale: The nurse should plan to include a safety response to hypoglycemia for the client taking insulin, which includes carrying oral glucose at all times. The client should be encouraged to wear a medical ID for emergency care. Clients should follow a prescribed dosing of insulin and not simply double dosages based on intake. Insulin should only be administered with an insulin syringe to ensure proper measurement of units.

   THIN Thinking: *Identify Safety Risk* – The nurse should always plan to include client safety in reinforcing client teaching. The client taking insulin is at risk for hypoglycemic episodes and should be instructed to carry oral glucose at all times.

4. **The nurse supports a group of women with gestational diabetes. To manage the challenges of diabetes while pregnant, what behaviors does the nurse encourage the women to implement? *Select all that apply.***
   a. Eat small meals at regular intervals.
   b. Monitor blood glucose 4-5 times/day.
   c. Count carbohydrates and document intake.
   d. Minimize physical activity and exercise.
   e. Eat three large meals per day.

   Topic/Concept: Hormonal **Subtopic:** Diabetes-Type I **Bloom's Taxonomy:** Applying **Clinical Problem-Solving Process:** Planning **NCLEX-PN®:** Physiological Adaptation **QSEN:** Evidence-based Practice **CJMM:** Generate Solutions

   Rationale: The nurse should instruct the client on ways to maintain stable glycemic control. This includes eating small meals at regular intervals throughout the day, counting carbohydrates, closely monitoring blood glucose levels, and keeping good records of intake and glucose levels. Mild to moderate physical activity should be encouraged as the client tolerates.

THIN Thinking: *Clinical Problem-Solving Process* – The nurse should provide the client with specific instructions on maintaining stable glucose levels for proper management of diabetes.

5. **The nurse cares for a client experiencing a hyperglycemic hyperosmolar state. The client has received 2 liters of 0.9% sodium chloride via rapid infusion. The client is responding well, and their current blood glucose is 362 mg/dL. Based on the client's current glucose level, what intravenous fluid does the nurse prepare to infuse?**
   a. The nurse continues rapid infusion of 0.9% sodium chloride.
   b. The nurse prepares to administer 0.45% sodium chloride.
   c. The nurse prepares to administer D5 0.45% sodium chloride.
   d. The nurse stops infusing all intravenous fluids at this time.

Topic/Concept: Hormonal **Subtopic:** Hyperglycemic syndrome **Bloom's Taxonomy:** Applying **Clinical Problem-Solving Process:** Implementation **NCLEX-PN®:** Pharmacological Therapies **QSEN:** Evidence-based Practice **CJMM:** Take Action

Rationale: Treatment of hyperglycemic hyperosmolar state (HHS) includes rapid infusion of isotonic fluids for fluid replacement followed by a switch to a hypotonic fluid to continue correcting hypovolemia. Once the blood glucose is in a manageable range (<250 mg/dL), the solution should be changed to include 5% dextrose to reduce the risk of cerebral edema and prevent hypoglycemia. Hydration is vital in managing HHS, and fluids should not be stopped suddenly.

THIN Thinking: *Clinical Problem-Solving Process* – The nurse should collect data from the client throughout treatment, monitoring fluid status, LOC, and blood glucose levels. Treatment progression is dependent on the client's response to fluid replacement and correction of hyperglycemia.

6. **The nurse cares for a client with hyperparathyroidism. The nurse instructs the client to avoid which foods in their diet? *Select all that apply.***
   a. Orange juice.
   b. Collard greens.
   c. Whole milk.
   d. Kiwi fruit.
   e. Lima beans.

Topic/Concept: Hormonal **Subtopic:** Hyperparathyroidism **Bloom's Taxonomy:** Applying **Clinical Problem-Solving Process:** Planning **NCLEX-PN®:** Health promotion and maintenance **QSEN:** Safety **CJMM:** Generate Solutions

Rationale: Management of hyperparathyroidism includes reducing intake of calcium and hydrating. Orange juice, green leafy veggies, and whole milk contain high levels of calcium and should be avoided.

THIN Thinking: *Clinical Problem-Solving Process* – The nurse should instruct the client on the need for a low calcium diet and plenty of water for hydration.

7. **The nurse cares for a client with hypoparathyroidism who is receiving intravenous calcium gluconate. Which findings alert the nurse that the client is now hypercalcemic?**
   a. Muscle cramps or spasms.
   b. Prolonged PR interval.
   c. Paresthesia of the hands.
   d. Hypotension.

Topic/Concept: Hormonal **Subtopic:** Hypoparathyroidism **Bloom's Taxonomy:** Analyzing **Clinical Problem-Solving Process:** Data Collection **NCLEX-PN®:** Reduction of Risk Potential **QSEN:** Patient-centered care **CJMM:** Analyze Cues

Rationale: A prolonged PR interval is associated with hypercalcemia, and the provider should be notified if it is observed during treatment with intravenous calcium. Muscle cramps, paresthesia of the hands, and hypotension are typically noted in hypocalcemia.

THIN Thinking: *Top Three* – Altered electrolytes can impact the cardiac rhythm. The nurse should monitor the client for a change from hypo- to hypercalcemia, which a lengthening PR interval may indicate.

8. **The nurse suspects the client is experiencing a thyroid storm. What priority items does the nurse ensure are in place at the bedside?**
   a. Beta-adrenergic blockers.
   b. Supplies for suction and intubation.
   c. Nasal cannula and portable oxygen.
   d. Levothyroxine and lactated ringers.

Topic/Concept: Hormonal **Subtopic:** Hyperthyroidism **Bloom's Taxonomy:** Applying **Clinical Problem-Solving Process:** Planning **NCLEX-PN®:** Coordinated Care **QSEN:** Teamwork and Collaboration **CJMM:** Prioritize Hypotheses

Rationale: Clinical manifestations of a thyroid storm include tachycardia, hyperthermia, tremors, and altered LOC. The nurse's priority is managing the client's airway, which includes suction equipment and supplies for intubation if necessary.

THIN Thinking: *Help Quick* – As the client is at risk for altered LOC, the patency of the client's airway may be compromised. The nurse must be prepared for the need for emergency equipment.

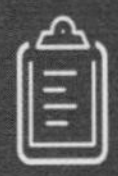

NurseThink® Quiz Answers

9. The nurse cares for a client with hypothyroidism who is one day post-op hip repair. The client is complaining of significant pain at the surgical site, and the nurse administers an opioid analgesic as prescribed. At this time, what follow-up does the nurse prioritize?

a. Monitoring changes in the client's cardiac rhythm.
b. Observing the client for respiratory depression.
c. Evaluating the client for signs of constipation.
d. Observing the client for changes in skin turgor.

Topic/Concept: Hormonal **Subtopic:** Cushing's syndrome **Bloom's Taxonomy:** Analyzing **Clinical Problem-Solving Process:** Evaluation **NCLEX-PN®:** Basic Care and Comfort **QSEN:** Patient-centered care **CJMM:** Evaluate Outcomes

Rationale: Clients with hypothyroidism have a decreased metabolism, thus increasing the need for close monitoring of signs of overmedication, such as respiratory depression or a change in responsiveness. Continued monitoring of cardiac function is also important with hypothyroidism but is not the priority. Constipation may occur with the use of opioids but is not the priority. Changes in skin turgor are not expected due to opioid use.

THIN Thinking: *Identify Risk to Safety* – The nurse should evaluate the care provided to each client. With a reduced metabolism, the client may metabolize medications slowly, placing them at risk for overmedication. The nurse should carefully monitor the client for signs of overdose and report changes to the provider.

10. The nurse reviews education with a client diagnosed with Cushing's syndrome. The nurse asks the client to indicate the area on the body, anteriorly, where fat is most likely to be distributed with this disease. Which location indicates the instruction was effective?

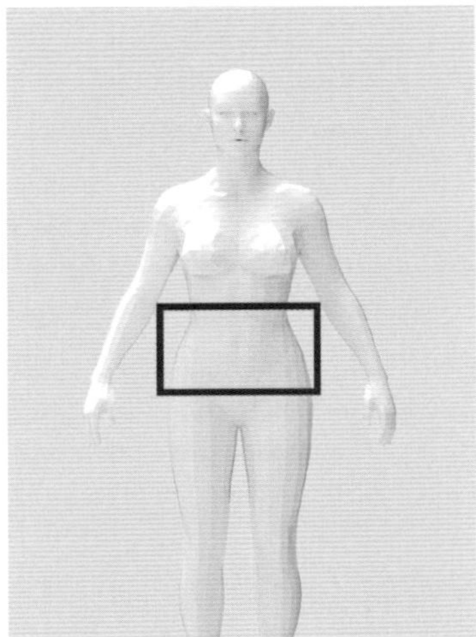

Topic/Concept: Hormones **Subtopic:** Cushing's syndrome **Bloom's Taxonomy:** Analyzing **Clinical Problem-Solving Process:** Evaluation **NCLEX-PN®:** Basic Care and Comfort **QSEN:** Patient-centered care **CJMM:** Evaluate Outcomes

Rationale: The client should indicate that fat is most likely distributed as truncal obesity. Other areas of extra fat distribution are not necessarily associated with Cushing's syndrome.

THIN Thinking: *Clinical Problem-Solving Process* – Effective instruction would lead the client to indicate the presence of truncal obesity and fat increases to the upper back/neck area. The nurse should evaluate for understanding that instruction was effective.

11. The nurse cares for a client experiencing an Addisonian crisis. The client reports nausea and vomiting, abdominal pain, and dizziness. What intervention does the nurse initiate first?

a. Place the client on their left side.
b. Apply oxygen via nasal cannula.
c. Call for an electrocardiogram.
d. Establish a peripheral intravenous and initiate infusion.

Topic/Concept: Hormonal **Subtopic:** Addison disease **Bloom's Taxonomy:** Applying **Clinical Problem-Solving Process:** Implementation **NCLEX-PN®:** Physiological Adaptation **QSEN:** Evidence-based Practice **CJMM:** Take Action

Rationale: Stabilization in this situation requires establishing an intravenous and initiating infusion of IVF and glucose, as well as administration of intravenous glucocorticoids. An ECG is indicated in this case but is not the priority. Oxygenation may be necessary but is not indicated based on the symptoms provided. The client may need to be placed on their left side to avoid aspiration of emesis, but this is not immediately indicated in this scenario as the priority.

THIN Thinking: *Help Quick* – An Addisonian crisis is a medical emergency. The nurse should immediately notify the provider of findings and gather the team to implement emergent care, including establishing good intravenous access.

12. The nurse cares for a client experiencing syndrome of inappropriate antidiuretic hormone (SIADH). What does the nurse include in the client's plan of care? *Select all that apply.*

a. Strict monitoring of intake and output.
b. Encourage 1000-2000 mL of water daily.
c. Initiate a low-sodium diet.
d. Daily weights at the same time each day.
e. Closely monitor serum sodium levels.

Topic/Concept: Hormonal **Subtopic:** SIADH **Bloom's Taxonomy:** Applying **Clinical Problem-Solving Process:** Planning **NCLEX-PN®:** Coordinated Care **QSEN:** Teamwork and Collaboration **CJMM:** Generate Solutions

Rationale: SIADH requires close monitoring for hyponatremia, strict I & O, fluid restriction, initiation and maintenance of seizure precautions, and monitoring for weight gain or fluid intoxication. 1-2 Liters of fluid per day is contraindicated with SIADH.

THIN Thinking: *Top Three* – The nurse should plan to closely monitor the client for signs of fluid retention, which may be evidenced by hypernatremia, weight gain, and increased intracranial pressure. The provider should be notified of any changes.

13. A client with diabetes insipidus (DI) is experiencing polyuria and polydipsia. What does the nurse plan to implement to maintain fluid balance?

a. Intravenous administration of isotonic fluids to correct hypovolemia.
b. Restriction of oral fluids to < 1000 mL/day.
c. Intravenous administration of hypotonic fluid to correct hypovolemia.
d. Intravenous administration of hypertonic fluids to correct hypervolemia.

Topic/Concept: Hormonal **Subtopic:** Diabetes insipidus **Bloom's Taxonomy:** Applying **Clinical Problem-Solving Process:** Planning **NCLEX-PN®:** Physiological Adaptation **QSEN:** Evidence-based Practice **CJMM:** Generate Solutions

Rationale: The client with DI is at risk for hypernatremia and hypovolemia related to the loss of free water. The nurse should plan to administer hypotonic solutions to replace lost volume and reduce serum sodium levels. Hypotonic solutions will move water from the vascular space into the cells, hydrating cells and diluting serum sodium levels. Isotonic solutions and hypertonic solutions are not indicated with DI. Restriction of fluid may worsen hypovolemia.

THIN Thinking: *Identify Safety Risk* – The nurse should plan to administer a hypotonic solution to the client with hypernatremia related to DI. Then, the nurse must continue monitoring serum sodium levels and observe the client for hypotension related to a fluid shift out of the vascular space.

14. The nurse cares for a child with a suspected Wilms' tumor. What physical finding does the nurse contribute to this diagnosis?

a. Hard, painless lump in the axillary.
b. Soft, reducible lump at neck base.
c. Lump at the waistband area.
d. Soft, painful lump behind the ear.

Topic/Concept: Hormonal **Subtopic:** Wilms tumor **Bloom's Taxonomy:** Analyzing **Clinical Problem-Solving Process:** Data Collection **NCLEX-PN®:** Health promotion and maintenance **QSEN:** Evidence-based Practice **CJMM:** Analyze Cues

Rationale: Wilms' tumor presents with a lump in the abdomen or at the waistband area. The area may be painful. Lumps or bumps in other areas are not indicative of Wilms' tumor.

THIN Thinking: *Clinical Problem-Solving Process* – During care of a client with a confirmed or suspected tumor, the nurse should avoid palpating, percussing, or massaging the area on or around the tumor as rupture could occur and may lead to metastasis.

15. The nurse reviews information with a client at high risk for metabolic syndrome. If followed, which instruction by the nurse is most likely to reduce the client's overall risk?

a. Implement diet changes to manage diabetes.
b. Consume foods to increase LDL levels.
c. Walk 15 minutes a day, three times a week.
d. Maintain fasting glucose >110 mg/dL.

Topic/Concept: Hormonal **Subtopic:** Metabolic syndrome **Bloom's Taxonomy:** Applying **Clinical Problem-Solving Process:** Evaluation **NCLEX-PN®:** Basic Care and Comfort **QSEN:** Evidence-based Practice **CJMM:** Evaluate Outcomes

Rationale: Metabolic syndrome has a cluster of risk factors. Management of metabolic syndrome is dependent on reducing modifiable risks, such as good glycemic control, management of diabetes, moderate exercise, and a healthy diet. LDL should be reduced, not increased. It is recommended to keep glucose levels <100mg/dL and engage in 30-60 minutes of activity daily.

THIN Thinking: *Clinical Problem-Solving Process* – Health education and health promotion are essential for clients with a high risk for metabolic syndrome. The nurse should provide timely, accurate information that encourages the client to manage the risk factors associated with challenging diagnoses.

16. The new nurse plans care for a client with Type II Diabetes. What statement by the new nurse indicates a lack of understanding of risk reduction in diabetes?

a. "It's important that the client closely monitor blood glucose levels."
b. "The client should exercise 30 minutes a day at least five days a week."
c. "Snacks should contain less than 45 grams of carbohydrates."
d. "The client should always avoid walking around barefoot."

Topic/Concept: Hormonal **Subtopic:** Diabetes-Type II **Bloom's Taxonomy:** Analyzing **Clinical Problem-Solving Process:** Evaluation **NCLEX-PN®:** Reduction of Risk Potential **QSEN:** Safety **CJMM:** Evaluate Outcomes

Rationale: The nurse should instruct the client to eat snacks containing less than 20 grams of carbohydrates. The other responses are correct and indicate a good understanding of risk reduction in diabetics.

THIN Thinking: *Clinical Problem-Solving Process* – The nurse must ensure that the client understands instruction related to a diagnosis of Diabetes. Positive outcomes are dependent on effective management of the disease.

17. The nurse reinforces education to a client newly diagnosed with Cushing's disease. Which statement by the client indicates the need for follow-up by the nurse?

a. "I may notice swelling in my legs if I don't keep them elevated."
b. "It's important that I urinate about the same amount that I drink."
c. "I need to weigh myself at least once a week."
d. "I should take my medications exactly as they are prescribed."

Topic/Concept: Hormonal **Subtopic:** Cushing's syndrome **Bloom's Taxonomy:** Analyzing **Clinical Problem-Solving Process:** Evaluation **NCLEX-PN®:** Coordinated Care **QSEN:** Teamwork and Collaboration **CJMM:** Evaluate Outcomes

Rationale: Close monitoring of I & O and daily weights are important to evaluate trends and fluid retention. The client should weigh themselves daily, at the same time, and without clothing (or with similarly weighted clothing) for the most accurate measurement. The other statements by the client are correct.

THIN Thinking: *Identify Risk to Safety* – The nurse should evaluate whether the client with Cushing's disease understands the importance of accurately documenting intake, output, and weight and provide further education as needed.

18. The home health nurse visits a client with Addison's disease. What instructions does the nurse review with the client for optimal disease management? *Select all that apply.*

a. Avoid becoming overheated.
b. Maintain a low-sodium diet.
c. Always carry emergency hydrocortisone.
d. Do not discontinue glucocorticoids abruptly.
e. Monitor and record weight accurately.

Topic/Concept: Hormonal **Subtopic:** Addison's Disease **Bloom's Taxonomy:** Applying **Clinical Problem-Solving Process:** Planning **NCLEX-PN®:** Health promotion and maintenance **QSEN:** Patient-centered care **CJMM:** Generate Solutions

Rationale: Management of care should include avoiding stress and becoming overheated, carefully monitoring I & O and weight, taking medications as prescribed, and carrying an emergency kit with hydrocortisone in case of Addisonian crisis. Clients with Addison's disease may use salt freely.

THIN Thinking: *Clinical Problem-Solving Process* – When planning care, the nurse should include the importance of managing cortisol and glucose levels and preparing for a potential crisis.

19. The nurse implements an oral glucose tolerance test for a client who is pregnant. Rank order the steps of implementation from first to last.

a. Have the client drink the oral glucose.
b. Obtain baseline fasting blood glucose.
c. Monitor blood glucose at 30-minute intervals.
d. Maintain NPO status 8-12 hours before the test.
e. Obtain blood glucose 2 hours after initiation.

Answer: D, B, A, C, E.

Topic/Concept: Hormonal **Subtopic:** Gestational diabetes **Bloom's Taxonomy:** Applying **Clinical Problem-Solving Process:** Implementation **NCLEX-PN®:** Reduction of Risk Potential **QSEN:** Patient-centered care **CJMM:** Take Action

Rationale: The client should be NPO 8-12 hours before the oral glucose tolerance test. Before the test, fasting blood glucose should be obtained. The client should then consume the oral glucose drink, and glucose levels should be obtained at 30-minute intervals for 2 hours. Final glucose should be obtained two hours after the start of the test. The client should be monitored closely for hypo- and severe hyperglycemia throughout the testing.

THIN Thinking: *Clinical Problem-Solving Process* – The nurse must implement the procedure correctly to elicit valid results.

20. The nurse cares for a client with newly diagnosed hypothyroidism who has been prescribed the medication in the image. What does the nurse ensure the client knows about this medication?

a. This medication should be held 36-48 hours prior to surgery.
b. This medication may be discontinued after the disease has resolved.
c. This medication must be taken at the same time each morning.
d. This medication should be taken in the evening, with food or milk.

Topic/Concept: Hormonal **Subtopic:** Hypothyroidism **Bloom's Taxonomy:** Applying **Clinical Problem-Solving Process:** Planning **NCLEX-PN®:** Pharmacological Therapies **QSEN:** Evidence-based Practice **CJMM:** Generate Solutions

Rationale: Levothyroxine is a lifelong treatment regimen. Dosages may be adjusted over time, but the medication should be taken in the morning and at the same time daily. This medication should not be abruptly discontinued and is generally not withheld prior to surgery.

THIN Thinking: *Top Three* – There are important details about some medications that the nurse should ensure the client knows to prevent complications from improper use.

CHAPTER

13

Movement

Mobility / Sensory / Nerve conduction

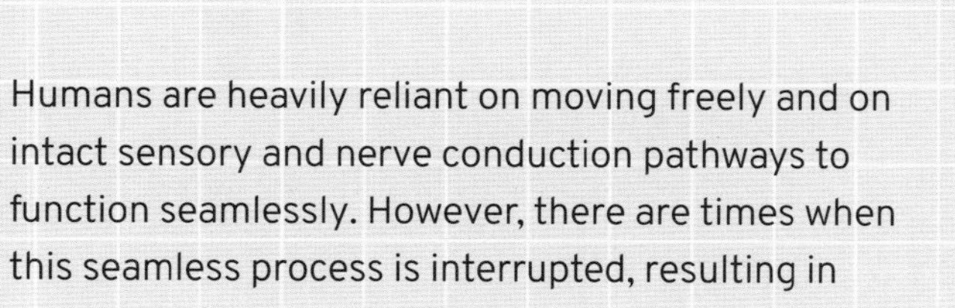

Humans are heavily reliant on moving freely and on intact sensory and nerve conduction pathways to function seamlessly. However, there are times when this seamless process is interrupted, resulting in problems with how humans function in their daily lives.

Many illnesses stem from impairments in mobility, sensory deficits, and problems with nerve conduction. Nurses should be knowledgeable about these illnesses and apply that knowledge to safe client care.

Priority Exemplars:

- Multiple sclerosis
- Fractures
- Cerebral palsy
- Seizures
- Osteoporosis
- Osteoarthritis
- Peripheral neuropathy
- Trigeminal neuralgia
- Carpal tunnel
- Amputation
- Amyotrophic lateral sclerosis
- Guillain-Barré syndrome
- Myasthenia gravis
- Parkinson's disease
- Cataracts
- Glaucoma
- Conjunctivitis
- Macular degeneration
- Hearing impairment
- Scoliosis
- Labyrinthitis/Meniere's disease
- Otitis media/externa
- Spina bifida
- Spinal cord injury

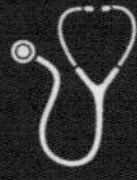

Go To Clinical

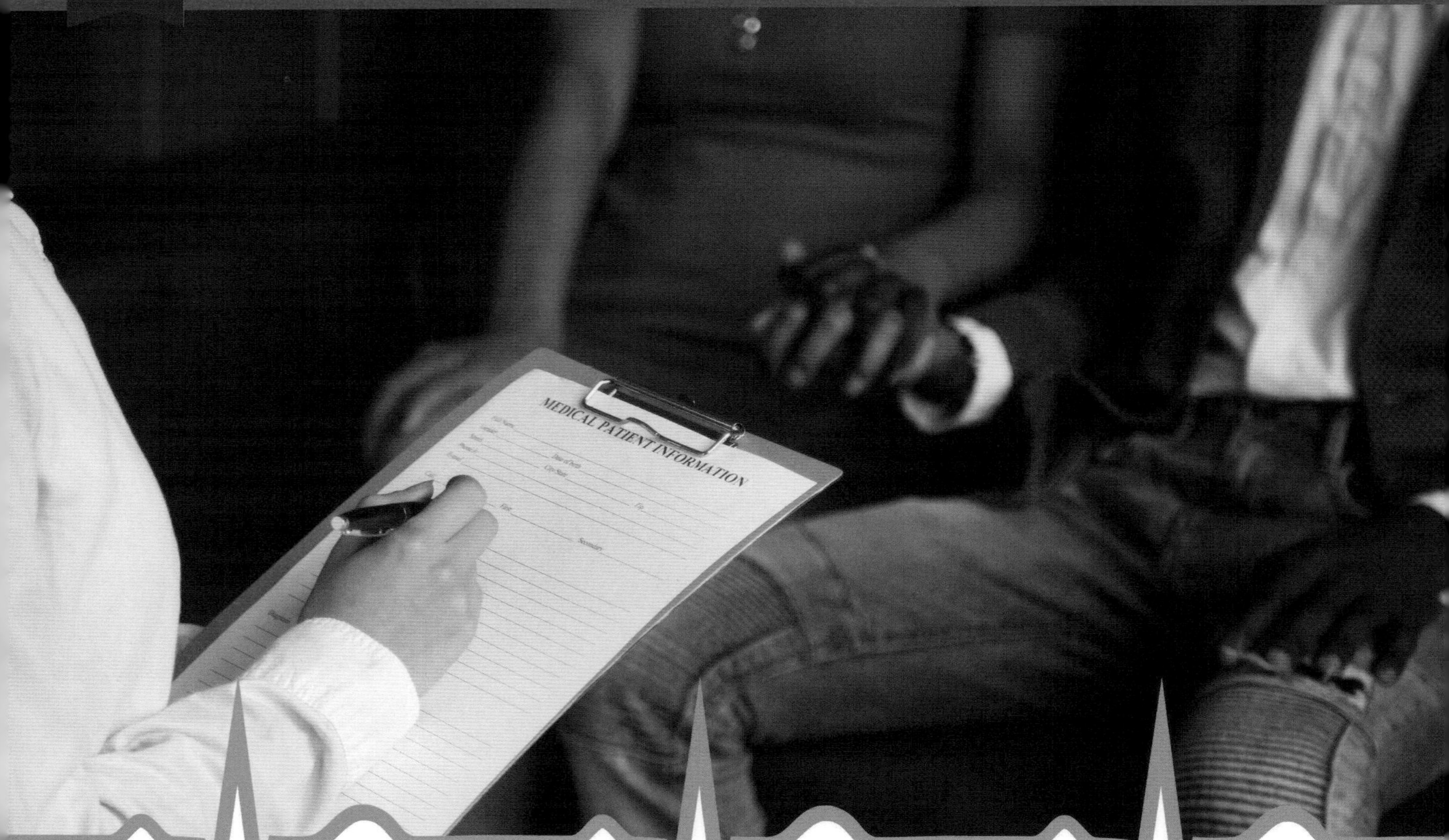

Go To Clinical Case 1

M.T. is a 32-year-old female who visits the clinic for new onset of symptoms that have persisted for over two months. M.T. is active with no significant medical history. M.T. reports noticing numbness and weakness in her left arm and both hands, causing writing and typing to be difficult and painful. She also reports visual disturbances and feeling increasingly fatigue. In the past few days, M.T. noted feeling "unbalanced" when standing and walking, causing her to seek medical attention.

M.T. discloses that she received a promotion two months prior and has been under a lot of stress trying to keep up with work demands. In addition, she reports having personal issues with a former friend. That individual believed they should have been awarded the promotion that M.T. received. This colleague became challenging and antagonizing at work.

M.T. is admitted to the medical-surgical unit with suspected multiple sclerosis. Establish priorities for M.T.

NurseThink® Time

Using the NurseThink® system, complete the priorities. Check your answers designated by 💡 in the Multiple sclerosis Priority Exemplar.

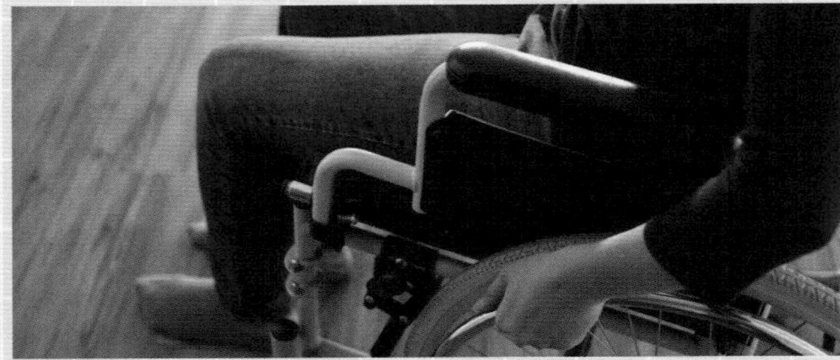

Image 13-1: How do numbness and weakness in the lower extremities contribute to the need for a wheelchair? What nursing care is required when a client requires a wheelchair?

NurseThink® Time

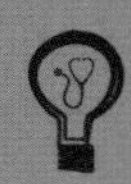

Priority Data Collection or Cues

1.

2.

3.

Priority Laboratory Tests/Diagnostics

1.

2.

3.

Priority Interventions or Actions

1.

2.

3.

Priority Potential & Actual Complications

1.

2.

3.

Priority Nursing Implications

1.

2.

3.

Priority Medications

1.

2.

3.

Reinforcement of Priority Teaching

1.

2.

3.

Multiple sclerosis

Pathophysiology/Description

- Multiple sclerosis (MS) is a chronic, progressive condition in which demyelination of neurons in the central nervous system occurs
- The disease may have a genetic tendency, with genetic factors seen in families that have more than one person with the disease
- The disease usually has an onset between the second to the fifth decade of life in more women than men
- Factors that precipitate MS
  - Pregnancy
  - Emotional stress
  - Infection
  - Trauma
  - Fatigue
  - Climate change

Priority Data Collection or Cues

- Monitor respiratory status to detect any early symptoms of respiratory compromise
- Ask client about energy level, MS causes muscle weakness and fatigue
- Check client's vision, may find double or blurred vision, or unilateral blindness
- Observe client's balance and coordination, may have poor balance and lack of coordination
- Monitor client's speech, may find difficulty speaking
- Ask client about bladder incontinence or retention and constipation of bowels
- Observe client's hearing
- Look for cognitive dysfunction such as processing of information, finding of words and memory which present in late-stage MS
- Observe for emotional lability such as euphoria and anger, which sometimes manifest with MS
- Examine client's eyes, may find nystagmus
- Monitor ambulation, client may trip while walking
- Ask client about falls at home
- Inquire whether client experiences numbness and tingling to extremities
- Observe client for spasticity to lower extremities
- Examine skin for pressure ulcers caused by immobility

Priority Laboratory Tests/Diagnostics

- Lumbar puncture to examine cerebrospinal fluid will indicate elevated gamma globulin level
- Evoked potential testing may show delayed response
- Computed tomography (CT) scan and magnetic resonance imaging (MRI) of brain and spinal cord may show tissue damage, inflammation and plaques

Priority Interventions or Actions

- For client with diplopia, cover the affected eye with a patch
- Provide proper skin care in acute exacerbation to prevent pressure ulcers
- Turn and reposition client
- Encourage bladder training to minimize incontinence
- Encourage coughing and deep breathing exercises to prevent respiratory compromise
- Encourage a well balanced, high-fiber diet
- Administer medications as prescribed
- Maintain client in a safe environment that is free of potential hazards for falling
- Provide foods that are easy to swallow to decrease risk of aspiration
- Initiate physical, occupational and speech consult as prescribed
- Assist client to make decisions about lifestyle modifications
- Encourage client and family to talk about the emotional aspect of the diagnosis. Provide psychological consult if needed

Priority Potential & Actual Complications

- Infections
- Respiratory conditions such as pneumonia
- Paralysis with total dependence for all activities of daily living (ADLs)
- Blindness
- Depression

Priority Nursing Implications

- Sexual functioning is severely compromised in clients with MS. Explore alternate means of intimacy
- With interferon, it is important to wear protective clothing and sunscreen lotion while taking the drug and the site of injection administration must be rotated with each dose. It is normal to experience flu-like symptoms when the drug is first started
- Dalfampridine must not be used in clients with seizure disorder as it may precipitate seizures
- Prednisone should not be stopped abruptly to avoid prednisone withdrawal symptoms, which include weakness, severe fatigue, and joint and body aches

Go To Clinical Answers

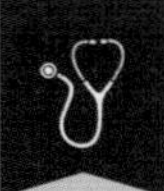

Text designated by are the top answers for the Go To Clinical related to Multiple sclerosis.

Priority Medications

- Drugs to treat MS are many and in various classes. Below are a few of the most common drugs used in each class
- Beta 1A interferon
  - Immunomodulator
  - Intramuscular once weekly
  - Dose can be titrated to prevent side effect of flu-like symptoms
- Mitoxantrone
  - Immunosuppressant
  - Intravenous infusion every 3 months
  - Serious side effects of cardiotoxicity, infertility and leukemia
- Alemtuzumab
  - Intravenous infusion
  - Monoclonal antibody
- Prednisone
  - Corticosteroid by oral route
  - Most beneficial when used to treat acute flare-ups
- Dalfampridine–oral administration
  - Enhances nerve conduction
  - Used to improve walking in MS

Reinforcement of Priority Teaching

- The long-term trajectory of the disease and how it progresses
- Help client to recognize triggers that worsen the symptoms
- Encourage client to avoid temperature extremes
- Early detection and treatment of infection
- Advise about the balance of rest and exercise
- Eat well-balanced nutritious meals
- Consume fiber to help treat constipation
- Measures to minimize injury due to sensory loss, such as decreasing water temperature
- Seek pharmacist or health care provider's opinion before taking over-the-counter medication
- Measures to make the home environment safe such as removing loose rugs and installing hand bars in showers
- Explain self-catheterization to the client as indicated
- Provide information on resources to assist client with coping such as The National Multiple Sclerosis Society
- Needed medications and administration guidelines

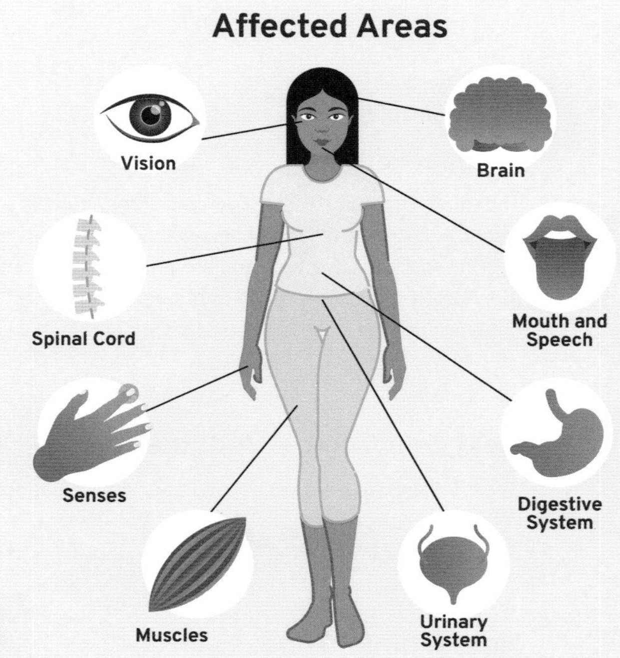

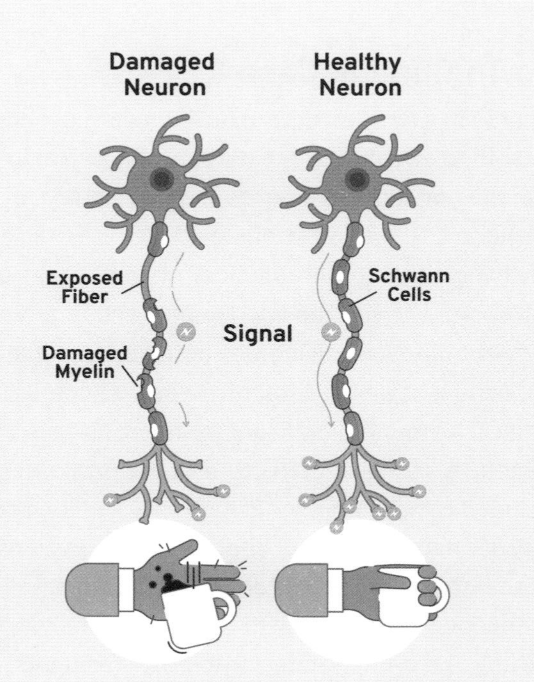

Image 13-2: What are several safety concerns for a client with MS based on these affected areas?

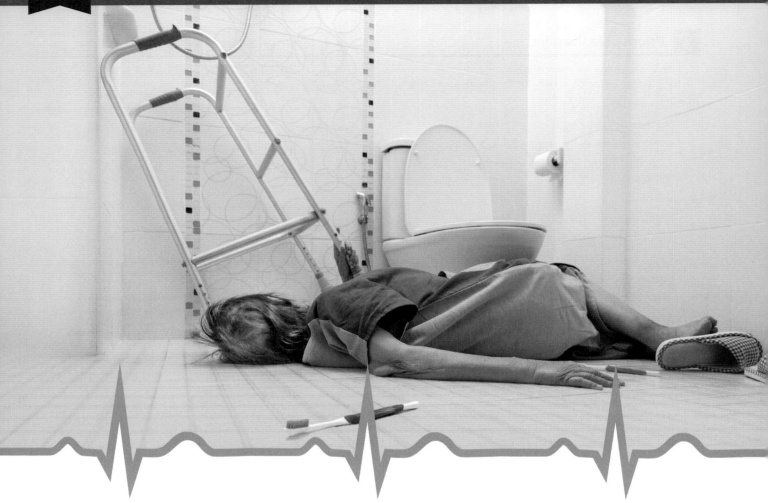

Go To Clinical Case 2

A nurse in a long-term care facility heard a loud crash and ran to investigate the noise. Upon arrival to room 312, the nurse found a resident in the bathroom on the floor. E.P., a 76-year-old resident of the facility, was lying on the bathroom floor of another resident's bathroom. She was moaning in pain and guarding her right hip. No bruising was noted upon initial inspection; however, a fracture was suspected. E.P.'s medical history is significant for heart disease, dementia, and several fractures. E.P.'s vital signs included temperature 97.2°F (36.2°C); blood pressure 154/89 mmHg; pulse 92 beats/min; respirations 22 breaths/min. E.P. was ambulatory with a walker but needed assistance with activities of daily living (ADLs). She often wanders into other residents' rooms and rummages in their belongings. Establish nursing priorities of care for E.P.

Clinical Hint

The most common fracture found in older adults is a hip fracture. Older adults experience changes in balance, decreased motor function, and are prone to osteoporosis (decreased calcium resulting in thinner and weaker bones) which increase their risk for fractures.

Next Gen Clinical Judgment

Consider the ways nurses evaluate neurovascular status in clients.

NurseThink® Time

Using the NurseThink® system, complete the priorities. Check your answers designated by the lightbulb icon in the Fractures Priority Exemplar.

NurseThink® Time

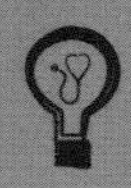

Priority Data Collection or Cues

1.

2.

3.

Priority Laboratory Tests/Diagnostics

1.

2.

3.

Priority Interventions or Actions

1.

2.

3.

Priority Potential & Actual Complications

1.

2.

3.

Priority Nursing Implications

1.

2.

3.

Priority Medications

1.

2.

3.

Reinforcement of Priority Teaching

1.

2.

3.

Fractures

Pathophysiology/Description

- A fracture is a break in the continuity of a bone that results from traumatic injuries or other disease processes
- There are many types of fractures classified in different ways
- Complete vs incomplete fractures: With incomplete fractures, the bone is still intact with the fracture only occurring across the shaft, while with a complete fracture, the bone is broken right through
- Open vs closed fracture: In an open fracture, bone is exposed through broken skin, while in a closed fracture, the skin is unbroken
- Displaced vs nondisplaced fracture: With displaced fractures, the bones are broken and separate, sometimes in fragments, while in nondisplaced fracture, the bone is broken but stays intact

Priority Data Collection or Cues

- Monitor for pain that is sudden and localized to the affected area
- Perform neurovascular data collection to include capillary refill, color, sensation, peripheral pulses, edema, and temperature
- Look for tenderness at the injury site
- Observe client for guarding of the affected area
- Monitor client's weight-bearing status. With a fracture bearing weight causes pain
- Examine the affected site for swelling, redness and deformity
- Determine type of fracture
- Complete history of injury occurrence
- Examine skin for bleeding and/or bone protrusion
- Monitor for muscle spasms because of involuntary muscle reflex
- Listen for crunching of bone fragments, can occur with fragmented fracture

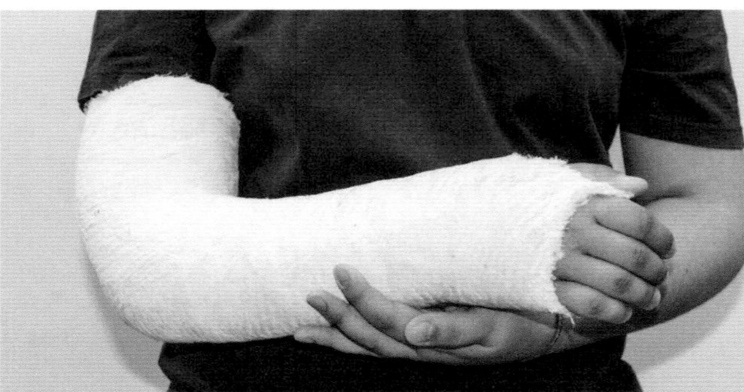

Image 13-3: List important data to collect when a client is to be discharged home with a cast. What data would indicate that the cast was too tight? What data, if detected, should be reported to the charge nurse or the health care provider? What should the nurse anticipate as part of the instruction plan for this client?

Priority Laboratory Tests/Diagnostics

- X-ray of the affected extremity will show the fracture
- Computed tomography (CT) scan and magnetic resonance imaging (MRI) will show fracture and any damage to surrounding structures

Priority Interventions or Actions

- Administer drug therapy as prescribed
- Immobilize the affected extremity to prevent movement that might cause further damage
- Cover open fracture wound with sterile dressing
- Interventions related to fixing fracture (traction, reduction, cast, fixation)
  - Inform client of the type of surgery and the device that will be used after surgery
  - Monitor neurovascular status of affected extremity
  - Provide proper alignment to promote comfort and prevent damage to fracture repair
  - Monitor drainage system used. Measure output
  - Monitor for bleeding and signs of infection on casts, dressings or at pin insertion sites
  - Plan client care with client's immobility status in mind
  - Provide adequate fluid to prevent constipation from immobility
  - Provide good skin care to prevent pressure ulcers as client is immobile
  - Check traction to ensure the weights are not touching any surfaces and are hanging freely
  - Manage internal fixation apparatus such as checking for intact screws, pins and plates
  - Monitor the traction ropes and pully mechanism to ensure no obstructions
  - Clean pin sites as prescribed
  - Provide measures to prevent a thromboembolism such as having client sit on side of bed and dangle feet, range of motion to unaffected extremity. Administer low dose anticoagulant as ordered
  - Have client perform deep breathing to prevent respiratory compromise
  - Monitor casted extremity to ensure cast is not too tight, causing circulatory compromise

Priority Potential & Actual Complications

- Infection
- Osteomyelitis
- Avascular necrosis
- Physical immobility
- Blood clots
- Compartment syndrome
- Fat embolism

Priority Nursing Implications

- A major and life-threatening complication of fractures is compartment syndrome, where the extremity gets swollen, increasing the pressure within the muscle compartment. Blood flow and nerves become compromised and capillary refill decreases drastically. Manifestations are pain in the limb that is not relieved by analgesics, loss of color, loss of sensation, loss of function, paleness, and inability to palpate distal pulses. A surgical procedure(fasciotomy) is used to correct compartment syndrome and the wound is left open to decompress the tissue

Priority Medications

- Carisoprodol
  - Muscle relaxant
  - Treat pain and stiffness caused by muscle spasms
  - Oral administration
- Cyclobenzaprine
  - Muscle relaxant
  - Treat pain caused by muscle spasms
  - Oral administration
- Methocarbamol
  - Muscle relaxant
  - Treat pain caused by muscle spasms
  - Administered via intravenous, IM, or orally

Reinforcement of Priority Teaching

- The importance of walking at least 30 minutes three times weekly to maintain bone mass
- Elevate extremity with cast above the heart level
- The need to examine the extremity below cast and report any abnormalities, such as numbness and tingling, cool to touch, paleness
- Encourage client not to place objects under the cast as in trying to scratch the skin under the cast
- Instructions on the need to report a foul odor associated with the cast
- How to clean pin sites with an external fixator and monitor for infection
- If an internal fixator was used, explain to the client about the need for frequent x-rays to determine alignment and healing
- Stress the importance for client to keep follow-up appointments
- Remove unsafe obstacles from home that might increase risk of falls, such as loose rugs
- Alert client to the fact that when a cast is removed, the extremity may appear shrunken but with time it will start to appear normal again
- The importance of keeping physical and occupational therapy appointments
- Explain to the client that modifications may need to be made in the home to accommodate the impaired mobility
- Encourage client to maintain the prescribed weight-bearing status
- Explain the use of assistive devices

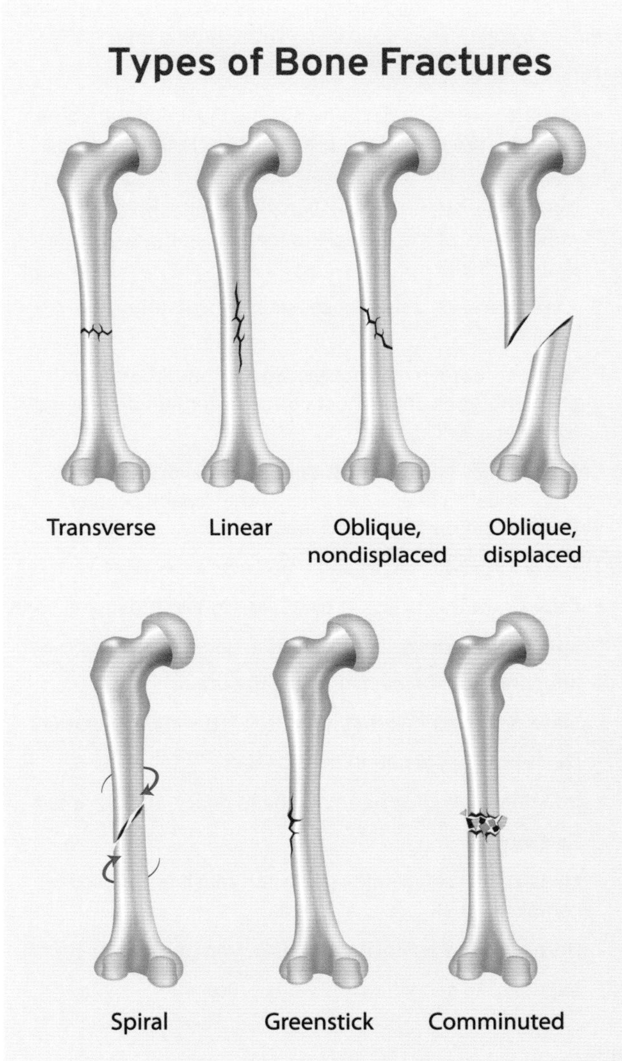

Image 13-4: Describe each type of bone fracture and the priority interventions for each.

Go To Clinical Answers

Text designated by (icon) are the top answers for the Go To Clinical related to Fractures.

Cerebral palsy

Pathophysiology/Description

- Cerebral palsy (CP) is a disorder that affects the ability of an individual to move and maintain proper posture. It generally results from damage to the neurons before, during, or early after birth
- While some persons with cerebral palsy are not able to walk or function independently, others are able to walk and perform activities of daily living without difficulty
- Types of cerebral palsy
  - Spastic cerebral palsy, which is the most common type. The person's body has increased muscle tone, causing stiffness
  - Dyskinetic cerebral palsy causes loss of control with movements of the hands and feet, making walking and sitting difficult
  - Ataxic cerebral palsy causes poor coordination and balance
  - Mixed cerebral palsy incorporates a combination of different types of CP, most common combination being dyskinetic and spastic
- Cerebral palsy has significant impact on every aspect of the individual's life and can cause other health problems. Seizures, deafness and blindness common
- There are several causes and risk factor associated with CP
  - Fetal stroke due to lack of blood flow to the developing brain
  - Mutation in genes
  - Infections in infancy that affect the brain
  - Maternal infections that affect the fetus in development
  - Decreased oxygenation during labor
  - Infant involved in a traumatic head injury, such as a fall
  - Zika virus
  - Measles and chickenpox (both can cause pregnancy complications)
  - Herpes, cytomegalovirus, syphilis from mother to infant
  - Exposure to certain toxins while pregnant

Priority Data Collection or Cues

- Look for variations in muscle tone and movement, such as floppiness, stiffness, exaggerated reflexes, tremors, involuntary movements
- Determine the child's attainment of developmental milestones
- Observe use of hands, child may favor one side of the body, using the same hand all the time
- Observe the child's gait (if able to walk), may observe a crouched walk, wide gait, tip-toe walking or knees crossing when walking
- Examine the child's mouth, may find drooling
- Observe eating, may see difficulty swallowing or with eating
- Observe the child's speech, may find that there is difficulty getting words out or delayed development of speech
- Observe child's fine motor skills, may find inability to pick up objects or use objects, such as using a crayon to color
- Monitor for seizure activity
- Monitor child for extreme irritability and crying
- Look for abnormal posture such as bent sideways or exaggerated arching of the back

Priority Laboratory Tests/Diagnostics

- Cranial ultrasound to provide baseline data
- Magnetic resonance imaging (MRI) to detect neurological abnormalities or lesions
- Computed tomography (CT) scan to determine the cause and time of the brain injury that may have contributed to the cerebral palsy
- Electroencephalogram (EEG) to monitor for seizures

Priority Interventions or Actions

- An interprofessional, long-term intervention is needed for a child with cerebral palsy
  - Physical therapist to help with muscle strength and gait
  - Occupational therapist to support activities of daily living and adaptive equipment
  - Speech therapist to manage speech problems and impaired swallowing
  - Mental health professional to assist child with coping skills
  - Orthopedic surgeon to diagnose and treat bone and muscle problems
  - Developmental therapist to assist with development of social skills and age-specific behaviors
  - Pediatric neurologist to manage the neurological symptoms associated with CP
  - Special education teacher to manage special learning needs

Priority Potential & Actual Complications

- Seizures
- Cognitive impairment, difficulty with vision and hearing
- Dental diseases
- Contractures, malnutrition
- Abnormal sensory perception
- Urinary incontinence
- Mental health conditions

Priority Nursing Implications

- Cerebral palsy is a long-term, life-altering condition that will change the lives of both parents and child. It is important to discuss the long-term social support that may be required, so that caregivers can cope well with caring for a child with this condition

Priority Medications

- Baclofen: muscle relaxant used to treat spasticity
    - Administered via spinal catheter, lumbar puncture, or implantable pump
    - Screening doses are given first and maintenance dose is not recommended unless screening dose criteria are met
- Onabotulinum toxin A
    - Administered via injection into affected muscles
    - Know widely under the brand name Botox
    - Used to treat when spasticity is localized to a single group of muscles

Reinforcement of Priority Teaching

- Importance of ensuring child keeps all appointments with the health professionals
- How to use adaptive equipment/devices with child. Check proper administration of medications
- Importance of communicating with child at the child's developmental level
- Explain the importance of reinforcing work done by the various therapists
- Encourage caregiver to intervene early on child's behalf so that severity of symptoms might be minimized
- Safety for the child, to include use of helmets, removal of sharp objects and ensuring the home is conducive to mobility of a child with CP. Explain seizure precautions and what to do if the child has a seizure
- Provide caregiver with information on cerebral palsy support groups

Clinical Hint

Therapy is an important aspect of the treatment plan for clients with cerebral palsy. Therapy may include physical, occupational, or speech therapy. Therapy may help to increase movement, strength, reduce pain, and help the client to be as independent as possible.

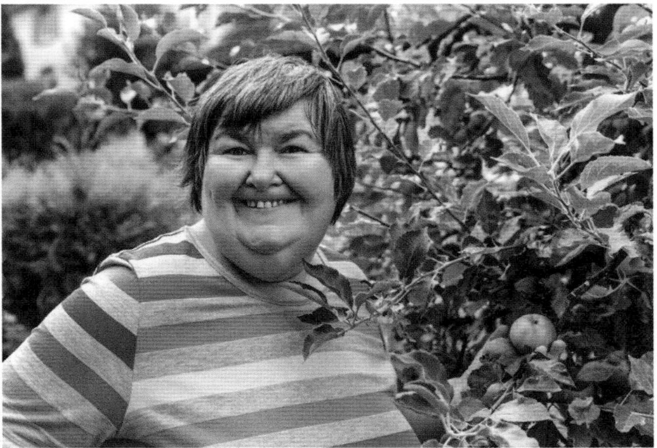

Image 13-5: Over 60% of patients with cerebral palsy live past the age of 50. Describe nursing actions to support clients with cerebral palsy across the lifespan

There are many disorders associated with cerebral palsy. For these 3 disorders, list 3 priority nursing concerns. Remember that a priority nursing concern can be either data collection or intervention.

DYSPHAGIA
1. ______
2. ______
3. ______
VISUAL IMPAIRMENT
1. ______
2. ______
3. ______
DECREASED MOTOR FUNCTION
1. ______
2. ______
3. ______

Table 13-1: Disorders associated with cerebral palsy

Seizures

Pathophysiology/Description

- Seizures are sudden, uncontrolled and excessive discharge of neurons within the brain. Epilepsy is chronic seizures
- Causes of seizures include brain injury, genetic factors, trauma, brain tumors, stroke, metabolic disorder and toxicity
- Most seizures are caused by brain dysfunction. Disorders outside the brain, such as hypertension, septicemia, kidney disease and others, can also cause seizures
- Seizures are classified as generalized and focal. With general seizures, both sides of the brain are involved, and the client usually loses consciousness. Focal seizures involve one side of the brain and may stay to that side only. Focal seizures can spread to involve other parts of the brain and eventually end in a generalized seizure
- There are several types of generalized seizures but tonic-clonic seizure is the most common of the generalized seizures. Clients usually lose consciousness and if standing, they fall to the ground

Priority Data Collection or Cues

- Complete health history, to include seizure history
- Ask client about period just before seizure activity, some clients experience an aura (a feeling that warns them a seizure is about to start)
- Seizure activity data collection
  - Type of seizure, generalized or focal
  - Onset, seizure activity, duration and client's status after the seizure
  - Factors that may have precipitated a seizure
  - Oral cavity after seizure to determine any damage, such as client biting tongue
  - Breathing during and after seizure, ensure no airway occlusion
  - Vital signs after a seizure
  - Incontinence, as some clients become incontinent of bladder and/or bowel during seizure
  - Client's behavior in the postictal phase
  - Closely monitor during status epilepticus

Priority Laboratory Tests/Diagnostics

- Electroencephalography (EEG), to examine the electrical activity of the brain
- Lumbar puncture to test cerebrospinal fluid (CSF)
- Complete blood cell count, liver and kidney function tests and blood chemistries to look for cause of seizures
- Computed tomography (CT) scan and Magnetic resonance imaging to determine structural lesions

Priority Interventions or Actions

- Remove any unsafe objects from client's immediate environment during a seizure. Gently place client on floor if seizure starts while client is standing or sitting. Never leave client during seizure
- In acute care setting, pad client's side rails. Do not restrain in active seizure
- Document details of seizure such as behavior before, onset, type of seizure, duration and postictal state
- Refrain from placing objects in client's mouth during a seizure
- Monitor client for loss of bowel and bladder continence
- Support client's airway, breathing and circulation. May need to open airway for suctioning after seizure. Administer oxygen if needed. Closely monitor client post-seizure
- Loosen clothing that is restrictive
- If status epilepticus occurs, assist in administering intravenous or rectal antiseizure medications

Priority Potential & Actual Complications

- Status epilepticus, which is continuous seizure activity with rapid spasms where the client does not experience consciousness between the seizures
- Injury to self
- May be fatal
- Mental issues, such as depression from ineffective coping

Priority Nursing Implications

- Seizures refractory to treatment may be treated with surgical extraction of the epileptic focus in the brain. Extensive evaluation needed to ensure safe surgical procedure

Priority Medications

- Phenytoin
  - Administered orally and via intravenous (slow, diluted)
  - Anticonvulsant drug to manage seizures
  - Monitor blood levels
- Carbamazepine
  - Oral and intravenous administration
  - An anticonvulsant that is also a mood stabilizer
  - Produces fewer adverse effects, it is a preferred drug for tonic-clonic and partial seizures
- Phenobarbital
  - Oral and intravenous administration (slow)
  - Barbiturate used in acute seizures and maintenance therapy

- A schedule intravenous drug that may cause dependence
  - Monitor for respiratory depression
- Clonazepam
  - Oral administration, some continuous subcutaneous use
  - Anticonvulsant drug to manage seizures
  - Gradually taper to reduce the dosage or to discontinue
- Lorazepam
  - Oral and intravenous administration
  - Benzodiazepine to manage status epilepticus
  - Usually serve as an adjunct to other antiseizure drugs for short-term seizure control

Reinforcement of Priority Teaching

- Importance of taking life-long medications to prevent seizures, taking medications as ordered and reporting any side effects to health care provider. Instruct on wearing a MedicAlert bracelet
- Identify events that trigger the seizures and how to avoid them
- Encourage avoidance of alcohol intake, poor sleep and excessive tiredness as they can trigger seizures
- Assist client to locate resources, whether online or on ground to get additional information on seizures
- Explain the importance of letting others in the immediate social circle know about their seizure disorder, in the event of an emergency
- Explain to the client that if seizure lasts more than 5 minutes, emergency medical care must be called
- Provide client with a list of how others should manage the client during and after a seizure, so client might share it with family members

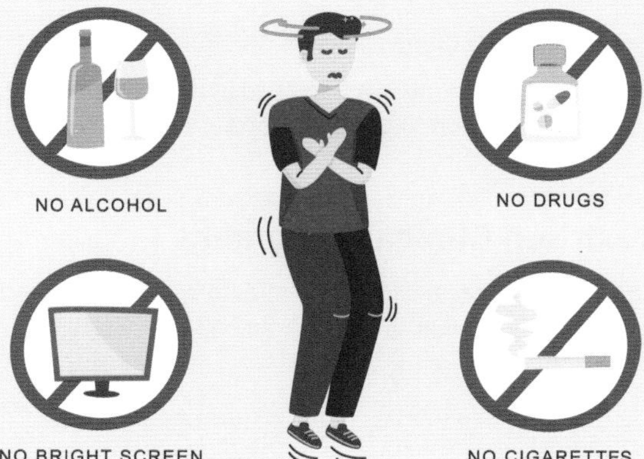
Epilepsy Seizure Prevention
NO ALCOHOL
NO DRUGS
NO BRIGHT SCREEN
NO CIGARETTES

Image 13-6: With a friend, discuss how each of these items identified in the image may precipitate seizure activity.

Clinical Hint

Clients taking phenytoin (Dilantin) to treat seizures should have their blood levels monitored at regular intervals. Phenytoin may cause gingival hyperplasia (overgrowth of the gums); therefore, the client should brush and floss their teeth and visit their dentist regularly.

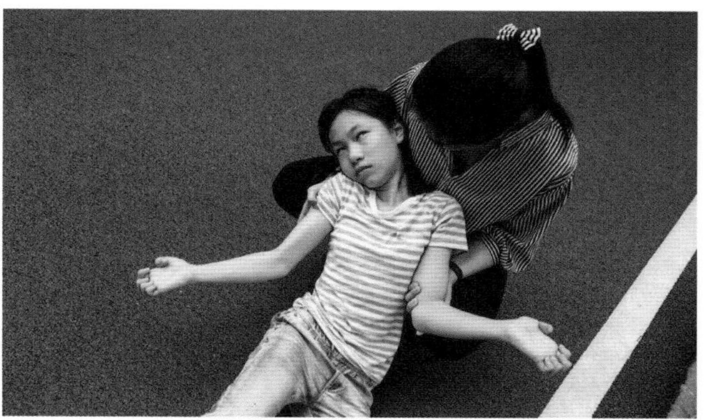

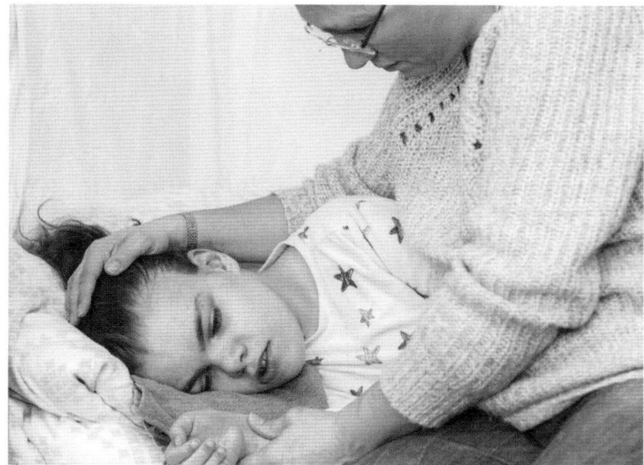

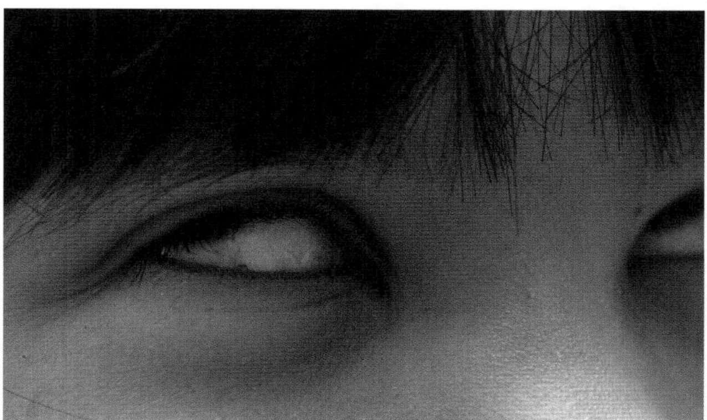

Image 13-7: These images depict clients during or after a seizure. List 5 nursing interventions appropriate for each of these clients.

Osteoporosis

Pathophysiology/Description

- Osteoporosis is a progressive metabolic disease that is marked by breakdown of bone tissue and demineralization of bone resulting in fragile bones that are susceptible to fractures
- Risk factors include female gender, estrogen deficiency in women, low calcium diet, long-term use of corticosteroid drugs, older age (older than 65) and family history
- Diseases associated with osteoporosis include kidney disease, cirrhosis, and rheumatoid arthritis

Priority Data Collection or Cues

- Brittle bones may lead to fractures and pain, especially in the vertebrea
- Ask about pain to hips that is made worse when standing or walking. Observe for poor balance
- Determine height and compare with past adult height, reduction in height might be seen from vertebral compression
- Bent shape, called dowager's hump, manifested by a humped look to the thoracic spine
- Correct usage of assistive devices, such as walkers. Client's awareness of home mobility safety

Priority Laboratory Tests/Diagnostics

- Bone mineral densitometry evaluates mineral density of bones and compares to bone mineral density of a healthy adult. Serum calcium, vitamin D, phosphorus and alkaline phosphatase
- Dual-energy X-ray absorptiometry (DXA) measures density of bones in hips, forearm and spine. A T-score of -2.5 or lower is indicative of osteoporosis

Priority Interventions or Actions

- Administer drug therapy as prescribed. Provide vitamin C, D, and calcium
- Provide diet high in protein to maintain muscle mass
- Instruct client in proper use of assistive devices. Encourage, and assist client with walking
- Provide range of motion exercises to client's tolerance to maintain functioning of joint
- Assist with application of orthotic device to protect areas of fracture

Clinical Hint

Lifestyle choices are critical in the prevention of osteoporosis.

Priority Potential & Actual Complications

- Fractures, physical immobility and hunched-over posture

Priority Nursing Implications

- With zoledronic acid therapy, client must have serum calcium and renal function tests before administration
- Kyphoplasty and vertebroplasty are two surgeries used to repair vertebral fractures from osteoporosis. They are minimally invasive surgeries

Priority Medications

- Alendronate
  - Used to treat and prevent osteoporosis
  - Given orally once a week
  - Stay in sitting position for at least 30 minutes after taking. Take 30 minutes prior to taking other drugs or food
- Ibandronate
  - Used to treat or prevent osteoporosis
  - Given once a month via the oral route
  - Stay in sitting position for at least 30 minutes after taking. Take 30 minutes prior to taking other drugs or food

Reinforcement of Priority Teaching

- Walk at least 30 minutes three times weekly to maintain bone mass
- Avoid activities that place excessive stress on the bones, such as running
- Smoking cessation, nicotine causes bone destruction
- Minimize alcohol intake, alcohol consumption contributes to bone destruction
- Encourage foods high in calcium, Vitamin C and D
- Encourage good body mechanics to avoid fractures and adequate hydration to decrease formation of kidney stones

Next Gen Clinical Judgment

What behaviors as a young and middle adult may prevent osteoporosis later in life (modifiable risk factors)?

What factors may not be changed (non-modifiable risk factors)?

Develop two to three statements the nurse may share with clients to prevent osteoporosis in later years.

Osteoarthritis

Pathophysiology/Description

- A progressive disorder marked by destruction of articular cartilage of the joints
- With time and further degeneration of cartilage, bone rubs on bone causing pain
- Causes of osteoarthritis: congenital disorders, repetitive use of joints, decreased estrogen, and damage to surrounding joint structures

Priority Data Collection or Cues

- Joint pain that is worsened by activity and alleviated by rest (this is in early stage)
- Determine factors that aggravate and relieve arthritis pain. Movement from sit to stand may be difficult
- Ability to complete daily activities. Joint pain prevents completion of activities of daily living
- Observe for redness and swelling around joints caused by osteophytes formation, called Heberden's nodes and cysts or bony outgrowths called Bouchard's nodes
- Monitor for asymmetry of affected extremities. OA usually impacts one side of the body
- Ask about stiffness of joints, usually occurs after client has been in one position for a long while
- Monitor for a grating sound (called crepitation) in joint caused by cartilage particles in the cavity of the joint
- Observe client's knees, may be bowlegged or knock-kneed

Priority Laboratory Tests/Diagnostics

- Computed tomography (CT) scan, magnetic resonance imaging (MRI) and bone scan are used to look for early arthritic chances to joint. X-rays used to stage the degree of damage to joints
- Synovial fluid analysis helps to differentiate OA from other types of arthritis. With OA, synovial fluid will be normal

Priority Interventions or Actions

- Administer drug therapy as prescribed. Assist with completion of activities of daily living
- Provide range of motion exercises. Initiate physical and occupational therapy consult as indicated
- Immobilize affected joint with brace or splint as prescribed, in acute phase of inflammation
- Use device such as a bed cradle to keep pressure from bed linens off client's affected feet
- Use moist heat to help with stiffness. Ensure client rests during acute flare-up

Priority Potential & Actual Complications

- Physical immobility, sleep disturbances, disability and social isolation
- Gout and bone death (called osteonecrosis)

Priority Nursing Implications

- Osteoarthritis may be debilitating in advanced stages
- Osteoarthritis may affect client's ability for self-care. Sensitivity and support are critically important

Priority Medications

- Non-steroidal anti-inflammatory drugs (NSAIDs)
  - There are several NSAIDs that can be used. Ibuprofen is one that is commonly used; oral administration
  - Most significant adverse effect of NSAIDs is gastrointestinal bleeding
- Capsaicin cream
  - Topical analgesic that blocks pain impulse
  - Available by prescription and over-the-counter
- Cortisone
  - Corticosteroids used to treat OA when joint is inflamed and swollen
  - Injected into the joint
  - Further intervention is needed if after 4 injections the pain and swelling are not relieved

Reinforcement of Priority Teaching

- Use heat to treat affected joints but use a cold compress with active inflammation
- Use of splints on affected joint as prescribed. Administration of drugs for pain
- Use of assistive device to assist with immobility, such as cane and walker
- Weight loss to minimize stress on the joints. End exercise and rest if pain starts in affected joint
- Importance of modifying the home environment to enhance safety

Next Gen Clinical Judgment

Irreparable damage can occur in a client with osteoarthritis. Identify two readily and easily recognizable signs of osteoarthritis and identify three interventions in treating clients with these two signs.

Peripheral neuropathy

Pathophysiology/Description

- Peripheral neuropathy results when there is damage to peripheral nerves. The peripheral nervous system controls signals between the body and the central nervous system. Impairment in this system causes disruptions of signals and clinical manifestations in parts of the body, depending on the nerves that are affected
- Causes of peripheral neuropathy are multifactorial
  - Diabetes mellitus, infections, trauma, vascular problems and tumors
  - Excessive alcohol intake, inherited and autoimmune diseases
- The overarching symptoms of peripheral neuropathy are muscle atrophy, weakness, diminished reflexes, loss of sensation, numbness and tingling to extremities

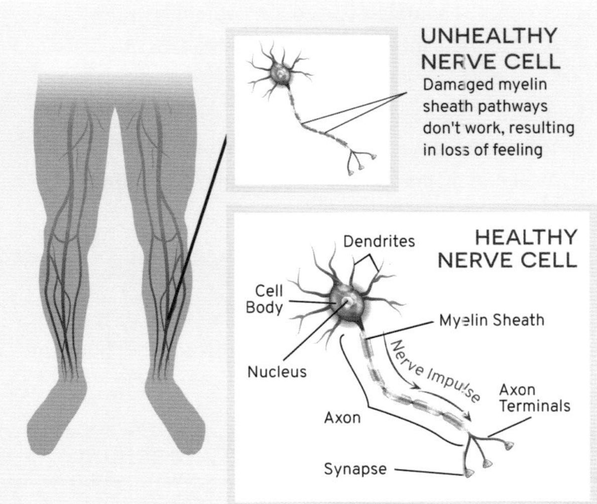

Image 13-8: What words might a client use to describe peripheral neuropathy in a foot or other area of the body?

Priority Data Collection or Cues

- Clinical manifestations and data collection relate to the nerves that are affected in the body
  - Bowel and/or bladder incontinence. Decreased sensation
  - Extremities (primarily feet) for weakness, numbness, tingling and open wounds
  - Ask about heat intolerance. Burning or sticking pain in extremities
  - Decreased or heightened sensitivity to pain and pressure
  - Involuntary muscle twitching. Diminished reflexes

Priority Laboratory Tests/Diagnostics

- Electromyography (EMG), and nerve conduction velocity tests check the electrical activity of nerves and muscles
- Quantitative Sensory Testing (QST) is used to determine small and large nerve ending damages
- Autonomic Testing used to determine functioning of the autonomic nervous system
- Computed tomography (CT) scan and magnetic resonance imaging (MRI) will look for tumors or other conditions causing nerve impairment
- Nerve biopsy to look for nerve abnormalities
- Some of the many laboratory tests used for peripheral neuropathy
  - Thyroid panel for hypothyroidism and blood glucose to determine control of diabetes
  - Comprehensive metabolic panel to determine metabolic conditions
  - Vitamin B12 for vitamin deficiencies and antinuclear nuclear antibody for autoimmune conditions

Priority Interventions or Actions

- Intervention is first directed toward controlling or alleviating the underlying cause
- Peripheral neuropathy is a common comorbidity with other disorders
  - Administer pain medication as prescribed
  - Minimize client's risk for injury by removing obstacles in immediate environment
  - Apply any special extremity devices, such as hand splint or orthotic shoes, if prescribed
  - Assist with ambulation and use of assistive devices, like walker or cane to minimize risk of falls
  - Check bath water to ensure correct temperature to avoid burning skin
  - If the client is hypersensitive to touch, use a bed cradle
  - Provide client with slippers or ask family members to bring slippers from home to avoid walking barefooted
  - Provide incontinent care or provide client with cleaning supplies
  - Perform range of motion to weakened muscles

Priority Potential & Actual Complications

- Trauma to skin, falls, and physical disability
- Infection, cellulitis, osteomyelitis

Priority Nursing Implications

- Peripheral neuropathy is often associated with diabetes. Inspect the feet and hands of clients with diabetes to find wounds or infections not felt by clients
- In the older client, it is challenging to diagnose peripheral neuropathy as many symptoms of the condition might be mistaken for the normal aging process

Priority Medications

- Non-steroidal anti-inflammatory drugs (NSAIDs)
  - There are several NSAIDs that can be used. Ibuprofen is one that is commonly used and is administered orally
  - Most significant adverse effect of NSAIDs is gastrointestinal bleeding, from platelet aggregation
- Gabapentin
  - Generally administered orally for neuropathic pain
  - Treat nerve pain, causes drowsiness and dizziness
- Pregabalin
  - Generally administered orally for neuropathic pain
- Capsaicin cream
  - Topical analgesic that blocks pain impulse
  - Available by prescription and over-the-counter
- Amitriptyline
  - Oral antidepressant that treats neuropathic pain by manipulating chemical processes in brain
- Nortriptyline
  - Oral antidepressant that treats neuropathic pain by manipulating chemical processes in brain
  - May cause crawling feeling and numbness

Reinforcement of Priority Teaching

- Smoking cessation since smoking constricts blood vessels which causes poor circulation
- Exercise to get more oxygen and blood flowing to nerves
- Good diabetes management, to include checking blood glucose, eating healthy and taking prescribed medications
- Instruct client to check feet daily for wounds. Demonstrate the use of a mirror to examine the plantar surface of feet
- Instruct client to wear shoes in and outside of the house to decrease risk of injury to feet
- Explain the importance of taking prescribed medications to manage conditions that cause peripheral neuropathy
- Explain that wearing splints and orthopedic shoes can help to take pressure off the nerves
- Direct client on taking pain medication to relieve pain
- Provide instructions on use of a Transcutaneous electrical nerve stimulation (TENS) device, if prescribed
- Explain importance of physical and/or occupational therapy to help improve function of impaired extremity
- Counsel client to limit alcohol intake

Clinical Hint

Clients with diabetes are at risk for neuropathy. Diabetic neuropathy is nerve damage most often in the legs and feet. Clients typically complain of pain and numbness. This condition is caused by uncontrolled blood glucose levels.

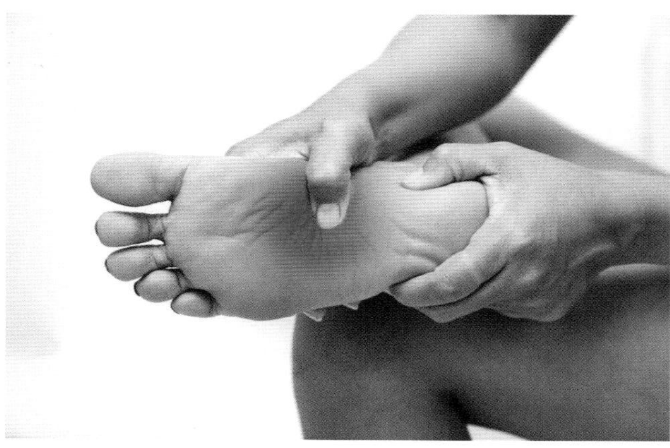

Image 13-9: What data should the nurse collect when a client presents with peripheral neuropathy?

Next Gen Clinical Judgment

Use the lines to list important nursing actions to keep clients with peripheral neuropathy safe.

Pathophysiology/Description

- Trigeminal neuralgia (TN) is a form of chronic neuropathic pain that affects the 5th cranial nerve, the trigeminal nerve. It causes severe, sudden, stabbing, shock-like episodes of facial pain. This is type 1 TN which is classified as classic TN. There is also an atypical aspect to the condition called type 2 TN
- Type 2 TN is characterized by burning, aching and stabbing pain that is constant, but the severity may be less intense than type 1 TN. Clients with TN can experience both types
- Causes of TN are multiple sclerosis, tumors that cause nerve compression, vascular compression of the trigeminal nerve and shingles
- Medications are used to control TN, but clients can choose to have surgery to treat TN if medication therapy fails or if they cannot tolerate the medications
- Types of surgery
  - Microvascular decompression: removing/displacing blood vessels that compress the nerve
  - Brain stereotactic radiosurgery (Gamma knife): use of radiation to damage trigeminal nerve
  - Balloon compression: a hollow needle inserted through face, flexible catheter with balloon on end threaded through the needle. Pressure from the inflated balloon damages the nerve
  - Glycerol injections: needle inserted in face and guided to spinal fluid that surrounds the trigeminal nerve ganglion. Sterile glycerol is injected to damage the nerve
  - Radiofrequency rhizotomy: hollow needle inserted through face and electrode is inserted via the needle. Through alternating wakefulness and sedation, the part of the nerve associated with the pain is located and heat from the electrode damages the nerve fibers

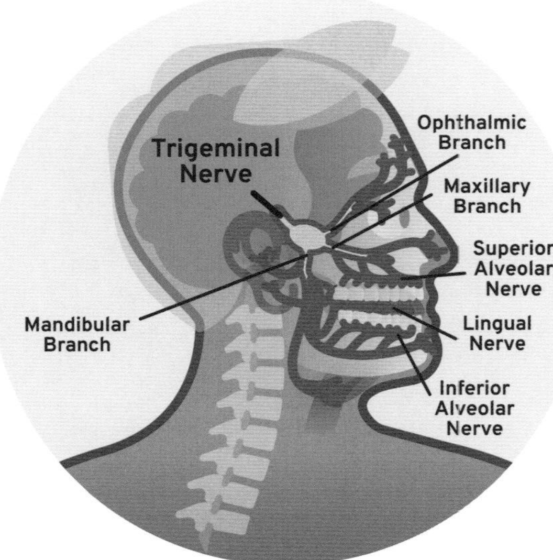

Image 13-10: The image depicts the nerves in the face and head. How do the locations of these nerves relate to the signs and symptoms of trigeminal neuralgia?

Priority Data Collection or Cues

- Ask client about onset of pain, usually described as sudden and abrupt
- Ask client to describe the pain, usually described as stabbing, burning, knife-like in type 1 TN or constant, aching and burning in type 2 TN
- Examine location of pain, usually pain is on the nose, lips, cheeks and gums
- Ask about triggers for the pain, clients usually state pain is triggered by touch, to a specific spot on the face, by actions such as yawning, washing the face, shaving, chewing, talking, wind exposure and applying makeup, among others
- Monitor for severity of symptoms, which can be episodic in the beginning but with shorter pain free episodes as the condition progresses
- Monitor sleep pattern as some clients will sleep excessively to avoid the pain
- Observe client to determine hygiene practices (especially facial, oral and hair care), as some clients may neglect hygiene care to avoid the pain

Priority Laboratory Tests/Diagnostics

- Magnetic resonance imaging (MRI) is done to see if there are other causes of the pain
- Complete neurologic examination

Priority Interventions or Actions

- Administer medications as prescribed
- Provide foods to client that are not at extremes of temperature
- Provide meals that are soft, where chewing is not needed
- Provide an environment that is not drafty/windy
- Provide hygiene care after client has been medicated to minimize pain
- Postoperative interventions
  - Monitor client's pain and compare with preoperative pain
  - Administer pain medication as prescribed
  - Monitor client's facial nerve, corneal reflex, hearing and extraocular muscles often to ensure no major damage
  - Apply cold compress/ice pack to face on the surgical side for 3 to 5 hours after a percutaneous radiofrequency rhizotomy
  - If surgery involved a small craniotomy, as with microvascular decompression procedure, monitor neurological status frequently, specifically intracranial pressure and level of consciousness
  - Monitor surgery site for bleeding and signs of infection

Priority Potential & Actual Complications

- Facial paralysis
- Depression and social isolation
- Weight loss from fear of eating (due to pain triggered by chewing)
- Poor personal hygiene, especially oral and facial

Priority Nursing Implications

- The pain from trigeminal neuralgia can be so excruciating that clients with the condition avoid the triggers that cause the pain, such as mouth care, facial care (shaving) and eating
- Clients withdraw from socialization because of fear of having attacks of pain in public

Priority Medications

- Gabapentin
  - Oral neuropathic pain agent
  - Treat nerve pain, causes drowsiness and dizziness
- Amitriptyline
  - Oral antidepressant that treats trigeminal neuralgia by manipulating chemical processes in brain
- Carbamazepine
  - Oral anti-seizure medication that treats pain by blocking the firing of nerves
- Clonazepam
  - Oral anti-seizure medication that treats pain by blocking the firing of nerves
  - Drowsiness and dizziness are common side effects

Reinforcement of Priority Teaching

- Chew foods on the side of the mouth that is not affected
- Need for a soft toothbrush
- Protect face from temperature extremes such as strong winds
- Importance of proper hygiene and that medicating self before hygiene activities will reduce the pain
- Advise client to avoid eating foods that are either too hot or too cold. Encourage lukewarm, soft foods that do not require much chewing
- Eat foods that have high caloric value and proteins
- Explain to clients that when having percutaneous procedures, they will be awake
- Counsel client not to chew foods on the surgery side of the face until sensation returns to the face
- Monitor surgery site for signs of infection
- If corneal damage occurred from surgery, instruct client to wear an eye shield. Reinforce importance of having regular eye exams

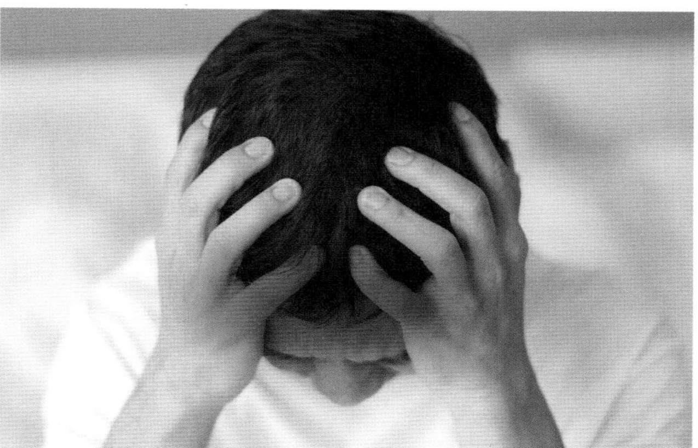

Image 13-11: List priority interventions that can be used to assist this client in treating trigeminal neuralgia pain.

Next Gen Clinical Judgment

A client has undergone surgery for trigeminal neuralgia pain. List 3 statements, made by the client, that would indicate a need for the client to contact their health care provider?

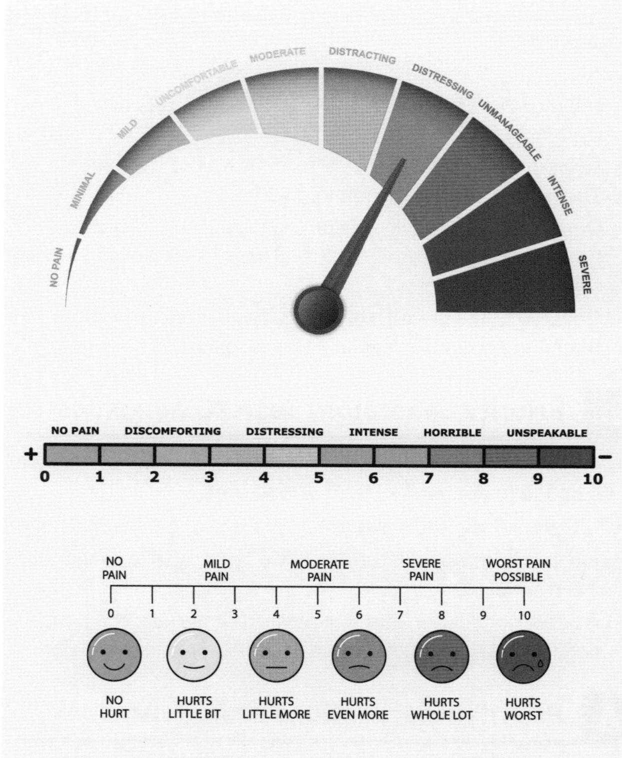

Image 13-12: How should the nurse use these tools to determine the level of pain a client is experiencing?

Carpal tunnel

Pathophysiology/Description

- Carpal tunnel syndrome (CTS) occurs when there is compression of the median nerve, the nerve that runs from the forearm into the palm of the hand via the carpal tunnel
- Persons who engage in occupations or hobbies that require repetitive wrist movement are at high-risk for getting CTS
- Additional contributing factors to CTS
  - Trauma to wrist
  - Hormonal involvement during pregnancy or menopause
  - Rheumatoid arthritis
  - Diabetes mellitus
  - Peripheral vascular disease
- For symptoms that persist longer than 6 months, carpal tunnel release surgery is recommended. This involves cutting a ligament around the wrist to take pressure off the median nerve. This is usually done in an outpatient setting

Priority Data Collection or Cues

- Observe for weakness in affected arm
- Ask client about numbness, impaired sensation, itching and pain in affected hand and fingers
- Ask about onset of pain. Pain and numbness may cause client to awaken from sleep at nights
- Ask client to form a fist. This is sometimes difficult to do with CTS
- Observe use of client's thumb. With chronic CTS, the muscles at the base of the thumb may become dysfunctional
- Monitor client's ability to perform fine hand movements. These are quite often impaired with CTS
- Observe for a positive Phalen's sign which manifests as tingling in the hands when the wrist is freely flexed for more than 60 seconds
- Observe for positive Tinel's sign, manifested as tingling in the hands when the medial nerve is tapped

Priority Laboratory Tests/Diagnostics

- X-rays of the arm and hand can show conditions that cause damage to the nerves, such as fractures
- Ultrasound will show abnormality in size of the median nerve
- Electromyography determines the severity of damage to the median nerve
- A nerve conduction study assesses the nerve's ability to send a signal along the nerve or to the muscle

Priority Interventions or Actions

- Administer medications as prescribed
- Immobilize the hand using a splint
- Postoperative interventions, if client opted for surgery
  - Monitor pain level and administer analgesics as prescribed
  - Monitor vital signs
  - Examine dressing for bleeding
  - Examine wound for signs of infection
  - Monitor neurovascular status of fingers
  - Referral to physical therapist

Priority Potential & Actual Complications

- Dysfunction of the affected hand, if no surgical intervention
- Complications related to surgery
  - Bleeding
  - Median nerve injury
  - Scarring that may be sensitive
  - Infection
  - Damage to blood vessels

Priority Nursing Implications

- Carpal tunnel release can take two approaches, open release surgery or endoscopic carpal tunnel release. The endoscopic approach affords for quicker recovery time and has less discomfort postoperatively

Priority Medications

- Non-steroidal anti-inflammatory drugs (NSAIDs) is choice of pain medication for CTS
  - There are several NSAIDs that can be used. Oral ibuprofen is one that is commonly used
  - Most significant adverse effect of NSAIDs is gastrointestinal bleeding

Reinforcement of Priority Teaching

- Encourage the use of a hand splint at night to decrease nighttime numbness and pain
- Instruct client to seek physical therapy care
- Be very careful when picking up objects that can slip from hand and cause damage, such as a cup with hot beverage
- Take frequent breaks from repetitive tasks
- Explain application of ice packs to wrist that becomes swollen and red
- Carpal tunnel release surgery
  - How to change dressing at the surgery site
  - How to monitor for infection
  - How to don and doff splint
  - Full recovery is not instantaneous and may take a few months
  - Strength is decreased after surgery but will improve with time
  - Plan on modifying work for a few weeks, especially if it involves repetitive hand movements
  - Consider changing jobs, if possible
  - May develop nerve damage from surgery
  - Wear fingerless gloves at work to keep hands warm
  - Use a work desk that keeps hands in a neutral position while working

Pathophysiology/Description

- Amputation is defined as removal of a body part, usually limb or part of a limb, due to trauma or by surgery
- Amputation is highest in older adults due to disease processes such as diabetes mellitus and peripheral vascular conditions. When younger individuals have amputations, it is quite often the result of trauma

Priority Data Collection or Cues

- Observe client's and family's emotional state regarding amputation
- Determine client's knowledge of pre and postoperative care
- If amputation is from sudden traumatic event, observe for bleeding and hemodynamic instability of client, such as hypotension, tachycardia, hypovolemic shock and stabilize for surgery

Priority Laboratory Tests/Diagnostics

- Arteriogram, venogram and Doppler studies will show blood flow through the arteries and veins of the extremity, usually poor circulation is identified
- Complete blood cell count will show elevated white blood cell count if infection results from the amputation

Priority Interventions or Actions

- If traumatic amputation, stabilize the client to minimize hemorrhage and maintain hemodynamic status
- Preoperative interventions
  - Ensure client's questions regarding surgery are answered
  - Discuss what will occur in the postoperative phase of care
  - Reinforce instructions on use of incentive spirometry and deep breathing exercises that will be used after surgery
  - Discuss phantom limb pain that might be experienced when the limb is removed
- Postoperative interventions
  - Monitor for bleeding and signs of infection at surgery site
  - Ongoing monitoring of vital signs to determine hemodynamic stability
  - Administer pain medications as prescribed
  - Encourage client and family to discuss feelings about loss of limb. Monitor for posttraumatic stress disorder and provide appropriate consultations as needed
  - Ensure that a surgical tourniquet is available in the event of excessive bleeding
  - Prevent flexion contractures (common in hip joint). Assist client to lie on abdomen with hip extended a few times throughout the day
  - Maintain sterility in dressing changes to prevent infection
  - Ensure physical and occupational therapists are involved in client's care
  - Assist client with ambulation
  - Apply compression bandage as ordered to decrease swelling, promote healing, shrink residual limb and decrease pain

Priority Potential & Actual Complications

- Hemorrhage
- Phantom pain
- Physical disability
- Mental disorders such as depression

Priority Nursing Implications

- Amputations that occur in upper extremities are usually more devastating because they usually happen because of traumatic events, giving the client no time to prepare for the loss. The role of the nurse here is crucial when it comes to helping the client cope with the sudden loss

Priority Medications

- Pain medication is per the choice of the surgeon and the client's needs

Reinforcement of Priority Teaching

- Explain to client that phantom pain from missing limb usually subsides
- Use mirror therapy for phantom limb sensation and pain. Looking at the remaining limb in the mirror sends a signal to the brain that the other limb is not there
- Discuss the importance of maintaining appointments for physical and/or occupational therapy
- Encourage client not to hang or dangle the residual limb over the side of the bed to prevent swelling
- Clean residual limb nightly with bacteriostatic soap and warm water and do not use lotions or oils on the limb unless prescribed
- Instructions not to elevate residual limb on pillow
- Assist client with performing active range of motion exercises, when tolerable
- When walking for the first time, the missing limb may distort their position in space, making them uncoordinated and increasing their risk of falling
- Demonstrate crutch walking
- Explain that full weight can be borne on the prosthesis about 90 days following amputation
- Demonstrate how to change dressings and look for infection
- Complications that warrant a call to health care provider
- How to keep the prosthesis socket clean by washing with water and soap and rinsing well
- Explain the importance of properly maintaining the prosthesis and wearing shoes that are properly fitted
- Explain importance of modifying the home environment to enhance safety

Pathophysiology/Description

- Amyotrophic lateral sclerosis (ALS), known as Lou Gehrig's disease. A progressive, degenerative neuromuscular disorder that involves death of motor neurons in the brain and spinal cord
- More common in men than women and onset is usually somewhere between age 50 and 75
- Causes and risk factors
  - Genetic mutation and hereditary, dysfunctional immune response, and environmental toxins
  - Excess levels of glutamate in the brain and having served in the military

Priority Data Collection or Cues

- Monitor respiratory status to detect any early respiratory compromise
- Monitor for fatigue and falls
- May find client's speech is slurred
- Observe the client's ability to ambulate, may see that client trips while walking
- Inquire whether client experiences muscle cramps and twitching. Observe for muscle wasting
- Ask if client has been dropping things, common with ALS. Observe for spastic muscles
- Client may have difficulty sleeping. Ask about bowel habits, constipation is common
- Observe when eating, may find difficulty swallowing and drooling
- Observe posture, may find that client has difficulty maintaining good posture

Priority Laboratory Tests/Diagnostics

- Electromyography determines the severity of damage to the median nerve. A nerve conduction study monitors the nerve's ability to send a signal along the nerve or to the muscle
- Magnetic resonance imaging (MRI) can show other conditions that may be causing the symptoms

Priority Interventions or Actions

- Administer medications as prescribed. Provide foods that are easy to swallow to prevent aspiration
- Assist with limb and trunk exercises to minimize spastic muscles. Maintain a safe environment
- Provide tracheostomy care if client has a tracheostomy
- Initiate physical, occupational, speech and psychological consults as prescribed

Priority Potential & Actual Complications

- Total dependence for all activities of daily living (ADLs), inability to speak
- Respiratory compromise from muscle paralysis, respiratory depression, and death

Priority Nursing Implications

- Riluzole causes liver function changes so monitor liver function while taking the drug
- Be empathetic as physical care is provided, understanding that client and family are likely very distressed with the diagnosis and the impending decline of client's status

Priority Medications

- Riluzole
  - Works by decreasing the release of glutamate, thus minimizing damage to motor neurons
  - Taken orally, must be taken at least an hour before, or two hours after, a meal
- Edaravone
  - Slows decline in daily functioning
  - May causes dizziness, tachycardia and skin rash
  - Administered intravenous according to protocol

Reinforcement of Priority Teaching

- Explain the long-term trajectory of the disease. Ensure completion of advance directives and end-of-life care
- Encourage exercise to reduce muscle spasticity. Foods that have high nutrition value and are easy to swallow
- Observe for signs and symptoms of respiratory muscle decline and explain when emergency help is to be sought
- A safe home environment to minimize risk of falls. Ensure access to speech, physical and occupational therapy
- Counsel clients that medications may slow, not cure, the disease process
- Discuss other medications to treat symptoms of ALS such as constipation and sleep problems
- Recommend a psychosocial consult to manage the long-term emotional, social and financial implications of ALS

Clinical Hint

Currently there is no cure for ALS and treatment is aimed at relieving symptoms and slow the disease progression. Most people with ALS will live between 3 and 5 years after symptoms appear.

Guillain-Barré syndrome

Pathophysiology/Description

- Guillain-Barré Syndrome (GBS) is an autoimmune, acute inflammation of peripheral and cranial nerves
- Myelin sheath is lost and the nerves that are affected become edematous and inflamed causing a slowing or inhibition of nerve impulses
- Guillain-Barré syndrome is usually seen after a person has had an infection of the respiratory or gastrointestinal tract

Priority Data Collection or Cues

- Observe respiratory status to detect symptoms of respiratory failure, a major complication of GBS
- Monitor results of arterial blood gasses and need for ventilator support. Look for cardiac dysrhythmias
- Monitor pain, which may be worse during the night. Numbness and tingling of the extremities. Absent reflexes
- Muscle strength shows weakness and/or paralysis. Energy level may be decreased
- Look for hypertension, orthostatic hypotension and bradycardia
- Monitor for paralytic ileus, drooling indicating inadequate gag reflex, and difficulty swallowing
- Ask client about sleep patterns. Client may report less sleep because of pain at nights
- Monitor bowel and bladder status, often see incontinence in both

Priority Laboratory Tests/Diagnostics

- Electromyography (EMG) shows cause of weakness. Lumbar puncture shows elevated protein level
- Nerve conduction tests response of the nerves and muscles to electrical impulses

Priority Interventions or Actions

- Have emergency equipment at bedside, cough and deep breathe, and monitor respiratory status
- Monitor for progression of paralysis. Perform activities when muscle strength is optimal
- Turn and reposition every two hours or more frequently. Use pressure relieving devices
- Perform meticulous skin care if incontinent of bladder and bowel
- Provide foods that are easy to swallow to prevent aspiration
- Administer nutrition via enteral or parenteral route if unable to eat orally
- Prepare client for plasmapheresis or intravenous immunoglobulin as prescribed
- Ensure referrals to speech, occupational and physical therapists

Priority Potential & Actual Complications

- Respiratory infection, respiratory failure, paralysis and death

Priority Nursing Implications

- The symptoms in GBS can move very quickly and progress to a life-threatening stage in a few hours. Clients with early symptoms must be treated rapidly before more muscle groups, such as those in the chest and diaphragm, are impacted causing respiratory and cardiac failure

Priority Medications

- Immunoglobulin (intravenous Ig), given at a high dose
  - Best effect is seen when administered to client within 14 days of symptoms starting
  - Blocks damaging antibodies. This is the preferred treatment over plasmapheresis

Reinforcement of Priority Teaching

- Recovery is slow, but most people usually recover fully
- Triggers that increase symptoms, when to seek healthcare, and signs and symptoms of infection
- Advise the client to get adequate rest and exercise and to eat a well balanced diet that is easy to swallow
- Resources that may help client and family cope with the condition

Next Gen Clinical Judgment

Identify the top three safety concerns related to the nursing care of the client with Guillain-Barré Syndrome.

____

____

____

____

____

____

Myasthenia gravis

Pathophysiology/Description

- Myasthenia gravis (MG) is an autoimmune, neuromuscular disease where significant weakness and fatigue of skeletal muscle groups occur
- The disease is characterized by an attack on acetylcholine by antibodies, resulting in decreased numbers of acetylcholine receptor sites at the neuromuscular junction
- Excessive secretion of cholinesterase, not enough secretion of acetylcholine, or muscle fibers that do not respond to acetylcholine are causes of MG
- Factors that precipitate MG
  - Pregnancy
  - Stress
  - Extremes of temperature
  - Certain drugs
  - Trauma
  - Menstruation
- The thymus gland, though small in adults, seems to foster the production of acetylcholine antibodies so clients can choose to have it removed in a procedure called a thymectomy

Priority Data Collection or Cues

- Monitor respiratory status to detect symptoms of respiratory compromise as MG can cause difficulty breathing and respiratory insufficiency
- Monitor breath sounds as client is at risk for respiratory infection
- Ask client about energy level, MG causes muscle weakness and fatigue
- Examine client's vision, may find double vision. Observe eyes, may find ptosis
- Observe client eating, may see difficulty chewing and swallowing
- Observe client's speech, may find difficulty speaking and/or client's voice fades away with continuous conversation, caused by progressive weakness to muscle
- Monitor client for infection as it can exacerbate MG, causing a myasthenic crisis

Priority Laboratory Tests/Diagnostics

- Edrophonium test (Tensilon test) elicits sudden improvement in muscle strength indicating MG
- Electromyography (EMG) examines electrical activity between client's brain and muscles, may find poor electrical activity
- Chest X-ray to look for respiratory involvement, such as pneumonia
- Computed tomography (CT) scan to examine the thymus gland for tumors or other abnormalities
- Acetylcholine receptor antibodies test will be positive for the antibodies

Priority Interventions or Actions

- Place emergency equipment at client's bedside in the event of a cholinergic or myasthenic crisis
- Monitor client's respiratory system. Ensure effective breathing. Encourage coughing and deep breathing. Monitor for respiratory failure
- Administer anticholinesterase drugs as prescribed and monitor for adverse effects
- Monitor for cholinergic crisis caused by excessive anticholinesterase drugs
- Monitor for myasthenic crisis caused by insufficient medication, infection, fatigue or progression of MG that was not identified
- Monitor muscles for improved strength, indicating therapeutic effect of drugs
- Ongoing monitoring of vital signs
- Encourage ambulation to prevent complications of immobility. Plan activities around times when client's muscle strength is optimal
- Balance activity and rest to prevent fatigue
- Provide foods that are easy to swallow to decrease risk of aspiration. Monitor for aspiration
- Prepare client for plasmapheresis if prescribed
- Prepare client for administration of intravenous immunoglobulin G, if prescribed

Priority Potential & Actual Complications

- Myasthenic crisis
- Cholinergic crisis
- Tumors of the thymus

Priority Nursing Implications

- Myasthenic crisis is an acute flare-up of weakness in the muscles that is triggered by certain illnesses, pregnancy, surgery or various other stressors. This crisis may cause respiratory insufficiency because of weakness to muscles that impact breathing and swallowing. Anticholinesterase medications must be increased to address this condition
- Cholinergic crisis occurs when too much anticholinesterase drug has been administered. The condition is manifested by nausea, vomiting, abdominal pain, increased bronchial secretions, blurred vision, sweating, pupillary miosis and hypotension. Stop anticholinesterase and administer atropine sulfate
- Myasthenia gravis is a balance of acetylcholine levels in the body. Weakness may be related to high and low levels of this neurotransmitter.

Priority Medications

- Pyridostigmine
  - Administered orally (may also be IM or intravenous)
  - Anticholinesterase to treat MG
  - Timing of medications is critical
- Neostigmine
  - Administered IM, intravenous or subcutaneously
  - Anticholinesterase
  - Dose titrated to individual client
- Atropine sulfate: Anticholinergic drug
  - Given intravenous or IM
  - Treat anticholinesterase toxicity/cholinergic crisis
  - Large doses of neostigmine should be accompanied by a dose of atropine
- Edrophonium
  - Used in tension test to diagnose myasthenia gravis
  - Positive for MG if client's muscle strength improves within seconds after administration
- Azathioprine
  - Given orally or via intravenous in clients with MG if other medications are ineffective
  - Immunosuppressant medication

Next Gen Clinical Judgment

Compare and contrast the appearance of a client with myasthenic crisis and one with cholinergic crisis.

Reinforcement of Priority Teaching

- Long-term trajectory of the disease and what the needs will be, living with the disease
- Help client to recognize triggers that worsen the symptoms of MG
- Explain to client signs and symptoms of an infection and to seek care immediately
- Importance of a good balance of rest and exercise
- Eat a well-balanced nutritious meal that is semisolid and easy to swallow
- Schedule medications for maximal muscle strength effect at time of activity, such as eating
- Signs and symptoms of cholinergic and myasthenic crisis
- Other options of treatment for myasthenia gravis beyond medications, such as plasmapheresis or surgery
- Importance of seeking pharmacist or health care provider's opinion before taking over-the-counter medications
- Administration of medications, adhering to the cautions with each drug and observing for side effects
- Provide information on resources that may assist client with coping with the disease such as Myasthenia Gravis Foundation

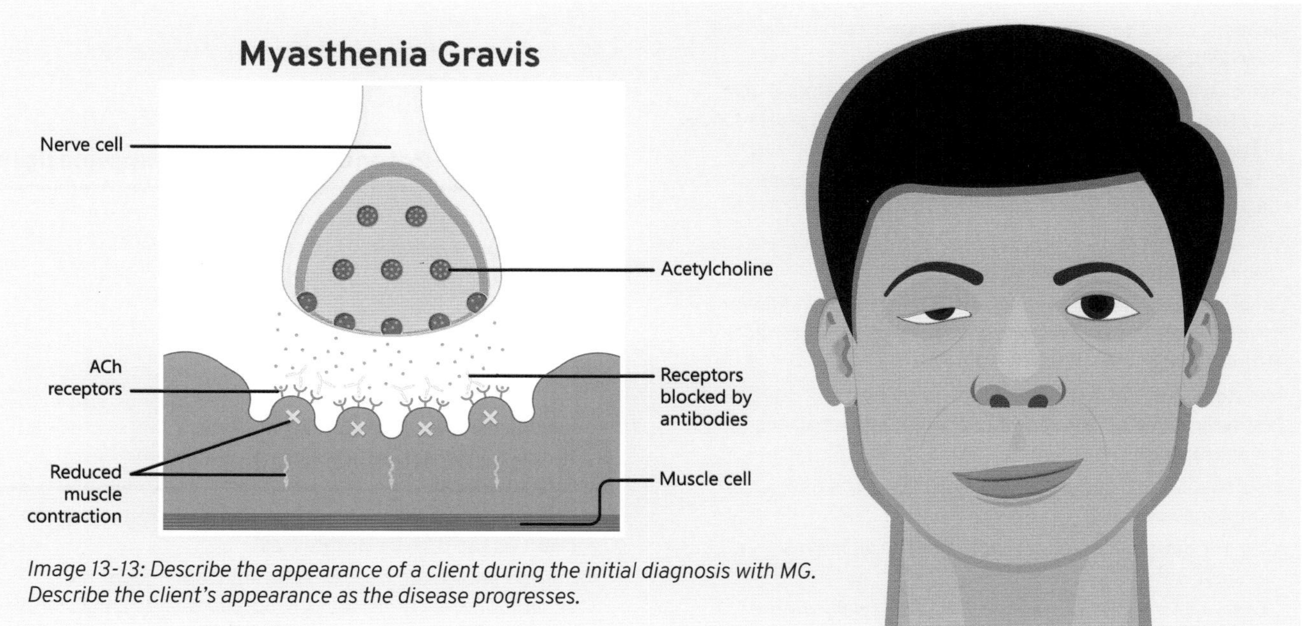

Image 13-13: Describe the appearance of a client during the initial diagnosis with MG. Describe the client's appearance as the disease progresses.

Parkinson's disease

Pathophysiology/Description

- Parkinson's disease is a chronic neurodegenerative disease that is characterized by lack of the chemical messenger, dopamine. Dopamine is needed for proper functioning of the extrapyramidal system so when dopamine is lacking, the extrapyramidal system malfunctions
- The main features of Parkinson's disease are gross slowness in starting and executing movement along with resting tremors and gait disturbance
- Parkinson's disease is seen mostly in men and diagnosis occurs as age increases. The disease slowly progresses, often ending in disability and total dependence for care needs
- Causes
  - Genetics
  - Environmental factors such as exposure to pesticides, well water, industrial chemicals
  - Residing in rural areas
  - Lewy bodies, which are clumps of protein found in brain of clients with Parkinson's disease
- Antiparkinsonian drugs are the mainstay of treating Parkinson's disease. Surgical therapy is also available. These include ablation (destruction of affected part of brain), deep brain stimulation (using electrodes to decrease activity produced by depletion of dopamine) and transplantation of fetal neural tissue in the brain of person with Parkinson's disease. Transplantation research is continuing

Priority Data Collection or Cues

- Monitor client's gait, may observe shuffling gait, classic of later stage Parkinson's disease
- Observe movement, will see bradykinesia. Look for purposeful movement, may find akinesia
- Examine client's stance, will find a stooped posture where trunk and head lean forward
- Ask client to write something and observe writing. Words may trail off the page and be smaller than when started, due to tremors
- Observe for tremors that increase at rest and decrease when hands are active
- Observe facial expression, may see a masklike expression (called deadpan expression)
- Observe client's posture, will see rigidity that can appear to have jerkiness (called cogwheel rigidity). Examine muscle strength, may find muscle weakness
- Monitor client for postural instability by performing the pull test (stand behind client and tug client backward, eliciting a backward fall)
- Listen to client's speech,which may be slurred and monotone speech
- Look for bowel and bladder incontinence which may manifest with Parkinson's disease
- Observe client eating, may see difficulty swallowing, as dysphagia is common as Parkinson's disease progresses. Look for drooling
- Monitor client for psychological complications of Parkinson's disease such as depression and apathy

Priority Laboratory Tests/Diagnostics

- Computed tomography (CT) scan and magnetic resonance (MRI) to rule out other conditions such as a brain tumor
- Response to antiparkinsonian drug test: improvement in symptoms when this drug is given, confirms the diagnosis of Parkinson's disease

Priority Interventions or Actions

- Administer antiparkinsonian drugs
- Perform range of motion to client's tolerance to maintain mobility of joints and muscles. Initiate consult with physical therapy to prevent contractures and muscle wasting
- Turn and reposition client every two hours or more frequently, to prevent pressure ulcers. Use pressure relieving devices on bed
- Perform meticulous skin care for client who is incontinent of bladder and bowel
- Provide assistive device to help with ambulation
- Have client use strategies to minimize risk of falls, such as rocking from side to side, stepping over a line on the floor and lifting toes when stepping
- Plan activities around times when client's muscle strength is optimal
- Balance activity and rest to prevent fatigue
- Provide foods that are easy to chew and swallow to decrease risk of aspiration, because of dysphagia. Ensure food is cleared from mouth to prevent aspiration
- Provide foods that are high in calories
- Monitor constipation. Provide high fiber in diet and adequate fluids
- Administer nutrition via enteral or parenteral route if client is unable to eat orally

Priority Potential & Actual Complications

- Involuntary movements (dyskinesias)
- Psychiatric problems such as depression
- Dementia
- Dysphagia with resulting malnutrition
- Muscle weakness
- Injuries from falls

Priority Nursing Implications

- Parkinson's disease will become very debilitating for the client as the disease progresses
- Caregivers should be fully knowledgeable about the expectations as the disease progresses and can better plan for care of the client

Priority Medications

- Levodopa
  - Oral dopaminergic/antiparkinsonian agent
  - Dose can be increased to reach desired effect
- Levodopa/carbidopa
  - Oral dopaminergic/antiparkinsonian agent
  - May cause dyskinesia (involuntary and uncontrolled movement)
  - Carbidopa ensures more medication is able to reach the brain and be effective
- Ropinirole
  - Administered orally
  - Dopamine receptor agonist
  - May have fewer side effects than other dopamine agonists
- Benztropine
  - Generally given orally with Parkinson's disease
  - Anticholinergic drug. Works by balancing cholinergic and dopaminergic activities
- Diphenhydramine
  - Generally given orally with Parkinson's disease
  - Antihistamine drug. Manages tremors in Parkinson's disease
- Selegiline
  - Generally given orally with Parkinson's disease
  - Monoamine Oxidase Inhibitor
  - Used with levodopa/carbidopa to prolong the half-life of levodopa/carbidopa and enhance the levels of dopamine

Reinforcement of Priority Teaching

- Discuss options with client and caregiver that will allow client to maintain independence
- Discuss use of adaptive devices and equipment, such as a wheelchair, long spoon, special mug, among others
- Explain ways to modify client's clothing and shoes to increase client's independence in manipulating them, such as using Velcro closure instead of buttons
- The importance of making modifications in the home to facilitate client's independence and minimize risk for injuries. These include, removal of loose rugs, installing grab bars in shower, placing bench in shower, getting an elevated toilet set, among others
- Instruct caregivers to be patient and not rush the client when completing tasks, as task completion will be much slower than usual with Parkinson's disease
- Explain the importance of administering antiparkinsonian medications
- Explain foods that are high in pyridoxine (vitamin B6) as pyridoxine hinders the effect of antiparkinsonian drugs
- Continued physical and occupational therapy for strengthening of muscles and use of adaptive strategies for activities of daily living
- Discuss eating foods that are easy to chew and swallow
- Encourage eating six small meals throughout the day instead of few large meals
- Provide information on resources that may help client and family cope with the condition, such as the American Parkinson Disease Association and referral to counseling
- Discuss the long-term burden of caring for someone with Parkinson's disease. Assist client and family with seeking alternate options for care outside of the home, such as a long-term care facility, if desired
- Have client use strategies to minimize risk of falls (mentioned in priority interventions)

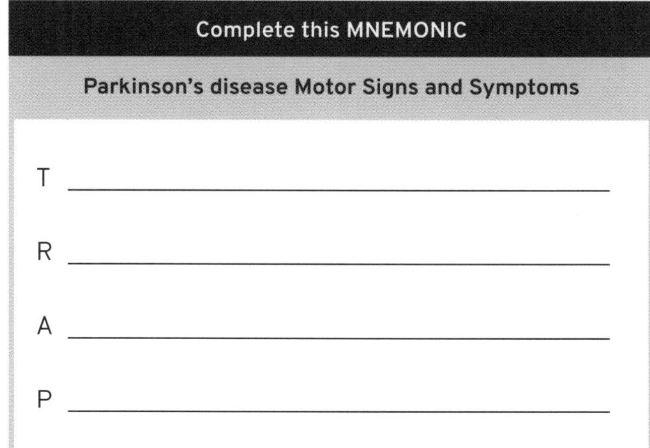

Complete this MNEMONIC
Parkinson's disease Motor Signs and Symptoms
T __________
R __________
A __________
P __________

Table 13-2: Use the image below to identify the motor signs and symptoms of Parkinson's disease.

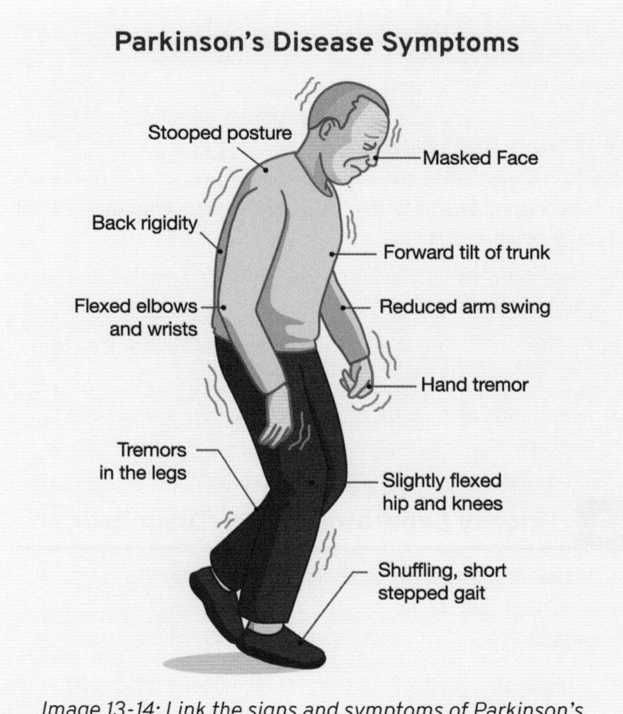

Image 13-14: Link the signs and symptoms of Parkinson's Disease with the pathophysiological changes.

Cataracts

Pathophysiology/Description

- Opacity of the lens that affects transparency, causing vision changes. Can occur in one or both eyes
- Causes include age related, eye trauma, congenital such as caused by maternal diseases, radiation and diabetes mellitus, among others
- Cataract surgery is usually done on one eye at a time. Most of the postoperative care is done by the client and/or caregiver at home

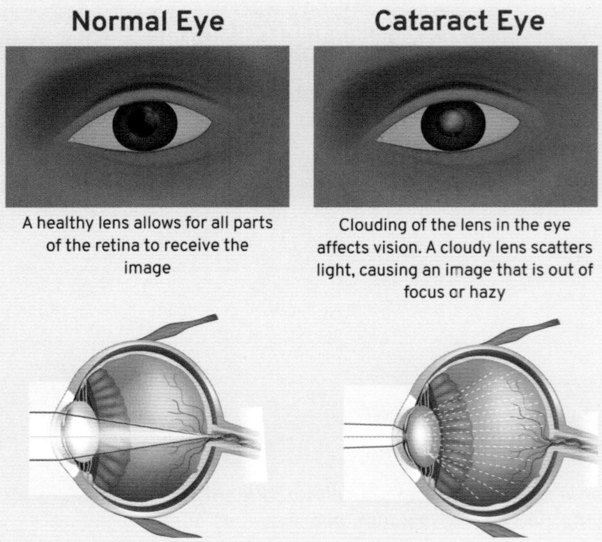

Normal Eye

A healthy lens allows for all parts of the retina to receive the image

Cataract Eye

Clouding of the lens in the eye affects vision. A cloudy lens scatters light, causing an image that is out of focus or hazy

Image 13-15: Relate the pathophysiology of cataracts with the signs and symptoms.

Priority Data Collection or Cues

- Decreased and/or blurred vision. Examine color perception, may be abnormal
- Glare from driving worsened by night driving. Double vision (diplopia)
- Redness and pain in eye, more prominent in age-related cataract
- Knowledge of surgical procedure. Ability to adhere to postoperative instructions

Priority Laboratory Tests/Diagnostics

- Visual acuity test shows vision impairment
- Slit lamp examination shows cataract on lens. Glare testing shows vision loss
- Pupil dilation test shows extent of cataract's impact on vision

Priority Interventions or Actions

- Preoperative interventions
    - Reinforce teaching on expectations of surgery and postoperative care. Administer eye medications
    - Decrease lighting to prevent photopia after administering mydriatic
- Postoperative interventions
    - Examine eye patch to ensure adequate coverage of eye. Elevate head of bed 30-40 degrees
    - Position off operative side. Administer analgesics if needed. Assist with ambulation
    - Prevent client actions that increase intraocular pressure, such as bending and coughing

Priority Potential & Actual Complications

- Infection, bleeding, vision loss and dislocation of implanted lens

Priority Nursing Implications

- Consider the impact of cataracts on older adults. Independence may be lost as poor vision allows them to be dependent on others to assist them with tasks such as driving. Be supportive and provide information on ways they might still maintain independence

Priority Medications

- Tropicamide (one of many drugs used to dilate the eye)
    - Cycloplegic drug administered as eye drops
    - Produces both paralysis and dilation
- Ketorolac ophthalmic solution (non-steroidal anti-inflammatory eye drops)
    - Used to reduce inflammation and decrease pain
    - A 0.5% ophthalmic solution can also be used

Reinforcement of Priority Teaching

- No actions that increase eye pressure. No lifting heavier than 5 pounds
- Wear sun shades to prevent photophobia. Expect eye discomfort for a few days
- No rubbing of eye, as it can result in an infection. Proper instilling of eye drops
- Notify health care provider of redness, unusual drainage, vision loss, floaters or light flashes
- Decreased depth perception while wearing the eye patch
- Visual acuity may not return to the operative eye until 1-2 weeks after surgery
- Importance of follow-up visits

Pathophysiology/Description

- A group of eye disorders that damage the optic nerve due to increased ocular pressure
- Two types of glaucoma
  - Primary open-angle glaucoma (POAG): drainage path for aqueous humor is blocked so outflow is decreased in the trabecular network. Most common type of glaucoma
  - Primary angle-closure glaucoma (PACG): angle closure causes reduction in the outflow of aqueous humor. Some causes of angle closure might be pupil dilation or bulging lens

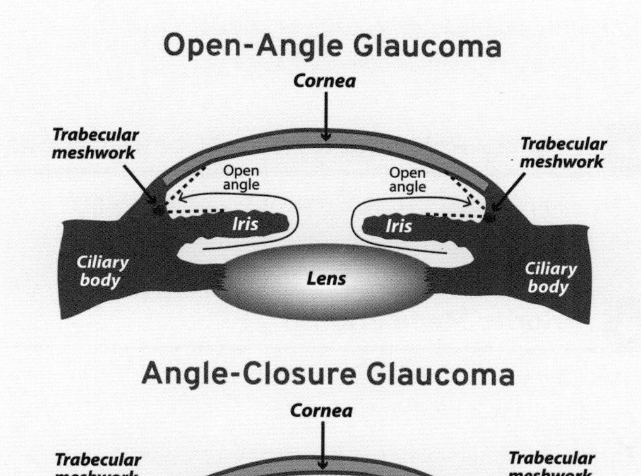

Image 13-16: Compare and contrast open-angle and angle-closure glaucoma. How do the signs and symptoms and management differ between the two types of glaucoma?

Priority Data Collection or Cues

- Accommodation diminished with glaucoma. Sudden, severe eye pain with PACG
- Peripheral vision loss, indicative of POAG. Nausea and vomiting with PACG
- Blurred vision and visualization of colored halos with PACG
- Client's understanding of condition and ability to follow the long-term treatment regimen

Priority Laboratory Tests/Diagnostics

- Visual acuity test shows vision impairment. Perimetry shows impairment in visual fields
- Slit lamp examination shows fixed pupil and flat anterior chamber angle with PACG and normal angle with POAG. Tonometry shows elevated intraocular pressure
- Ophthalmoscopy shows a deeper and wider optic disc with POAG

Priority Interventions or Actions

- Eye medications to decrease intraocular pressure
- Preoperative interventions for PACG
  - Instruction regarding expectation of iridectomy surgery and postoperative care
  - Administer intravenous or oral hyperosmotic drugs to decrease intraocular pressure
- Postoperative interventions
  - Examine eye patch to ensure adequate coverage of eye. Elevate head of bed 30-40 degrees
  - Position off operative side. Administer analgesics if needed. Assist with ambulation
  - Prevent client actions that increase intraocular pressure, such as bending and coughing

Priority Potential & Actual Complications

- Infection, bleeding, loss of vision and recurrence of glaucoma

Priority Nursing Implications

- Primary angle-closure glaucoma is an emergency that must be addressed immediately

Priority Medications

- Dipivefrin
  - A-Adrenergic agonist opthalmic solution
  - Decreases production of aqueous humor
- Carbachol
  - Cholinergic agent opthalmic solution
  - Causes iris sphincter to contract and trabecular meshwork to open, allowing aqueous outflow

Reinforcement of Priority Teaching

- No actions that increase eye pressure. No lifting heavier than 5 pounds
- Wear sun shades to prevent photophobia. Expect eye discomfort for a few days
- No rubbing of eye, as it can result in an infection. Proper instilling of eye drops
- Notify health care provider of redness, unusual drainage, vision loss, floaters or light flashes
- Decreased depth perception while wearing the eye patch
- Visual acuity may not return to the operative eye until 1-2 weeks after surgery
- Importance of follow-up visits. Regular eye exams. MedicAlert Identification

Clinical Hint

Early diagnosis of glaucoma is critical to preserve vision.

Conjunctivitis

Pathophysiology/Description

- Conjunctivitis is inflammation or infection of the conjunctiva. Conjunctivitis caused by bacteria is contagious and good handwashing must be done to prevent the spread
- Causes: bacteria, viruses, chemical irritants, trauma, foreign body in eye and chlamydia
- Most cases of conjunctivitis get better on their own
- Keratitis, infection or inflammation of the cornea, can also impact the conjunctiva resulting in a condition called keratoconjunctivitis

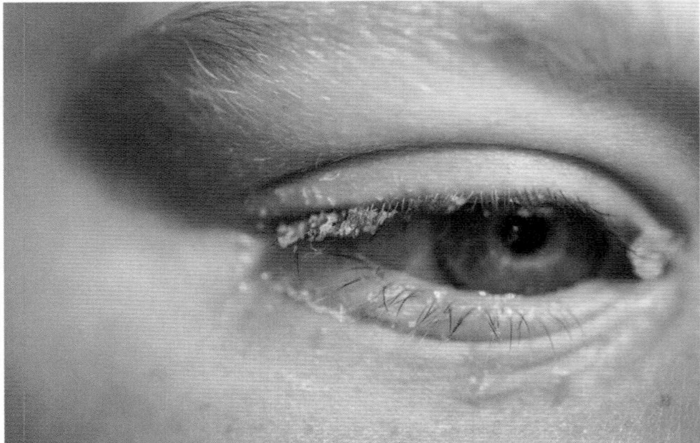

Image 13-17: Bacterial Conjunctivitis.

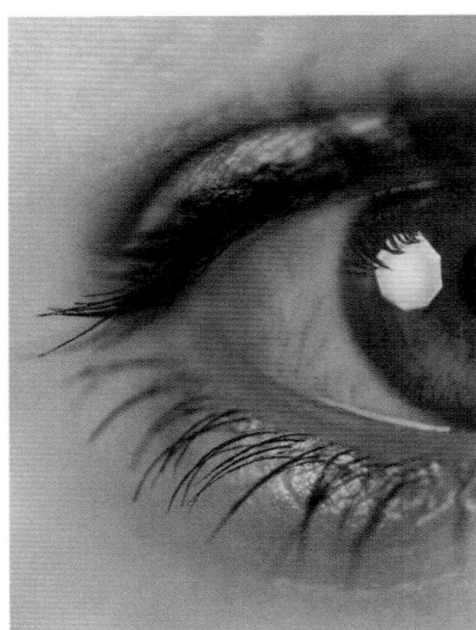
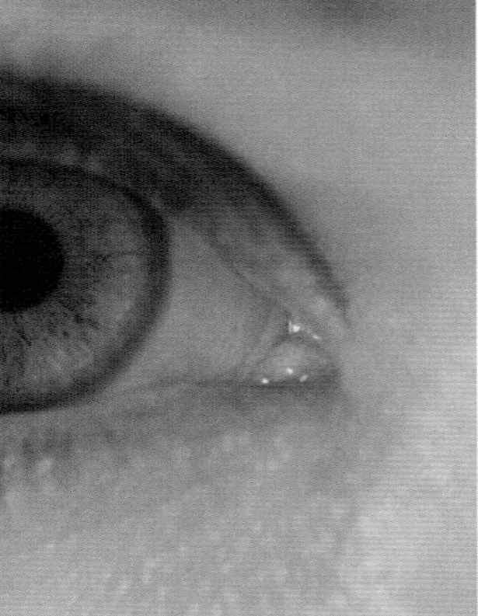

Image 13-18: Viral Conjunctivitis. Compare and contrast client symptoms and interventions for bacterial and viral conjunctivitis.

Priority Data Collection or Cues

- Observe client for itchy, burning, teary and red eyes. Observe for swelling to the eyelids
- Examine eyes for drainage. Mucopurulent drainage usually indicates bacterial or chlamydial causes
- Ask client about tolerance to light as conjunctivitis may cause mild photophobia
- Ask client to describe feeling in the eyes, usually described as gritty or sandy feel to eyes

Priority Laboratory Tests/Diagnostics

- Visual acuity test to determine if conjunctivitis has affected vision
- Slit lamp examination is used to examine small sections of structures of the eye to detect small abnormalities. Conjunctivitis will be seen
- Eye culture to determine if cause of conjunctivitis is bacterial

Priority Interventions or Actions

- Administer eye drops as prescribed
- Maintain proper infection control practice
- Apply cold or warm compress

Priority Potential & Actual Complications

- Meningitis, if bacterial conjunctivitis is left untreated
- Keratitis

Priority Medications

- Moxifloxacin (for bacterial conjunctivitis)
  - Quinolone opthalmic antibiotic
  - Used to treat conjunctivitis caused by bacteria
- Ocular lubricant
  - Can be bought over-the-counter
  - Used to moisten the eye and alleviate dryness and irritation
  - Must not be used to treat a bacterial eye infection

Reinforcement of Priority Teaching

- Proper handwashing to prevent spread of the condition
- Advise to not share make-up and to discard remaining make-up
- Counsel client to stop wearing contact lens until conjunctivitis is resolved and to discard current lens
- Encourage client not to rub or scratch eyes
- Advise client not to share towels and washcloths
- Proper administration of eye drops without touching eye
  - Hold head back and pull lower eyelid down to form a pocket
  - Dropper held above the eye without touching the eye
  - Gaze up and look away from dropper. Squeeze drops into pocket of eye
  - Finger pressed for 1 minute to the inside corner of eye, so fluid does not get into the tear duct

Macular degeneration

Pathophysiology/Description

- Macular degeneration (MD) occurs when the macula, which is the central part of the retina, deteriorates
- The vision loss from macular degeneration is irreversible. Though MD rarely causes complete blindness, the physical disability that limited vision causes can be life-altering
- The condition is seen as individuals age and so it is often referred to as age-related macular degeneration
- Risk factors
  - Genetics
  - Ethnicity: more common in Caucasians than other ethnic groups
  - Cardiovascular disease
  - Smoking or smoke exposure
- Types of macular degeneration
  - Dry MD: yellow deposits in the retinal pigment epithelium, called drusen, increase in numbers and size causing distorted vision. Dry MD is the most common type and is not curable
  - Wet MD: growth of abnormal blood vessels leaks fluid and blood into the retina causing scars to form. The scars result in distortion of vision

Priority Data Collection or Cues

- Check for blurred, darkened and distorted vision
- Check for floaters or spots in field of vision, called scotomas. This is common in MD
- Check for decreased central vision
- Ask about the need for brighter light when working, which is a consistent finding with MD
- Observe client's ability to read print, may find that words are blurred

Priority Laboratory Tests/Diagnostics

- Ophthalmoscopy shows drusen deposits and other changes consistent with MD
- Optical coherence tomography examines the anatomy of the retina and appearance of the macula
- Scanning laser ophthalmoscopy examines anatomy of the retina and appearance of the macula
- Amsler grid tests the integrity of the retina
- Fundus photography, indocyanine green dyes and intravenous angiography clarifies the extent of MD and whether it is wet or dry

Priority Interventions or Actions

- Assist with administration of intraocular injected medications to slow vision loss and monitor for side effects such as eye irritation, photosensitivity and eye pain
- If client had photodynamic therapy, ensure no part of their body is exposed before leaving to go home as sunlight on any part of the body can activate the drug used in the therapy, causing sunburn

Priority Potential & Actual Complications

- Progression from dry to wet macular degeneration
- Visual hallucinations
- Physical disability due to vision loss

Priority Nursing Implications

- Loss of central vision from macular degeneration can be very devastating for the client and family. It is important to understand the implications of this loss when it comes to caring for the client and interacting with the family. Help them to determine the best ways to cope with the vision loss and lifestyle changes that will need to be made

Priority Medications

- Ranibizumab via eye injection
  - Selective inhibitors of endothelial growth factor
  - Slows vision loss in wet MD
- Aflibercept via eye injection
  - Selective inhibitors of endothelial growth factor
  - Slows vision loss in wet MD
- Pegaptanib via eye injection
  - Selective inhibitors of endothelial growth factor
  - Slows vision loss in wet MD

Reinforcement of Priority Teaching

- Explain the use of visual aids to maximize current vision, such as electronic hand-held magnifiers, E-readers, image zooming, among others
- Explain that taking high doses of vitamins and minerals can help to decrease the risk of vision loss
- Reinforce education on the side effects of medications that are injected in the eye
- Explain that injections are administered every 4 to 6 weeks
- Explain that the health care provider will determine response to medication therapy using the optic coherence tomography test
- If client had photodynamic therapy, encourage to avoid intense light and sunlight for 5 days after the procedure as the drug used can be activated by light
- Explain that smoking cessation helps to slow vision loss

Next Gen Clinical Judgment

Consider the life changes associated with visual impairment. What community resources may assist a client to deal with changes in vision?

Hearing impairment

Pathophysiology/Description

- Hearing loss is the inability to hear sounds
- There are various factors that cause hearing loss. Impacted cerumen, foreign items in the ear, otitis media, damage to tympanic membrane, presbycusis and ototoxicity are just a few of the causes
- Types of hearing loss
  - Sensorineural: occurs due to functional defect of inner ear, such as noise causing trauma over time. This type of hearing loss is usually permanent
  - Conductive: transmission of sound waves to the inner ear is hindered because of conditions in the middle or outer ear such as impacted cerumen
  - Mixed: hearing loss results from a combination of both sensorineural and conductive factors
  - Central: the inability to interpret speech and sound due to problem occurring in the brain
  - Functional: psychological factors seem to cause functional hearing loss. The person does not hear or respond even though there are no physical reasons for the hearing loss

Priority Data Collection or Cues

- Determine onset of client's symptoms
- Determine history of ear infections or other ear injuries
- Ask about exposure to constant loud noise
- Engage client in speech to determine if client asks to repeat statements, as is common in hearing loss
- Observe to see if the client responds incorrectly to questions asked
- Observe if client turns head to one side to hear, as if favoring one ear
- Observe the client to see if they cannot respond when spoken to unless looking directly at the speaker's lips
- Examine client for ringing in the ear (tinnitus), among the first signs of hearing loss
- Listen to client's tone of voice in conversation, shouting is usual
- Observe if the client increases the sound level on equipment, such as television or radio, when others in the room are hearing the sound perfectly
- Ask client about withdrawal from large or social gatherings. This is usually because of fear of being engaged in a conversation
- Examine the impact hearing loss has on client's quality of life

Priority Laboratory Tests/Diagnostics

- Tuning fork tests to determine hearing loss and the type (sensorineural vs conduction)
- Audiometer test determines degree of hearing loss and how best to treat it
- Whisper test determines if client is able to hear spoken words from a certain distance

Priority Interventions or Actions

- Get the client's full attention before speaking. Speak into the client's better ear
- Do not cover face or mouth with hand when speaking to client. Maintain eye contact
- Ensure there is no food in the mouth or chewing of gum when speaking
- Stand close to client and ensure speech is slow and words are properly formed
- Use written words if needed
- Ensure the room is quiet and there are no distractors, such as television on or other people speaking
- Decrease the decibel of the voice when speaking as shouting does not help the client
- Ensure the room is well lit
- Ensure non-verbal expression matches spoken words as client who lip reads relies on a match of words with non-verbal expressions
- Rephrase sentences if needed

Priority Potential & Actual Complications

- Complete hearing loss
- Social isolation

Priority Nursing Implications

- Some older adults with hearing loss due to presbycusis, may believe that their hearing loss results from the aging process and so they simply accept it as such and believe that nothing can be done to aid their hearing. As nurses, it is important to present all options for hearing assistive devices and techniques to older adults with hearing loss

Reinforcement of Priority Teaching

- Face the person with whom a conversation is being had
- Instruct client to have conversations in good lighting so lip reading might be easier and ensure there is no background noise as distraction
- Ask others with whom a conversing is being held to speak clearly and into the unaffected ear
- Avoid high noise levels
- Provide information to client about types of hearing aids, listening devices and the cochlear implant procedure
- Provide information to client on the use of sign language (usually for clients who have severe hearing loss)
- Keep audiologist appointments

Scoliosis

Pathophysiology/Description

- Scoliosis is a deformity of the spine that is characterized by an S-shaped curvature of the lumbar and thoracic spine, occurring quite often during a child's growth spurts just before puberty (called idiopathic scoliosis), or seen at birth (called congenital scoliosis). The condition is seen more in girls than boys
- Some causes of scoliosis might be muscular dystrophy, cerebral palsy, defects from birth that affect spinal bone development and other factors such as infection or injuries to the spine
- The condition can be mild where there is no significant physical impairment or functioning, or so severe that it limits the child's physical functioning
- Scoliosis must be monitored as the child grows to determine any changes in spinal curvature
- Monitoring of scoliosis
  - With spinal curvature of 10-20 degrees (mild) the child must be evaluated every 3 months and X-rays done every 6 months, with prescribed exercises to increase muscle strength and improve posture
  - Spinal curvature 20-40 degrees(moderate), brace worn for 23 hours daily to prevent further curvature
  - Spinal curvature greater more than 40 degrees (severe), spinal fusion surgery with instrumentation is needed

Priority Data Collection or Cues

- Have client bend over at the waist, will observe asymmetry of the trunk
- Inspect client from behind, uneven shoulders, scapula, hips and waist will be seen
- Ask caregiver about appearance of client's clothing. Caregiver may report uneven appearance in length of client's skirt
- Examine leg length when client is standing, will notice asymmetry
- Determine client and caregiver's understanding of various options for treatment depending on the degree of child's curvature

Priority Laboratory Tests/Diagnostics

- Scoliometer to measure symmetry of the trunk
- X-ray to confirm the diagnosis of scoliosis
- Magnetic resonance imaging (MRI) to detect underlying conditions that may be impacting scoliosis

Priority Interventions or Actions

- Prepare client for testing that will measure curvature and determine treatment protocol
- Explain course of treatment to client and caregiver
- Reinforce exercises to treat client who has mild curvature
- Apply prescribed brace to client with moderate curvature
- Inspect skin under brace for signs of skin breakdown. Wash and dry skin before reapplying brace
- Encourage client in proper use of assistive devices. Prepare client for surgery, if severe scoliosis
- Postoperative interventions
  - Monitor dressing to surgical site for bleeding and infection. Administer analgesics
  - Perform log rolling when turning and repositioning client
  - Keep client's body in proper alignment. Do not twist or bend client's body
  - Prevent respiratory compromise by allowing client to cough and deep breathe. Have client use incentive spirometry
  - Use compression devices to minimize risk of blood clots. Assist with ambulation
  - Perform good skin care to prevent pressure ulcers. Place thoracolumbar sacral orthosis (TLSO) on client
  - Keep client nothing by mouth until able to eat oral foods, as prescribed
  - Monitor neurological and cardiac status

Priority Potential & Actual Complications

- Back problems such as pain. Cardiac and respiratory problems
- Physical appearance and physical disability
- Mental problems, such as depression and social isolation

Priority Nursing Implications

- As nurses, it is crucial that the emotional status of a client who must wear a brace for 23 of 24 hours in a day be considered as this is usually a child who might experience body image issues when socializing with peers

Reinforcement of Priority Teaching

- Demonstrate to client how to don and doff the brace
- Explain that wearing of the brace will be discontinued after bones have stopped growing
- Explain to wear brace for 23 hours daily and importance of washing and drying skin under brace before reapplying. Encourage the client to wear t-shirt under brace for skin protection
- Perform prescribed exercises daily to prevent further curvature
- Explain to client how to log roll and get on and off the bed after surgery
- Encourage not to bend or twist body. Encourage to sit straight in chairs and not to slump
- Explain importance of maintaining restrictions on activity for up to 8 months after surgery as prescribed. Encourage not to engage in sports that increase the risk of falls
- Explain that if a rod is placed in the spine, it will be lengthened every 6 months as the client grows
- Explain surgery site monitoring for bleeding, signs of infection and when to contact health care provider

Labyrinthitis/Meniere's disease

Pathophysiology/Description

- Labyrinthitis and Meniere's disease are both disorders of the inner ear that cause dizziness and affect balance
- When one of the two vestibular nerves in the inner ear becomes inflamed, for various reasons, labyrinthitis occurs
- Meniere's disease has no known cause but with the disease, excessive amounts of endolymph is observed in the membranous labyrinth, causing the labyrinth to rupture. There is usually poor reabsorption or overproduction of the endolymph fluid. Meniere's disease is also known as endolymphatic hydrops
- Factors causing labyrinthitis: bacterial and viral infections of middle and inner ear, respiratory and gastrointestinal tract
- In some cases, viral and bacterial infections, head injury, allergic reactions, stress and biochemical issues may have an association with Meniere's disease
- Most people with these conditions do not require surgical intervention. However, when attacks from Meniere's disease becomes incapacitating, surgery is an option

Priority Data Collection or Cues

- Collect data. Client may report symptoms that have lasted for hours or days
- Observe client for vertigo and dizziness. In Meniere's disease client may describe intense vertigo even when lying down. Observe for loss of balance
- Monitor for headaches, that may be severe with Meniere's disease. Monitor for nausea and vomiting
- Test client's hearing and may find hearing loss on affected side
- Examine client's eyes, may see nystagmus. Client may have difficulty focusing the eyes
- Observe client's stance, may see that client is unbalanced
- Ask client about ringing in the ear as this is common with labyrinthitis
- Ask client to describe feeling in ears, may say there is a feeling of fullness in the ear with Meniere's
- Examine client's spatial awareness, may describe a feeling of spinning in space or being pulled to the ground with Meniere's disease

Priority Laboratory Tests/Diagnostics

- Audiometer test determines if hearing loss is being experienced
- Electronystagmography (ENG) balance test. With Meniere's disease reduced balance response will be manifest in one ear
- Vestibular testing examines the inner ear to try and isolate the symptoms to a specific cause
- Glycerol test: the client is given an oral dose of glycerol and audiograms are performed. Diagnosis of Meniere's disease is supported if improvement in hearing and speech discrimination occurs
- Electroencephalogram, used to look at electrical activity in brain to rule out other causes of symptoms, in labyrinthitis

Priority Interventions or Actions

- In an acute attack, administer medications such as antihistamines, antivertigo, antiemetics and benzodiazepines. Diuretic may also be prescribed for Meniere's disease
- Maintain a safe environment to prevent client from falls
- Allow client to stay in bed in a room that is dark, that has reduced stimulation
- Ensure client does not make sudden head movements or changes position suddenly as these actions will worsen vertigo
- Provide client with an emesis basin as vomiting is expected
- Keep the wheels of the bed locked, side rails up and the bed in a low position
- Encourage client to call for assistance before getting out of bed
- Ensure client gets diet low in sodium, helps to decrease fluid in the ear in Meniere's disease
- Surgical interventions (endolymphatic sac decompression and placement of a shunt, vestibular nerve section or labyrinthectomy)
    - Monitor neurological system
    - Monitor dressing to affected ear. Monitor packing for bleeding and signs of infection
    - Administer medications for vertigo and nausea
    - Place bedside commode in client's room and encourage client to use it rather than attempting to walk to the bathroom
    - Ensure call bell is within client's reach and reinforce the importance of calling for assistance before getting up
    - Do not allow client to ambulate alone, as dizziness may persist after surgery
    - When conversing with client, speak on the nonoperative side

Priority Potential & Actual Complications

- Meningitis (with labyrinthitis)
- Hearing loss
- Loss of balance
- Social isolation

Priority Nursing Implications

- Prednisone should not be stopped abruptly as client will experience prednisone withdrawal symptoms which include weakness, severe fatigue, and joint and body aches

Priority Medications

- Diphenhydramine
  - Oral antihistamine
- Lorazepam
  - Oral administration
  - Benzodiazepine used to decrease sensations in both conditions
- Meclizine
  - Oral administration
  - Used to treat vertigo associated with both conditions
  - Exact dose depends on client's clinical response
- Prednisone
  - Corticosteroid used to control swelling in labyrinthitis
  - Dosage to be tapered, oral medications with these diagnoses
- Hydrochlorothiazide
  - Oral diuretic
  - Works by reducing fluid in inner ear
- Prochlorperazine
  - May be given orally, IM, intravenous, or rectally
  - Antiemetic used to treat nausea and vomiting in both conditions

Reinforcement of Priority Teaching

- Take medications as prescribed and report adverse effects to health care provider
- Encourage the client who had surgery to monitor packing to ear for signs of bleeding or abnormal drainage and report to health care provider
- Change positions slowly and avoid making jerking and quick motions with the head
- Maintain safety with attacks. Do not walk alone
- Explain importance of removal of fall hazards from home, such as loose area rugs. Encourage use of nonslip mats in the shower
- Explain to client about dietary factors that may help with Meniere's disease, such as limiting salt, monosodium glutamate (MSG), alcohol and caffeine
- Rest and decrease environmental stimulation during an attack of Meniere's disease and labyrinthitis
- Stop smoking and avoid allergens as both are irritants that may worsen the conditions
- Explain importance of follow-up appointments

Compare and Contrast		
	Similarities:	**Differences:**
Meniere's Disease (vs. Labyrinthitis and Benign Paroxysmal Positional Vertigo)		
Labyrinthitis (vs. Meniere's Disease and Benign Paroxysmal Positional Vertigo)		
Benign Paroxysmal Positional Vertigo (vs. Meniere's Disease and Labyrinthitis)		

Table 13-3: Compare and contrast these three conditions

Pathophysiology/Description

- Otitis media is an infection of middle ear that results in inflammation
- Otitis media is caused by a blockage of the eustachian tube because of swelling that occurs from allergies, colds or bacteria. An effusion can also occur with otitis media, which manifests as purulent or mucoid fluid, accumulating in the middle ear space following conditions such as trauma from pressure change and a sinus infection
- Children are particularly vulnerable to getting otitis media as they have shorter and flatter eustachian tubes than that of an adult's, making this condition a childhood disease
- Otitis media can become chronic with recurrent multiple attacks, causing cholesterol and epithelial cells to form in the middle ear leading to mastoiditis. These cholesterol formations must be surgically removed
- While otitis media is a middle ear infection, otitis externa (external otitis), also called swimmer's ear, is an inflammation or infection of the outer ear and ear canal. Swelling that occurs with otitis externa can lead to conductive hearing loss
- Otitis externa can be caused by several factors, such as swimming in contaminated water, trauma to the ear, fungi, bacteria or placing objects inside the ear to scratch the ear (such as a hairpin). Otitis externa is also more common in children than adults

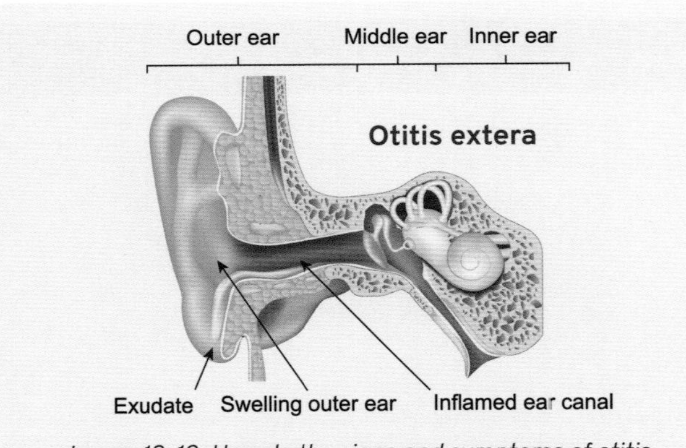

Image 13-19: How do the signs and symptoms of otitis externa relate to the pathophysiology of this condition?

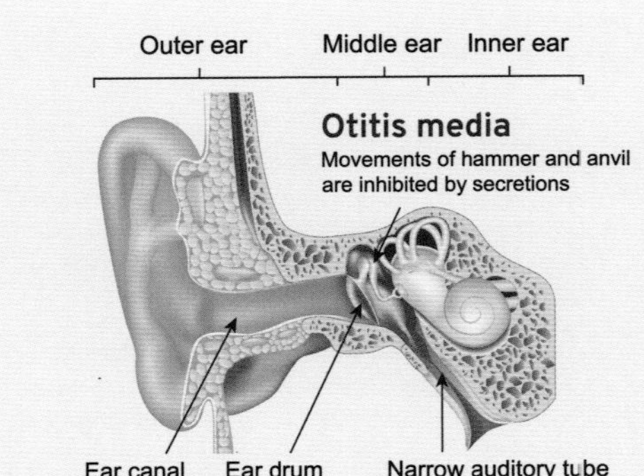

Image 13-20: How do the signs and symptoms of otitis media relate to the pathophysiology of this condition?

Priority Data Collection or Cues

- Monitor vital signs, will likely find increased temperature as fever is common in otitis media and in otitis externa if the infection has spread to adjacent tissues
- Observe for ear pain as this is one of the first signs with both conditions
- Monitor client for crying and fussiness because of the pain and discomfort. Client will be tugging and rubbing on the ear or placing finger in the ear
- Observe client's head movement, may see head moving from side to side
- Monitor client for hearing loss or muffled hearing that can occur in both conditions
- Ask caregiver about client's eating, may find loss of appetite
- Examine ear for drainage, blood-tinged or purulent drainage may be seen in otitis externa. Purulent drainage in chronic otitis media
- Observe client's chewing, may find that chewing causes significant discomfort with otitis externa
- Monitor for redness and edema, seen more with otitis externa

Priority Laboratory Tests/Diagnostics

- Otoscopic examination will reveal a bulging tympanic membrane with redness
- Tympanometry to measure the pressure in the ear and see if there is a ruptured eardrum
- X-ray, computed tomography (CT) scan and magnetic resonance imaging (MRI) of the mastoid, to look for bone involvement and a mass (with chronic otitis media)
- Culture and sensitivity of ear drainage to determine bacterial growth and best treatment course

Priority Interventions or Actions

- Apply moist heat for both conditions as prescribed
- Administer analgesics, antipyretics, antiemetics and antibiotics as prescribed
- Manipulate client's pinna gently when examining ear or instilling ear drops
- Monitor for therapeutic effect of medications
- Prepare client for surgery, if indicated
- Postoperative interventions for otitis media (myringotomy, tympanoplasty)
  - Monitor dressing to affected ear. Monitor packing for bleeding and signs of infection
  - Ensure use of proper infection control practices such as hand hygiene
  - Prevent client from making quick, sudden movements of the head
  - Encourage client not to cough or strain (as in having a bowel movement)
  - Do not offer client a straw to use for drinking

- Clean hair by wiping with a clean washcloth to avoid wetting the head. Keep ear dry

Priority Potential & Actual Complications

- Facial paralysis from tympanoplasty surgery and hearing loss

Priority Nursing Implications

- When caring for older adults with ear infections, be aware of malignant external otitis, which is an infection caused by a serious pathogen and usually afflicts older adults with diabetes. It can be potentially fatal if not treated because it can migrate from the external ear to the temporal bone causing osteomyelitis. Antibiotics must be administered to treat this infection

Priority Medications

- Several antibiotics are used to treat otitis media and otitis externa and dosages vary based on the age and weight of the child. Below are some examples
- Amoxicillin
  - Oral antibiotic to treat otitis media
  - Treat both otitis media and external otitis
- Amoxicillin/clavulanate
  - Oral antibiotic
  - Pediatric dosage is based on the age and weight of the child
- Ciprofloxacin and dexamethasone (combination drug)
  - Antibiotic and steroid medication instilled in the affected ear
  - Treat otitis externa and otitis media in adults and children older than 6 months
- Finafloxacin
  - Antibiotic otic suspension
  - Treat otitis externa in adults and children older than 12 months

Reinforcement of Priority Teaching

- Take medications as prescribed and report adverse effects to health care provider
- Notify the health care provider if the tympanoplasty tubes fall out
- Explain the proper administration of ear drops
- Finish all prescribed antibiotics even if client starts to feel better
- Monitor packing to ear and dressing for signs of bleeding or abnormal drainage and report to health care provider
- Demonstrate to client/caregiver on proper/safe cleaning of drainage
- Explain that while packing is in the ear, client may experience impaired hearing
- Change positions slowly and avoid making jerking and quick motions with the head
- Avoid forceful coughing and to not wash hair for 1 week
- Encourage not to travel by air in the weeks following surgery
- Explain not to blow the nose for about 1 week after surgery but if needed to blow, do so with 1 nostril at a time and with the mouth open
- Encourage the use of earplugs when client returns to swimming or other water activities that involve submerging in water
- Explain importance of follow-up appointments

Next Gen Clinical Judgment

Compare and contrast the symptoms and treatments for otitis externa and otitis media.

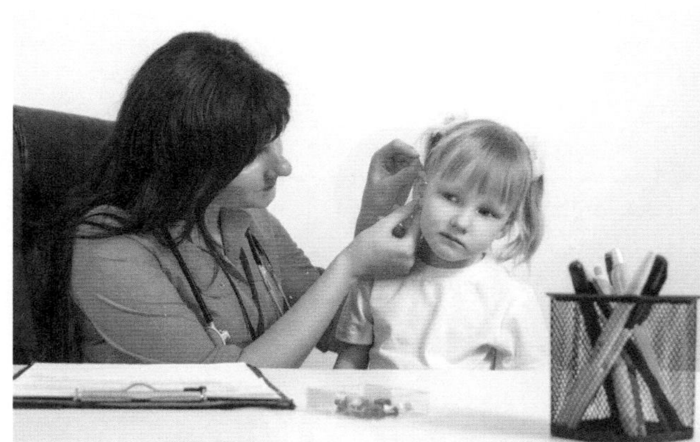

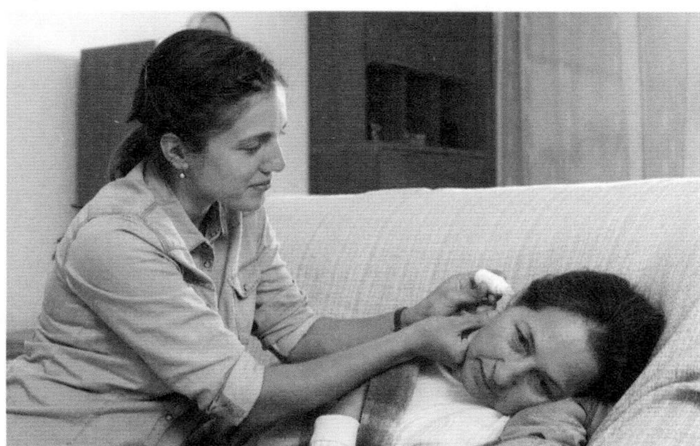

Image 13-21: Compare and contrast how medication is administered in the ears of children and adults.

Spina bifida

Pathophysiology/Description

- Neural tube forms in early pregnancy and usually closes around 4 weeks after conception. Spina bifida is a neural tube defect that occurs because the neural tube fails to close during development of the embryo
- Causes include maternal malnutrition, radiation, chemicals and a genetic mutation
- Risk factors include maternal obesity, low vitamin B12 and folate in pregnancy, and maternal diabetes, family history of neural tube defects, use of antiseizure medications in pregnancy
- The condition is seen more in females than males and among Caucasians and Hispanics than other ethnic groups
- There are two types of spina bifida, spina bifida cystica and spina bifida occulta
    - Spina bifida occulta: a mild form of the condition. There is no protrusion of meninges and only a small separation exists in the vertebrae. It usually goes undiagnosed as there are no neurologic deficits
    - Spina bifida cystica: spinal cord and meninges protrude and form a sac on the lumbar or sacral area. There are two types of spina bifida cystica, meningocele and myelomeningocele (myelomeninogocele is characterized by nerve fibers in the sac)

Priority Data Collection or Cues

- Look for flaccid paralysis of lower extremities
- Monitor bowel and bladder status, may find incontinence of both
- Observe joints, may find deformities of joints primarily hip subluxation and dislocation
- Examine back, will see protruded sac in back. Check sac for rupture, bleeding and signs of infection
- Examine posture, may see kyphosis and scoliosis
- Examine reflexes, may find missing deep tendon reflexes
- Look for nuchal rigidity, somnolence and fussiness which may indicate meningitis
- Observe child's fontanels, bulging fontanel might indicate increased intracranial pressure
- Monitor vital signs, elevated temperature may indicate an infection. Measure axillary temperature as a rectal thermometer might cause a rectal prolapse

Priority Laboratory Tests/Diagnostics

- Ultrasound scan of uterus, may show meningocele
- Maternal serum alpha-fetoprotein (MSAFP) test shows significantly high alpha-fetoprotein (AFP) levels
- Blood test to confirm the high AFP level, further evaluation is done if AFP is still high
- Amniocentesis, showing high levels of AFP

Priority Interventions or Actions

- Perform thorough neurological data collection
- Prevent meningocele from drying, cover with saline moistened sterile gauze. Change gauze dressing every 2-4 hours to prevent infection

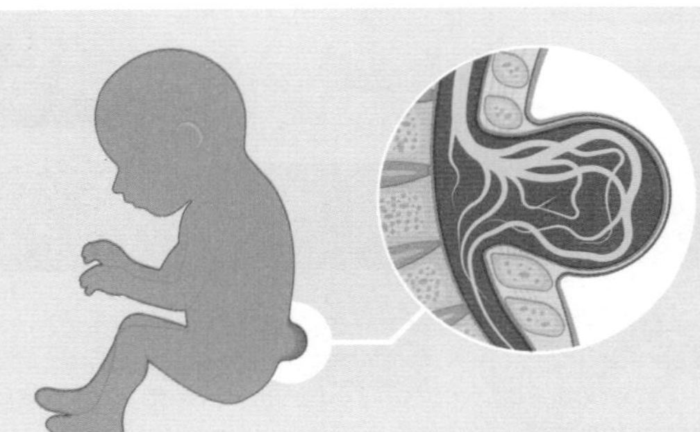

Spina Bifida

A birth defect that happens when a baby's backbone (spine) does not form normally

Image 13-22: Consider how the level of the defect dictates the impact of spina bifada.

Types of Spina Bifida

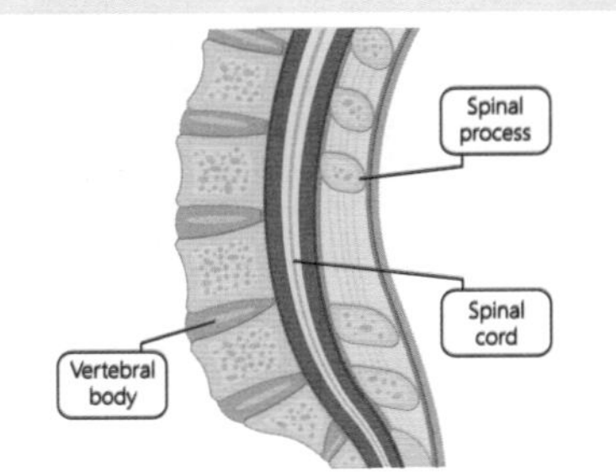

Spina bifida occulta

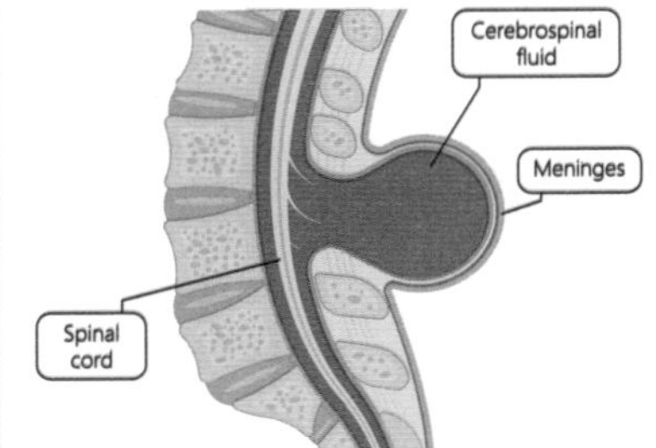

Meningocele

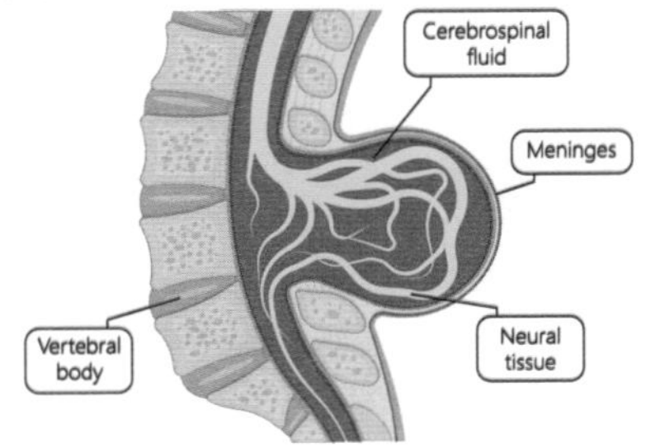

Myelomeningocele

- Measure child's head circumference as hydrocephalus can occur
- Maintain aseptic technique when caring for meningocele
- Position child in prone position to take pressure off the meningocele
- Do not place diaper on child before surgery as it may cover the meningocele
- Measure intake and output
- Use measures to prevent stool from soiling the meningocele
- Provide gentle range of motion to prevent contractures and muscle wasting
- Prepare child for surgery. Initiate nothing by mouth
- Ensure caregivers' questions are answered preoperatively
- Postoperative interventions
    - Monitor surgery site for bleeding signs of infection and cerebrospinal fluid leak
    - Administer pain medication as prescribed
    - Place child in a prone or side-lying position as prescribed
    - Continue bowel and bladder care as preoperatively
    - Continue neurological data collection as completed preoperatively
    - Resume feedings as prescribed when child is awake and alert from anesthesia
    - Involve caregivers in child's care

Priority Potential & Actual Complications

- Immobility
- Bowel and bladder incontinence
- Meningitis
- Orthopedic issues
- Sleep disorders
- Hydrocephalus
- Restricted or tethered spinal cord (spinal nerves become bound to the scar where surgery occurred)

Priority Nursing Implications

- In most cases of spina bifida, surgery occurs after the infant is born. However, when spina bifida is detected in pregnancy, prenatal surgery can be done to repair the spinal cord. Surgery must occur before week 26 of pregnancy

Reinforcement of Priority Teaching

- Show caregiver how to perform dressing changes and monitor surgical site for infection
- Proper positioning of child, prone or side-lying as prescribed
- Perform proper skin care and to avoid stools getting to the surgery site
- Show caregiver how to perform intermittent urinary catheterization, if prescribed
- Show how to perform gentle range of motion on child joints to prevent contractures
- Explain signs of complications and who to call if complications occur
- Explain the importance of feeding child a diet that has high fiber and fluids to prevent constipation
- Explain to caregiver that child may have latex allergy because of repeated exposure to latex in the acute care setting
- Demonstrate to caregiver how to use mobility aids for child, as prescribed
- Explain to caregiver on the trajectory of spina bifida and the long-term needs of the child
- Explain to caregiver that child may need ongoing care from several professionals such as neurology, orthopedics, urology, physical/occupational/speech therapy and special education professionals
- Assist caregiver with resources for support groups, if needed. Provide information for the Spina Bifida Association of America

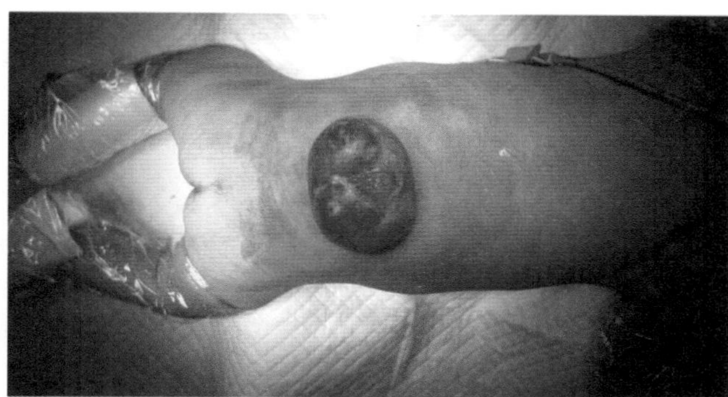

Image 13-23: This client is scheduled for a myelomeningocele repair. List 5 nursing interventions to keep the client safe in the preoperative period. List 5 nursing interventions to keep the client safe in the postoperative period.

Next Gen Clinical Judgment

A client with spinal bifida is being discharged home after a successful surgery. The PN/VN follows up on teaching done by the RN with the parents on when to seek immediate medical care. List 3 statements made by the parents that would indicate teaching was effective?

Spinal cord injury

Pathophysiology/Description

- Spinal cord injury (SCI) is caused by damage to the spinal cord, usually from a traumatic event, which causes temporary or permanent changes in function
- Classified as primary vs secondary injury. Primary refers to the initial injury caused by a specific event, such as a gunshot. Secondary refers to the ongoing damage that continues after the initial injury has occurred. There are many factors that can impact secondary injury, among them are cellular necrosis and vascular changes
- Characterized by the level of injury, degree of injury and mechanism of injury
- Level of injury
    - Tetraplegia (used to be called quadriplegia): trunk, arms, hands, pelvic organ and legs all impacted by the spinal cord injury
    - Paraplegia: all or part of the trunk, legs and pelvic organs are affected
- Degree of injury
    - Complete injury: sensory and motor function are lost below the level of injury
    - Incomplete injury: there is some motor or sensory function below the level of injury
- Mechanism of injury: Hyperflexion, flexion, extension-rotation, flexion-rotation and compression

Priority Data Collection or Cues

- Respiratory issues, likely with cervical injuries, especially above C4
- Vital signs and oxygen saturation. Ensure saturation is greater than 90%
- Cause of trauma, open wounds and signs of internal injuries
- Neurologic system, using the American Spinal Injury Association (ASIA) Impairment Scale
- Cardiovascular system, hypotension and bradycardia due to deficit in sympathetic nervous system
- Absence of reflexes and other deficits below the injury
- Neurogenic bladder and bowel, common in SCI. Treat as prescribed
- Paralysis in all four extremities or in lower extremities only
- Nutritional status. Client will have significant nutritional needs
- Neuropathic pain, often described as tingling, burning, or shooting
- Catheter-associated urinary tract infection because of the extended usage of urinary catheters

Priority Laboratory Tests/Diagnostics

- Computerized tomography (CT) scan showing degree and location of injury. X-ray, viewing spinal column
- Magnetic resonance imaging (MRI) showing neurological changes and any soft tissue damages

Priority Interventions or Actions

- Immobilize client and maintain a patent airway. Ensure oxygen saturation greater 90%
- Assist in the placement of endotracheal tube as needed. Monitor arterial blood gasses and determine need for client to be placed on a mechanical ventilator
- Monitor intravenous fluids as prescribed. Place nasogastric tube to suction
- Ensure client receives nutrition via alternate routes in the initial days of the injury
- Head in neutral position. Do not place in sitting position. Move with log roll technique
- Maintain normal body temperature. Monitor for signs of respiratory infection
- Perform ongoing monitoring of all systems. Provide prophylaxis for stress ulcers as prescribed
- Sequential compression devices to prevent venous thromboembolism. Low-dose heparin as prescribed
- Pressure ulcer prevention protocol, ensuring meticulous skin care
- Monitor for signs indicating spinal shock and/or autonomic dysreflexia/hyperreflexia
- Consultations for speech, occupational and physical therapists
- If autonomic hyperreflexia occurs: raise head of bed, loosen tight clothing, monitor for cause and relieve the cause. Most often it occurs because of a full bladder or bowel. Perform urinary catheterization and bowel evacuation if needed. Administer antihypertensive and monitor blood pressure every 15 minutes
- Postoperative interventions (skeletal traction for cervical or upper thoracic injuries)
    - Weights to the traction. Check to ensure weights hang freely without touching
    - Client's body in good alignment. Maintain use of Stryker frame or other types of special bed
    - Monitor proper fit of the halo jacket. Ensure 1 finger fits under the jacket
    - Place foam or fleece at pressure points under halo vest to prevent pressure ulcers
    - Clean pin sites on halo and skull tongs daily and monitor for signs of infection
    - High-protein, calcium-rich diet to promote bone healing and prevent muscle wasting
    - Wrench at the bedside that can open the halo in an emergency if needed
- Postoperative interventions (laminectomy or spinal fusion for thoracic, lumbar and sacral injuries)
    - Monitor circulation and motor function in lower extremities. Monitor respiratory function
    - Monitor surgery site for bleeding and infection. Provide cast care for full-body casts

- Client flat and in good alignment. Turn and reposition every 2 hours using log rolling
    - Encourage incentive spirometry and coughing and deep breathing
    - Nothing by mouth until bowel sounds return. Monitor intake and output

Priority Potential & Actual Complications

- Autonomic dysreflexia/hyperreflexia, spinal shock, neurogenic shock
- Complete or partial paralysis, total dependence, depression and social isolation

Priority Nursing Implications

- During the first 2 days of a spinal cord injury, edema may cause severe respiratory dysfunction, placing client at risk for respiratory failure. Respiratory problems are the main cause of death in persons who sustain a spinal cord injury
- When reflexes for a client with thoracic spinal injury at T6 or higher has returned after a spinal shock, autonomic hyperreflexia can occur. This is manifested as significantly high blood pressure, severe headache, bradycardia, flushing and sweating above the injury, blurred vision and nausea. Autonomic hyperreflexia is a medical emergency to avoid a stroke

Priority Medications

- Several drugs are used for various aspects of spinal cord injury. Below are some examples
- Enoxaparin
    - Low molecular weight heparin administered subcutaneously
    - Used to prevent venous thromboembolism
- Phenylephrine
    - Vasopressor drug administered IM or subcutaneously
    - Used to maintain mean arterial pressure at a level that improves perfusion to spinal cord
- Oxybutynin
    - Oral medication
    - Anticholinergic drug used to treat neurogenic bladder
- Nifedipine
    - Oral medication
    - Calcium channel blocker: one of many used to treat autonomic dysreflexia

Reinforcement of Priority Teaching

- Nutritional intake and bowel management
    - Eat 3 well-balanced meals daily that consist of high protein, and 20-30 grams of daily fiber to prevent constipation. Drink adequate fluids. Exercise as able
    - Determine schedule for bowel movements and manual rectal stimulation
- Care of halo vest
    - Clean pin sites as prescribed and apply antibiotic ointment. Report signs of infection
    - Open vest one side at time while lying down, clean, inspect, dry skin and replace brace
    - Dry vest with hair dryer if wet
    - Do not twist body. Always keep wrench close. Wear sheepskin pad under vest
- Autonomic hyperreflexia
    - Signs of autonomic hyperreflexia (aforementioned) and report immediately
    - Raise head of bed, check for bowel impaction or full bladder and relieve cause
- Skin care
    - Change position in bed every 2 hours, at least. Shift position in wheelchair every 15 minutes. Use pressure relief mattress and chair cushion
    - Cut fingernails short. Examine skin daily for skin breakdown
- Trajectory of spinal cord injury and the long-term care needs
- Need for ongoing care from several professionals. Resources for support groups

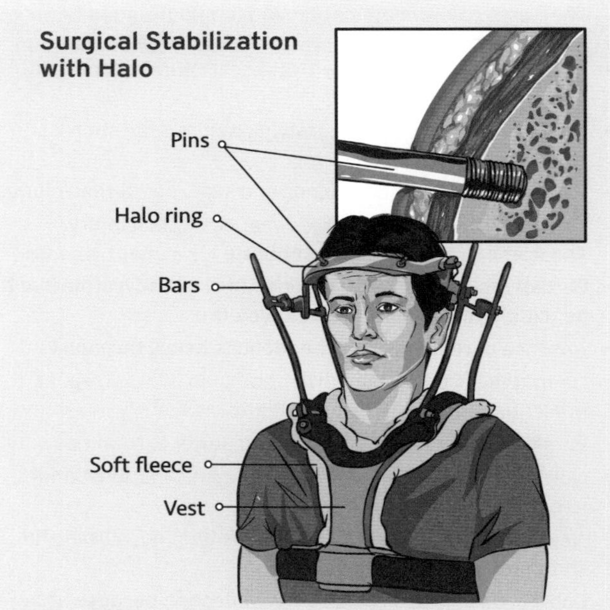

Image 13-24: Clients with spinal cord injury may have their spinal column stabilized using a halo traction with vest. List several nursing interventions indicated when a client is in halo traction with a vest.

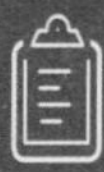

NurseThink® Quiz Questions

1. **The nurse cares for a client with cerebral palsy who wears orthotic devices 16 hours per day. Which finding best indicates the client is outgrowing the orthotic device?**
   a. Callused heel and ball of foot.
   b. Toes extend beyond the device.
   c. Blistering at the ankles.
   d. Inability to lift foot off the ground.

2. **The nurse cares for a pediatric client experiencing a clonic seizure. Which action does the nurse prioritize?**
   a. Determining the source of post-ictal confusion.
   b. Comforting the child with soothing words.
   c. Placing an oral airway to maintain airway access.
   d. Placing the child on their side in case of vomiting.

3. **A client is returning to a skilled nursing facility, and the nurse provides handoff report. To reduce the risk of seizures, which component of the care plan does the nurse emphasize?**
   a. The client should always wear a medical identification bracelet.
   b. The client should never be without intravenous access.
   c. A strict medication regimen is necessary to maintain therapeutic levels.
   d. The client should refrain from ambulating to avoid the risk of fall.

4. **The nurse reviews education with a middle-aged female about the risk for osteoporosis. Which recommendation does the nurse reinforce?**
   a. Reduce protein intake.
   b. Increase calcium consumption.
   c. Limited exercise.
   d. Sun tanning therapy.

5. **The nurse evaluates understanding for a client who was recently diagnosed with osteoarthritis. Which statement by the client requires follow-up by the nurse?**
   a. "Lidocaine and capsaicin creams should be applied using gloves."
   b. "I should inform my provider of any dietary supplements I take."
   c. "NSAIDs are nephrotoxic and should only be taken as directed."
   d. "Opioids are helpful treatments for mild to moderate pain."

6. **The nurse cares for an adolescent client with a tibial fracture. Which intervention does the nurse prioritize after the application of a temporary leg cast?**
   a. Check the area closest to injury for redness and swelling.
   b. Neurovascular evaluation above and below the injury.
   c. Ensure the casting materials are drying appropriately.
   d. Provide crutch walking education and demonstration.

7. **A client presents to the emergency room with chest wall trauma. The nurse suspects fractured ribs and flail chest. What data is most consistent with flail chest?**
   a. Paradoxical chest wall movement.
   b. Pain with respirations.
   c. Fractured rib protruding from the chest wall.
   d. Weak cough and hemoptysis.

8. **The nurse plans home care for the client with peripheral neuropathy secondary to uncontrolled Type II Diabetes. When reviewing the plan of care with the home health aide, which instructions does the nurse include? *Select all that apply.***
   a. Limit exercise to 30 minutes weekly.
   b. Check feet for injury or infection daily.
   c. Apply lotion to feet and between toes, twice daily.
   d. Avoid walking barefoot, even inside the home.
   e. Ensure shoes are well-fitting and supportive.

9. **The nurse cares for a client with suspected carpal tunnel syndrome (CTS). What does the nurse instruct the client to avoid?**
   a. Wrist splints at night.
   b. Wrist splints while working.
   c. Anti-inflammatory medications.
   d. Repetitive hand/wrist motions.

10. **The nurse cares for a client with a recent left below-the-knee amputation following a motorcycle accident. The nurse shares information with the spouse about what the client may experience post-amputation. Which statement by the spouse indicates understanding?**
   a. "Complaints about pain to an area that has been amputated are psychological."
   b. "The tissue above the amputation will remain pale and cool to touch."
   c. "Phantom limb pain is a real complication and can often be treated."
   d. "I should avoid asking my spouse about the injury and amputation."

11. **The nurse reinforces teaching with the caregiver of a client with amyotrophic lateral sclerosis (ALS). Which intervention does the nurse highlight to reduce the client's risk of aspiration?**
   a. Turn client and reposition every two hours.
   b. Administer all medications through a gastric tube.
   c. Crush medications and mix in food for administration.
   d. Elevate the head of the bed at least 45° when eating and drinking.

12. **The nurse cares for a client experiencing an acute exacerbation of multiple sclerosis (MS) and documents this in the electronic health record. Which issue requires priority intervention?**

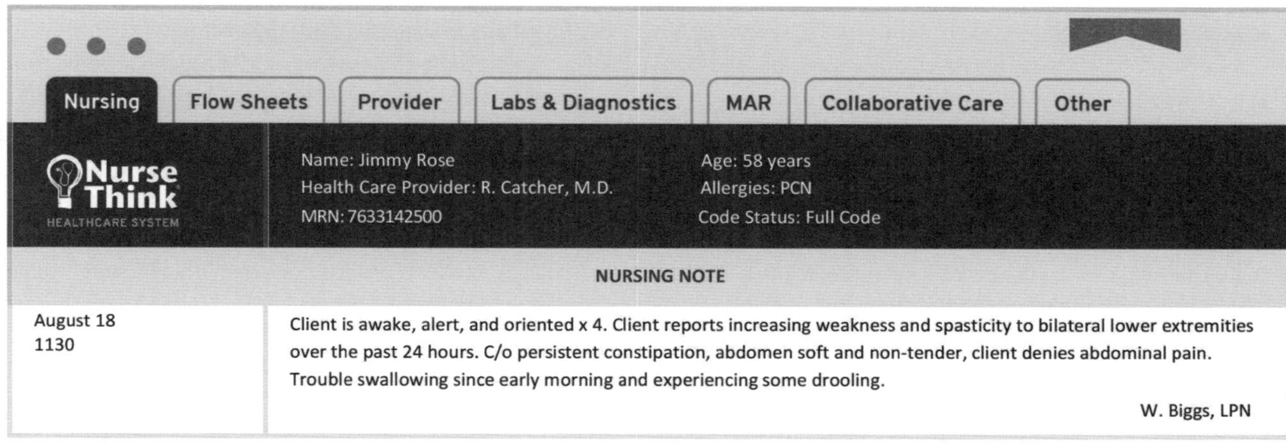

Nursing | Flow Sheets | Provider | Labs & Diagnostics | MAR | Collaborative Care | Other

Nurse Think HEALTHCARE SYSTEM

Name: Jimmy Rose
Health Care Provider: R. Catcher, M.D.
MRN: 7633142500

Age: 58 years
Allergies: PCN
Code Status: Full Code

NURSING NOTE	
August 18 1130	Client is awake, alert, and oriented x 4. Client reports increasing weakness and spasticity to bilateral lower extremities over the past 24 hours. C/o persistent constipation, abdomen soft and non-tender, client denies abdominal pain. Trouble swallowing since early morning and experiencing some drooling. W. Biggs, LPN

a. Dysphagia.
b. Bilateral lower extremity spasticity.
c. Fatigue.
d. Constipation.

13. **The nurse evaluates a client with a history of Parkinson's Disease and expects to see which clinical manifestations of the disease? *Select all that apply.***
   a. Muscle flaccidity.
   b. Unilateral tremors.
   c. Bradykinesia.
   d. Mask-like face.
   e. Flexed knees and elbows.

14. **An older adult client presents to the office with reports of blurry vision, difficulty seeing at night, and a halo appearance around lights. The nurse suspects cataracts. The client is concerned about the risk for injury related to changes in vision. What does the nurse instruct the client to avoid?**
   a. Wearing sunglasses.
   b. Nighttime driving.
   c. Regular eye examinations.
   b. Handrails for stairs.

15. **The nurse cares for a client with diabetes and administers a beta-blocker prescribed for the client's glaucoma. What potential complication does the nurse monitor for after giving the medication?**
   a. Bronchodilation.
   b. Hypoglycemia.
   c. Increased intracranial pressure.
   d. Hyperglycemia.

16. **The nurse cares for a 60-year-old client with a 15-year, two pack per day smoking history, hypertension, and obesity. The nurse reviews the risk factors for macular degeneration. Which statement by the client warrants follow-up by the nurse?**
   a. "Macular degeneration may be a complication of uncontrolled diabetes."
   b. "I should wear protective eyewear in the sun to protect my eyes from the light."
   c. "I should stop smoking to reduce my risk of macular degeneration."
   d. "I can't do anything about macular degeneration since it's an aging issue."

17. **A 2-year-old client has bilateral otitis media and a temperature of 103.2°F (39.6°C) . The provider has prescribed one dose of oral acetaminophen 10 mg per kg. The client weighs 22 pounds. How much acetaminophen does the nurse prepare to administer?**
   a. 160 mg.
   b. 100 mg.
   c. 220 mg.
   d. 484 mg.

18. The nurse cares for a client with a spinal cord injury who is experiencing spinal shock. Which intervention does the nurse implement to prevent skin breakdown in this client?

a. Regular repositioning to reduce pressure on dependent areas.
b. Avoid moving the client more than twice per shift for safety.
c. Always keep the client's head of bed > 45 degrees.
d. Change the client's position slowly using a slide board.

19. The nurse cares for a client with a spinal cord injury at L2-L3. The nurse plans care that anticipates flaccidity/ paralysis in which area of the body?

a. Unilateral extremities.
b. Mid-torso and below.
c. Bilateral lower extremities.
d. All four extremities.

20. The nurse cares for a pediatric client with conjunctivitis. The client is complaining of itching and tenderness to the eye and surrounding area. What is the nurse's best action to relieve the client's symptoms?

a. Application of a hot, moist cloth to the affected eye.
b. Administration of an oral antihistamine.
c. Encouraging the client to sleep in the prone position.
d. Application of a cool compress to the affected eye.

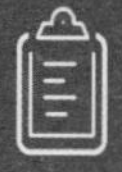

NurseThink® Quiz Answers

1. **The nurse cares for a client with cerebral palsy who wears orthotic devices 16 hours per day. Which finding best indicates the client is outgrowing the orthotic device?**
   a. Callused heel and ball of foot.
   b. Toes extend beyond the device.
   c. Blistering at the ankles.
   d. Inability to lift foot off the ground.

   Topic/Concept: Movement **Subtopic:** Cerebral Palsy **Bloom's Taxonomy:** Applying **Clinical Problem-Solving Process:** Data Collection **NCLEX-PN®:** Basic Care and Comfort **QSEN:** Evidence-based Practice **CJMM:** Analyze Cues

   Rationale: Orthotic devices are commonly used in the client with cerebral palsy to increase mobility, provide a stable base for movement, and control muscular imbalances. Toes extending beyond the length of the device, as with shoes, indicates the client has outgrown the current orthotic size. As the client grows, orthotics will need to be refitted. Blisters and calluses indicate pressure and friction in an area, not length issues. Immobility is not likely to be associated with the orthotic device but with the client's physical function.

   THIN Thinking: *Clinical Problem-Solving Process* – When collecting data related to orthotics, the nurse must understand the device's function and potential complications. Determining fit and skin integrity are important data collection points for the client with issues related to mobility.

2. **The nurse cares for a pediatric client experiencing a clonic seizure. Which action does the nurse prioritize?**
   a. Determining the source of post-ictal confusion.
   b. Comforting the child with soothing words.
   c. Placing an oral airway to maintain airway access.
   d. Placing the child on their side in case of vomiting.

   Topic/Concept: Movement **Subtopic:** Seizures (peds) **Bloom's Taxonomy:** Applying **Clinical Problem-Solving Process:** Implementation **NCLEX-PN®:** Safety and Infection Control **QSEN:** Safety **CJMM:** Take Action

   Rationale: Clonic seizures involve repetitive, rhythmic jerking movements. During seizure activity, the nurse's priority is to protect client safety. Placing the child on their side during a seizure will help the airway remain open and allow saliva and emesis to drain from the mouth, reducing the risk of aspiration. Post-ictal confusion can be expected for a short time after seizure activity. Though soothing communication can comfort children, this is not the priority and will have little impact on seizure activity. Nothing should be placed in the mouth of a person having a seizure.

   THIN Thinking: *Help Quick* – Actions that promote client safety and prevent further injury are priority actions in the case of seizure. It is important for the nurse to understand common and expected symptoms of seizures and how best to protect the client until the seizure resolves.

3. **A client is returning to a skilled nursing facility, and the nurse provides handoff report. To reduce the risk of seizures, which component of the care plan does the nurse emphasize?**
   a. The client should always wear a medical identification bracelet.
   b. The client should never be without intravenous access.
   c. A strict medication regimen is necessary to maintain therapeutic levels.
   d. The client should refrain from ambulating to avoid the risk of fall.

   Topic/Concept: Movement **Subtopic:** Seizures (Adult) **Bloom's Taxonomy:** Applying **Clinical Problem-Solving Process:** Planning **NCLEX-PN®:** Reduction of Risk Potential **QSEN:** Evidence-based Practice **CJMM:** Generate Solutions

   Rationale: Therapeutic levels of antiepileptics are necessary to reduce the risk of seizures. A strict medication schedule is the best approach to ensuring medication is taken at the same time daily. A medical identification bracelet is helpful for the client with seizures but will not reduce the overall risk for seizures. Clients outside of the hospital are not likely to maintain intravenous access; this is not a reasonable expectation. Avoiding ambulation is not a reasonable expectation. Client mobility should be maintained whenever possible.

   THIN Thinking: *Top Three* – When planning care for the client with seizures, the nurse must stress the importance of a medication regimen and serum testing for therapeutic antiepileptic medication levels. Sub-therapeutic levels will increase the risk of seizure activity.

4. **The nurse reviews education with a middle-aged female about the risk for osteoporosis. Which recommendation does the nurse reinforce?**
   a. Reduce protein intake.
   b. Increase calcium consumption.
   c. Limited exercise.
   d. Sun tanning therapy.

   Topic/Concept: Movement **Subtopic:** Osteoporosis **Bloom's Taxonomy:** Applying **Clinical Problem-Solving Process:** Planning **NCLEX-PN®:** Physiological Adaptation **QSEN:** Evidence-based Practice **CJMM:** Generate Solutions

Rationale: Calcium and vitamin D consumption is crucial for the prevention and treatment of osteoporosis. Protein intake should be increased to support the strengthening of the musculoskeletal system. Limited exercise is not recommended for healthy bone growth and maintenance. Exposure to sunlight for 15 minutes a day is helpful with vitamin D and calcium absorption; however, sun tanning therapy may increase the risk for some skin cancers and should not be recommended.

THIN Thinking: *Clinical Problem-Solving Process* –Vitamin D and calcium are important for healthy bone growth and maintenance. In the aging adult female, osteoporosis is a risk. The nurse should be prepared to help clients understand and reduce risks by addressing physiologic changes that occur with age.

5. **The nurse evaluates understanding for a client who was recently diagnosed with osteoarthritis. Which statement by the client requires follow-up by the nurse?**
   a. "Lidocaine and capsaicin creams should be applied using gloves."
   b. "I should inform my provider of any dietary supplements I take."
   c. "NSAIDs are nephrotoxic and should only be taken as directed."
   d. "Opioids are helpful treatments for mild to moderate pain."

Topic/Concept: Movement **Subtopic:** Osteoarthritis **Bloom's Taxonomy:** Analyzing **Clinical Problem-Solving Process:** Evaluation **NCLEX-PN®:** Pharmacological Therapies **QSEN:** Patient-centered Care **CJMM:** Evaluate Outcomes

Rationale: Opioids should be reserved for moderate to severe pain. Acetaminophen and NSAIDs are typically used for mild to moderate pain. As topicals, lidocaine and capsaicin creams should be applied with gloves to reduce absorption. Supplements may interact with other prescribed medications. Therefore, the provider should be aware of all supplements and OTC products the client is taking. NSAIDs should be taken as directed, and kidney function should be monitored.

THIN Thinking: *Clinical Problem-Solving Process* –It is important for the nurse to evaluate education provided to the client and family. The nurse should follow up when misunderstandings are noted and respond in affirmation when information is clearly understood.

6. **The nurse cares for an adolescent client with a tibial fracture. Which intervention does the nurse prioritize after the application of a temporary leg cast?**
   a. Check the area closest to injury for redness and swelling.
   b. Neurovascular evaluation above and below the injury.
   c. Ensure the casting materials are drying appropriately.
   d. Provide crutch walking education and demonstration.

Topic/Concept: Movement **Subtopic:** Fractures (Peds) **Bloom's Taxonomy:** Applying **Clinical Problem-Solving Process:** Planning **NCLEX-PN®:** Safety and Infection Control **QSEN:** Evidence-based Practice **CJMM:** Prioritize Hypotheses

Rationale: Data Collection of the area should occur before application of casting materials. Neurovascular monitoring, including sensation, pulses, pain, and pallor, should occur before and after applying casting materials to ensure that circulation is not compromised. Casting materials take time to dry; this is not the priority action after application of the cast. Crutch walking education may be needed, but this is not the priority action.

THIN Thinking: *Identify Risk to Safety* – The safety of the client is always the priority. If issues related to airway and breathing are not present, the next priority is circulation. The nurse must collect data on the injured extremity's baseline neurovascular status before application of casting, splinting, or any other orthopedic or restrictive device and immediately monitor neurovascular status after application to ensure circulation has not been compromised.

7. **A client presents to the emergency room with chest wall trauma. The nurse suspects fractured ribs and flail chest. What data is most consistent with flail chest?**
   a. Paradoxical chest wall movement.
   b. Pain with respirations.
   c. Fractured rib protruding from the chest wall.
   d. Weak cough and hemoptysis.

Topic/Concept: Movement **Subtopic:** Fractures (Adult) **Bloom's Taxonomy:** Applying **Clinical Problem-Solving Process:** Data Collection **NCLEX-PN®:** Physiological Adaptation **QSEN:** Evidence-based Practice **CJMM:** Recognize Cues

Rationale: Paradoxical chest wall movement is classic evidence of flail chest. Pain with respirations can be noted with any chest wall trauma. Protrusion of the bone indicates an open fracture and may result in a pneumothorax. Weak cough and hemoptysis may be present with various respiratory infections but are not expected findings with flail chest.

THIN Thinking: *Clinical Problem-Solving Process* –The nurse should conduct a thorough respiratory and trauma data collection when managing chest wall trauma. Flail chest is a common complication associated with chest wall trauma.

8. **The nurse plans home care for the client with peripheral neuropathy secondary to uncontrolled Type II Diabetes. When reviewing the plan of care with the home health aide, which instructions does the nurse include? *Select all that apply.***
   a. Limit exercise to 30 minutes weekly.
   b. Collect data on feet for injury or infection daily.
   c. Apply lotion to feet and between toes, twice daily.
   d. Avoid walking barefoot, even inside the home.
   e. Ensure shoes are well-fitting and supportive.

Topic/Concept: Movement **Subtopic:** Peripheral Neuropathy **Bloom's Taxonomy:** Applying **Clinical Problem-Solving Process:** Planning **NCLEX-PN®:** Coordinated Care **QSEN:** Teamwork and Collaboration **CJMM:** Generate Solutions

Rationale: Peripheral neuropathy and diabetes mellitus do not warrant a limitation in exercise. Exercise is encouraged as tolerated at 30 minutes a day, five days a week. Routine monitoring of skin, especially feet, is important in avoiding wounds and infections. Lotion should not be applied between toes in the diabetic client as this may facilitate the growth of bacteria/fungus in dark, cool places and lead to infection. Clients with peripheral neuropathy should avoid walking barefoot, even inside the home, to avoid injury. Clients with diabetes, especially those with peripheral neuropathy, should ensure footwear fits well and is supportive to avoid blisters and other injuries to the feet.

THIN Thinking: *Top Three* – For the client with diabetes, especially with known peripheral neuropathy, foot care is essential in preventing injury and infection. The nurse should be well-informed of evidence-based practices in proper foot care and delegate appropriately to unlicensed assistive personnel.

9. **The nurse cares for a client with suspected carpal tunnel syndrome (CTS). What does the nurse instruct the client to avoid?**
   a. Wrist splints at night.
   b. Wrist splints while working.
   c. Anti-inflammatory medications.
   d. Repetitive hand/wrist motions.

Topic/Concept: Movement **Subtopic:** Carpal Tunnel **Bloom's Taxonomy:** Applying **Clinical Problem-Solving Process:** Implementation **NCLEX-PN®:** Reduction of Risk Potential **QSEN:** Evidence-based Practice **CJMM:** Take Action

Rationale: Splinting at night and with symptoms (at work) is encouraged. Anti-inflammatory medications help reduce pain and inflammation. Repetitive motions are the likely cause of CTS symptoms. Rest and reduction of those motions are likely to eliminate pain and inflammation.

THIN Thinking: *Identify Risk to Safety* – The nurse should understand the physiologic processes involved in CTS and offer education for reducing risks. Reducing pain and inflammation by limiting repetitive movements and supporting the extremity are the best non-invasive treatments for CTS.

10. **The nurse cares for a client with a recent left below-the-knee amputation following a motorcycle accident. The nurse shares information with the spouse about what the client may experience post-amputation. Which statement by the spouse indicates understanding?**
    a. "Complaints about pain to an area that has been amputated are psychological."
    b. "The tissue above the amputation will remain pale and cool to touch."
    c. "Phantom limb pain is a real complication and can often be treated."
    d. "I should avoid asking my spouse about the injury and amputation."

Topic/Concept: Movement **Subtopic:** Amputation **Bloom's Taxonomy:** Analyzing **Clinical Problem-Solving Process:** Evaluation **NCLEX-PN®:** Physiological Adaptation **QSEN:** Evidence-based Practice **CJMM:** Evaluate Outcomes

Rationale: Phantom limb pain is most common in clients with chronic limb pain prior to amputation but can occur with traumatic amputations as well. This pain is real and physiological and can be treated in multiple ways. The tissue above the amputation should be warm to touch if adequate tissue perfusion is taking place. Pallor and coolness should be reported to the provider immediately. Grieving is likely after amputation, and the client should be encouraged to speak freely. Counseling may be necessary to facilitate adaptation to a change in body image and functioning.

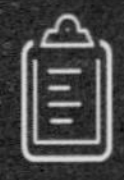

THIN Thinking: *Clinical Problem-Solving Process* – The nurse must consider the expected psychosocial and physiological responses to injuries, disease processes, and interventions to plan effective care and anticipate client concerns.

11. **The nurse reinforces teaching with the caregiver of a client with amyotrophic lateral sclerosis (ALS). Which intervention does the nurse highlight to reduce the client's risk of aspiration?**
    a. Turn client and reposition every two hours.
    b. Administer all medications through a gastric tube.
    c. Crush medications and mix in food for administration.
    d. ● Elevate the head of the bed at least 45° when eating and drinking.

Topic/Concept: Movement **Subtopic:** Amyotrophic lateral sclerosis **Bloom's Taxonomy:** Applying **Clinical Problem-Solving Process:** Planning **NCLEX-PN®:** Safety and Infection Control **QSEN:** Safety **CJMM:** Generate Solutions

Rationale: Turning and repositioning are important for preventing skin breakdown. Clients in the early stages of ALS may still eat and drink orally or may not yet have a gastric tube placed. Clients who can eat and drink orally may not need medications crushed and administered in medications. Additionally, not all medications can be crushed or opened. Elevating the head of the bed during eating, drinking, and brushing teeth will reduce the risk of aspirating food, drink, or body fluids.

THIN Thinking: *Identify Risk to Safety* – The nurse should plan care for the client with ALS that focuses on reducing the risk of aspiration, maintaining the airway, and preventing skin breakdown as a result of immobility and neurological complications.

12. **The nurse cares for a client experiencing an acute exacerbation of multiple sclerosis (MS) and documents this in the electronic health record. Which issue requires priority intervention?**
    ba. ● Dysphagia.
    b. Bilateral lower extremity spasticity.
    c. Fatigue.
    d. Constipation.

Topic/Concept: Movement **Subtopic:** Multiple Sclerosis **Bloom's Taxonomy:** Applying **Clinical Problem-Solving Process:** Planning **NCLEX-PN®:** Safety and Infection Control **QSEN:** Patient-centered Care **CJMM:** Prioritize Hypotheses

Rationale: Dysphagia is difficulty swallowing and may compromise the client's airway or result in aspiration; it is the priority concern at this time. Spasticity is expected with exacerbation of MS and can be treated with corticosteroids and muscle relaxants. It is an annoying complication but is not the priority. Fatigue is an expected clinical manifestation of MS. Constipation is a common treatable complication of MS. Without evidence of an intestinal blockage, constipation is not the priority.

THIN Thinking: *Identify Risk to Safety* – Airway compromise is the priority concern here, especially since the client is also experiencing drooling and is at risk for aspiration of saliva.

13. **The nurse evaluates a client with a history of Parkinson's Disease and expects to see which clinical manifestations of the disease? *Select all that apply.***
    a. Muscle flaccidity.
    b. ● Unilateral tremors.
    c. ● Bradykinesia.
    d. ● Mask-like face.
    e. ● Flexed knees and elbows.

Topic/Concept: Movement **Subtopic:** Parkinson's Disease **Bloom's Taxonomy:** Analyzing **Clinical Problem-Solving Process:** Data Collection **NCLEX-PN®:** Psychosocial Integrity **QSEN:** Evidence-based Practice **CJMM:** Analyze Cues

Rationale: Rigidity, not flaccidity, is characteristic of Parkinson's Disease. Other manifestations include unilateral tremors to the upper and lower extremities, bradykinesia (slow movements), mask-like face, and flexed elbows, knees, and wrists.

THIN Thinking: *Clinical Problem-Solving Process* –The nurse should anticipate the clinical manifestations of Parkinson's Disease when evaluating this client. Typical findings include slowed movements, muscle rigidity, tremors, stooped posture, flexed joints, dementia, and dysphagia.

14. **An older adult client presents to the office with reports of blurry vision, difficulty seeing at night, and a halo appearance around lights. The nurse suspects cataracts. The client is concerned about the risk for injury related to changes in vision. What does the nurse instruct the client to avoid?**
    a. Wearing sunglasses.
    b. ● Nighttime driving.
    c. Regular eye examinations.
    b. Handrails for stairs.

Topic/Concept: Movement **Subtopic:** Cataracts **Bloom's Taxonomy:** Applying **Clinical Problem-Solving Process:** Planning **NCLEX-PN®:** Coordinated Care **QSEN:** Teamwork and Collaboration **CJMM:** Generate Solutions

Rationale: The client may have cataracts and should avoid driving after dusk. The client should wear protective eyeglasses when in the sun and have regular, at least annual, eye examinations. To reduce the risk of falls, the client should use handrails when going up and down stairs.

THIN Thinking: *Identify Risk to Safety* – The nurse should instruct the client on ways to manage risks and reduce the impact of cataracts and vision changes on client safety.

15. **The nurse cares for a client with diabetes and administers a beta-blocker prescribed for the client's glaucoma. What potential complication does the nurse monitor for after giving the medication?**
    a. Bronchodilation.
    b. Hypoglycemia.
    c. Increased intracranial pressure.
    d. Hyperglycemia.

Topic/Concept: Movement **Subtopic:** Glaucoma **Bloom's Taxonomy:** Analyzing **Clinical Problem-Solving Process:** Evaluation **NCLEX-PN®:** Pharmacological Therapies **QSEN:** Evidence-based Practice **CJMM:** Evaluate Outcomes

Rationale: Beta-blockers result in bronchoconstriction and decreased intracranial pressure. Beta-blockers may place the client at a higher risk for hypoglycemia.

THIN Thinking: *Top Three* – When administering medication, the nurse should review information about potential complications of pharmaceutical treatments and monitor the client accordingly.

16. **The nurse cares for a 60-year-old client with a 15-year, two pack per day smoking history, hypertension, and obesity. The nurse reviews the risk factors for macular degeneration. Which statement by the client warrants follow-up by the nurse?**
    a. "Macular degeneration may be a complication of uncontrolled diabetes."
    b. "I should wear protective eyewear in the sun to protect my eyes from the light."
    c. "I should stop smoking to reduce my risk of macular degeneration."
    d. "I can't do anything about macular degeneration since it's an aging issue."

Topic/Concept: Movement **Subtopic:** Macular Degeneration **Bloom's Taxonomy:** Analyzing **Clinical Problem-Solving Process:** Evaluation **NCLEX-PN®:** Reduction of Risk Potential **QSEN:** Evidence-based Practice **CJMM:** Evaluate Outcomes

Rationale: Diabetes and excessive exposure to the sun are risk factors for macular degeneration. Smoking is a risk factor, and clients should be encouraged to quit. Advanced age is a risk factor, but other risk factors can be reduced in attempts to prevent the disorder.

THIN Thinking: *Clinical Problem-Solving Process* –The nurse should follow up on client teaching when the client communicates incorrect information or lacks understanding.

17. **A 2-year-old client has bilateral otitis media and a temperature of 103.2°F (39.6°C) . The provider has prescribed one dose of oral acetaminophen 10 mg per kg. The client weighs 22 pounds. How much acetaminophen does the nurse prepare to administer?**
    a. 160 mg.
    b. 100 mg.
    c. 220 mg.
    d. 484 mg.

Topic/Concept: Movement **Subtopic:** Otitis media (peds) **Bloom's Taxonomy:** Applying **Clinical Problem-Solving Process:** Implementation **NCLEX-PN®:** Pharmacological Therapies **QSEN:** Patient-centered care **CJMM:** Take Action

Rationale: Convert the client's weight to kg, then multiply the dose by the weight. 22 lbs/2.2 = 10 kg X 10 mg = 100 mg

THIN Thinking: *Help Quick* – Verifying medication calculations is a quick and critical action the nurse must take to ensure safe and effective care of every client.

18. **The nurse cares for a client with a spinal cord injury who is experiencing spinal shock. Which intervention does the nurse implement to prevent skin breakdown in this client?**
    a. Regular repositioning to reduce pressure on dependent areas.
    b. Avoid moving the client more than twice per shift for safety.
    c. Always keep the client's head of bed > 45 degrees.
    d. Change the client's position slowly using a slide board.

Topic/Concept: Movement **Subtopic:** Spinal cord injury **Bloom's Taxonomy:** Applying **Clinical Problem-Solving Process:** Implementation **NCLEX-PN®:** Health promotion and maintenance **QSEN:** Evidence-based Practice **CJMM:** Take Action

Rationale: Gentle, regular repositioning can help prevent skin breakdown. Keeping the head of bed higher than 45 degrees is not indicated for spinal shock and is not likely to significantly impact skin breakdown. A slide board is not indicated for this situation or purpose.

THIN Thinking: *Top Three* – Care should be taken to reduce pressure areas in the immobile or bedridden client. This is best achieved with gentle and frequent changes in position.

19. The nurse cares for a client with a spinal cord injury at L2-L3. The nurse plans care that anticipates flaccidity/ paralysis in which area of the body?

a. Unilateral extremities.
b. Mid-torso and below.
c. Bilateral lower extremities.
d. All four extremities.

Topic/Concept: Movement **Subtopic:** Spinal cord injury **Bloom's Taxonomy:** Applying **Clinical Problem-Solving Process:** Data Collection **NCLEX-PN®:** Physiological Adaptation **QSEN:** Evidence-based Practice **CJMM:** Analyze Cues

Rationale: Unilateral paraplegia is not consistent with a specific spinal cord injury. Paraplegia at the mid-torse and below is consistent with injury at T6. Paraplegia of the lower extremities is consistent with injury at L2-L3. Quadriplegia is consistent with a cervical injury.

THIN Thinking: *Clinical Problem-Solving Process* –The nurse should plan client-specific care. For this client, the plan should anticipate paralysis of the bilateral lower extremities.

20. The nurse cares for a pediatric client with conjunctivitis. The client is complaining of itching and tenderness to the eye and surrounding area. What is the nurse's best action to relieve the client's symptoms?

a. Application of a hot, moist cloth to the affected eye.
b. Administration of an oral antihistamine.
c. Encouraging the client to sleep in the prone position.
d. Application of a cool compress to the affected eye.

Topic/Concept: Movement **Subtopic:** Conjunctivitis **Bloom's Taxonomy:** Applying **Clinical Problem-Solving Process:** Implementation **NCLEX-PN®:** Physiological Adaptation **QSEN:** Safety **CJMM:** Take Action

Rationale: A cool compress should be applied to reduce inflammation and itching. A warm compress may help remove dried crust, but hot compresses should be avoided. Antihistamines may be used to help with itching, but this is not the best action. The prone position is not indicated with conjunctivitis.

THIN Thinking: *Help Quick* – The nurse should initially provide independent, non-invasive, non-pharmacological care to relieve the client's symptoms.

CHAPTER

14

Comfort

Pain / Pressure / Fatigue

This chapter discusses a variety of Priority Exemplars addressing alterations in comfort. Pain and pain management; skin disorders (including burns), and sleep issues. The skin is the key protective barrier to infection, pain is the fifth vital sign. People spend about one-quarter of their lives sleeping. These validate the importance of this chapter in studying for NCLEX®!

Priority Exemplars:

- Pressure ulcers
- Sleep disorders
- Acute pain
- Burns
- Chronic pain
- Fatigue
- Contact dermatitis/impetigo

Clinical Hint

All pain is uncomfortable, unwanted, and unpleasant. Pain can range from mild to severe. Pain can be acute or chronic. Nurses must understand that pain is whatever the client says it is.

Next Gen Clinical Judgment

Consider the number of clients you have cared for in pain. Compare and contrast the nursing care of clients with acute versus chronic pain.

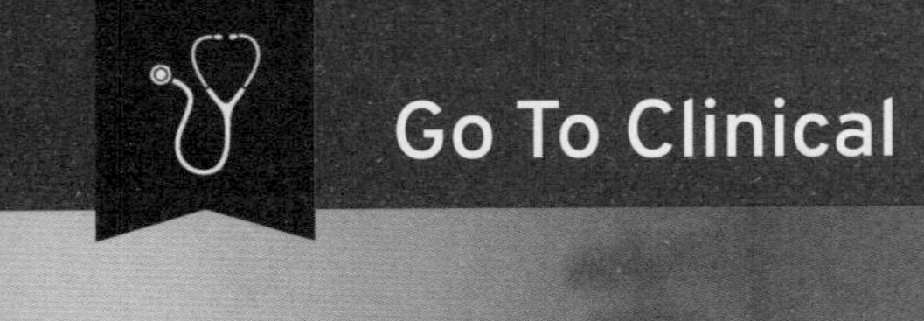

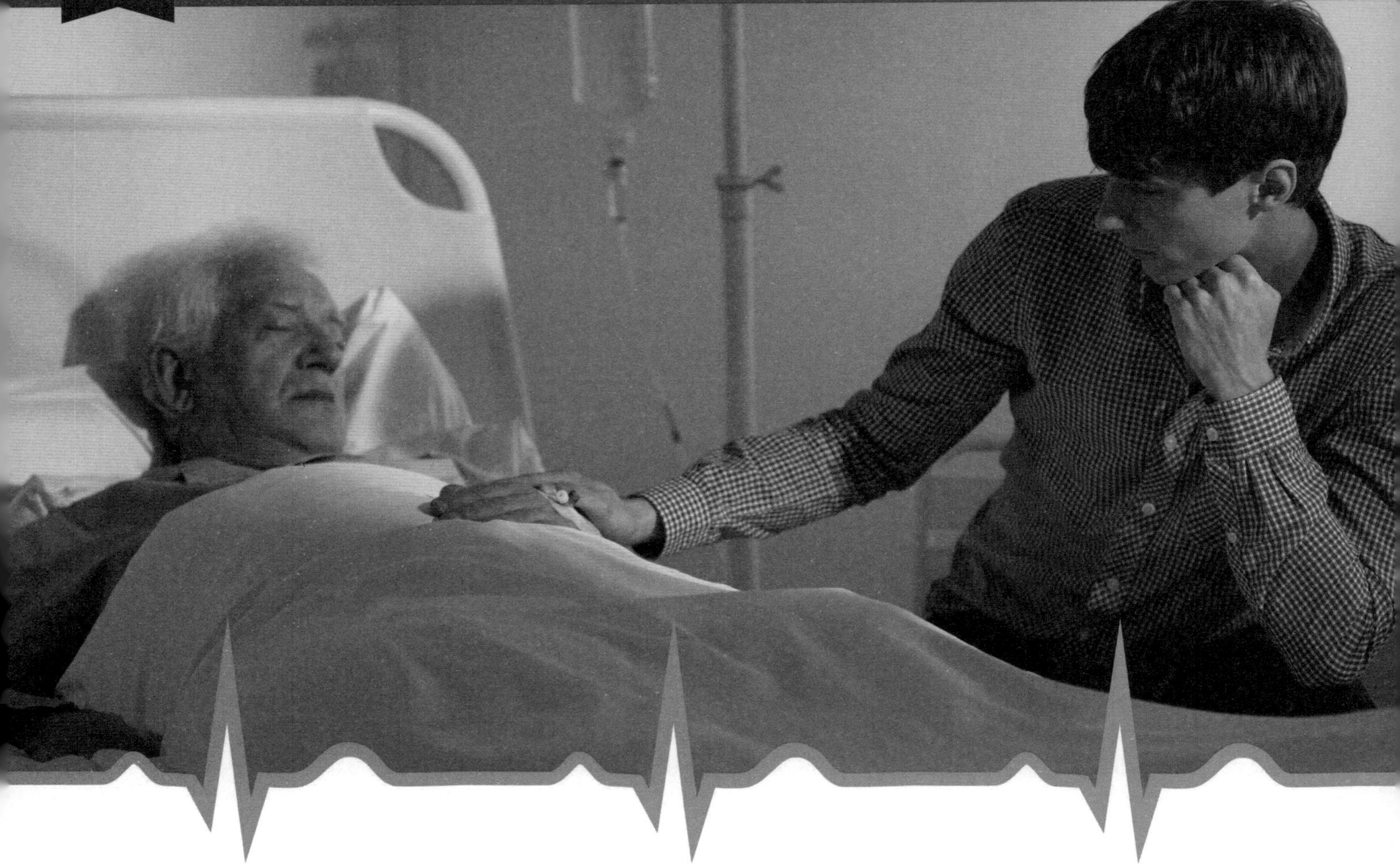

Go To Clinical

Go To Clinical Case 1

W. V., an 80 year old man lives alone. W.V.'s wife died 5 years ago; since then, W.V. has been living independently. His son calls him every day and visits once every two weeks. One day, the son receives a call from a neighbor. The neighbor is concerned that he has not seen W.V. in quite a while. The son visits his father and finds that he is lying in bed and is weak and confused. The father is lying in urine and can not recall when he last left the bed or ate a meal. The son attempts to get his father out of bed and is unable to assist him. The son and father discuss options and both realize that he needs long-term care. The son accesses a bed at a local facility and the client is transported via ambulance. W.V. is admitted as a resident with a diagnosis of malnutrition and weight loss. The nurse makes the client comfortable in the bed and is cleaning the resident's perineal area. When rolling the client to his side, the nurse notices a red spot forming on the resident's sacral area and is concerned about pressure ulcers. The nurse proceeds to set priorities for the resident.

NurseThink® Time

Using the NurseThink® system, complete priorities. Check your answers designated by in the Pressure ulcers Priority Exemplar.

Next Gen Clinical Judgment

Search the Internet and identify 5 best practices designed to prevent pressure ulcers in older adult clients who are immobile.

NurseThink® Time

Priority Data Collection or Cues

1.

2.

3.

Priority Laboratory Tests/Diagnostics

1.

2.

3.

Priority Interventions or Actions

1.

2.

3.

Priority Potential & Actual Complications

1.

2.

3.

Priority Nursing Implications

1.

2.

3.

Priority Medications

1.

2.

3.

Reinforcement of Priority Teaching

1.

2.

3.

Pathophysiology/Description

- The local injury to tissue created by pressure or a combination of shearing forces (friction of tissue pulling against a surface) and pressure. Most commonly found on bony prominences where pressure is exerted by chairs, beds, or equipment. May also be impacted by the presence of moisture
- Severity of pressure ulcer is associated with amount of pressure (client weight, location of pressure point), length of time area is exposed to pressure, and client tissue characteristics
- The heels and sacrum are the most common sites for pressure ulcers
- Protruding tissues or those prone to being a pressure point may also be at risk, including ears, shoulders, hips, ankles, chin, elbows, and sides of knees

Priority Data Collection or Cues

- Look for risk factors associated with pressure ulcers/poor perfusion including increased age, immobility/bedrest, poor wound healing, diabetes mellitus, conditions causing poor perfusion, incontinence, confusion/disorientation, neurological compromise, spinal cord injury/paralysis, anemia, pain, poor nutrition, obesity, contractures, long surgical procedures, and hyperthermia
- Look for characteristics of pressure ulcers associated with each stage
    - Suspected deep tissue injury described as a local area, purple or maroon in color, skin may blister or be intact, be painful, warm or cool, firm or mushy
    - **Stage I** described as intact skin with non-blanching redness, darker areas at location of injury, may be different from peripheral coloring of skin
    - **Stage II** described as a fluid-filled blister with a red-pink wound bed or open shallow ulcer, partial loss of dermis
    - **Stage III** described as a full thickness tissue erosion, may see subcutaneous fatty layer, may show beginnings of undermining and tunneling
    - **Stage IV** described as full thickness tissue loss with exposure of bone, tendons, or muscle tissue. May include eschar and necrotic tissue, undermining and tunneling present
- Look for signs of pressure ulcer infection including fever, redness, swelling, and drainage
- Wounds are described in detail, measured by width and depth of the wound, and this information is carefully documented in the medical record to determine severity and response to treatment. Ulcers are described by stage, size, location, type of wound, drainage, and presence of signs of infection or pain

Priority Laboratory Tests/Diagnostics

- Wound cultures should be done. Wounds may be contaminated or colonized with bacteria but the chronicity of wound or client immunosuppression may mask the signs of infection

Priority Interventions or Actions

- Address health status and conditions increasing risk for pressure ulcers
- Ensure adequate nutrition for healing. Oral, enteral or parenteral feedings, with supplementary proteins and vitamins, are often needed
- Monitor and manage pain
- Ensure adequate hygiene and cleanliness of tissues
- Wound care includes debridement and removal of dead tissue, wound cleaning via gentle irrigation with non-cytotoxic solutions, application of moist dressings (wet to dry dressing should not be used as they may disrupt healing tissue), and ensuring area is not experiencing pressure
- Wounds may require advanced healing mechanisms, wound vacuums, skin grafting, skin flaps, or surgical repair

Priority Potential & Actual Complications

- Cellulitis and chronic infection
- Sepsis
- May be fatal

Priority Nursing Implications

- Clients should be examined on admission for risk for skin breakdown. The Braden scale is a validated tool often used for this purpose. Assist in a full head to toe assessment of the skin
- Nurses should be aware of the challenges in examining variations in skin colors for changes and pressure areas
- Significant emphasis may be on prevention through basic processes such as turning/repositioning, not pulling clients along sheets to avoid shearing forces, positioning, splints, position changes when seated, providing supports/cushions/specially designed pads, and encouraging activity/ambulation when appropriate
- Clients most at risk for pressure ulcers may benefit from special beds which provide varying exposure to pressure/air movement mattresses, facilitate turning and movement, and relieve pressure areas. Wheelchair cushions, padded toilet seats, foam mattresses, overbed lifts, and lift sheets may be indicated; never position on the pressure ulcer

- Pressure ulcers commonly recur in the same or similar areas, warranting vigilant monitoring and nursing care
- Serial pictures or images of pressure ulcers are often helpful in comparing the wound to previous time periods and monitoring response to treatment
- Massage of pressure ulcers is contraindicated to prevent further skin breakdown
- Although most eschar (dry, necrotic tissue) must be removed (debrided), the dry tissue on the heels should remain to protect those areas
- Referral to a wound care specialist is often indicated

Priority Medications

- Pain medications as indicated

Reinforcement of Priority Teaching

- The risk factors and means to prevent pressure ulcers, along with locations of bony prominences. Reinforce teaching with caregivers on positioning strategies and the use of pads, pillows, and equipment to periodically move the client. Use strategies such as timers and turning logs to ensure frequent turning
- Awareness of assistive devices for lifting, moving, and positioning clients
- The importance of hygiene, cleanliness, hydration, and adequate nutrition
- Use of community resources and respite services to relieve caregiver role strain
- The signs and symptoms of pressure ulcers and infection with caregivers such that they may be detected early

Pressure Sore Areas On Human Body Parts

Pressure sores often form over bony prominences in fixed patients

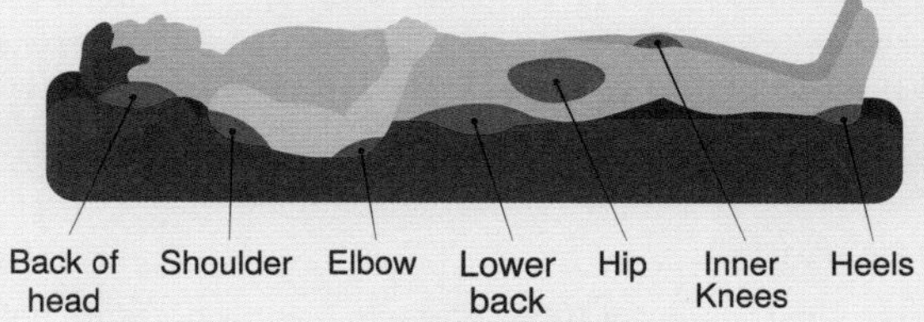

Image 14-1: Describe ways to prevent pressure ulcer formation for each of the areas identified.

Go To Clinical Answers

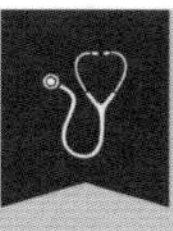

Text designated by the icon are the top answers for the Go To Clinical related to Pressure ulcers.

Bedsores (Pressure Ulcers)

Injuries of the skin and underlying tissue resulting from prolonged pressure on the skin

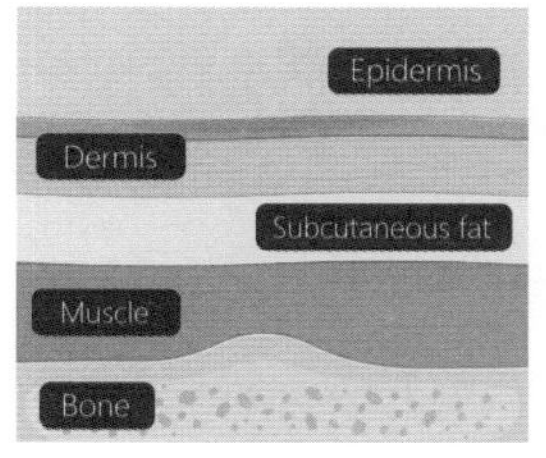

Stage 1

Skin is reddened and may be warm to the touch, may either feel firmer or softer than the surrounding skin.

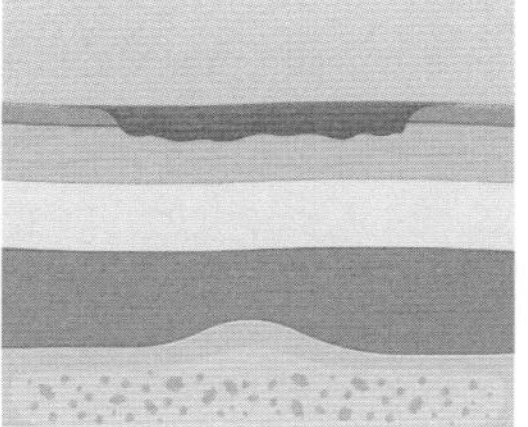

Stage 2

Skin breaks open exposing the epidermis or dermis. The lesion will be superficial and may resemble an abrasion or a popped blister.

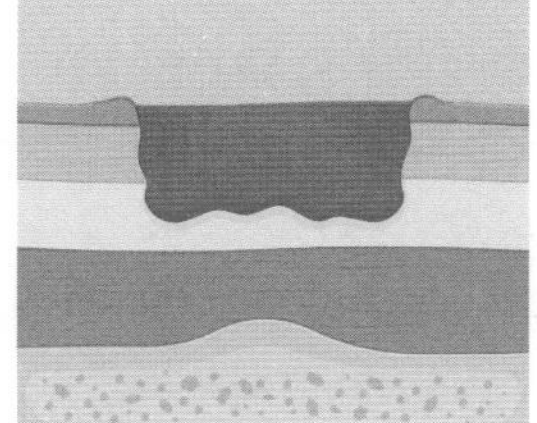

Stage 3

Lesion extends into the dermis and may extend to the subcutaneous layer. At this stage, the lesion will form a small crater. Fat may begin to show in the open sore.

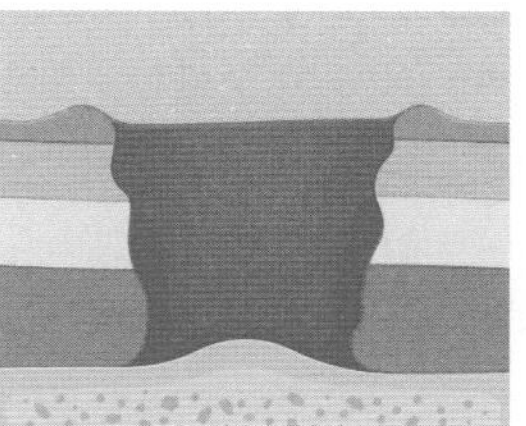

Stage 4

Subcutaneous layer and underlying fascia are breached, exposing muscle and bone.

Image 14-2: List treatment regimens for each pressure ulcer stage. Using this chart, search for pressure ulcer images on the internet and stage them.

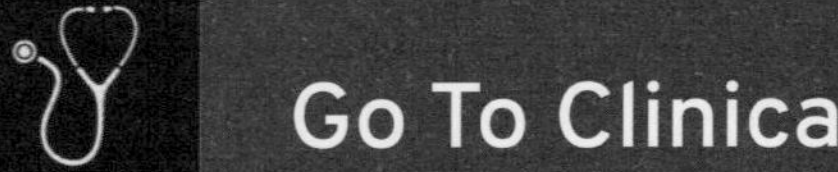

Go To Clinical

Go To Clinical Case 2

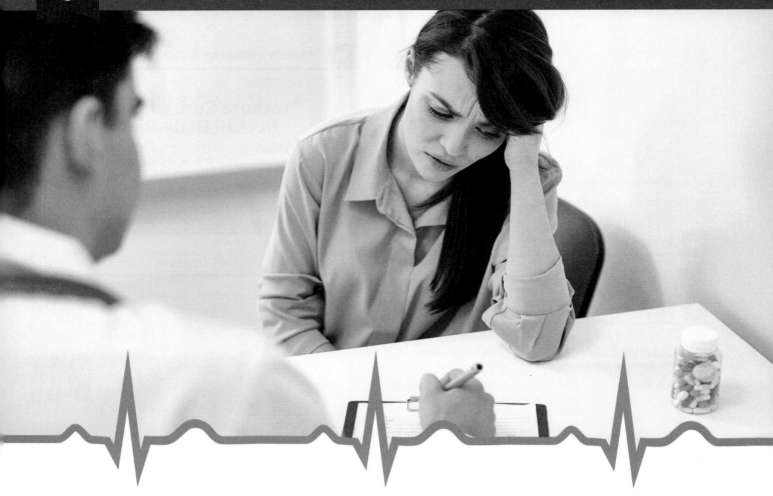

Y.P. is a 45-year-old female that presents to the clinic with difficulty falling and staying asleep. She noticed the problem in the last six months after several family members and friends died due to complications from the COVID-19 virus. Y.P. reports not being able to fall asleep until at least one hour after going to bed, and when she does fall asleep, she wakes up several times throughout the night. Y.P. denies previous sleep problems. Y.P. stated since she has been having these difficulties falling asleep, she has been self-medicating with over-the-counter remedies that helped temporarily. Recently, Y.P. feels that nothing is helping. Y.P. states, "I am really worried about this. I am tired all the time. It has started to impact my work. I almost fell asleep on the drive home last week. I don't have the energy for friends or family." Y.P.'s husband reports he notices that his wife tosses and turns throughout the night, and occasionally he notices she has some leg jerking. Begin setting priorities for Y.P.'s care.

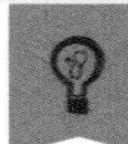

NurseThink® Time

Using the NurseThink® system, complete priorities. Check your answers designated by 💡 in the Sleep disorders Priority Exemplar.

Next Gen Clinical Judgment

Each individual has an internal clock that follows the pattern of day and night to affect the sleep-wake cycle. This internal clock is referred to as the biological clock. The biological clock is controlled by a part of the brain called the suprachiasmatic nucleus, a group of cells in the hypothalamus that respond to light and dark signals. Take a few moments to think of factors that may interfere with a client's biological clock.

NurseThink® Time

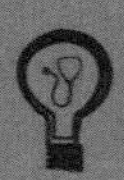

Priority Data Collection or Cues

1.

2.

3.

Priority Laboratory Tests/Diagnostics

1.

2.

3.

Priority Interventions or Actions

1.

2.

3.

Priority Potential & Actual Complications

1.

2.

3.

Priority Nursing Implications

1.

2.

3.

Priority Medications

1.

2.

3.

Reinforcement of Priority Teaching

1.

2.

3.

Pathophysiology/Description

- Defined as a group of disorders associated with sleep or times of rest, conditions may lead to poor quality sleep
- Sleep deprivation may lead to moodiness, cognitive impairment, obesity, depressed immune response, hypertension, GERD, and increased insulin resistance/type 2 diabetes
- About 70 million people in American suffer from sleep disorders
- Insomnia is the difficulty falling asleep, waking during sleep and having difficulty falling back asleep, or waking early. May be acute or chronic; may be primary or secondary
- Restless leg syndrome is the unpleasant sensory/motor activity of one or both legs. May be primary or secondary. May be associated with diabetes, hypertension, anemia, pregnancy, renal failure, or rheumatoid arthritis
- Narcolepsy is the disordered sleep pattern in a client which causes uncontrolled, spontaneous sleep during waking hours, may occur during activities. Clients may pass immediately into rapid eye movement sleep from the awake state. Clients with narcolepsy are protected by the Americans with Disabilities Act. May be triggered by a head trauma, change in sleep patterns, or an infection
- Obstructive sleep apnea (OSA) is the partial or complete obstruction of the airway during sleep

Priority Data Collection or Cues

- Monitor for symptoms of sleeplessness including sleep patterns, fatigue level, and impact of sleep issues on social, personal, and occupational functioning
- Monitor for chronic disorders that disturb sleep (COPD, heart failure)
- Monitor for difficulties falling asleep, waking during sleep and having difficulty falling back asleep, or waking early
- Use standardized measures to monitor sleep
- Determine if client takes medications that may cause or increase sleep disorders
- Monitor for symptoms of restless leg syndrome including the uncontrollable urge to move/involuntary movement of legs, paresthesias, creeping/crawling sensations in the legs, numbness/tingling, restlessness, or pain at rest
- Monitor for symptoms of narcolepsy including witnessed or experienced periods of sudden sleep states, sleep paralysis, hallucinations, or cataplexy (falling during sudden sleep episodes)
- Monitor clients at risk for OSA including clients older than 65 years, or with a BMI > 28 kg/m^2, neck circumference > 17 inches, acromegaly, history of smoking, craniofacial abnormalities, and COPD
- Look for signs/symptoms of OSA including insomnia, audible snoring, startling during sleep, daytime sleepiness, morning headaches, and irritability

Priority Laboratory Tests/Diagnostics

- Complete blood count to look for anemia
- Serum ferritin levels
- Renal function (BUN, creatinine)
- Actigraphy to monitor sleep, rest, and activity levels
- Polysomnography (PSG) monitors muscle tone (EMG), eye movements (EOG), and brain activity (EEG) to look for narcolepsy and other sleep disorders. May include chest/abdominal movement sensors and oral/nasal airflow measurements to diagnose OSA
- Multiple sleep latency tests/sleep studies for narcolepsy
- Overnight oxygen saturation measurement for OSA

Priority Interventions or Actions

- Treat underlying cause of sleep disorder
- Institute sleep hygiene measures (see below)
- Consider cognitive behavioral therapy or other counseling to deal with stressors
- Restless leg syndrome may be relieved by activity (walking, stretching, kicking, rocking)
- Narcolepsy is most successfully treated with a combination of medications and behavioral therapies
- OSA
  - If mild, client is instructed to sleep on side or elevate head of bed/use pillows
  - Avoid alcohol or sedatives 3-4 hours before sleep
  - Weight loss
  - Use an oral appliance to maintain an open airway
  - If these measures unsuccessful, clients are recommended to use continuous positive airway pressure (CPAP) or bilevel positive airway pressure (BiPAP) via mask to open airways. Clients are encouraged to select a mask most comfortable for them. Adherence to nightly CPAP or BiPAP is often poor due to the mask, noise, the interference with partner sleep, and the fact that the machine needs to be transported with the client for overnight stays. Client may complain of nasal stuffiness after use
  - Surgical repair or radiofrequency ablation may be effective for clients with refractory OSA

Priority Potential & Actual Complications

- Social, personal, and occupational dysfunction from sleep disorders/disturbed sleep
- Social withdrawal/isolation/depression
- Motor vehicle and work-related injuries related to lack of attentiveness/sleepiness/falling asleep
- Untreated sleep apnea may lead to hypertension, heart failure, dysrhythmias, and impotence

Priority Nursing Implications

- Prolonged sleep deprivation in hospitalized clients may lead to delirium and prolonged recoveries. Nurses need to employ measures to foster sleep in clients, including rest times so clients have uninterrupted times of restful sleep. In intensive care and other environments, dim lights at night, limit nighttime activities, group interventions, provide comfort measures, and establish quiet hours may assist in attaining restful sleep and quiet rest periods
- Many sleep disorders go untreated, nurses have an important role in detecting and assisting clients to manage sleep disorders
- Support groups are often helpful for clients with sleep disorders
- For clients with OSA, nurses need to use caution when administering central nervous system depressants or opioids to avoid respiratory depression

Priority Medications

- Melatonin–oral, subligual, intranasal, and dermal administration
    - Available over-the-counter as a sleep aid/supplement
    - Relieves insomnia associated with jet lag and shift work
    - May lower blood pressure and interact with warfarin and CNS depressants
- Zolpidem
    - First line agents for insomnia
    - May be safely used for one year under close medical surveillance
    - Available as oral pills, dissolvable oral tablets, and sublingual tablets
- Carbidopa/levodopa–oral administration
    - Antiparkinsonian medication to increase dopamine
    - May relieve restless leg syndrome
- Enacarbil–oral administration
    - Anticonvulsant
    - May relieve the sensory symptoms of restless leg syndrome
- Modafinil–oral administratio
    - First line agent for narcolepsy
    - Non-amphetamine wake-promotion drug

Next Gen Clinical Judgment

A client has a sleep disorder and is hospitalized. Which priority interventions should be included in the client's plan of care to promote sleep during the hospitalization?

Reinforcement of Priority Teaching

- Sleep hygiene practices including going to bed only when sleepy, getting out of bed if haven't fallen asleep in 20 minutes, limiting liquids at night, quiet reading (not screen time) prior to sleep, warm baths or showers just prior to sleep, limiting exercise before bedtime (at least 6 hours prior to) but getting adequate exercise during the day, limiting caffeine/stimulants/nicotine/alcohol before bed, having a small protein snack/warm milk prior to sleep to avoid hunger, reducing light and noise if sleeping time is not at night, keeping bed for sleeping and only sleeping activities, staying out of bed during the day, set a regular sleep and wake up time, limiting day-time naps, limiting use of hypnotics, and stress reducing strategies to avoid anxiety at sleep time
- Keep a sleep diary to maintain an accurate account of sleep, encourage sleep partners to participate in recording sleep activity

Next Gen Clinical Judgment

Explain how these drugs affect sleep.

Hypnotics: ______________________________

Diuretics: ______________________________

Antidepressant & stimulants: ______________________________

Beta-Adrenergic Blockers: ______________________________

Anticonvulsants: ______________________________

Alcohol: ______________________________

Nicotine: ______________________________

Go To Clinical Answers

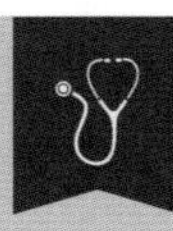

Text designated by ● are the top answers for the Go To Clinical related to Sleep disorders.

Pathophysiology/Description

- Pain is one of the most prominent healthcare issues today, with subjective and objective interpretations, current management controversies, and debilitating consequences
- Pain was described by Margot McCaffery as "whatever the person experiencing the pain says it is, existing whenever the person says it does." Other definitions discuss unpleasant sensory and emotional experiences related to actual or potential tissue damage
- Two types of pain (these may be acute or chronic)
  - Nociceptive pain
    - May be superficial somatic (skin/mucous membranes), deep somatic (muscles/bones/tendons), or visceral (deep organs/GI tract/bladder)
    - Pain perception is impacted by physiologic, affective, cognitive, behavioral, and sociocultural dimensions
    - Nociception processing of pain includes transmitting message from site of tissue damage to central nervous system and is made up of 4 processes including transduction (release of chemicals in response to tissue damage), transmission (message transferred from periphery to spinal cord/dorsal root to thalamus and cortex), perception (personal interpretation of message), and modulation (descending messages that inhibit or facilitate effects of pain transmission)
    - Causes include trauma, surgery, injury, burns, disease, or necrosis
    - Usually responsive to opioid and non-opioid drugs
    - Nociceptive pain may be described as sharp, aching, dull, or cramping
  - Neuropathic pain
    - Including central pain (lesion in CNS), peripheral neuropathies (related to diabetes/alcoholism), deafferentation pain (loss of afferent transmission as in phantom pain), and sympathetically maintained pain (complex regional pain syndrome)
    - Causes include trauma, infection, metabolic disease, infection, alcoholism, tumors, toxins, or neurologic diseases
    - Treatment usually requires adjuvant drugs
    - Neuropathic pain may be described as burning, shooting, itching, or stabbing
- Acute pain is defined as lasting less than three months, may be mild to severe levels, pain is generally associated with a specific event, decreases over time and generally goes away. Acute pain may signal tissue damage and allow for adaptation. Unremitting acute pain may become chronic in nature but goal of management of acute pain is relief of pain. Relief may not be total, but pain is reduced to a tolerable level

Priority Data Collection or Cues

- Screen all clients for pain (pain is the fifth vital sign)
- Use standardized pain data collection tools
- Look for risk factors for acute pain experiences including injury/trauma, surgery, pathophysiological changes in the body (necrosis of myocardial tissue, ischemia to peripheral extremities, acute degeneration of bone/muscle, vascular changes of cerebral vessels), labor/delivery, or infection
- Ask clients about personal interpretation of the meaning of pain
- Monitor self-report of pain (as client is able), including:
  - Onset (clients with acute pain may recall event or injury)
  - Pattern (may increase with activity or change based on medication dosing/duration of medication effects)
  - Duration
  - Location/radiation (more often specific rather than generalized)
  - Intensity
  - Quality (nature and characteristics)
  - Associated factors (pain may increase or decrease with activity, increases or decreases during sleep)
  - Previous and current management strategies/healthcare seeking/utilization/previous experiences
  - Impact on social and occupational functioning
  - Impact on sleep, activity, function, emotions, sexual libido/performance, and relationships with others
- Look for objective signs of acute pain including how they hold their body/positioning, sitting very still or restless, pallor, elevated heart rate/respiratory rate/blood pressure, fatigue, anxiety, agitation, diaphoresis, confusion, facial expressions/gestures, moaning, or urinary retention
- Monitor for breakthrough pain, procedural/incident pain, or end-of-dose failure

Priority Laboratory Tests/Diagnostics

- Diagnostic tests to detect underlying causes

Priority Interventions or Actions

- Ensure accurate documentation of data collection and treatments
- Treat underlying cause (antibiotics for infections, splint postoperative surgical site, cast fractured limb, manage cardiovascular function)
- Non-pharmacologic methods should accompany pharmacologic methods, including application of heat/cold, acupuncture, relaxation strategies, distraction, imagery, hypnosis, transcutaneous electrical nerve stimulation, massage, and use of complementary/alternative strategies
- Frequently monitor pain levels and evaluate effectiveness of management strategies
- Acute pain management may be facilitated by implantable pain pumps, patient-controlled analgesia, and alternative administrations routes, including transmucosal, buccal, intranasal, transdermal, and rectal routes

Priority Potential & Actual Complications

- Untreated pain is associated with prolonged healing, immunosuppression, emotional/physical discomfort/dysfunction, depression, and sleep disorders
- Physiological complications may include weight loss, hypertension, hyperglycemia/glucose intolerance, atelectasis/pneumonia, paralytic ileus/constipation, immobility/deep vein thromboses, weakness/fatigue, infections, confusion/poor decision-making, fluid and electrolyte imbalance, social withdrawal, and isolation

Priority Nursing Implications

- Nurses may use standardized pain data collection tools, body maps to pinpoint pain location and radiation, and scales/analogs/FACES/ranking tools to measure pain intensity. These tools are valuable with clients with developmental/cognitive/communication barriers
- Self-report and description (rating) is critical, but often nurses must use other methods to monitor pain for those who are unable to participate (clients who are non-verbal, unconscious, or who have communication disorders)
- Clients in acute pain often benefit from around-the-clock analgesia, rather than PRN scheduling. This prevents pain from getting to a level too high/difficult to manage
- Multimodal analgesia dictates that two or more agents are used together to manage pain, thereby increasing pain medication effectiveness, increasing client perceptions of pain management, and decreasing potential side effects of each medication (opioid-sparing effect of acetaminophen when delivered with hydrocodone)
- Nurses need to vigilantly look for respiratory depression in clients receiving opioid agents and carefully monitor during first doses, when dose is increased, or when multiple agents are used to manage pain

Priority Medications

- Acetaminophen
  - Oral, per rectum, intravenous; sustained-release oral medications available
  - For mild to moderate pain and is an antipyretic, no antiplatelet or anti-inflammatory effects
  - Long-term use or high doses may impair liver function, cause liver toxicity
- Ibuprofen
  - Orally
  - May cause GI side effects (bleeding, perforation, or ulceration, especially in older adults)
  - May increase hypertension, myocardial infarction, and stroke
- Ketorolac
  - May be given via oral, IM or IV routes
  - For < 5 days
  - Ensure hydration to avoid kidney dysfunction
- Celecoxib–oral administration
  - Inhibits COX-2, not COX-1, and creates less GI side effects (risk still exists)
  - May be associated with cardiovascular thrombosis, MIs, and CVAs (increased risk with long-term use or CV risk factors)
- Codeine with acetaminophen
  - Associated with high incidence of nausea and constipation
  - Oral agent for moderate pain relief, acetaminophen has opioid-sparing effects
  - 5-10% of European Americans lack the enzymes needed to metabolize codeine to endogenous morphine
- Hydrocodone with acetaminophen
  - Oral combination of opioid with co-analgesics
  - Used for moderate to severe pain
  - Short-term management of acute pain
- Morphine
  - Oral, per rectum, intravenous, subcutaneous, epidural, intrathecal, sublingual
  - For moderate to severe pain
- Lidocaine
  - Topical local anesthetic
  - Used for painful procedures (venipuncture, lumbar puncture, bone marrow aspiration)
  - Takes about 30 minutes to achieve effect, lasts about 60 minutes
- Naloxone
  - Reverses effects of opioids
  - IV, Subq, nasal spray
  - If opioids used for pain management for several days, client may experience severe pain and/or withdrawal symptoms when naloxone administered

Reinforcement of Priority Teaching

- All components of data collection and management of pain
- The side effects of medications, including constipation, sedation, nausea, itchiness, and respiratory depression associated with opioids, dose or agent limiting side effects, adverse reactions, and scheduling. Side effects are major causes of poor pain control and non-adherence in cases of acute and chronic pain

Clinical Hint

Infants may experience pain even if they are not able to express their discomfort. The American Academy of Pediatrics (2020) statement suggests that health care providers lessen the pain newborns experience. To do so:

1. Avoid painful procedures that are not necessary.
2. Hold and swaddle the newborn or infant during painful procedures.
3. Provide oral sucrose solution 2 minutes before a procedure.
4. Have the mom breastfeed before or during the procedure.

Pathophysiology/Description

- One of the leading causes of morbidity and mortality due to trauma
- Defined as injury to body caused by heat/fire (thermal/ smoke inhalation), chemicals, electricity, or radiation
- Impact of burn dependent on client characteristics, burning agent, length of exposure, and temperature of the burning agent

Priority Data Collection or Cues

- Check the impact on airway/breathing and circulation; monitor vital signs
- Check the impact of burns on clients with selected co-morbidities (very young, older adults, poor nutrition, those with chronic illness, those with other injuries)
- Check the severity of burn as dictated by depth, extent, and location
  - Depth including superficial partial thickness (epidermis), partial thickness (dermis), and full thickness (into the layers of fat, muscle, and bone)
  - Extent guided by the Rule of Nines or Lund Browder formula
  - Location of the burn, including burns in areas that may impact breathing (face, neck, head, around chest), impair self-care (eyes, hands, feet, joints), or increase risk for infection (nose, ears, and perineum)
- Monitor response to treatment (work of breathing, urine output, heart rate, blood pressure, mean arterial pressure (> 65 mmHg)
- Monitor body temperature frequently to detect hypothermia or infection

Priority Laboratory Tests/Diagnostics

- Hemoglobin and hematocrit including elevated hematocrit with hemoconcentration during emergent and acute phases
- Electrolytes including serum sodium (decreased serum sodium in emergent; increased sodium in acute phase due to high sodium fluids/enteral feedings); hyperkalemia in emergent phases due to cellular destruction or hypokalemia in acute phase due to loss from wounds
- Bronchoscopy to monitor airway for damage or edema
- ABGs to monitor oxygenation and ventilation
- Monitor kidney function/potential for acute tubular necrosis
- Chest X-Ray to detect smoke inhalation

Priority Interventions or Actions

- Prehospital
  - Maintain patent airway/provide oxygen as indicated
  - Remove from source/remove clothing
  - Smaller burns may be covered with tap-water dampened soaks, larger burns should be covered for shorter periods to avoid hypothermia
  - For chemical burn, remove the agent and flush with water
  - Check for other injuries and transport as needed
- Emergent (up to 72 hours after the burn)
  - Continued airway management/assist with intubation and ventilation as indicated, monitor for airway edema and progressing respiratory distress
  - Fluid shifts from blood vessels into interstitial and other third spaces due to increased capillary permeability and protein levels require fluid resuscitation
    - Assist in establishing 2 intravenous sites
    - Use the Parkland formula (4 mL lactated ringers X weight in Kg X % of total body surface area); ½ the first fluids in first 8 hours, ¼ in second 8 hours, ¼ in third 8 hours
  - Ensure pain management via intravenous route dependent upon the severity of pain, the extent of the burn, and client perceptions of pain
  - Provide wound care including showering, dressing changes, debridement/enzymatic debridement, escharotomies/fasciotomies, grafting (allografting, artificial skin, cultured epithelial autografts)
  - Prevent contractures, prevent deficits / maintain functioning including splinting/positioning, physical/ occupational therapies, turning, range-of-motion exercises, and encourage participation in self-care
  - Examine readiness for and toleration of feedings (bowel sounds, abdominal tenderness/distension/firmness, bowel function, vomiting/nausea)
- Rehabilitation (weeks to months after the burn)
  - Continue measures to prevent contractures and skin breakdown
  - Evaluate wound healing and subsequent treatments (reconstructive surgeries, use of water-based moisturizers, antihistamines for itching skin)
  - Provide encouragement during slow healing process
- Monitor psychosocial responses to trauma, pain, body image changes, treatments, and recovery

Clinical Hint

Burns may be some of the most painful injuries experienced by clients.

Priority Potential & Actual Complications

- Upper/lower airway burns with or without smoke inhalation
- Hypovolemic shock
- Infection/sepsis
- Metabolic asphyxiation (carbon monoxide/hydrogen cyanide)
- Reduction of circulation to affected extremities
- Curling's ulcers
- Hyperglycemia with insulin resistance
- Heart failure/pulmonary edema
- Pneumonia
- Delirium
- Venous thromboembolism
- Acute tubular necrosis

Priority Nursing Implications

- Nurses have a significant role in the prevention of burns, providing education, and monitoring safety
- Burns are very painful and cause anxiety, nurses are active in managing pain, fear, anxiety, and the physiological status
- Implement venous thromboembolism prophylaxis procedures as prescribed
- Because burns create a hypermetabolic/hypercatabolic state, nutrition is key to promote wound healing and health. Early initiation of oral or enteral feedings is now recommended to ensure adequate nutrition and positive nitrogen balance. Nurses need to ensure safe enteral feedings to avoid aspiration

Priority Medications

- Enoxaparin
  - Administered subcutaneously
  - Venous thromboembolism prophylaxis
  - Monitor for perfusion to subcutaneous tissues during fluid shifts
- Ranitidine
  - Intravenous or oral
  - Prevent Curling's and stress ulcers
  - Monitor for occult blood in stools and other signs of ulceration
- Morphine
  - Management of severe pain
  - Intravenous (IM poorly absorbed with fluid shifts)
  - Monitor for respiratory depression and constipation
- Tetanus toxoid
  - Administered intramuscularly
  - Given to all burn victims to prevent tetanus
  - If the client has not had an immunization in 10 years, administer tetanus immunoglobulin
- Silver sulfadiazine
  - Silver containing topical ointment to decrease microbial growth
  - More effective than systemic antibiotics in early stages when perfusion is poor
  - Monitor for allergy to sulfur

Reinforcement of Priority Teaching

- Resources to cope with a potentially long, painful, and difficult healing period
- Emotional support related to changes in body appearance and function, including sexuality, self-esteem, and perceptions of self-worth
- Support systems and community resources to aid in rehabilitation
- Wound care, physical/occupational therapies, diet, medications, signs of infection, pain management, and follow-up
- Potential for itching, sensitivity, pigmentation changes, contractures, scarring, and hypersensitivity of burn sites
- Burn prevention information is available to the client and family

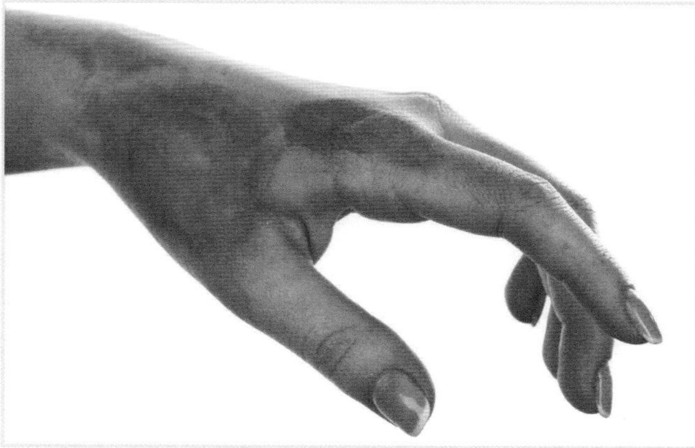

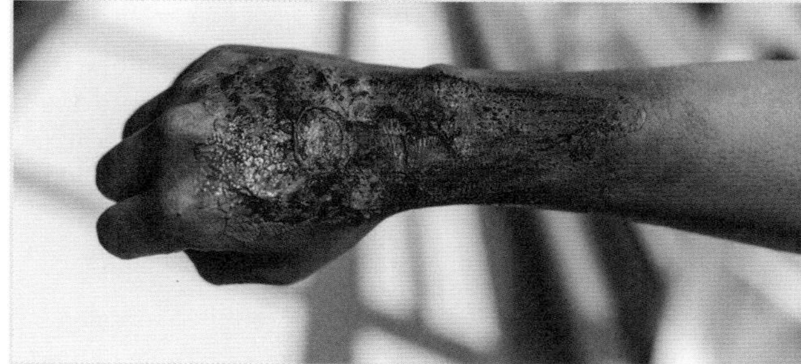

Image 14-3: Explain burn depth, clinical manifestations, and treatment for each burn type identified in these images.

Pathophysiology/Description

- Chronic pain is defined as mild to severe pain lasting more than three months, may appear gradually or suddenly, onset may not be traced to a stimulating event, cause may or may not be known, continues past the anticipated time of relief, usually not adaptive in nature, does not go away, and may increase and decrease throughout the day despite analgesia. May or may not be eliminated but interventions are focused on reduction of disability and resumption of function
- There are concerns that chronic pain is often undertreated, especially associated with cancer and end-of-life care. Conversely, chronic pain management is often associated with the prevailing opioid crisis, calling into question some current practices
- Pain is one of the most prominent healthcare issues today, with subjective and objective interpretations, current management controversies, and debilitating consequences
- Pain was described by Margot McCaffery as "whatever the person experiencing the pain says it is, existing whenever the person says it does." Other definitions discuss unpleasant sensory and emotional experiences related to actual or potential tissue damage
- Two types of pain (these may be acute or chronic)
  - Nociceptive pain
    - May be superficial somatic (skin/mucous membranes), deep somatic (muscles/bones/tendons), or visceral (deep organs/GI tract/bladder)
    - Pain perception is impacted by physiologic, affective, cognitive, behavioral, and sociocultural dimensions
    - Nociception processing of pain includes transmitting message from site of tissue damage to central nervous system and is made up of 4 processes including transduction (release of chemicals in response to tissue damage), transmission (message transferred from periphery to spinal cord/dorsal root to thalamus and cortex), perception (personal interpretation of message), and modulation (descending messages that inhibit or facilitate effects of pain transmission)
    - Causes include trauma, surgery, injury, burns, disease, or necrosis
    - Usually responsive to opioid and non-opioid drugs
    - Nociceptive pain may be described as sharp, aching, dull, or cramping
  - Neuropathic pain
    - Including central pain (lesion in CNS), peripheral neuropathies (related to diabetes/alcoholism), deafferentation pain (loss of afferent transmission as in phantom pain), and sympathetically maintained pain (complex regional pain syndrome)
    - Causes include trauma, infection, metabolic disease, infection, alcoholism, tumors, toxins, or neurologic diseases
    - Treatment usually requires adjuvant drugs
    - Neuropathic pain may be described as burning, shooting, itching, or stabbing
- Chronic pain may cause significant and long-term suffering, perceptions of lack of self-control, anxiety, depression, and insecurity

Priority Data Collection or Cues

- Screen all clients for pain (pain is the fifth vital sign)
- Use standardized pain data collection tools
- Look for risk factors for chronic pain experiences including pathophysiological changes in the body (joint and musculoskeletal changes leading to arthritis and back pain, vascular changes related to chronic migraine headaches, muscle aches due to fibromyalgia), or age/physiological deterioration
- Ask clients about personal interpretation of the meaning of pain
- Observe for self-report of pain (as client is able), including onset (clients with chronic pain may not know exact initiation of pain), pattern (chronic pain may increase or decrease over time, may increase or decrease with sleep cycles or during times of activity), duration (may be less specific than acute pain), location/radiation (may be specific or more generalized), intensity, quality (nature and characteristics, may be less able to describe with chronic pain), associated factors (chronic pain may be associated with depression/emotional factors that increase pain perception, pain may increase or decrease with activity), previous and current management strategies/healthcare seeking/utilization/previous experiences, impact on social and occupational functioning, and impact on sleep, activity, function, emotions, sexual libido/performance, and relationships with others (more significant impacts with chronic pain)
- Look for objective signs of chronic pain which may be similar to and/or different from those with acute pain; client may state pain is severe without objective signs due to the body's adaptation to the pain state (may not reflect sympathetic nervous system stimulation). Additional classic symptoms include flat affect, depression, irritability, reduced level of activity and social interaction, and fatigue
- Monitor for breakthrough pain, procedural/incident pain, or end-of-dose failure. Clients with chronic pain may struggle to cope with the additional pain associated with procedures, lack of management, or experiences associated with fear or apprehension

Priority Laboratory Tests/Diagnostics

- Diagnostic tests to detect underlying causes

Priority Interventions or Actions

- Ensure accurate documentation of data collection and treatments and compare with previous data collection at each healthcare encounter

- Treat underlying cause (back pain may indicate need for physical therapy, exercises and stretching, or surgical repair, chronic migraines may benefit from identification and elimination of triggers)
- Non-pharmacologic methods should accompany pharmacologic methods, including application of heat/cold, acupuncture, relaxation strategies, distraction, imagery, hypnosis, transcutaneous electrical nerve stimulation, massage, and use of complementary/alternative strategies
- Frequently monitor pain levels and evaluate effectiveness of management strategies
- New chronic pain interventions include therapeutic nerve blocks, neuroablative procedures, neuroaugmentation, and surgical intervention

Priority Potential & Actual Complications

- Untreated pain is associated with prolonged healing, immunosuppression, emotional/physical discomfort/dysfunction, depression, and sleep disorders
- Physiological complications may include weight loss, hypertension, hyperglycemia/glucose intolerance, atelectasis/pneumonia, paralytic ileus/constipation, immobility/deep vein thromboses, weakness/fatigue, infections, confusion/poor decision-making, fluid and electrolyte imbalance, social withdrawal, and isolation
- Chronic pain may lead to significant decreases in social, self-care, and occupational functioning

Priority Nursing Implications

- Nurses may use standardized pain data collection tools, body maps to pinpoint pain location and radiation, and scales/analogs/FACES/ranking tools to monitor pain intensity. These tools are valuable with clients with developmental/cognitive/communication barriers
- Multimodal analgesia dictates that two or more agents are used together to manage pain, thereby increasing pain medication effectiveness, increasing client perceptions of pain management, and decreasing potential side effects of each medication (opioid-sparing effect of acetaminophen when delivered with hydrocodone)
- Nurses need to vigilantly look for respiratory depression in clients receiving opioid agents and carefully monitor during first doses, when dose is increased, or when multiple agents are used to manage pain
- Nurses need to be aware of opioid-induced hyperalgesia wherein clients appear to be more sensitive to pain following pharmacological pain management strategies
- Clients with chronic pain often find relief in use of the cannabinoids. These medications, whether smoked or in oral/pill form, provide pain relief, decrease nausea, increase appetite, are opioid-sparing, and reduce the impact of opioid withdrawal. Their use in pain management continues to be researched and current legislation demonstrates the value of these medications for some clients
- Chronic pain management is often made more complex by tolerance, physical dependence, pseudoaddiction, and addiction
- Providing pain management for clients with opioid and other addictions may be complex, but these clients deserve respectful and high-quality pain data collection and management

Priority Medications

- See medications in Acute pain Priority Exemplar
- Clients with chronic pain may receive adjuvant medications to support pain management, including corticosteroids, antiseizure medications, antidepressants, adrenergic agonists, GABA receptor agonists, or local anesthetics
- Fentanyl
  - Very potent analgesic
  - Transdermal route indicated for chronic pain
  - Watch for symptoms of overdose, including decreased respirations, excessive sleepiness, confusion, or lethargy
- Tapentadol
  - For moderate to severe chronic pain, available in sustained-release formula, given orally for chronic pain
  - Less nausea and constipation than other opioids
- Clonidine–oral administration for chronic pain
  - Alpha-adrenergic agonist
  - Used for chronic headaches or neuropathic pain
- Mexiletine
  - Oral/systemic anesthetic for neuropathic pain
  - Watch for nausea, dizziness, paresthesias, tremoring, and seizures
  - Avoid with clients with cardiac disorders
- Trolamine salicylate
  - Topical, locally absorbed aspirin-containing cream
  - Used for muscle and joint pain
  - Avoids GI irritation
- Dronabinol
  - Cannabinoid medication approved for medical use
  - May be smoked or in a prepared oral form
  - Enhance endogenous opioid system, alleviates nausea, and increases appetite
  - May be effective in decreasing the impact of withdrawal

Reinforcement of Priority Teaching

- Components of data collection and management of pain
- Side effects of medications, including constipation, sedation, nausea, itchiness, and respiratory depression associated with opioids, dose or agent limiting side effects, adverse reactions, and scheduling. Side effects are major causes of poor pain control and non-adherence in cases of acute and chronic pain

Pathophysiology/Description

- Described as the ongoing, persistent feeling of tiredness; lasting more than a few days or weeks
- Subjective description of lack of energy that hampers functioning in the social, personal, and occupational areas
- May be a symptom of an underlying healthcare issue (such as cancer) or may be unexplained
- May indicate a sleep deficit or may be associated with the increased energy required in the healing process or the body's response to disease
- Fatigue may be associated with end-of-life, may be an early sign of other illnesses, such as heart failure or chronic obstructive pulmonary disease, or may be the most significant side effect of treatment and last for a long period after treatments for cancer
- Chronic fatigue syndrome is described as debilitating fatigue along with other symptoms. Although the cause is unknown, may be triggered by stress/stressful event and illnesses with flu-like symptoms, or triggered by organisms such as Epstein-Barr virus, cytomegalovirus, and others
- Fibromyalgia is described as a chronic disorder associated with fatigue, pain, morning stiffness, depression, difficulty coping with stress, anxiety, inflammatory bowel syndrome, and non-restful sleep; thought to be associated with neurotransmitter dysregulation

Priority Data Collection or Cues

- Look for risk factors associated with fatigue, including depression, anxiety, dehydration, hypothyroidism, insomnia, infection, or concurrent or chronic disease or disorders (diabetes, heart failure, respiratory illnesses)
- Monitor for reversible causes of fatigue (poor sleep, dehydration, illness)
- Observe client's tolerance to activities and determine those activities/interests in which the client most wants to participate
- Fatigue is a subjective symptom. Ask the client to describe fatigue, use numeric scales to quantify level of fatigue, or administer standardized fatigue scales
- Look for pallor, adequacy of perfusion, oxygenation, and ventilation
- Determine if client takes medications that may cause or increase fatigue
- Administer standardized depression or anxiety scales, if indicated
- Look for risk factors for chronic fatigue syndrome including significant stress, trauma, or illness
- Monitor for symptoms of chronic fatigue syndrome including fatigue not associated with exertion and not relieved by rest, changes in memory function and ability to concentrate, sore throat, muscle and joint pain, headache, and malaise
- Look for risk factors associated with fibromyalgia including familial history of this and other sleeping disorders, or a recent trauma or illness that may trigger the illness
- Monitor for symptoms of fibromyalgia including fatigue, malaise, burning pain, facial/head/neck pain, joint tenderness/point tenderness at 11 of the 18 identified and specific body points associated with fibromyalgia, cognitive changes and changes in level of consciousness, and diarrhea, constipation, bloating, and pain associated with irritable bowel syndrome

Priority Laboratory Tests/Diagnostics

- Complete blood count—monitor for anemia, a potential causal factor of fatigue and elevations in white blood cells which may indicate infection
- With fibromyalgia, ANA levels (antinuclear antibodies) may be low
- Muscle biopsies with fibromyalgia may demonstrate muscle atrophy

Priority Interventions or Actions

- Determine and manage underlying cause for fatigue; if cause is unknown, treatment is often symptomatic
- Balance time for activity with time for rest, discuss favorite activities with client and create a plan to create time for each, determine and maximize activities during the time of day when the client feels most energetic. Ensure adequate rest prior to periods of activity
- Ensure client is awake and active, as able, during the day to optimize nighttime sleep
- Ensure adequate hydration. Many believe dehydration is a root cause of fatigue in otherwise healthy individuals
- Encourage optimal nutrition, including foods high in protein, iron, and whole fiber, some recommend limiting sugar, caffeine, and alcohol which may disrupt sleep and irritate muscles
- Develop progressive exercise programs, as able, to increase time and intensity of exercise
- In hospitalized clients, reduce disruption during nighttime sleep and group activities to allow for uninterrupted rest
- Implement strategies to reduce stress, including coping strategies, biofeedback, cognitive behavioral therapy, psychotherapy, massage, yoga, progressive relaxation, Tai Chi, walking and low-impact exercise programs, use of hot and cold therapies, mindfulness strategies, and sleep hygiene practices

Priority Potential & Actual Complications

- Social withdrawal/social isolation/depression/anxiety
- Immobility/disuse syndrome

Priority Nursing Implications

- Many clients experience fatigue and pain. Make sure pain is managed and analgesics are used to ensure adequate pain relief. Once pain is managed, then consider hypnotic agents and other sleep-inducing strategies
- For hospitalized clients, nurses may advocate for rest times so clients have uninterrupted times of restful sleep. In intensive care and other environments, dim lights at night, limit nighttime activities, group interventions, provide comfort measures, and establish quiet hours to assist in attaining restful sleep and quiet rest periods
- Chronic fatigue syndrome and fibromyalgia may be extremely frustrating for clients and families; clients may not be "believed" or their symptoms and limitations may not be deemed as credible by others in their social or occupational circles

Priority Medications

- Oral NSAIDS
  - Manage mild to moderate pain levels
  - These may allow for restful sleep by addressing the pain that disturbs sleep
- Ferrous sulfate
  - Oral forms of iron should be enteric coated or sustained-release to ensure absorption in the duodenum for optimal absorption
  - Liquid oral-forms of iron will stain the teeth so a straw and diluting the solution is recommended
- Zolpidem–oral administration with fatigue
  - Short-term hypnotic; long-term use should be closely monitored
  - May be used with severe sleep problems (including to fibromyalgia and chronic fatigue syndrome)
- Clonazepam–oral administration with fatigue
  - Anticonvulsant agent
  - Effective with stimulating sleep and reducing anxiety
- Duloxetine–oral administration with fatigue
  - Antidepressant
  - Administer early in the day to avoid insomnia
  - Used with fibromyalgia
- Pregabalin–oral administration
  - Used to treat the pain associated with fibromyalgia
- Cyclobenzaprine–oral administration with fatigue
  - Muscle relaxant with sedative effects
  - May increase productive sleep

Reinforcement of Priority Teaching

- Sleep hygiene practices including going to bed only when sleepy, getting out of bed if haven't fallen asleep in 20 minutes, limiting liquids at night, quiet reading (not screen time) prior to sleep, warm baths or showers just prior to sleep, limiting exercise before bedtime (at least 6 hours prior to) but getting adequate exercise during the day, liming caffeine/stimulants/nicotine/alcohol before bed, having a small protein snack/warm milk prior to sleep to avoid hunger, reducing light and noise if sleeping time is not at night, keeping bed for sleeping and only sleeping activities, staying out of bed during the day, set a regular sleep and wake up time, limiting day-time naps, limiting use of hypnotics, and stress reducing strategies to avoid anxiety at sleep time
- Importance of a balance of sleep, rest, and activity in their lives
- Short-term use of hypnotic agents to attain restful sleep, consider melatonin or lavender oil via diffuser
- Fibromyalgia and chronic fatigue syndrome may interfere with working, attaining health insurance, and receiving needed healthcare. Encourage clients to use available resources to meet basic and healthcare needs
- Fatigue disorders have an unknown course, some resulting in a long recovery period or a lack of full recovery. Client needs to deal with the anger, frustration, and sadness felt by clients and the skepticism or negative reactions of those in the client's world

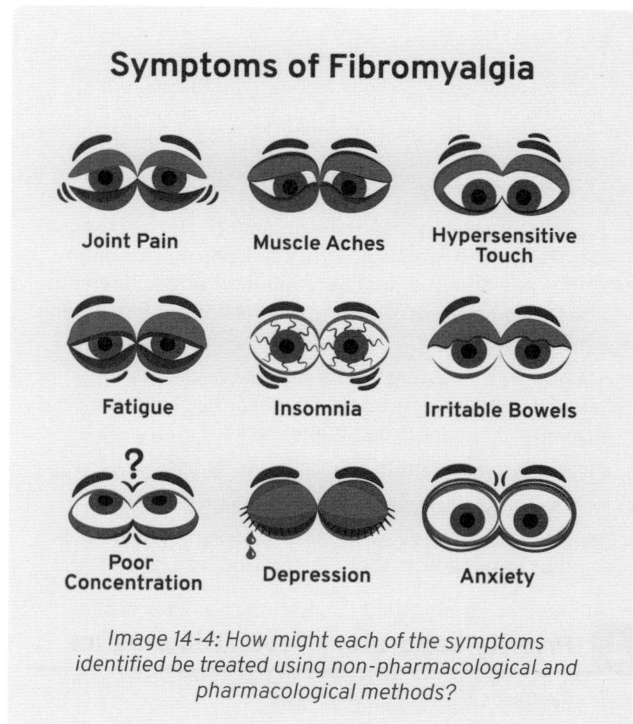

Image 14-4: How might each of the symptoms identified be treated using non-pharmacological and pharmacological methods?

Pathophysiology/Description

- Atopic dermatitis is an inflammatory response to environmental allergens, may be chronic and recurrent, may occur with asthma and nasal congestion
- Allergic contact dermatitis is a delayed hypersensitivity reaction of the skin after a chemical has penetrated the skin and becomes antigenic. After 7-10 days, memory cells form an antibody response. Subsequent exposures yield skin lesions within 48 hours. Often related to exposure to metal, rubber, oils associated with plants, and some cosmetics or dyes
- Latex allergies yield a contact dermatitis related to the chemical processes of making gloves
- Impetigo is a bacterial infection of the skin, often associated with Group A Beta-hemolytic streptococcus or Staphylococcus. May be a primary or secondary infection

Priority Data Collection or Cues

- Examine the characteristics of atopic dermatitis including acute phase (erythema, seeping vesicles, and pruritis). During subacute phase, lesions may become scaly with red/brown plaques. Chronically, skin may become thickened, hyperpigmented, dry, and scaled
- Look for allergic contact dermatitis including red papules or vesicles, may be pruritic, burn or cause pain. If rash is extended over a period of time, the skin may become thick and scaly
- Monitor for response to latex which may be 6-48 hours after exposure including symptoms of drying, mild swelling, fissuring, and cracking of the skin. May progress to redness, marked swelling, and crusting. May lead to scaling and hyperpigmentation
- Impetigo may be associated with poor hygiene. Examine client's hygiene practices. With children, look for open lesions and potential for contamination with scratching, lack of hygiene, and exposure to infectious agents (stools, urine, etc.)
- Other risk factors to be noted that are associated with impetigo include obesity, diabetes mellitus, moist skin folds, history of atopic dermatitis, and treatment with corticosteroids, immunosuppressants, or antibiotics
- Look for appearance of impetigo, including vesicular-papular rash with yellow-brown drainage. Redness noted around the edges and are often pruritic

Priority Laboratory Tests/Diagnostics

- Skin cultures if drainage is accessible
- Other diagnostic procedures for associated risk factors/ illnesses
- In severe cases, allergy testing to determine hypersensitivities

Priority Interventions or Actions

- Use moisturizers on dry skin areas
- Topical immunomodulators and corticosteroids
- Phototherapy sometimes used to dry skin and allow for healing
- Identify and limit exposure to allergic or latex stimulators of skin change
- Impetigo is often treated with systemic antibiotics
- Topical care of impetigo includes warm saline compresses followed by gentle washing to remove exudate and crusting. Areas are left open to air to dry and heal. May be treated with topical antiinfectives

Priority Potential & Actual Complications

- Secondary bacterial infections (impetigo) may occur with untreated skin irritations that are exposed to infectious agents
- Untreated impetigo may lead to bacterial acute glomerulonephritis

Priority Nursing Implications

- Nurses need to be cognizant of their personal risk for contact dermatitis, especially latex, related to extensive and long-term exposure. Many agencies have latex exposure policies or latex free practices

Priority Medications

- Pimecrolimus–topical administration
  - Immunosuppressant/suppresses the inflammatory response
  - Used to treat atopic and contact dermatitis
- Mupirocin
  - Topical antibiotic
  - Used to treat impetigo
- Penicillin
  - Oral medication administered for impetigo
  - Provides systemic treatment to reduce severity and spread of impetigo

Reinforcement of Priority Teaching

- Encourage clients to avoid agents that cause allergic contact dermatitis
- Emotional stress may exacerbate skin reactions
- Clients who are prone to contact and allergic dermatitis as they may experience hypersensitivity reactions, allergic reactions, and drug intolerances/allergies
- The importance of hygiene and effective handwashing
- Impetigo may be contagious, ensure that clients and family are aware of means to prevent spread of infection

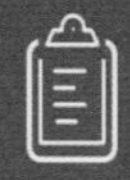

NurseThink® Quiz Questions

1. **The emergency room nurse triages a pediatric client with second and third-degree burns to the bilateral upper extremities, hands, and anterior torso after tripping and falling into a bonfire. The nurse documents the burns in the triage note. Using the rule of nines, what percentage of the total body surface area (BSA) does the nurse calculate has been burned?**
   a. 36%.
   b. 18%.
   c. 27%.
   d. 54%.

2. **The nurse cares for a client recovering from second-degree burns to 30% of their body. What does the nurse incorporate in the client's plan of care to reduce the risk of infection? *Select all that apply.***
   a. Limit visitors, especially those who may be ill.
   b. Consider limiting consumption of fresh vegetables.
   c. Place the client on fluid restriction < 1000 mL daily.
   d. Administer tetanus toxoid as prescribed.
   e. Perform wound care only in a sterile environment.

3. **The nurse cares for a client in the rehabilitative phase of second and third-degree burns. Which action by the client does the nurse encourage to prevent the development of contractures?**
   a. Autografting.
   b. Pressure garments.
   c. Splinting.
   d. Limited activity.

4. **The nurse evaluates pain in an older child with a suspected fracture to the right wrist. The child is quiet and guarding the wrist but is not crying or visibly distressed. Which statement by the child indicates the child does not understand the pain measurement scale?**

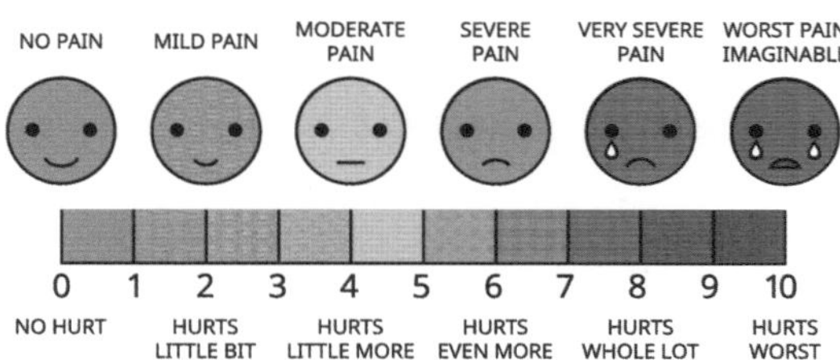

   a. "I only want to cry when I move it, so I pick the yellow face."
   b. "If it didn't hurt at all, I would pick the blue face."
   c. "If I were crying, I would pick one of the faces with tears."
   d. "Since I'm not crying, I should pick the blue or green face."

5. **The nurse cares for a client with acute pain related to a fractured ankle. The nurse prepares the client for application of a temporary cast for discharge from the emergency room. What is the nurse's next best action?**
   a. Inform the client that the procedure will be painful.
   b. Provide analgesics in preparation for the procedure.
   c. Avoid discussing pain until the client brings it up.
   d. Begin wrapping the injured ankle with cast padding.

6. **The nurse cares for a client with acute pain related to a sprained ankle. The client rates the pain 6/10 on a Likert Scale and asks if there is anything they can do to help the pain that does not involve medication. The nurse plans to include which interventions in the client's discharge plan of care?**
   a. Rest, ice, compression, and elevation of the injured ankle.
   b. Radiology, ice, cold, and elevation of the injured ankle.
   c. Rest, ice, contracture, and ecchymoses of the injured ankle.
   d. Radiology, ice, compression, and elevation of the injured ankle.

7. **The nurse collects a thorough medical history on an older adult client with a history of back pain and osteoarthritis. Which question is most important for the nurse to ask when considering chronic pain management?**
   a. "Do you take over-the-counter medications, and if so, how often?"
   b. "Do you have a history of diarrhea or constipation?"
   c. "How long have you been diagnosed with osteoarthritis?"
   d. "Do you have a history of kidney or liver disease?"

8. **The nurse cares for a client with newly diagnosed fibromyalgia. To reduce pain exacerbations, what does the nurse instruct the client to avoid?**
   a. Cold packs.
   b. Heating pads.
   c. Complementary therapies.
   d. High-impact exercise.
   The nurse should instruct the client to avoid activities that may exacerbate symptoms.

9. **The nurse cares for a client with chronic pain related to lupus erythematosus (lupus). When administering corticosteroids, the nurse ensures that the client is not also receiving which medication?**
   a. Acetaminophen.
   b. NSAIDs.
   c. Docusate sodium.
   d. Capsaicin cream.

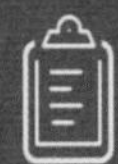

NurseThink® Quiz Questions

10. **The nurse cares for a client with contact dermatitis secondary to poison ivy. Which action by the nurse is the best approach to applying topical ointment to the skin?**
    a. Only allow the client to apply the ointment.
    b. Wear gloves and wash hands before and after application.
    c. Do not use topical ointments for the treatment of poison ivy.
    d. Only apply ointment using a sterile-tipped applicator.

11. **A client has been prescribed diphenhydramine to reduce pruritis associated with contact dermatitis. Which medication instruction does the nurse reinforce with the client?**
    a. "It may cause drowsiness."
    b. "It is a useful stimulant."
    c. "It has an unlimited dosage."
    d. "It should be taken with alcohol."

12. **A client presents to the health care provider's office with complaints of chronic fatigue secondary to fibromyalgia and states, "I just want to live my life without feeling bad all of the time." What is the nurse's best response?**
    a. "Sometimes we just have to power past our pains and discomforts."
    b. "Please tell me more about how fatigue impacts your daily life."
    c. "Have you considered exercise to increase your mood and energy level?"
    d. "Maybe you should consider seeing a psychologist or therapist."

13. **The nurse cares for a female client with complaints of chronic fatigue and tachycardia. The client completes outpatient testing and is diagnosed with iron deficiency anemia. The nurse plans to increase which foods in the client's nutrition plan?**

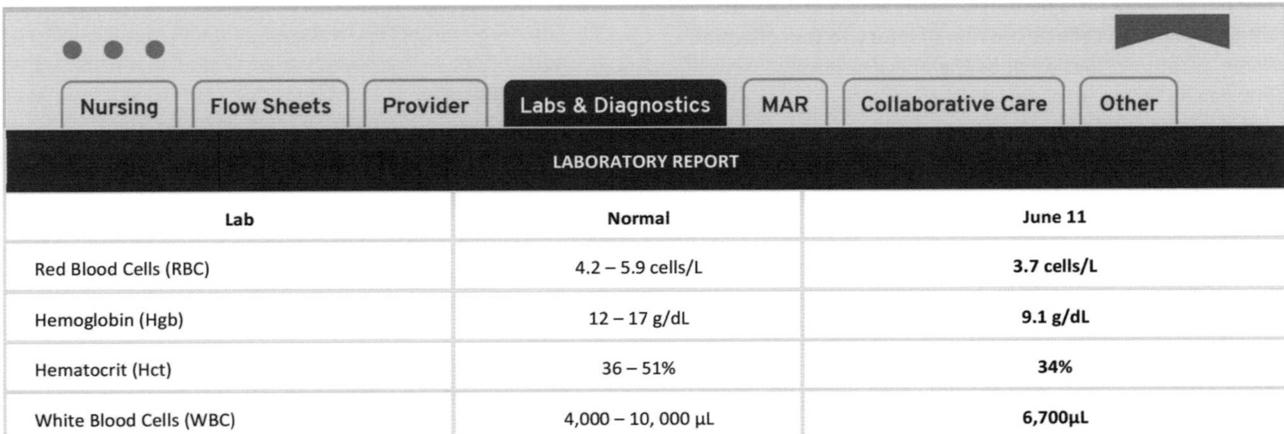

LABORATORY REPORT

Lab	Normal	June 11
Red Blood Cells (RBC)	4.2 – 5.9 cells/L	**3.7 cells/L**
Hemoglobin (Hgb)	12 – 17 g/dL	**9.1 g/dL**
Hematocrit (Hct)	36 – 51%	**34%**
White Blood Cells (WBC)	4,000 – 10, 000 µL	**6,700µL**

    a. Cabbage, cauliflower, and eggs.
    b. Citrus fruits, tomatoes, and strawberries.
    c. Lima beans, spinach, and dried nuts.
    d. Green leafy vegetables and whole grains.

14. **The nurse and client discuss nonpharmacologic therapies for fibromyalgia. Which statement by the client requires follow-up by the nurse?**
    a. "Gentle aerobic exercise may reduce stiffness and discomfort."
    b. "Cognitive behavioral therapy may reduce my response to pain."
    c. "Developing a regular sleeping pattern may reduce insomnia."
    d. "Regular exercise may exacerbate pain and discomfort."

15. **The nurse cares for a client taking duloxetine for depression and insomnia associated with fibromyalgia. The nurse informs the client of which common side effects of duloxetine?**
    a. Dry mouth, somnolence, and nausea.
    b. Insomnia, dizziness, and weight gain.
    c. Headaches and nervousness.
    d. Nausea, vomiting, and constipation.

16. **An older adult client asks the nurse about pharmacologic treatment options for chronic insomnia. Which information does the nurse consider when planning a response?**
    a. Alprazolam is often a good choice for insomnia in the elderly.
    b. The risk for addiction to sleeping medications is very high.
    c. Benzodiazepines should be used cautiously in older clients.
    d. Tylenol PM is the drug of choice for insomnia in the elderly.

17. **A client with narcolepsy reports feeling drowsy around 2 pm. What intervention does the nurse implement?**
    a. Administer a stimulant to keep the client awake during the day.
    b. Take the client for a walk around the facility to promote alertness.
    c. Provide a safe environment for the client to take a nap.
    d. Offer the client a drink and a high-protein snack.

18. **The nurse cares for a pediatric client with a history of sleepwalking. To reduce the risk of injury to this client at home, what information does the nurse collect?**
    a. Family history of sleepwalking behaviors.
    b. Concurrent history of restless leg syndrome.
    c. Style of home and the presence of stairs.
    d. Use of electronic devices close to bedtime.

19. **The school nurse prepares a presentation for teachers on communicable diseases frequently seen in schools. What priority information does the nurse include?**
    a. It's often spread by contact with unwashed hands contaminated with feces.
    b. Infected children should stay home for 5-7 days to prevent spread to others.
    c. Impetigo is only contagious to those with weakened immune systems.
    d. It is highly contagious, so careful hand and surface cleaning is necessary.

20. **The nurse cares for a client with repeated occurrences of impetigo to the chin. The client voices concern about spreading the infection to their roommate. What is the most appropriate information for the nurse to obtain?**
    a. Does the client share a razor or linens with the roommate?
    b. Does the client or roommate have a weakened immune system?
    c. Does the client or roommate have medical knowledge?
    d. Does the roommate have another place to live during outbreaks?

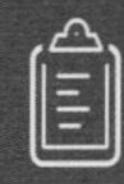

NurseThink® Quiz Answers

1. **The emergency room nurse triages a pediatric client with second and third-degree burns to the bilateral upper extremities, hands, and anterior torso after tripping and falling into a bonfire. The nurse documents the burns in the triage note. Using the rule of nines, what percentage of the total body surface area (BSA) does the nurse calculate has been burned?**
   a. 36%.
   b. 18%.
   c. 27%.
   d. 54%.

   Topic/Concept: Comfort **Subtopic:** Burns (peds) **Bloom's Taxonomy:** Applying **Clinical Problem-Solving Process:** Data Collection **NCLEX-PN®:** Coordinated Care **QSEN:** Teamwork and Collaboration **CJMM:** Recognize Cues

   Rationale: The pediatric rule of nines indicates 9% for each upper extremity and 18% for the anterior torso. 18 + 9 + 9 = 36%

   THIN Thinking: *Clinical Problem-Solving Process* – The nurse must understand the Rule of Nines for pediatric and adult clients, noting the changes in the surface area of the head and lower extremities based on the age of the pediatric client.

2. **The nurse cares for a client recovering from second-degree burns to 30% of their body. What does the nurse incorporate in the client's plan of care to reduce the risk of infection? *Select all that apply.***
   a. Limit visitors, especially those who may be ill.
   b. Consider limiting consumption of fresh vegetables.
   c. Place the client on fluid restriction < 1000 mL daily.
   d. Administer tetanus toxoid as prescribed.
   e. Perform wound care only in a sterile environment.

   Topic/Concept: Comfort **Subtopic:** Burns (adult) **Bloom's Taxonomy:** Applying **Clinical Problem-Solving Process:** Planning **NCLEX-PN®:** Safety and Infection Control **QSEN:** Safety **CJMM:** Generate Solutions

   Rationale: Visitors should be limited to reduce the risk of infection in the compromised client. Consumption of fresh fruits and vegetables may be limited to reduce exposure to contaminants. Fluid should be increased for burn victims. Tetanus toxoid is an expected order for burns and other injuries of the skin. Wound care should be strict aseptic technique, not necessarily sterile.

   THIN Thinking: *Identify Risk to Safety* – The nurse should be familiar with care of the burn client and implement care that reduces the risk of infection and promotes client safety.

3. **The nurse cares for a client in the rehabilitative phase of second and third-degree burns. Which action by the client does the nurse encourage to prevent the development of contractures?**
   a. Autografting.
   b. Pressure garments.
   c. Splinting.
   d. Limited activity.

   Topic/Concept: Comfort **Subtopic:** Burns **Bloom's Taxonomy:** Applying **Clinical Problem-Solving Process:** Planning **NCLEX-PN®:** Physiological Adaptation **QSEN:** Evidence-based Practice **CJMM:** Generate Solutions

   Rationale: Autografting is used for burns covering large areas and is not a client-implemented intervention. Pressure garments are often used to reduce scarring, not contractures. Splinting may be used to maintain range of motion of involved joints and prevent contractures. Limited activity will worsen immobility in a client with burns.

   THIN Thinking: *Clinical Problem-Solving Process* –The nurse should implement care promoting range of motion and flexibility and preventing contractures and stiffening.

4. **The nurse evaluates pain in an older child with a suspected fracture to the right wrist. The child is quiet and guarding the wrist but is not crying or visibly distressed. Which statement by the child indicates the child does not understand the pain measurement scale?**
   a. "I only want to cry when I move it, so I pick the yellow face."
   b. "If it didn't hurt at all, I would pick the blue face."
   c. "If I were crying, I would pick one of the faces with tears."
   d. "Since I'm not crying, I should pick the blue or green face."

   Topic/Concept: Comfort **Subtopic:** Acute pain (peds) **Bloom's Taxonomy:** Analyzing **Clinical Problem-Solving Process:** Evaluation **NCLEX-PN®:** Psychosocial Integrity **QSEN:** Patient-centered care **CJMM:** Evaluate Outcomes

   Rationale: Based on the client's demeanor, their pain likely ranges from mild to severe, so statement A is reasonable. The explanations of the blue face and the faces with tears are accurate: blue is 0-1/10 or no pain, very severe pain and worst pain imaginable are both indicated on the faces with tears. Faces without tears range from no pain to severe pain and do not just include blue or green, so statement D is inaccurate.

   THIN Thinking: *Clinical Problem-Solving Process* –The faces pain scale should be explained thoroughly to the older pediatric client. The nurse should evaluate the client's understanding before asking the client to rate their pain.

5. **The nurse cares for a client with acute pain related to a fractured ankle. The nurse prepares the client for application of a temporary cast for discharge from the emergency room. What is the nurse's next best action?**
   a. Inform the client that the procedure will be painful.
   b. Provide analgesics in preparation for the procedure.
   c. Avoid discussing pain until the client brings it up.
   d. Begin wrapping the injured ankle with cast padding.

   Topic/Concept: Comfort **Subtopic:** Acute pain (adult) **Bloom's Taxonomy:** Applying **Clinical Problem-Solving Process:** Implementation **NCLEX-PN®:** Pharmacological Therapies **QSEN:** Evidence-based Practice **CJMM:** Take Action

   Rationale: Analgesics should be provided before painful procedures to limit the severity during the procedure. The nurse should inform the client that the procedure may be uncomfortable, encouraging them to express their pain, but this is not the priority action. Cast padding application occurs immediately before application of casting materials.

   THIN Thinking: *Help Quick* – The nurse should implement care that limits pain. By providing pain medication before the procedure, the client can complete the procedure in anticipation of pain being controlled.

6. **The nurse cares for a client with acute pain related to a sprained ankle. The client rates the pain 6/10 on a Likert Scale and asks if there is anything they can do to help the pain that does not involve medication. The nurse plans to include which interventions in the client's discharge plan of care?**
   a. Rest, ice, compression, and elevation of the injured ankle.
   b. Radiology, ice, cold, and elevation of the injured ankle.
   c. Rest, ice, contracture, and ecchymoses of the injured ankle.
   d. Radiology, ice, compression, and elevation of the injured ankle.

   Topic/Concept: Comfort **Subtopic:** Acute pain **Bloom's Taxonomy:** Applying **Clinical Problem-Solving Process:** Planning **NCLEX-PN®:** Basic Care and Comfort **QSEN:** Patient-centered Care **CJMM:** Generate Solutions

   Rationale: The acronym RICE (rest, ice, compression, elevation) should be included in the client's discharge plan of care. Radiology is not part of the RICE plan of care; cold is duplicative of ice. Contracture and ecchymoses (bruising) are not interventions.

   THIN Thinking: *Help Quick* – The nurse should include basic principles for musculoskeletal injury in the client's discharge plan of care. This includes the acronym RICE (rest, ice, compression, elevation) for sprains and other musculoskeletal injuries to reduce inflammation, associated pain, and edema.

7. **The nurse collects a thorough medical history on an older adult client with a history of back pain and osteoarthritis. Which question is most important for the nurse to ask when considering chronic pain management?**
   a. "Do you take over-the-counter medications, and if so, how often?"
   b. "Do you have a history of diarrhea or constipation?"
   c. "How long have you been diagnosed with osteoarthritis?"
   d. "Do you have a history of kidney or liver disease?"

   Topic/Concept: Comfort **Subtopic:** Chronic pain (older adult) **Bloom's Taxonomy:** Applying **Clinical Problem-Solving Process:** Planning **NCLEX-PN®:** Coordinated Care **QSEN:** Teamwork and Collaboration **CJMM:** Prioritize Hypotheses

   Rationale: All of this information is helpful, but identifying a history of kidney or liver disease is the most important. Analgesics, especially opioids and NSAIDs, can have toxic effects on the kidneys and liver. Therefore, it's important to identify the presence of these conditions before initiating treatment.

   THIN Thinking: *Identify Risk to Safety* – A thorough medical history, including medications, is important for all clients. Polypharmacy and comorbidities increase the risks associated with medications, and the nurse must carefully consider these variables.

8. **The nurse cares for a client with newly diagnosed fibromyalgia. To reduce pain exacerbations, what does the nurse instruct the client to avoid?**
   a. Cold packs.
   b. Heating pads.
   c. Complementary therapies.
   d. High-impact exercise.

   Topic/Concept: Comfort **Subtopic:** Chronic pain (adult) **Bloom's Taxonomy:** Applying **Clinical Problem-Solving Process:** Planning **NCLEX-PN®:** Health promotion and maintenance **QSEN:** Evidence-based Practice **CJMM:** Generate Solutions

   Rationale: Cold packs may help reduce inflammation and discomfort. Heating pads are helpful for muscular pain. Complementary therapies may help reduce pain or change the client's response to pain. Low-impact exercise is recommended for the client with fibromyalgia.

   THIN Thinking: *Clinical Problem-Solving Process* – The nurse should instruct the client to avoid activities that may exacerbate symptoms.

9. **The nurse cares for a client with chronic pain related to lupus erythematosus (lupus). When administering corticosteroids, the nurse ensures that the client is not also receiving which medication?**
   a. Acetaminophen.
   b. NSAIDs.
   c. Docusate sodium.
   d. Capsaicin cream.

Topic/Concept: Comfort **Subtopic:** Chronic pain **Bloom's Taxonomy:** Analyzing **Clinical Problem-Solving Process:** Planning **NCLEX-PN®:** Pharmacological Therapies **QSEN:** Evidence-based Practice **CJMM:** Prioritize Hypotheses

Rationale: NSAIDs are contraindicated for use alongside corticosteroids and may increase the risk for gastritis or gastric bleeding. Acetaminophen, docusate sodium, and capsaicin cream are not contraindicated for use with corticosteroids.

THIN Thinking: *Identify Risk to Safety* – The nurse should evaluate the client's risk for injury when taking medications concurrently.

10. **The nurse cares for a client with contact dermatitis secondary to poison ivy. Which action by the nurse is the best approach to applying topical ointment to the skin?**
   a. Only allow the client to apply the ointment.
   b. Wear gloves and wash hands before and after application.
   c. Do not use topical ointments for the treatment of poison ivy.
   d. Only apply ointment using a sterile-tipped applicator.

Topic/Concept: Comfort **Subtopic:** Contact dermatitis **Bloom's Taxonomy:** Applying **Clinical Problem-Solving Process:** Implementation **NCLEX-PN®:** Safety and Infection Control **QSEN:** Patient-centered Care **CJMM:** Take Action

Rationale: The nurse should wash hands before and after client care. Gloves are necessary when applying ointment to skin issues that may spread with direct contact. The client may not be able to apply the ointment independently, and a sterile-tipped applicator is not required.

THIN Thinking: *Identify Risk to Safety* – The nurse should understand the implications of applying topical medications and include precautions for preventing the spread of infection.

11. **A client has been prescribed diphenhydramine to reduce pruritis associated with contact dermatitis. Which medication instruction does the nurse reinforce with the client?**
   a. "It may cause drowsiness."
   b. "It is a useful stimulant."
   c. "It has an unlimited dosage."
   d. "It should be taken with alcohol."

Topic/Concept: Comfort **Subtopic:** Contact dermatitis **Bloom's Taxonomy:** Applying **Clinical Problem-Solving Process:** Planning **NCLEX-PN®:** Pharmacological Therapies **QSEN:** Safety **CJMM:** Generate Solutions

Rationale: The risk for drowsiness is increased with diphenhydramine, and the nurse should share this with the client to reduce the risk for injury. Clients must follow prescribed dosing instructions. Diphenhydramine should not be taken with alcohol as it will worsen drowsiness and may lead to injury.

THIN Thinking: *Identify Risk to Safety* – The nurse should include accurate information about the use of diphenhydramine, including information that may increase the client's risk for injury.

12. **A client presents to the health care provider's office with complaints of chronic fatigue secondary to fibromyalgia and states, "I just want to live my life without feeling bad all of the time." What is the nurse's best response?**
   a. "Sometimes we just have to power past our pains and discomforts."
   b. "Please tell me more about how fatigue impacts your daily life."
   c. "Have you considered exercise to increase your mood and energy level?"
   d. "Maybe you should consider seeing a psychologist or therapist."

Topic/Concept: Comfort **Subtopic:** Fatigue **Bloom's Taxonomy:** Applying **Clinical Problem-Solving Process:** Implementation **NCLEX-PN®:** Coordinated Care **QSEN:** Patient-centered Care **CJMM:** Take Action

Rationale: Asking the client to share more about their concern is an open-ended question that will encourage expression by the client. The nurse should avoid being dismissive or implying the issue is psychological.

THIN Thinking: *Clinical Problem-Solving Process* –The nurse should use open-ended questions to encourage dialogue with the client.

13. **The nurse cares for a female client with complaints of chronic fatigue and tachycardia. The client completes outpatient testing and is diagnosed with iron deficiency anemia. The nurse plans to increase which foods in the client's nutrition plan?**
    a. Cabbage, cauliflower, and eggs.
    b. Citrus fruits, tomatoes, and strawberries.
    c. Lima beans, spinach, and dried nuts.
    d. Green leafy vegetables and whole grains.

    Topic/Concept: Comfort **Subtopic:** Fatigue (chronic) **Bloom's Taxonomy:** Applying **Clinical Problem-Solving Process:** Planning **NCLEX-PN®:** Physiological Adaptation **QSEN:** Evidence-based Practice **CJMM:** Generate Solutions

    Rationale: Cabbage, cauliflower, and eggs are foods high in Vitamin K; Citrus fruits, tomatoes, and strawberries are high in Vitamin C; Green leafy vegetables and whole grains are high in Vitamin B6. Lima beans, spinach, and dried nuts lists foods that are good sources of iron and will benefit the client with iron deficiency anemia.

    THIN Thinking: *Top Three* – The nurse should increase the deficient nutrient in the client's diet. With iron deficiency anemia, the nurse should plan to increase iron-rich foods, including meats, hearts and livers, lima beans, spinach, dried nuts, and whole-grain cereals.

14. **The nurse and client discuss nonpharmacologic therapies for fibromyalgia. Which statement by the client requires follow-up by the nurse?**
    a. "Gentle aerobic exercise may reduce stiffness and discomfort."
    b. "Cognitive behavioral therapy may reduce my response to pain."
    c. "Developing a regular sleeping pattern may reduce insomnia."
    d. "Regular exercise may exacerbate pain and discomfort."

    Topic/Concept: Comfort **Subtopic:** Fibromyalgia **Bloom's Taxonomy:** Analyzing **Clinical Problem-Solving Process:** Evaluation **NCLEX-PN®:** Health Promotion and Maintenance **QSEN:** Patient-centered Care **CJMM:** Evaluate Outcomes

    Rationale: Gentle aerobic exercise should be encouraged and will not exacerbate pain. Cognitive behavioral therapy may impact the client's response to pain. The development of regular sleeping patterns may be beneficial to the client with fibromyalgia and insomnia.

    THIN Thinking: *Help Quick* – If the client has misunderstood important information, the nurse should offer gentle correction and ensure the client understands their condition and plan of care.

15. **The nurse cares for a client taking duloxetine for depression and insomnia associated with fibromyalgia. The nurse informs the client of which common side effects of duloxetine?**
    a. Dry mouth, somnolence, and nausea.
    b. Insomnia, dizziness, and weight gain.
    c. Headaches and nervousness.
    d. Nausea, vomiting, and constipation.

    Topic/Concept: Comfort **Subtopic:** Insomnia **Bloom's Taxonomy:** Applying **Clinical Problem-Solving Process:** Data Collection **NCLEX-PN®:** Pharmacological Therapies **QSEN:** Evidence-based Practice **CJMM:** Recognize Cues

    Rationale: Common side effects of duloxetine (Cymbalta) include nausea, dry mouth, constipation, and somnolence. Weight gain and dizziness are often side effects of pregabalin (Lyrica); headache, constipation, and nervousness are common side effects of fluoxetine (Prozac); nausea, vomiting, and constipation are common side effects of milnacipran (Savella).

    THIN Thinking: *Top Three* – The nurse should help the client understand the purpose and potential side effects of any pharmacological interventions.

16. **An older adult client asks the nurse about pharmacologic treatment options for chronic insomnia. Which information does the nurse consider when planning a response?**
    a. Alprazolam is often a good choice for insomnia in the elderly.
    b. The risk for addiction to sleeping medications is very high.
    c. Benzodiazepines should be used cautiously in older clients.
    d. Tylenol PM is the drug of choice for insomnia in the elderly.

    Topic/Concept: Comfort **Subtopic:** Sleep disorders (older adult) **Bloom's Taxonomy:** Applying **Clinical Problem-Solving Process:** Planning **NCLEX-PN®:** Pharmacological Therapies **QSEN:** Patient-centered Care **CJMM:** Prioritize Hypotheses

    Rationale: Benzodiazepines like alprazolam are risky in older adults and should be used cautiously. Some medications used for insomnia can be addictive, but many medications can be used in the short term and will not lead to addiction. Tylenol PM can be purchased over the counter and contains acetaminophen and diphenhydramine. Both medications may not be needed, and overuse of acetaminophen can cause liver damage.

    THIN Thinking: *Identify Risk to Safety* – The nurse should plan to include relevant and accurate information while addressing specific risks to the older adult client.

17. A client with narcolepsy reports feeling drowsy around 2 pm. What intervention does the nurse implement?

a. Administer a stimulant to keep the client awake during the day.
b. Take the client for a walk around the facility to promote alertness.
c. Provide a safe environment for the client to take a nap.
d. Offer the client a drink and a high-protein snack.

Topic/Concept: Comfort **Subtopic:** Narcolepsy **Bloom's Taxonomy:** Applying **Clinical Problem-Solving Process:** Implementation **NCLEX-PN®:** Psychosocial Integrity **QSEN:** Patient-centered Care **CJMM:** Take Action

Rationale: Rest is important for clients with narcolepsy, and the client should be encouraged to nap when sleepy. Walking may increase the risk for injury in the drowsy client. Protein is useful in improving energy, but eating should not routinely be used to promote alertness as it can also promote weight gain. Administering a stimulant is not recommended in most cases and would be determined on an individual basis.

THIN Thinking: *Help Quick* – The nurse should focus on implementing appropriate and safe care for the client. Right now, rest is necessary to reduce episodes of narcolepsy and avoid injury.

18. The nurse cares for a pediatric client with a history of sleepwalking. To reduce the risk of injury to this client at home, what information does the nurse collect?

a. Family history of sleepwalking behaviors.
b. Concurrent history of restless leg syndrome.
c. Style of home and the presence of stairs.
d. Use of electronic devices close to bedtime.

Topic/Concept: Comfort **Subtopic:** Sleep disorders (peds) **Bloom's Taxonomy:** Applying **Clinical Problem-Solving Process:** Data Collection **NCLEX-PN®:** Reduction of Risk Potential **QSEN:** Safety **CJMM:** Recognize Cues

Rationale: Multi-story homes with stairs increase the risk of injury for the sleepwalker; therefore, the nurse must gather this information to determine plans to reduce that risk. Family history is important information but does not reduce the risk of injury. History of restless leg syndrome and the use of electronic devices do not influence the risk of injury.

THIN Thinking: *Identify Risk to Safety* – The nurse should collect data that will help reduce the future risk for injury in the sleepwalker.

19. The school nurse prepares a presentation for teachers on communicable diseases frequently seen in schools. What priority information does the nurse include?

a. It's often spread by contact with unwashed hands contaminated with feces.
b. Infected children should stay home for 5-7 days to prevent spread to others.
c. Impetigo is only contagious to those with weakened immune systems.
d. It is highly contagious, so careful hand and surface cleaning is necessary.

Topic/Concept: Comfort **Subtopic:** Impetigo **Bloom's Taxonomy:** Applying **Clinical Problem-Solving Process:** Planning **NCLEX-PN®:** Safety and Infection Control **QSEN:** Evidence-based Practice **CJMM:** Prioritize Hypotheses

Rationale: Impetigo is very contagious in all populations, and careful cleaning is necessary to prevent the spread of infection. Children can return to school 24 hours after beginning antibiotics. Hand, foot, and mouth disease is spread by fecal contamination.

THIN Thinking: *Top Three* – To reduce the spread of infectious diseases, understanding the mode of transmission is key.

20. The nurse cares for a client with repeated occurrences of impetigo to the chin. The client voices concern about spreading the infection to their roommate. What is the most appropriate information for the nurse to obtain?

a. Does the client share a razor or linens with the roommate?
b. Does the client or roommate have a weakened immune system?
c. Does the client or roommate have medical knowledge?
d. Does the roommate have another place to live during outbreaks?

Topic/Concept: Comfort **Subtopic:** Impetigo **Bloom's Taxonomy:** Analyzing **Clinical Problem-Solving Process:** Data Collection **NCLEX-PN®:** Psychosocial Integrity **QSEN:** Patient-centered Care **CJMM:** Analyze Cues

Rationale: Impetigo is highly contagious regardless of weakened immunity; thus, it is important to determine if the roommates share items that may spread the infection. There is no need for the roommates to live separately if other infection control measures are taken.

THIN Thinking: *Identify Risk to Safety* – When determining safety risks, the nurse must consider both the client and those in contact with the client.

CHAPTER

15

Adaptation

Stress / Violence / Coping / Addiction

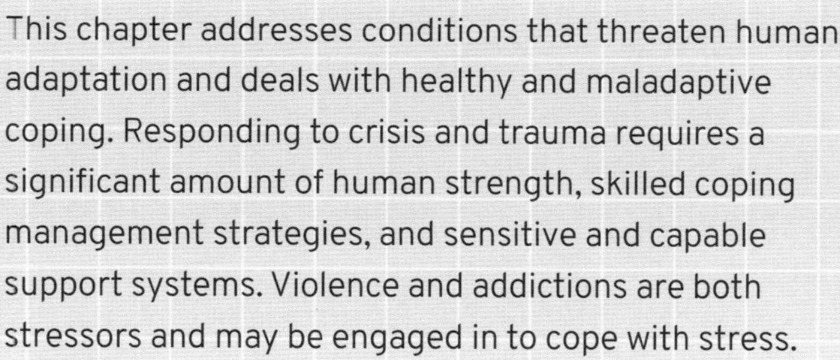

This chapter addresses conditions that threaten human adaptation and deals with healthy and maladaptive coping. Responding to crisis and trauma requires a significant amount of human strength, skilled coping management strategies, and sensitive and capable support systems. Violence and addictions are both stressors and may be engaged in to cope with stress.

Nurses have an important role in assisting clients to cope with stressors, recover from trauma, and deal with the ramifications and recovery from addiction. The challenge for the new nurse is that adaptation-related issues and concerns can arise at anytime. The nurse must be ready to address these concerns by collecting Priority Data and Cues and implementing Priority Interventions or Actions. As you care for the clients on the following pages, consider the safety issues related to each exemplar. Remember, NCLEX® is about safety!

Next Gen Clinical Judgment

Consider the clients for whom you have provided care in the past. Think about those with physiological **and** emotional disorders.

1. How did the client's emotional state impact the client's physiological status?
2. How did management of the physical illness or condition impact the client's emotional health?
3. What nursing care was indicated?

Priority Exemplars:

- Eating disorders
- Substance abuse
- Post-traumatic stress disorder (PTSD)
- Trauma: Abuse, rape, and sexual assault
- Crisis intervention
- Obsessive-compulsive disorder

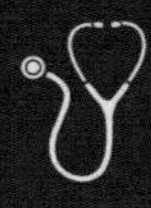

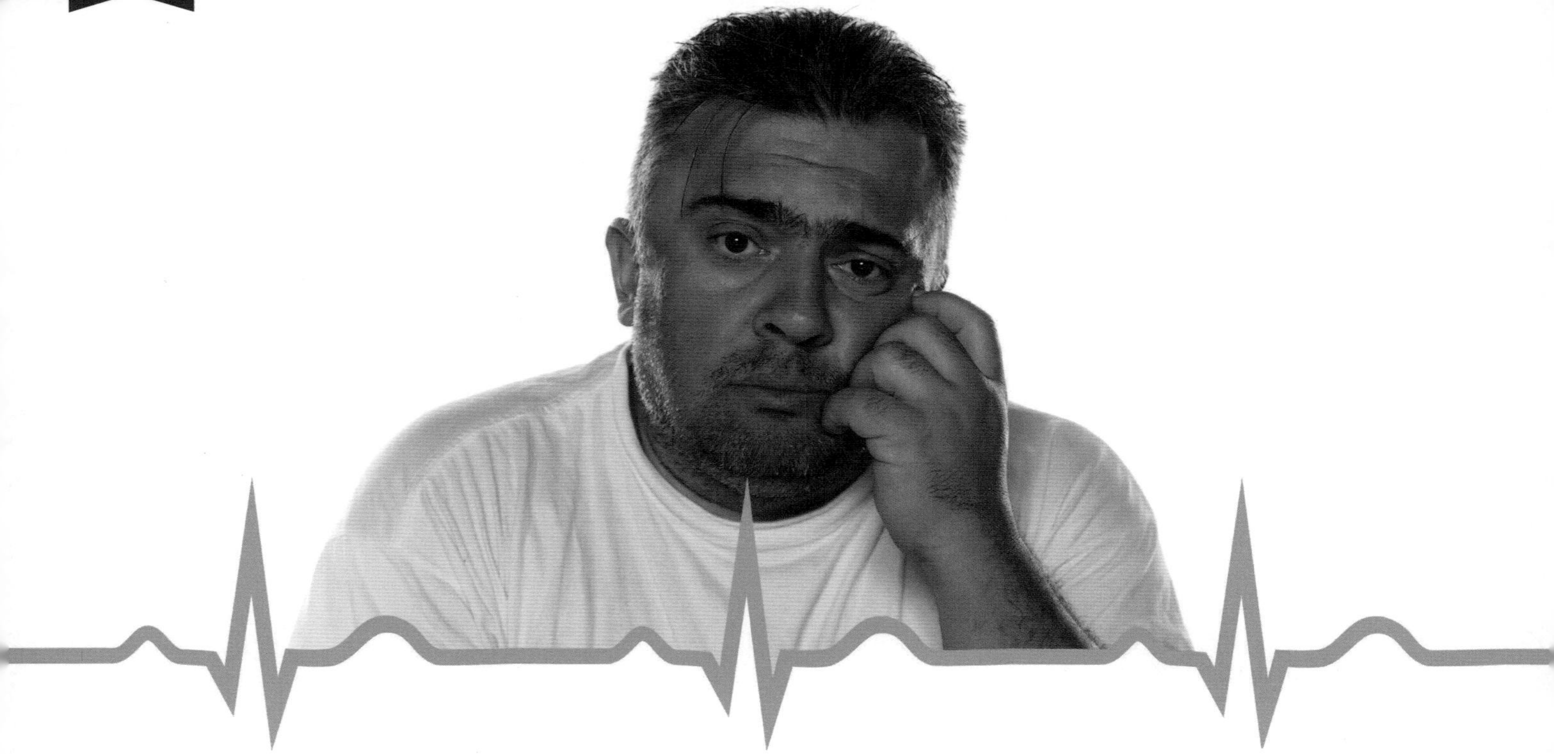

Go To Clinical Case 1

J.C. is a 49-year-old Latino man who presents to the primary health care provider's office with his wife. J.C.'s wife states "He just sits around and watches television and eats. Ever since he lost his job 6 months ago, he seems so depressed. Every so often he'll get mad and yell but usually he just sits in his chair. He will go into the kitchen and eat a whole bag of potato chips or a whole box of cookies. Last night he ate a half-gallon of ice cream. Today he said, 'Who cares how much I weigh? Who cares about anything? I will probably die soon, anyway'." J.C. appears unclean and is dressed in a sloppy manner with frank body odor. He refuses to answer questions and will not engage in eye contact. J.C.'s wife states "My husband was always a hard worker and loved his job as a construction engineer. When he was laid off from his job, he really had trouble coping. We do not have a bathroom scale at home, but I think he has gained about 50 pounds. He was neat and trim before." J.C. refused to answer questions about drug or alcohol intake. J.C.'s wife stated "He drinks beer but not every day. Sometimes he will drink 10 beers at a sitting, but then not drink for a few days. Sometimes I worry about him hurting himself, but he told me that he doesn't have the courage to kill himself."

The nurse takes the client's vital signs which include: Temperature 98.7°F (37°C), 94 beats/minute, 22 breaths/minute, blood pressure 172/88 mmHg. J.C.'s weight is 286 lbs (130 kg) and his height is 5 feet 11 inches (71 inches). His current BMI is 39.9. J.C.'s wife reports that J.C.'s weight was previously around 200-210 pounds. J.C. walks with his head down and a slow-shuffling gait but cooperates with the nurse. J.C.'s wife states "I don't know whether to be more worried about his eating and his physical health or his depression."

NurseThink® Time

Using the NurseThink® system, complete priorities. Check your answers designated by 💡 in the Eating disorders Priority Exemplar. You may also check out the exemplar on Depression to assist you with NurseThink® time!

Next Gen Clinical Judgment

Depression and eating disorders are frequent co-morbidities. What other mental health disorders often occur together? How might a co-morbidity impact the nursing care of clients with these disorders?

NurseThink® Time

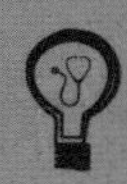

Priority Data Collection or Cues

1.

2.

3.

Priority Laboratory Tests/Diagnostics

1.

2.

3.

Priority Interventions or Actions

1.

2.

3.

Priority Potential & Actual Complications

1.

2.

3.

Priority Nursing Implications

1.

2.

3.

Priority Medications

1.

2.

3.

Reinforcement of Priority Teaching

1.

2.

3.

Pathophysiology/Description

- Anorexia nervosa
  - Fear of obesity with a distortion of body image, preoccupation with food, and refusal to eat
  - Perception of being overweight despite being emaciated
  - May or may not be accompanied by a loss of appetite
  - Reduced food intake/fasting, extensive exercising, and self-induced vomiting/use of laxatives or diuretics
  - Increased incidence in western cultures, societal and cultural pressures on appearance and weight
  - Primarily in women ages 12-30 years, male rate may be underestimated
  - May be restricting (weight loss achieved through not eating and increased exercise) or binge-eating/purging
- Bulimia nervosa
  - Episodic, uncontrolled, rapid, and compulsive eating of large quantities of food over a short period of time followed by attempts to rid the body of calories (vomiting, laxatives, diuretics, exercise, fasting)
  - Report of lack of control during eating episodes
  - Most common in women during late adolescence/early adulthood
- Binge eating disorder
  - Recurrent eating of large amounts of food
  - Usually eat alone and may feel guilty and depressed after episode
  - Does not include purging
  - More common in women than men
  - May be related to obesity
  - May increase risk for type 2 diabetes, hypertension, and cancer
  - Most common in adults ages 46-55
  - Binge eaters have high rates of impulsivity and are more likely to abuse drugs and alcohol
- Co-morbidities of eating disorders with substance use and mood/anxiety disorders (bulimia with anorexia nervosa; binge eating with depression)
- Conditions associated with physiological, environmental, familial, psychodynamic, and individual characteristics

Priority Data Collection or Cues

- Monitor vital signs. Client may be bradycardic, hypotensive, and hypothermic. May have marked hypotension with position changes
- Weigh client. With anorexia, may be less than 85% of normal weight, may be normal or fluctuating weight with bulimia, binge eating may lead to substantial weight gain and obesity
- Ask about eating patterns including lack of eating with anorexia, binging with bulimia and binge eating (often sweet, high-calorie, soft foods – rapid eating without chewing)
- Ask about or observe purging methods including diuretics, laxatives, exercise, self-induced vomiting, fasting
- Ask about what stops food binges including abdominal distension and discomfort, self-induced vomiting, self-blame/disgust, or other activities
- Physical data collection:
  - Observe for lanugo (downy-like body hair) with anorexia, peripheral edema from low serum protein levels
  - With self-induced vomiting, observe client for erosion of tooth enamel, calluses on fingers (Russell's sign), history of esophagitis, mouth ulcers, parotid enlargement, dental caries
  - Monitor hydration status
- History may include menstrual irregularities or amenorrhea, orthostatic hypotension, obsession with food and preparation, compulsive hand-washing
- Monitor for depression, anxiety, guilt, self-blame, preoccupation with appearance, boredom, stressors, low self-esteem
- Observe client's perceptions of their body and appearance
- Use standardized screening tests including the Eating Disorders Inventory, Body Attitude Test, Eating Attitudes Test, or Diagnostic Survey for Eating Disorders

Priority Laboratory Tests/Diagnostics

- Serum electrolytes (purging, dehydration, poor nutrition)
- Obtain ECG for ST segment and T wave changes associated with electrolyte changes
- CBC: Elevated hematocrit (dehydration); anemia (poor nutrition)
- Urine specific gravity for dehydration
- Serum protein levels to determine nutritional status. Clients who binge eat often do not eat nutritious foods

Priority Interventions or Actions

- Hospitalization indicated in cases of
  - Malnutrition
  - Dehydration with electrolyte disturbances
  - Bradycardia and cardiac dysrhythmias, hypotension, hypothermia
  - Suicidal ideations
- To address nutritional needs
  - If refusing PO, may require nasogastric feedings (may also be required if condition deteriorates)
  - If taking PO, work with dietitian to slowly increase calories

- Small, frequent feedings
- Encourage a high fiber diet low in sodium and caffeine
- Focus on weight gained, not food eaten—weigh daily and establish weight gain goals—use behavior modification strategies (privileges and consequences)
- Monitor intake and output
- Contract for a set time period for meals and stay with client during and after meals, look for stashed or discarded food

- To address emotional needs
  - Explore feelings of inadequacy, coping mechanisms, and fears that lead to eating disorder, family issues/feelings of control or lack of control
  - Discuss body image and credibility of distorted perceptions
  - Examine areas of personal self-worth other than appearance
  - Refer for group, family, or individual therapy
- To address overeating
  - Establish a food diary
  - Discuss feelings and thoughts related to overeating
  - Create an eating and exercise plan that allows for reasonable weight loss

Priority Potential & Actual Complications

- Malnutrition/emaciation
- Electrolyte disturbance/cardiac dysrhythmias
- Heart disease and other consequences of obesity
- Obesity (binge eating)
- Renal failure
- May be fatal

Priority Nursing Implications

- Nurses may be instrumental in building relationship with client, ensuring that manipulative behaviors are limited
- Focus on healthy eating to meet body needs and the consequences of over or under-eating
- Nurses may play a key role in collecting data on and assisting clients and families to address issues such as control, coping, stress, and healthy communication
- Nurses may advocate for policies and programming to promote the development of healthy body images and levels of self-esteem with a focus on health and optimal functioning

Priority Medications

- Fluoxetine
  - SSRI antidepressant; oral administration
  - Assist with depression, bulimia (may decrease craving for carbohydrates) and anorexia
  - May take 1-2 weeks to take effect
  - May increase risk of suicide
  - In conjunction with counseling/therapy

Clinical Hint

Eating disorders are often physical means to exert control when the client feels out of control emotionally.

Reinforcement of Priority Teaching

- About the nature of the illness, the management of the illness, and potential support services
- Refer to community organizations for all forms of eating disorders
- The chronic nature of eating disorders and the complexity of the emotional and physical issues

Go To Clinical Answers

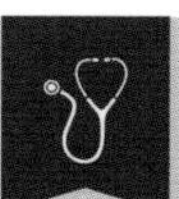

Text designated by are the top answers for the Go To Clinical related to Eating disorders.

Next Gen Clinical Judgment

1. How may the appearances of clients with anorexia nervosa, bulimia nervosa, and binge-eating disorder differ?
2. How may clients with these disorders appear the same?
3. Review the Priority exemplar and list common interventions for these disorders.

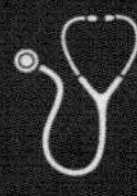

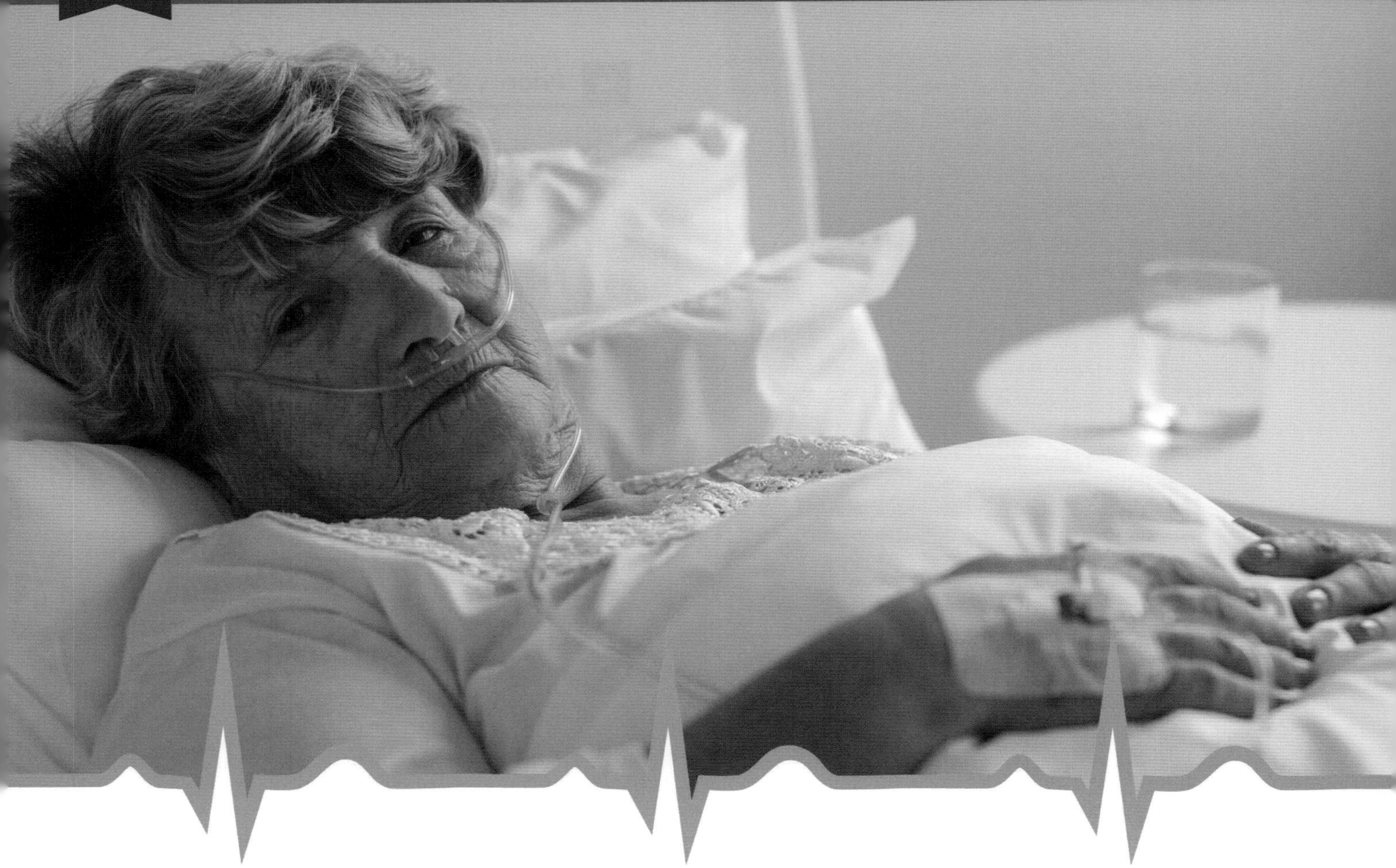

Go To Clinical

Go To Clinical Case 2

D.L. is a 68-year-old Caucasian female admitted for abdominal pain, nausea and vomiting, and signs of dehydration. D.L. reports that these symptoms began three days ago, although she claims she has been "able to keep fluids down." D.L. was afebrile on admission with her vital signs within normal limits, except her heart rate which was slightly above baseline.

The nurse enters the client's room on day 2 and finds D.L. agitated, diaphoretic, and irritable. D.L. claims she has a "terrible headache" and that she "needs a drink." Upon admission, D.L. denied alcohol use. Further questioning revealed that D.L. consumes 8-10 alcoholic drinks per day and that she has had this drinking pattern for 9 years, since the death of her husband. D.L.'s hands are trembling with a weak hand grasp bilaterally. D.L. states she only eats snacks at home and "drinks her meals."

D.L. is unemployed and supports herself on savings, social security, and her husband's insurance monies. She reports she has few friends and is estranged from her immediate family.

D.L.'s current vital signs: Temperature 99°F (37.2°C), 132 beats/minute, 28 breaths/minute, and blood pressures 164/94 mmHg.

The health care provider is contacted and safety precautions initiated.

NurseThink® Time

Using the NurseThink® system, complete priorities. Check your answers designated by 💡 in the Substance abuse Priority Exemplar.

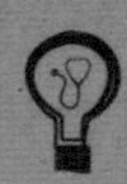

Priority Data Collection or Cues

1.

2.

3.

Priority Laboratory Tests/Diagnostics

1.

2.

3.

Priority Interventions or Actions

1.

2.

3.

Priority Potential & Actual Complications

1.

2.

3.

Priority Nursing Implications

1.

2.

3.

Priority Medications

1.

2.

3.

Reinforcement of Priority Teaching

1.

2.

3.

Pathophysiology/Description

- A complex set of issues and disorders characterized by legal or illegal substance use, addiction, intoxication, and withdrawal
  - Addiction is a chronic disease associated with use of a substance that stimulates the reward and motivation regions of the brain, leading to pathological seeking of more substance. Characterized by tolerance where greater amounts of substance are needed, may impair social and occupational functioning
  - Substance use disorder is when use of a substance impairs social and occupational function
  - Intoxication is a state of euphoria, exhilaration, lethargy, or stupor as a result of substance ingestion, may have physical and emotional dimensions
  - Withdrawal is physical and emotional readjustment after addictive substances are discontinued abruptly
- Symptoms depend upon the substance used, amount of substance used, and the duration of usage
- Substance use disorder and addiction have physical, genetic, environmental, and cultural etiological factors
- Alcohol and other substances have significant impact on the nervous, hepatic, cardiac, and renal systems

Priority Data Collection or Cues

- Client's safety status, potential for injury to self and others
- Vital signs during withdrawal include tachycardia, hypertension
- Vital signs with sedative/opioid use/overdose include hypotension, respiratory depression, and poor perfusion
- Monitor for substance and substance-specific effects
  - Alcohol—socially and culturally approved substance, potential for misuse
  - Caffeine—readily available and used stimulant
  - Cannabis—marijuana
  - Opioids—prescription drug misuse
  - Sedatives, hypnotics, anxiolytics—benzodiazepine, prescription drug misuse, illegally obtained substances
  - Stimulants—cocaine, crack cocaine
  - Others—hallucinogens, inhalants, tobacco
- Standardized tools for substance use
  - Clinical Institute Withdrawal Assessment of Alcohol Scale
  - Michigan Alcoholism Screening Test
  - CAGE (Ever felt you need to Cut down drinking? People Annoyed you by criticizing your drinking? Ever felt Guilty about your drinking? Ever had an Eye-opener in the morning?)(May be modified for other substances)
  - Drug Abuse Screening Test (DAST)
  - Clinical Opiate Withdrawal Scale (COWS)
- Determine potential for dual diagnosis in all mental health clients
- Determine patterns of usage
- Observe for symptoms of withdrawal including diaphoresis, tremor of eyelids, hands, or tongue, nausea and vomiting, irritability or depressed mood, weakness, anxiety, hallucinations, headache, insomnia, illusions (dependent on substance)

Priority Laboratory Tests/Diagnostics

- Blood alcohol level in which intoxication occurs between 100 to 200 mg/dL
- Breathalyzer for alcohol in most states, 0.08% legal intoxication
- Serum toxicology levels for substances
- Monitor CBC and serum protein
- Obtain liver function studies

Priority Interventions or Actions

- Care during withdrawal
  - Monitor vital signs and neurological status, re-orient client as needed
  - Remove objects that they may harm themselves with
  - Provide one-on-one supervision as appropriate
  - Institute seizure precautions, determine the need for restraints, security devices
  - Administer medications to control symptoms
  - Maintain client hygiene
- Addressing addiction/misuse
  - Develop nurse-client relationship
  - Convey an attitude of acceptance, discouraging manipulation, rationalization, denial, and projection
  - Address misconceptions about substance use with objective facts
  - Reinforce teaching with client about the impact of substances on the body
  - Encourage group participation
  - Use motivational interviewing to allow client to set goals for personal recovery, identify assets of goal attainment, collect data on personal strength to facilitate change, determine obstacles to change, and develop strategies for goal attainment
  - Provide referrals to self-help, crisis intervention, and counseling services
- Provide nutritional support and consult a dietitian, limit protein with liver impairment, decrease dietary sodium to prevent fluid overload, provide small, frequent meals of non-irritating food if gastritis or esophagitis exists, thiamine supplements as indicated
- Individual counseling and group therapy

Priority Potential & Actual Complications

- Peripheral neuropathy, alcoholic myopathy, alcoholic cardiomyopathy, esophagitis, gastritis, pancreatitis, alcoholic hepatitis, cirrhosis, leukopenia, thrombocytopenia, sexual dysfunction
- Wernicke's encephalopathy/ Korsakoff's psychosis (thiamine deficiency-confusion, memory loss, lethargy, stupor)
- In pregnant women, fetal alcohol syndrome (craniofacial abnormalities, developmental delays, learning disabilities, organ dysfunction)
- Alcohol withdrawal delirium (see Delirium Priority Exemplar)
- Sedatives/hypnotics/opioids-respiratory depression/cough suppression
- May be fatal
- Stimulants-myocardial infarction, cardiac dysrhythmias

Priority Nursing Implications

- Safety is a critical need for clients using and abusing substances, during intoxication, during delirium, or in withdrawal
- No safe alcohol use has been determined during pregnancy, therefore nurses need to instruct pregnant women to abstain during pregnancy
- During withdrawal from sedatives/opioids-clients may experience rapid eye movement (REM) rebound with insomnia and dreaming
- Nurses should be aware of potential drug diversion in the workplace and chemically-impaired co-workers
- Nurses may observe clients who enter clinical agency for other diagnoses/procedures who demonstrate signs of withdrawal
- With older adults, the use of alcohol, drug interactions, or polypharmacy may impact functional ability, sleep patterns, urinary continence, and cognitive function, including increased risk for falls

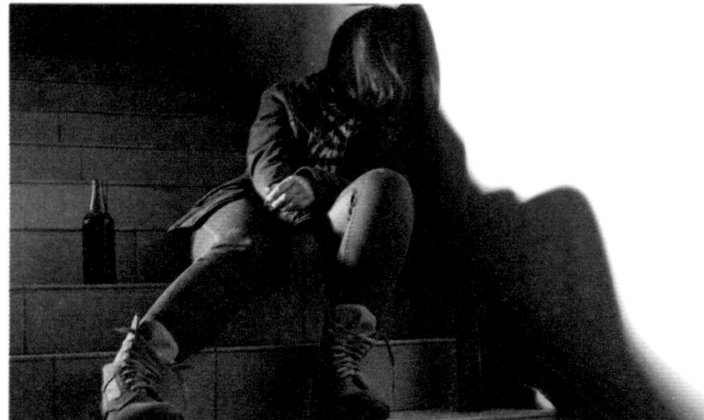

Image 15-1: What are the health implications of binge drinking? What are the long-term implications of alcoholism? What are the long term complications associated with other types of substance abuse?

Priority Medications

- Naloxone–administered IV, IM, Subcutaneous, or intranasal routes
  - Antagonist to narcotic agents
  - May stimulate withdrawal
- Disulfiram–oral administration
  - Alcohol deterrent
  - Generates symptoms if alcohol is ingested
  - Range of symptoms from nausea/vomiting to death based on amount of alcohol ingested and individual sensitivity
  - Should not be started until 12 hours after alcohol abstinence
  - Instruct client about alcohol in selected over-the-counter medications and substances
- Naltrexone–oral or IM
  - Opiate antagonist
  - To treat alcohol and heroin addiction
- Lorazepam–oral, IV, or IM
  - Benzodiazepine–anti-anxiety agent
  - To reduce withdrawal symptoms
  - High doses provided routinely, with bolus doses for breakthrough symptoms
- Vitamin supplementation–oral
  - Folic acid, multivitamins, thiamine
  - With long-term alcohol use
- Flumazenil–administered IV
  - Antidote
  - Benzodiazepine overdose
- Methadone–generally oral, may be buccal or rectal in rare instances; also IV, IM, or subcutaneously in some clients
  - Prevents withdrawal in clients addicted to opioids
  - Part of a comprehensive cessation program

Reinforcement of Priority Teaching

- Use of alternative coping strategies to using substances: Reading, hobbies, exercise, meditation, music, relaxation techniques, and physical activity
- The need for abstinence, the impacts of substance use, their role in enabling substance use, management of substance use, and community resources to support recovery (Alcoholics Anonymous, etc.)
- Employ motivational interviewing to enhance client engagement in behavior change

Go To Clinical Answers

Text designated by the icon are the top answers for the Go To Clinical related to Substance abuse.

Post-traumatic stress disorder (PTSD)

Pathophysiology/Description

- Trauma—an extremely stressful and distressing experience that leads to emotional shock and incurs significant and long-lasting psychological effects
- Classified as:
  - Post-traumatic stress disorder (stress response to an event outside the usual human experience and of significant magnitude such as rape, war, disasters)
    - Diagnosis with PTSD is based on severity of symptoms, persistence of more than a month, and significant impact on social or occupational functioning
  - Acute stress disorder (symptoms are similar to PTSD, but resolution occurs within one month)
  - Adjustment disorder (stress reactions from routine daily events, such as failure, rejection, or divorce, disorder usually resolved within six months of stressor)
    - May occur with or without anxiety or depressed mood
    - May occur with or without conduct disturbance
- Based on client history (or family observations), client may exhibit a pattern of difficulty accepting change or ineffective coping skills
- Symptoms may occur immediately post-trauma or may be delayed
- Adjustment disorders, as well as PTSD, may occur across the lifespan
- Emotional reactions may include guilt, anger, aggression
- Individual response to a trauma/disaster: Influenced by the severity and scope of the event and the individual's ego-strength, coping resources, temperament, previous experiences with stress
- Coping may be influenced by individual perception of the event

Next Gen Clinical Judgment

A nurse assigned to care for a client with post-traumatic stress disorder. The client is a 78-year-old veteran who was in active combat during the Vietnam conflict. Search the Internet for best practices for communicating with this client. Write down 5 communication interventions recommended for clients with PTSD:

1. ______________________
2. ______________________
3. ______________________
4. ______________________
5. ______________________

Priority Data Collection or Cues

- General
  - Use standardized tools to determine levels of depression and anxiety
  - Determine client's risk for harm to self or others
  - Elicit client history from family and others as needed
  - Ask about and observe for substance use and abuse
- Post-traumatic stress disorder
  - Determine the impact of the trauma on client's abilities for self-care, socialization, work, engagement in activities
  - Determine the event causing symptoms, the client's role in the event, and current factors related to the event
  - Observe for intrusive memories, dissociative reactions (flashbacks) or dreams/nightmares
  - Determine if client experiences high level of anxiety or arousal
  - Ask about support systems and other coping mechanisms
  - Ask about avoidance behaviors of experiences or stimuli (noises, reminders of event)
  - Explore psychotic behaviors, distorted thoughts, and self-blame
  - Ask about sleep and sleep disturbances
- Acute stress disorder
  - Ask about recurrent memories, distressing dreams, dissociative reactions, and intense reactions
  - Monitor for depression, dissociative symptoms, and avoidance behaviors
  - Observe for hypervigilance or hyperarousal
- Adjustment disorder
  - Monitor for ability to work, engage in social activities
  - Collect data on mood level, tearfulness, feelings of hopelessness, nervousness, worry, and restlessness
  - Ask about history of conduct disorders, including truancy, vandalism, reckless driving, fighting

Priority Laboratory Tests/Diagnostics

- Determine serum alcohol levels or drug toxicology screens

Priority Interventions or Actions

- Encourage safety-related behaviors and provide precautions as needed
- Create a non-threatening environment with consistent caregivers
- Ensure a therapeutic, trusting relationship
- Stay with client during flashbacks, nightmares, and intrusive memories
- Encourage client communication about experiences and emotions at client's pace

- Explore coping mechanisms and support systems, discuss with client the coping mechanisms that were effective before the trauma
- Address client's feelings of guilt or self-blame
- Promote healthy grieving (see Bereavement Priority Exemplar)
- Allow for expression of pent-up anger, guilt, and frustration including physical exercise, walking, work, crafts, routes of expression (artwork, poetry)
- Use role-play to act out stressful situations and potential responses
- Refer client for therapy, including cognitive behavioral therapy, prolonged exposure therapy (like flooding or implosion therapy), group and family therapy, self-help groups, crisis intervention, eye movement desensitization and reprocessing (allows client to understand traumatic events as they are explored during rapid eye movement initiated by watching therapist's finger)

Priority Potential & Actual Complications

- Suicide or harm of others
- Debilitating social and/or occupational dysfunction

Priority Nursing Implications

- Nurses' roles implementing trauma-informed care: ***Realize*** the increased prevalence of trauma-related incidents, ***Recognize*** signs/symptoms in clients, families, and others, ***Respond*** in practice, and avoid ***Retraumatization***
- Current attention is focused on the impact of war and sexual assault victims and the need for increased awareness and resources in the community. Nurses have a key role in advocating for clients with these experiences as they work through their trauma
- Nurses may encounter clients who experienced a variety of traumas in their lives and nurses should employ sensitive and astute means to collect data to ensure clients receive the help they need to cope with physical, emotional, and sexual traumatic events

Priority Medications

- Paroxetine–oral administration
  - SSRI
  - Found to be effective with PTSD
  - May take 1-4 weeks to be effective
- Amitriptyline–oral administration
  - Tri-cyclic antidepressant
  - Effective with PTSD
- Carbamazepine–generally given orally, limited IV use
  - Anticonvulsant
  - Reduces intrusive thoughts and flashbacks
- Cannabinoids– inhalation, oral, sublingual, topical, rectal, or via oromucosa
  - May be helpful in calming client and controlling symptoms
  - Clients with PTSD have low endogenous cannabinoid levels
- Prazosin–oral administration
  - Antihypertensive
  - Used to manage recurrent nightmares

Reinforcement of Priority Teaching

- The nature of the traumatic response, the methods of intervention, and supports
- Community resources to provide support, self-help groups, peer counseling, education, protective respite care, and other resources
- Past coping mechanisms that have proven effective
- Relaxation techniques and anxiety-reducing strategies

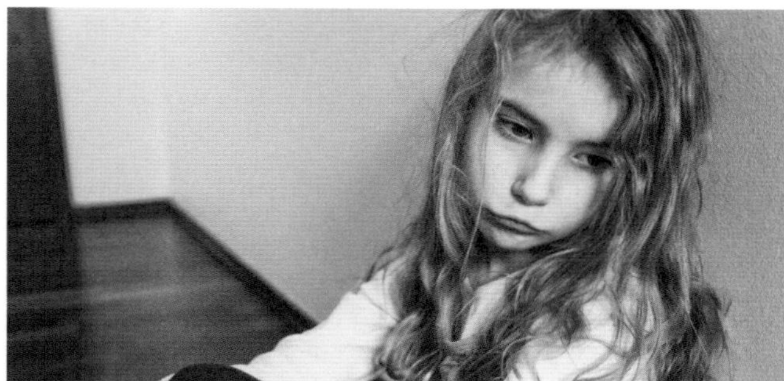

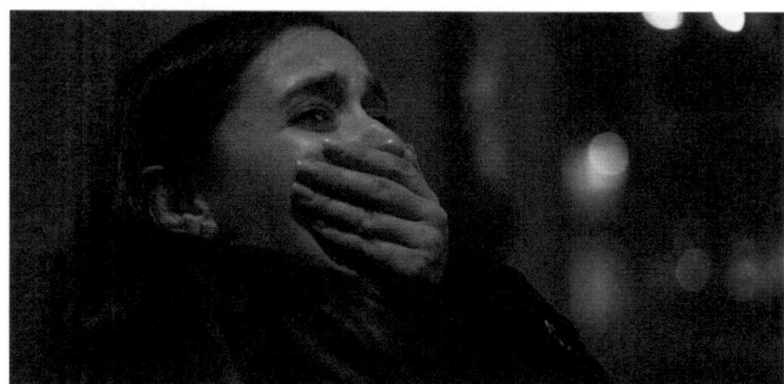

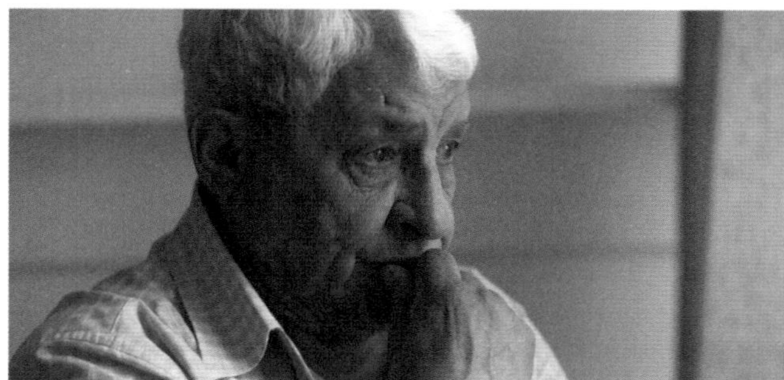

Image 15-2: Trauma-informed care may differ among clients of various ages. How would nursing interventions differ based on the ages of the clients in these images?

Pathophysiology/Description

- Abuse is the maltreatment of a person by another
- Etiologies of violence/abusive behaviors have biological, psychological, and sociocultural dimensions. Organic brain syndromes, mental health disorders, role modeling of violent behaviors, poverty, and other conditions may predispose an individual to violence perpetration
- May involve intimate partner violence (violence between intimate partners, domestic violence, battering), child abuse and neglect, elder abuse, and sexual violence, including sexual trafficking
- Battering is a pattern of physical, emotional, and sexual violence to exert coercive control over an intimate partner
    - Victims of battering often have a low self-esteem, guilt/self-blaming for the violence, are socially isolated, may have experienced violence in childhood, may wish to protect children and keep family intact, may be financially dependent, fear retaliation, fear losing custody of children, lack a support network, or ascribe to social/cultural beliefs about marriage, role of women/men, and power
    - Perpetrators of battering are often jealous, maintain two demeanors (outside world, in home as abuser), highly stressed with limited coping, often emotionally degrading and controlling, withhold opportunities, money, and transportation to keep the victim under control
    - Cycle of battering includes Tension/building phase, Acute battering incident, Honeymoon phase (calm, apologetic, loving)
- Child abuse is maltreatment that may include physically, emotionally, or sexually violent acts imposed on a child by a caregiver, may result in physical injury and emotional consequences
- Elder abuse is physical, sexual, or emotional violence against elder adults, may include neglect or economic exploitation, older adults may be vulnerable due to illness, dependency, immobility, or altered mental status
- Neglect may be physical (denying physical needs, such as food, shelter, healthcare, or supervision) or emotional (failure to meet individual's needs for love and support)
- Sexual exploitation is when a child or dependent individual is induced or coerced to engage in sexual conduct to promote a business, performance, or adult's sexual pleasure
- Sexual violence may include rape (use of power and violence over a sexual partner), sexual assault (sexual act in which the individual is coerced or forced), sexual coercion, unwanted sexual contact, acquaintance/date rape, statutory rape (between a person above the age of consent and a person less than the age of consent), marital rape (spousal rape if against the partner's will)

Priority Data Collection or Cues

- Observe threats to client safety
- Monitor vital signs and client's physiological level of stability
- Signs of physical abuse
    - Unexplained bruises, marks, black eyes, burns, or broken bones
    - Inconsistent or conflicting recounting of experiences
    - Changes in behavior including aggressiveness, excessive fears, hyperactivity, apathy, withdrawal
    - Marks or bruises at various stages of healing
    - Marked reactions to abuser including fear, withdrawal, or ignoring
    - Caregiver/perpetrator reports conflict with victims, describe victim as bad or deserving, harsh discipline, perpetrators may have history of abuse in their life
- Signs of emotional abuse
    - Emotional lability
    - Emotional developmental delay
    - Lack of attachment to caregiver
    - Suicidal ideations or attempts
    - Caregiver belittles/berates individual, rejects the person
- Signs of neglect
    - Absence from school/work, lack of home involvement in school/work
    - Lack of healthcare and hygiene, not meeting nutritional and shelter needs
    - Caregiver may be a substance abuser, may be depressed or indifferent
- Signs of sexual abuse
    - Difficulty walking, sitting, or increased reaction to touching by others
    - Reports of regressive behaviors, including bed wetting, and refuses to change in front of others
    - Torn or stained clothes/underwear
    - Unusual sexual knowledge or behaviors
    - May become pregnant, contract an STI, or demonstrate unusual behaviors
    - Perpetrator may be over-protective, isolative, or controlling
- Signs of elder abuse
    - Similar to those above
    - Observe for financial abuse or medication overdose

Priority Laboratory Tests/Diagnostics

- Tests to determine physical status based on abuse and symptoms
- Pregnancy test
- Sexually transmitted infection testing

Priority Interventions or Actions

- Maintain safety of client/victim
- Convey comfort, safety, and acceptance of victim
- Explain all interactions and treatments explicitly
- Photograph all injuries if permitted by the client
- Do not bathe or change clothes until after examination to preserve evidence
- Engage a sexual assault nurse examiner as indicated
- Ensure privacy during history and physical
- Allow client to pace their discussion of the assault
- Ensure client has support and refer, as indicated, to community resources

Priority Potential & Actual Complications

- Violent behaviors may breed additional violence and subsequent generations of abusers
- Serious physical and emotional sequelae from rape, abuse, and assault
- Violence may be extreme causing morbidity and mortality
- Rape trauma syndrome-see PTSD Priority Exemplar

Priority Nursing Implications

- Nurses must focus on the safety of the client/victim
- Current attention is devoted to the need for explicit consent prior to participation in sexual activity. Consent can only be received when an individual is sober, conscious, at age of consent and aware of the circumstance/consequences. Nurses are involved in educating and reinforcing positive relationship skills and about the concept of consent
- Nurses are often a front-line, sensitive intervener with victims. Providing support, caring, and thoughtful communication are critical to gain client's trust and ensure atraumatic care
- State laws differ about an abused victim's ability to report and press charges against a perpetrator. Maltreatment of children (< 18 years) and elders are, in most states, subject to mandatory reporting laws. Victims not covered by these parameters have the choice to disclose abuse. Nurses need to be aware of local and national laws related to abuse
- Play, art, games, and creative therapies may be used to elicit information from children about abuse episodes
- Nurses should be sensitive to ensuring a safe environment when interviewing a client for potential abuse. For example, away from partner/spouse if intimate partner violence is suspected
- Nurses may need to collaborate with law enforcement to obtain evidence (photographs, specimens)

Reinforcement of Priority Teaching

- Lists of community resources including self-help groups, crisis hotlines, shelters, support groups, the civil/criminal justice system, and counseling services
- Information to parents/caregivers about the realistic abilities of children, providing resources and information on healthy parenting, ensuring methods to relieve stress, and encourage seeking services for mental health issues
- Rape is a crime of violence, not of passion. Advise about bystander advocacy and methods to promote stress management, reduction in alcohol and substance abuse, and gender equity to promote primary prevention of rape and sexual abuse
- Finding alternative residences for older adults who are victims and respite services to reduce stress levels when caregiving

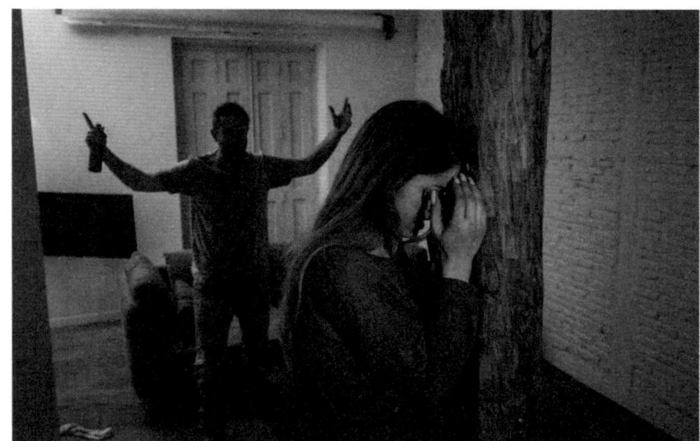

Image 15-3: A female client reveals to the nurse that she is the victim of intimate partner violence. List two immediate priorities of care. List two long-term priorities of care.

The client divulges that she was sexually assaulted last night. What additional data should be collected? What additional actions should be included in caring for this client?

Clinical Hint

Sexual Assault Nurse Examiners (SANE) nurses are especially educated and certified to care for a victim in a sensitive and respectful manner while employing best practices in securing evidence and ensuring safety.

Crisis intervention

Pathophysiology/Description

- Crisis is a sudden event that impacts the individual and current coping mechanisms prove inadequate to address issues and problem solving
- Hospitalization may be indicated if client expresses potential to harm self or others
- Characteristics
  - All people, at some time, experience a crisis
  - Crises are connected to a precipitating event
  - Crises are interpreted and perceived by the individual (a crisis for one person may not be for another)
  - Crises are, by definition, resolved in a short period of time (1-3 months)
  - Crises provide the opportunity for personal growth or may erode at individual's coping for subsequent problems and crises
- Human responses to crisis include feeling powerless, overwhelmed, and anxious. May perceive coping strategies are inadequate and may become obsessive, solely directed on addressing crisis. May experience physical manifestations of anxiety
- Crisis response is based on individual's perception of the event, availability of supports, and availability of coping strategies
- Phases of crisis
  - Phase 1 Exposure to the stressor
  - Phase 2 Current coping mechanisms fail, anxiety increases
  - Phase 3 Client seeks assistance and/or uses all coping and resources to resolve conflict/crisis
  - Phase 4 If unresolved, leads to psychological distress, panic, and disordered thinking
- Types of crises
  - Dispositional: acute response to an external stressor
  - Anticipated life transitions: lack of coping to normal times of transition
  - Crisis from traumatic stress: response to an external stressor over which the client has no control
  - Maturational/developmental: response to lack of coping with normal developmental stressors
  - Psychiatric emergencies: severe impairments secondary to the stressor. These may include overdose, suicide attempts, anger episodes, or intoxication

Priority Data Collection or Cues

- Determine the client's capacity for harming self or others. Ask if client has a plan
- Encourage the client to talk about the precipitating event and describe the event and when it occurred
- Ask client about personal capacity to cope with this and previous crises / determine pre-crisis functioning
- Collect preliminary data on the client's physical and emotional status / observe for pre-existing psychiatric issues
- Determine previous experiences with this crisis/coping mechanisms employed
- Ask about current coping mechanisms and their effectiveness
- Determine the existence and adequacy of support systems
- Monitor for use of substances

Priority Interventions or Actions

- Management is focused on short-term identification and mobilization of resources
- Focus of management is problem-solving and productive change to restore functioning and achieve personal growth
- Establish a therapeutic relationship based on acceptance and active listening
- Set limits on aggressive, hostile, impulsive, or violent behavior
- Clarify the current crisis/problem, explore causes, and compare nurse's perceptions with the client's
- Discuss feelings of anger, resentment, guilt, or disappointment
- Discuss potential changes and coping mechanisms/ alternative strategies to deal with the crisis. Deliberate the pros and cons of different coping options / assist client to select coping strategies
- Clarify those components of the crisis that cannot be changed and feelings those evoke
- Identify and refer to resources and support systems

Priority Laboratory Tests/Diagnostics

- Serum blood alcohol levels and drug/toxicology screens

Priority Potential & Actual Complications

- Unresolved crisis may lead to anxiety, depression, and post-traumatic stress disorder
- May harm self or others

Priority Nursing Implications

- Nurses may work with peer-support teams including those with personal experience in dealing with crisis
- Crisis intervention skills may be used by nurses to help individuals after a disaster, diagnosis with a life-threatening illness, or any significant life change
- As clients learn to cope with current crisis, nurses may be instrumental in fostering new coping mechanisms and ways to deal with future crises

Reinforcement of Priority Teaching

- Awareness of crisis hotlines, crisis centers, and hospital/ agency resources focused on crisis intervention

Obsessive-compulsive disorder (OCD)

Pathophysiology/Description

- Characterized as one of the anxiety disorders
- Obsessions are intrusive thoughts that are recurrent and stressful, may be recognized as irrational, but are so powerful and repetitive that they cannot be ignored, may try to repress/ignore them, but "giving" into the obsession allows for stress relief
- Compulsions are repetitive and ritualistic behaviors or mental acts that individuals feel driven or forced to perform, are completed in order to reduce the associated anxiety that is generated by obsession, significant dread of a negative event exists if the compulsions cannot be carried out
- Obsessive-compulsive disorder (OCD)includes either obsessions, compulsions, or both and can be so significant that it causes social and/or occupational dysfunction and the behaviors take up more than one hour per day
- Engaging in obsessive-compulsive behaviors is stress-relieving for the client
- Common compulsions include handwashing, checking, ordering, praying, counting, and repeating words silently
- Equally common in men and women
- May be associated with hoarding disorder
- Usually begins in adolescence or early adulthood, but may begin earlier
- Usually a chronic illness, may be made more complex by substance use or episodes of depression
- Causes-changes in the anatomy and physiology of the brain, along with changes in brain biochemistry, are associated with OCD

Priority Data Collection or Cues

- Observe client's level of anxiety using standardized scales
- Review client's and family's reports of ritualistic behavior, obsessive thoughts, inability to meet basic needs, inability to meet responsibilities, or levels of anxiety
- Monitor level of anxiety when client is unable to engage in OCD behaviors
- Determine client's ability to engage in alternative coping strategies to replace ritualistic behaviors
- Determine risk for suicide

Priority Interventions or Actions

- Establish a trusting environment, reassure client that they are safe and use open-ended questions
- Stay with client when in a panic or highly anxious
- Use brief messages—stay calm and describe agency routines
- Manage hyperventilation—take several breaths in a paper bag, then slow deep abdominal breaths, repeat as needed
- Decrease environmental stimuli
- Use sedation as needed
- Explore sources of anxiety once "attack" has subsided
- Assist client to identify triggers or early onset of anxiety and how to deal with these including deep breathing, imagery, prayer, meditation, or exercise
- For specific OCD behaviors consider use of controlled systematic desensitization (gradual exposure to stimuli) or implosion therapy (flooding with stimuli)
- Explore coping strategies and anxiety-management methods to replace ritualistic behavior

Priority Potential & Actual Complications

- Substance use/abuse as self-medication
- Generalized anxiety disorder
- Major depressive disorder

Priority Nursing Implications

- Times of stress, such as illness or trauma, may cause client to revert to OCD behaviors and require the nurse to assist with coping mechanisms or refer as indicated for a psychiatric consultation or counseling
- Methods to deal with stress that may be explored include progressive muscle relaxation, yoga, exercise, music, meditation, imagery, prayer, or affirmations

Priority Medications

- Fluoxetine, paroxetine, sertraline
  - SSRIs–oral administration
  - May require higher doses than those with depression
  - Side effects: Sleep disturbance, headache, and restlessness
- Clomipramine–oral administration
  - Tricyclic antidepressant
  - Side effects: Orthostatic hypotension, sedation, sexual side effects
  - May lower seizure threshold

Reinforcement of Priority Teaching

- Recognize and avert rising anxiety levels that cause client to resort to OCD behaviors
- Healthy coping mechanisms to replace ritualistic behavior
- The nature of the illness, the management of the illness, and community support services/potential for ongoing counseling

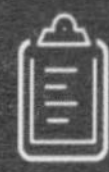

NurseThink® Quiz Questions

1. **The nurse cares for a client with an eating disorder. What treatment is most likely to be used as it is appropriate for all forms of eating disorders?**
   a. Cognitive-based therapy (CBT).
   b. Family therapy.
   c. Antidepressant therapy.
   d. Group therapy.

2. **The nurse collects data for a client with potential bulimia nervosa. Which finding does the nurse correlate with the disorder?**
   a.
   b. 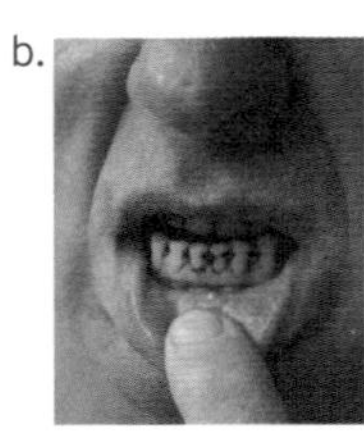
   c. 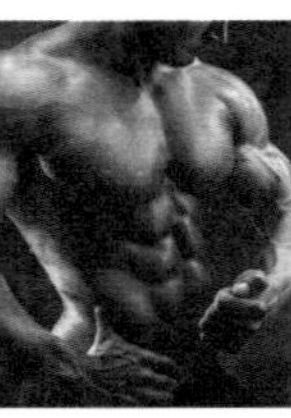
   d. 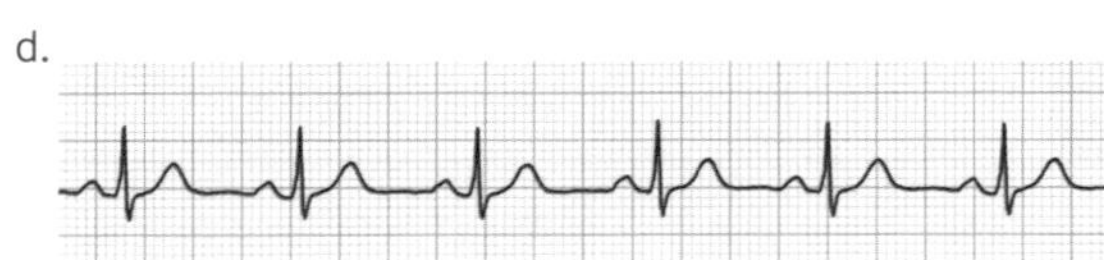

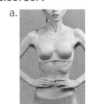

3. **The nurse cares for a client with binge-eating disorder. What complications does the nurse attribute to this diagnosis? *Select all that apply.***
   a. Diabetes mellitus II.
   b. Hypotension.
   c. Hyperlipidemia.
   d. Heart disease.
   e. Central sleep apnea.

4. **The nurse observes a child's legs. Which image does the nurse report as a sign of suspected child abuse?**
   a.
   b. 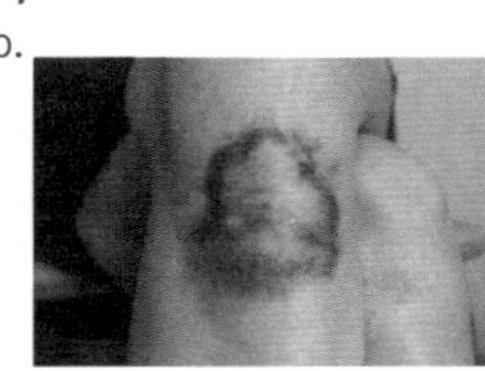

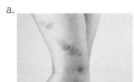

5. **The nurse prepares a presentation on rape prevention for a group of teens. What risk factors for being raped does the nurse include? *Select all that apply.***
   a. Delinquency.
   b. Strong parental relationship.
   c. Low socioeconomic status.
   d. Drug and alcohol use.
   e. Lack of sexual abuse history.

6. **The nurse cares for a client who was sexually assaulted. What finding suggests the client is in the reorganization phase of rape-trauma syndrome?**
   a. They need to talk to resolve their feelings.
   b. They go about life activities superficially.
   c. They experience somatic symptoms.
   d. They are experiencing flashbacks and nightmares.

7. **The nurse cares for a client during a crisis. What goals does the nurse expect to be included in their plan of care?**
   a. Prepare for hospitalization through the crisis.
   b. Avoid relying on the individual's strengths during the crisis.
   c. Cope with immediate stressors to lessen suffering.
   d. Return the individual to a lesser functioning level.

8. **The nurse plans care for a client experiencing a crisis. What intervention does the nurse prioritize?**
   a. Encourage effective coping strategies.
   b. Connect with the client and establish a therapeutic relationship.
   c. Develop a support plan with adequate follow-up.
   d. Explore the client's perception of the crisis.

9. **The nurse evaluates the effectiveness of the local community crisis counseling center. What component does the nurse expect to find if the crisis counseling available is appropriately focused?**
   a. Allows survivors to seek out their services.
   b. Strengthens existing community support systems.
   c. Conducted in traditional settings.
   d. Functions within established standard hours.

10. The nurse cares for a client who has overdosed on multiple substances and administers naloxone intravenously to reverse the side effects from the overdose. Based on the reported information, what substance does the nurse report to the provider to obtain an additional prescription to reverse?

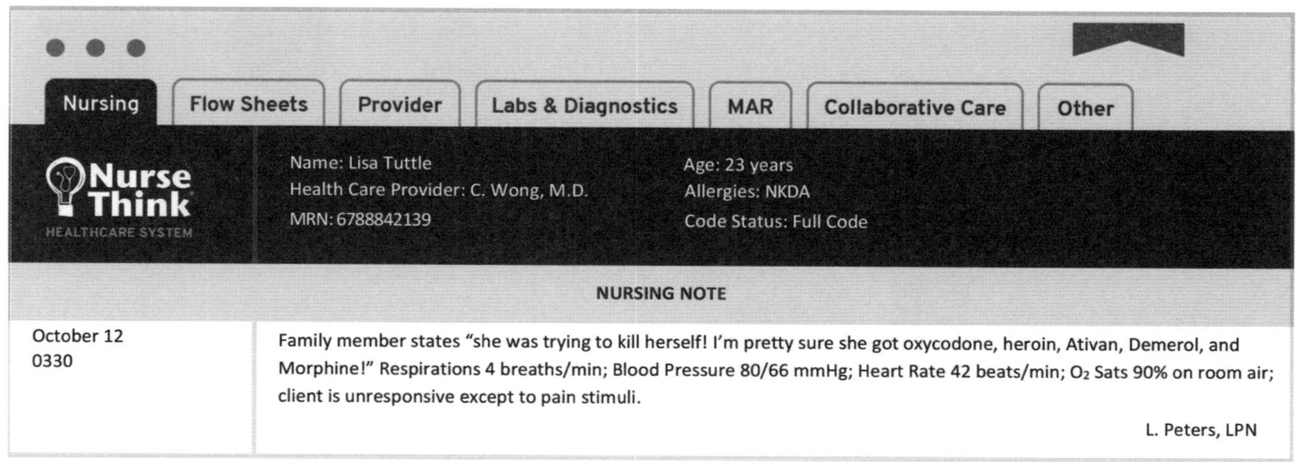

Nursing | Flow Sheets | Provider | Labs & Diagnostics | MAR | Collaborative Care | Other

Nurse Think HEALTHCARE SYSTEM

Name: Lisa Tuttle
Health Care Provider: C. Wong, M.D.
MRN: 6788842139

Age: 23 years
Allergies: NKDA
Code Status: Full Code

NURSING NOTE	
October 12 0330	Family member states "she was trying to kill herself! I'm pretty sure she got oxycodone, heroin, Ativan, Demerol, and Morphine!" Respirations 4 breaths/min; Blood Pressure 80/66 mmHg; Heart Rate 42 beats/min; O_2 Sats 90% on room air; client is unresponsive except to pain stimuli. L. Peters, LPN

a. Heroin.
b. Methadone.
c. Oxycodone.
d. Lorazepam.

11. The nurse reviews education with a pregnant client on the effects of substance abuse on her unborn child. What does the nurse include as an effect of marijuana use?
   a. Withdrawal symptoms.
   b. Chromosomal breakage.
   c. Intrauterine growth restriction (IUGR).
   d. Cleft palate.

12. The nurse reviews the EKG of a client who has overdosed on cocaine. Which strip illustrates the likely effect this overdose has on the client's heart?

a.
ST Elevation Myocardial Infarction (STEMI)

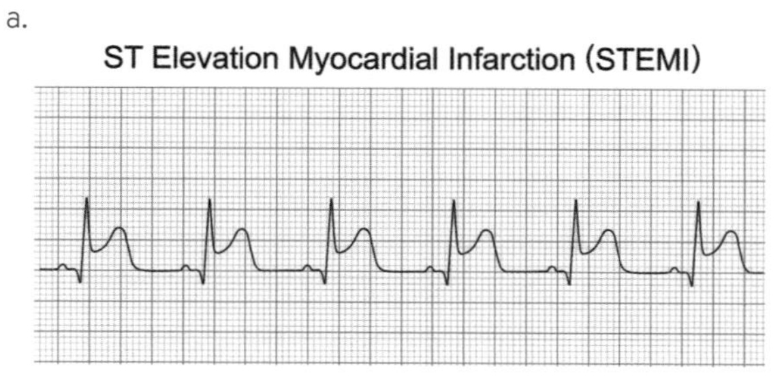

b.
Sinus Bradycardia

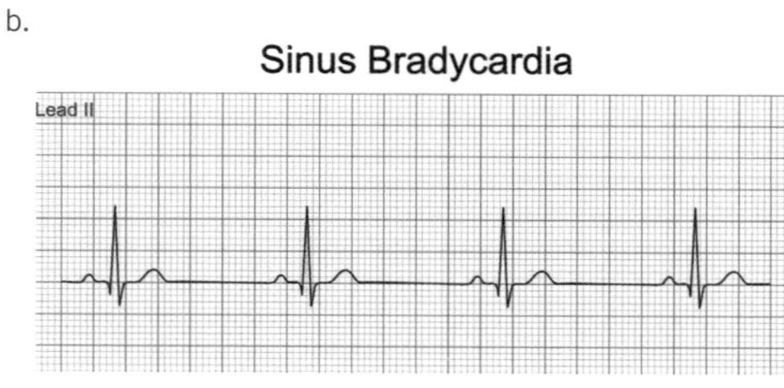

c.
Normal Sinus Rhythm

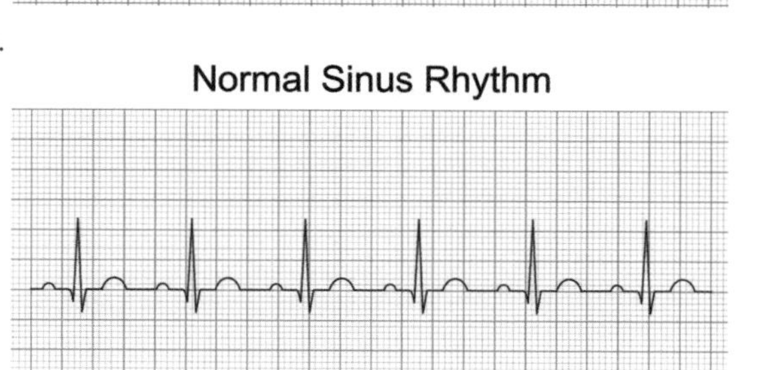

d.
First Degree AV Block

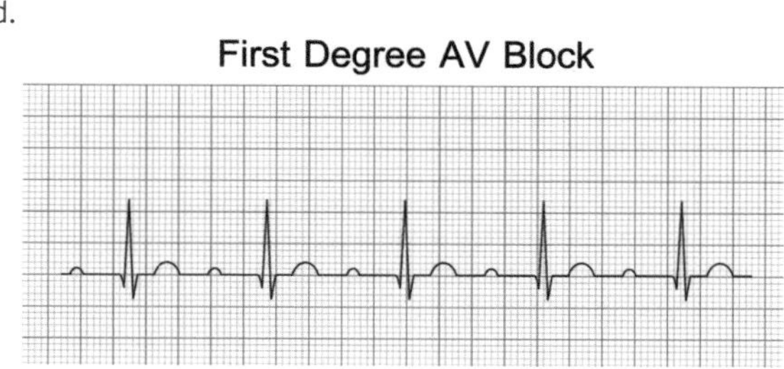

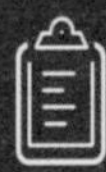

NurseThink® Quiz Questions

13. **Place in order the steps in the continuum of substance addiction. All responses may not be used.**
    a. Tolerance.
    b. Occasional use.
    c. Physical dependence.
    d. Frequent use.
    e. Abusive use.

14. **The nurse cares for the spouse of a recovering alcoholic. What does the nurse expect to find if the spouse is experiencing co-dependency due to their spouse's alcohol abuse? *Select all that apply.***
    a. Overinvolvement with the spouse.
    b. Obsessively trying to control the spouse's behaviors.
    c. Discouraging behavior related to alcohol use.
    d. No desire to get approval from others.
    e. Personal sacrifices to cure the spouse.

15. **The nurse cares for a client withdrawing from alcohol. When does the nurse expect to see the onset of delirium tremens (DTs) if the client experiences them?**
    a. 6-24 hours.
    b. 1-2 days.
    c. 36-48 hours.
    d. 3-5 days.

16. **The nurse cares for a client who has been sexually assaulted. When planning care, which intervention is not included by the nurse?**
    a. Prove rape with evidence.
    b. Provide comfort.
    c. Treat physical injuries.
    d. Empower the client.

17. **The nurse conducts an admission interview with a client who has obsessive-compulsive disorder (OCD). The client is pacing and counting the floor tiles and will not sit down to answer the admission questions. What is the nurse's best response to these actions?**
    a. Tell the client to answer the questions, and then they can continue.
    b. Continue to ask questions while they count the tiles.
    c. Allow them to continue until they are comfortable enough to sit.
    d. Demand they stop or will be physically restrained.

18. **Which shape is most likely to cause increased anxiety in a client with severe obsessive-compulsive disorder (OCD)?**
    a. b.  c. 

19. **When caring for a client with obsessive-compulsive disorder (OCD), what does the nurse expect to be part of the treatment plan? *Select all that apply.***
    a. Selective serotonin reuptake inhibitors.
    b. Antipsychotics.
    c. Cognitive behavior therapy.
    d. Deep brain stimulation.
    e. Benzodiazepines.

20. **The nurse cares for a 9-month-old client with suspected abusive head trauma (AHT) or shaken baby syndrome. Which finding does not support this diagnosis?**
    a. Irritable and hard to comfort.
    b. Difficulty feeding.
    c. Unable to lift head.
    d. Tracking objects with eyes.

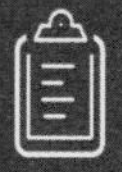

NurseThink® Quiz Answers

1. **The nurse cares for a client with an eating disorder. What treatment is most likely to be used as it is appropriate for all forms of eating disorders?**
   a. Cognitive-based therapy (CBT).
   b. Family therapy.
   c. Antidepressant therapy.
   d. Group therapy.

   Topic/Concept: Adaptation **Subtopic:** Eating disorders **Bloom's Taxonomy:** Applying **Clinical Problem-Solving Process:** Planning **NCLEX-PN®:** Pharmacological Therapies **QSEN:** Patient-centered Care **CJMM:** Generate Solutions

   Rationale: All forms of eating disorders can use antidepressants as a part of their therapy regimen. Family therapy, group therapy, and CBT can be used in one or more eating disorders, but not all types as antidepressants can.

   THIN Thinking: *Top Three* – Anticipation of treatment needs will prepare the nurse to create the treatment plan for their client and understand the desired outcomes.

2. **The nurse collects data for a client with potential bulimia nervosa. Which finding does the nurse correlate with the disorder?**

   Answer: b.

   Topic/Concept: Adaptation **Subtopic:** Eating disorders **Bloom's Taxonomy:** Analyzing **Clinical Problem-Solving Process:** Data Collection **NCLEX-PN®:** Psychosocial Integrity **QSEN:** Evidence-based Practice **CJMM:** Analyze Cues

   Rationale: Bulimia nervosa frequently causes tooth decay as the stomach acid from induced vomiting erodes the teeth. It can weaken muscles and cause cardiac dysrhythmias. Most clients with this illness are harder to diagnose because they are overweight or normal weight and not underweight.

   THIN Thinking: *Clinical Problem-Solving Process* – The nurse must understand that just because a client is a normal weight or overweight does not mean they do not have an eating disorder. Eating disorders need to be recognized and treated to prevent long-term effects, permanent damage, and even death.

3. **The nurse cares for a client with binge-eating disorder. What complications does the nurse attribute to this diagnosis? *Select all that apply.***
   a. Diabetes mellitus II.
   b. Hypotension.
   c. Hyperlipidemia.
   d. Heart disease.
   e. Central sleep apnea.

   Topic/Concept: Adaptation **Subtopic:** Eating disorders **Bloom's Taxonomy:** Analyzing **Clinical Problem-Solving Process:** Data Collection **NCLEX-PN®:** Physiological Adaptation **QSEN:** Evidence-based Practice **CJMM:** Analyze Cues

   Rationale: Due to the extreme weight gained in this illness, the client will exhibit complications related to their obesity or even morbid obesity. They may have hypertension, obstructive sleep apnea, diabetes mellitus type II, hyperlipidemia, and heart disease, among other problems. Central sleep apnea is not related to weight gain and, therefore, not related to this disease.

   THIN Thinking: *Top Three* – The nurse must be careful not to add bias into their data collection. An overweight client can also have an eating disorder and be malnourished just as easily as an underweight one. Both cases require intervention.

4. **The nurse observes a child's legs. Which image does the nurse report as a sign of suspected child abuse?**

   Answer: a.

   Topic/Concept: Adaptation **Subtopic:** Trauma: Abuse **Bloom's Taxonomy:** Applying **Clinical Problem-Solving Process:** Implementation **NCLEX-PN®:** Coordinated Care **QSEN:** Teamwork and Collaboration **CJMM:** Take Action

   Rationale: Patterns of bruising in child abuse can be determined by extent, shape, number, and location. Often, there will be multiple bruises in different stages of healing that resemble objects or finger marks on areas of the body that do not normally get bumped or fallen on. The first image is a large bruise, but it is a single bruise on the knee, which most likely resulted from a bump or fall and does not resemble an object or finger.

   THIN Thinking: *Help Quick* – It is imperative that a nurse recognizes and reports any suspected child abuse to prevent further injury and death of that child as these situations escalate without intervention.

5. **The nurse prepares a presentation on rape prevention for a group of teens. What risk factors for being raped does the nurse include? *Select all that apply.***
   a. Delinquency.
   b. Strong parental relationship.
   c. Low socioeconomic status.
   d. Drug and alcohol use.
   e. Lack of sexual abuse history.

   Topic/Concept: Adaptation **Subtopic:** Trauma: Rape **Bloom's Taxonomy:** Applying **Clinical Problem-Solving Process:** Planning **NCLEX-PN®:** Basic Care and Comfort **QSEN:** Patient-centered Care **CJMM:** Prioritize Hypotheses

Rationale: Poverty, alcohol and drug use, delinquency, history of sexual abuse, and poor child-parent relationships increase the risk of being raped.

THIN Thinking: *Identify Risk to Safety* – Identifying risks and educating on those risks is one way to help prevent issues. A person at risk is more likely to take extra precautions if they understand they are at higher risk of a particular issue.

6. **The nurse cares for a client who was sexually assaulted. What finding suggests the client is in the reorganization phase of rape-trauma syndrome?**
   a. ● They need to talk to resolve their feelings.
   b. They go about life activities superficially.
   c. They experience somatic symptoms.
   d. They are experiencing flashbacks and nightmares.

Topic/Concept: Adaptation **Subtopic:** Trauma: Sexual Assault **Bloom's Taxonomy:** Analyzing **Clinical Problem-Solving Process:** Data Collection **NCLEX-PN®:** Psychosocial Integrity **QSEN:** Patient-centered Care **CJMM:** Recognize Cues

Rationale: During the reorganization phase, clients with rape-trauma syndrome desire to talk to resolve their feelings. In the acute phase, they may experience somatic symptoms and go about life mechanically or superficially. If they do not recover from the event and develop PTSD, they will likely have nightmares and flashbacks.

THIN Thinking: *Clinical Problem-Solving Process* – Understanding the expected healing pattern helps the nurse identify ineffective healing and intervene at the earliest point possible.

7. **The nurse cares for a client during a crisis. What goals does the nurse expect to be included in their plan of care?**
   a. Prepare for hospitalization through the crisis.
   b. Avoid relying on the individual's strengths during the crisis.
   c. ● Cope with immediate stressors to lessen suffering.
   d. Return the individual to a lesser functioning level.

Topic/Concept: Adaptation **Subtopic:** Crisis Intervention **Bloom's Taxonomy:** Applying **Clinical Problem-Solving Process:** Planning **NCLEX-PN®:** Coordinated Care **QSEN:** Teamwork and Collaboration **CJMM:** Generate Solutions

Rationale: When planning for care in a crisis, the nurse should use the individual's strengths and available resources to get through, avoid hospitalization if at all possible, return the individual at or above pre-crisis functioning, and cope with the immediate stressors to lessen suffering.

THIN Thinking: *Clinical Problem-Solving Process* – Any person at any stage in life can experience a personal crisis that disrupts their ability to function. These crises can be different for everyone as each individual has different values and coping mechanisms. It is the nurse's job to meet the client where they are to help them, despite what they feel about what the client deems a crisis in their life.

8. **The nurse plans care for a client experiencing a crisis. What intervention does the nurse prioritize?**
   a. Encourage effective coping strategies.
   b. ● Connect with the client and establish a therapeutic relationship.
   c. Develop a support plan with adequate follow-up.
   d. Explore the client's perception of the crisis.

Topic/Concept: Adaptation **Subtopic:** Crisis Intervention **Bloom's Taxonomy:** Applying **Clinical Problem-Solving Process:** Implementation **NCLEX-PN®:** Reduction of Risk Potential **QSEN:** Evidence-based Practice **CJMM:** Take Action

Rationale: It is important to make a genuine connection while a person is in crisis. Once a therapeutic relationship is established, the client will be more receptive to other nursing interventions.

THIN Thinking: *Help Quick* – The nurse must constantly be aware that a client in crisis is at high risk for self-violence and must quickly identify the need for immediate intervention if this is imminent.

9. **The nurse evaluates the effectiveness of the local community crisis counseling center. What component does the nurse expect to find if the crisis counseling available is appropriately focused?**
   a. Allows survivors to seek out their services.
   b. ● Strengthens existing community support systems.
   c. Conducted in traditional settings.
   d. Functions within established standard hours.

Topic/Concept: Adaptation **Subtopic:** Crisis Intervention **Bloom's Taxonomy:** Analyzing **Clinical Problem-Solving Process:** Evaluation **NCLEX-PN®:** Health Promotion and Maintenance **QSEN:** Patient-centered Care **CJMM:** Evaluate Outcomes

Rationale: A community crisis counseling program should be outreach-oriented, meaning it reaches out and does not wait for survivors to seek out their services. It should supplement and strengthen community support systems. It should be conducted in nontraditional settings like the clients' homes and during off-hours to accommodate participants' lives.

THIN Thinking: *Top Three* – Proper services need to be provided to work with the busy and demanding lives of those who need the services. Mental health is often set as a secondary need over physical health problems. As a result, clients are less likely to prioritize stopping everyday life activities to seek psychological help. More convenient options increase the likelihood that clients will get the help they need.

10. The nurse cares for a client who has overdosed on multiple substances and administers naloxone intravenously to reverse the side effects from the overdose. Based on the reported information, what substance does the nurse report to the provider to obtain an additional prescription to reverse?

a. Heroin.
b. Methadone.
c. Oxycodone.
d. Lorazepam.

Topic/Concept: Adaptation **Subtopic:** Substance abuse **Bloom's Taxonomy:** Applying **Clinical Problem-Solving Process:** Implementation **NCLEX-PN®:** Pharmacological Therapies **QSEN:** Patient-centered Care **CJMM:** Take Action

Rationale: Heroin, methadone, oxycodone, morphine, and meperidine are all opiates that can be reversed with naloxone. Lorazepam is a benzodiazepine that will require the use of flumazenil to reverse.

THIN Thinking: *Help Quick* – It is important to understand the reversal agents for overdosed substances so the nurse can appropriately utilize them in an emergency.

11. The nurse reviews education with a pregnant client on the effects of substance abuse on her unborn child. What does the nurse include as an effect of marijuana use?

a. Withdrawal symptoms.
b. Chromosomal breakage.
c. Intrauterine growth restriction (IUGR).
d. Cleft palate.

Topic/Concept: Adaptation **Subtopic:** Substance abuse **Bloom's Taxonomy:** Applying **Clinical Problem-Solving Process:** Data Collection **NCLEX-PN®:** Pharmacological Therapies **QSEN:** Evidence-based Practice **CJMM:** Recognize Cues

Rationale: Marijuana can cause IUGR. Cleft palate can be from amphetamine use, chromosomal breakage from LSD use, and withdrawal symptoms from multiple other drugs.

THIN Thinking: *Identify Risk to Safety* – The nurse must inform the client not only of the risks to the fetus if they continue to use drugs but to their likelihood of being charged with child abuse if they continue to use while pregnant and harm does come to the child.

12. The nurse reviews the EKG of a client who has overdosed on cocaine. Which strip illustrates the likely effect this overdose has on the client's heart?

Answer: a.

Topic/Concept: Adaptation **Subtopic:** Substance abuse **Bloom's Taxonomy:** Applying **Clinical Problem-Solving Process:** Data Collection **NCLEX-PN®:** Basic Care and Comfort **QSEN:** Evidence-based Practice **CJMM:** Analyze Cues

Rationale: Cocaine is a stimulant that speeds up the heart rate and can cause clamping of the coronary arteries resulting in an AMI and showing elevation in the ST segment.

THIN Thinking: *Top Three* – It is important to understand the effects a drug will have on the body to anticipate the client's needs and complications that could arise and need to be addressed so that the nurse is vigilant in watching for these issues.

13. Place in order the steps in the continuum of substance addiction. All responses may not be used.

a. Tolerance.
b. Occasional use.
c. Physical dependence.
d. Frequent use.
e. Abusive use.

Answer: B, D, E, C–A is not used.

Topic/Concept: Adaptation **Subtopic:** Substance abuse **Bloom's Taxonomy:** Applying **Clinical Problem-Solving Process:** Data Collection **NCLEX-PN®:** Psychosocial Integrity **QSEN:** Patient-centered Care **CJMM:** Recognize Cues

Rationale: Tolerance can build to a substance anywhere on the continuum but is not an actual step in the addiction continuum.

THIN Thinking: *Clinical Problem-Solving Process* – Understanding the stages in a process helps the nurse identify where a client is in that process to determine what level of help that client needs.

14. The nurse cares for the spouse of a recovering alcoholic. What does the nurse expect to find if the spouse is experiencing co-dependency due to their spouse's alcohol abuse? *Select all that apply.*

a. Overinvolvement with the spouse.
b. Obsessively trying to control the spouse's behaviors.
c. Discouraging behavior related to alcohol use.
d. No desire to get approval from others.
e. Personal sacrifices to cure the spouse.

Topic/Concept: Adaptation **Subtopic:** Substance abuse **Bloom's Taxonomy:** Analyzing **Clinical Problem-Solving Process:** Evaluation **NCLEX-PN®:** Psychosocial Integrity **QSEN:** Safety **CJMM:** Evaluate Outcomes

Rationale: A co-dependent person will display overinvolvement with the person, obsession over trying to control their behaviors, enabling behaviors, desire to get approval from others, and personal sacrifices in the hopes of getting the person cured of their problem. Principles of Psychiatric Nursing (10th ed.). St. Louis, Missouri: Elsevier Mosby. Chapter 23)

THIN Thinking: *Top Three* – Co-dependency is a psychiatric illness that can be seen in the significant other or the children of the alcoholic who live in the household and needs to be treated.

15. The nurse cares for a client withdrawing from alcohol. When does the nurse expect to see the onset of delirium tremens (DTs) if the client experiences them?

a. 6-24 hours.
b. 1-2 days.
c. 36-48 hours.
d. 3-5 days.

Topic/Concept: Adaptation **Subtopic:** Substance abuse **Bloom's Taxonomy:** Applying **Clinical Problem-Solving Process:** Data Collection **NCLEX-PN®:** Physiological Adaptation **QSEN:** Patient-centered Care **CJMM:** Recognize Cues

Rationale: DTs is a serious medical emergency expected to occur around 3-5 days after the last consumption of alcohol. Early withdrawal symptoms can be expected in 6-24 hours, peaking at 1-2 days, and hallucinations can be expected between 36-48 hours.

THIN Thinking: *Clinical Problem-Solving Process* – Delirium tremens is a medical emergency that includes disorientation, delusions (usually paranoid), and visual hallucinations. Earlier withdrawal symptoms become much more pronounced, including increased pulse, blood pressure, temperature, and seizures.

16. The nurse cares for a client who has been sexually assaulted. When planning care, which intervention is not included by the nurse?

a. Prove rape with evidence.
b. Provide comfort.
c. Treat physical injuries.
d. Empower the client.

Topic/Concept: Adaptation **Subtopic:** Trauma: Sexual Assault **Bloom's Taxonomy:** Applying **Clinical Problem-Solving Process:** Planning **NCLEX-PN®:** Coordinated Care **QSEN:** Teamwork and Collaboration **CJMM:** Prioritize Hypotheses

Rationale: The nurse will facilitate evidence collection but not be expected to prove rape with evidence. They will also provide comfort, treat physical injuries, treat STDs, empower the client, and discuss resources and a safety plan for them.

THIN Thinking: *Top Three* – Providing comfort and treating injuries are the primary responsibilities of the nurse with an adult victim. Do not force the client to allow for collecting evidence, as this can further traumatize them.

17. The nurse conducts an admission interview with a client who has obsessive-compulsive disorder (OCD). The client is pacing and counting the floor tiles and will not sit down to answer the admission questions. What is the nurse's best response to these actions?

a. Tell the client to answer the questions, and then they can continue.
b. Continue to ask questions while they count the tiles.
c. Allow them to continue until they are comfortable enough to sit.
d. Demand they stop or will be physically restrained.

Topic/Concept: Adaptation **Subtopic:** Obsessive-compulsive disorder (OCD) **Bloom's Taxonomy:** Applying **Clinical Problem-Solving Process:** Implementation **NCLEX-PN®:** Basic Care and Comfort **QSEN:** Evidence-based Practice **CJMM:** Take Action

Rationale: Compulsive behaviors relieve anxieties in clients with OCD. Allowing them to finish these rituals until they relieve their anxiety in a new environment will allow them to relax and be more receptive to being cooperative and answer the admission questions. Forcing them to stop or interrupting them will do nothing but increase their anxiety, lessen compliance, and destroy the nurse-client relationship.

THIN Thinking: *Help Quick* – The nurse has to understand the needs of each psychiatric disease and how to intervene appropriately to ensure effective nurse-client relationships are established.

18. **Which shape is most likely to cause increased anxiety in a client with severe obsessive-compulsive disorder (OCD)?**

Answer: c.

Topic/Concept: Adaptation **Subtopic:** Obsessive-compulsive disorder (OCD) **Bloom's Taxonomy:** Analyzing **Clinical Problem-Solving Process:** Data Collection **NCLEX-PN®:** Psychosocial Integrity **QSEN:** Patient-centered Care **CJMM:** Recognize Cues

Rationale: Asymmetrical shapes are more likely to add to a client's anxiety as most clients with OCD strive to achieve matching and symmetry in design and other things.

THIN Thinking: *Clinical Problem-Solving Process* – Understanding what increases symptoms of OCD will help the nurse avoid these things when caring for specific clients, keeping them calmer.

19. **When caring for a client with obsessive-compulsive disorder (OCD), what does the nurse expect to be part of the treatment plan? *Select all that apply.***
    a. Selective serotonin reuptake inhibitors.
    b. Antipsychotics.
    c. Cognitive behavior therapy.
    d. Deep brain stimulation.
    e. Benzodiazepines.

Topic/Concept: Adaptation **Subtopic:** Obsessive-compulsive disorder (OCD) **Bloom's Taxonomy:** Applying **Clinical Problem-Solving Process:** Planning **NCLEX-PN®:** Pharmacological Therapies **QSEN:** Safety **CJMM:** Generate Solutions

Rationale: SSRIs, antipsychotics, CBT, and deep brain stimulation may be used to treat OCD. Benzodiazepines are usually reserved for severe panic disorders and not anxiety related to OCD.

THIN Thinking: *Clinical Problem-Solving Process* – The nurse should understand potential treatment paths expected to inform and prepare their client for the treatment planned.

20. **The nurse cares for a 9-month-old client with suspected abusive head trauma (AHT) or shaken baby syndrome. Which finding does not support this diagnosis?**
    a. Irritable and hard to comfort.
    b. Difficulty feeding.
    c. Unable to lift head.
    d. Tracking objects with eyes.

Topic/Concept: Adaptation **Subtopic:** Trauma: Abuse (child) **Bloom's Taxonomy:** Applying **Clinical Problem-Solving Process:** Data Collection **NCLEX-PN®:** Basic Care and Comfort **QSEN:** Patient-centered Care **CJMM:** Recognize Cues

Rationale: Infants with abusive head trauma often will not be able to follow objects with their eyes. However, with so many other positive symptoms—unable to lift head, difficulty feeding, and irritability—it's very likely the child is suffering from an injury of this type.

THIN Thinking: *Clinical Problem-Solving Process* – Infants under two years old are at high risk of shaken baby syndrome. It is important to recognize the signs and address them to avoid advancement of their symptoms.

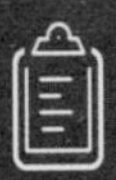

CHAPTER

16

Emotion

Mood / Anxiety / Grief

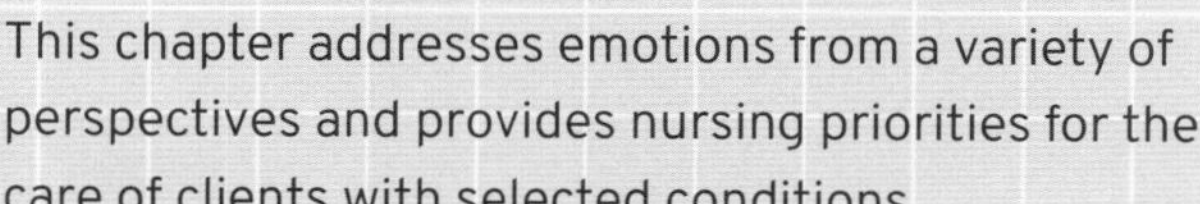

This chapter addresses emotions from a variety of perspectives and provides nursing priorities for the care of clients with selected conditions.

This chapter will review several conditions across the continuum of mental health to illness. No matter where a nurse works they will encounter clients with stress, alterations in emotional health, or persistent/debilitating mental health disorders. The nurse will often confront clients with mental health issues as co-morbidities with physical, social, or interpersonal situations, requiring sensitive and empathic caring. All nurses need to have a working knowledge of and the clinical judgment skills needed to work with clients with mental health alterations. As discussed in Chapter 15, adaptation in response to stress and crisis, the impact of trauma, and enhancing coping are all nursing priorities.

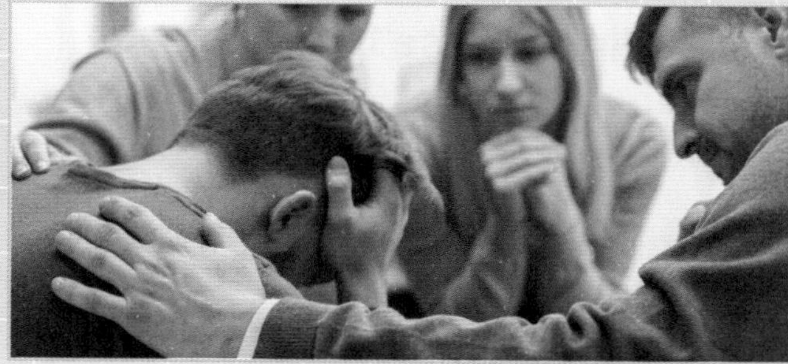

Image 14-1: How might nurses assist clients and families deal with mental health issues, such as those addressed in this chapter?

Priority Exemplars:

- Depression
- Death and dying
- Bereavement
- Anxiety disorders
- Bipolar disorders
- Schizophrenia
- Postpartum depression (PPD)

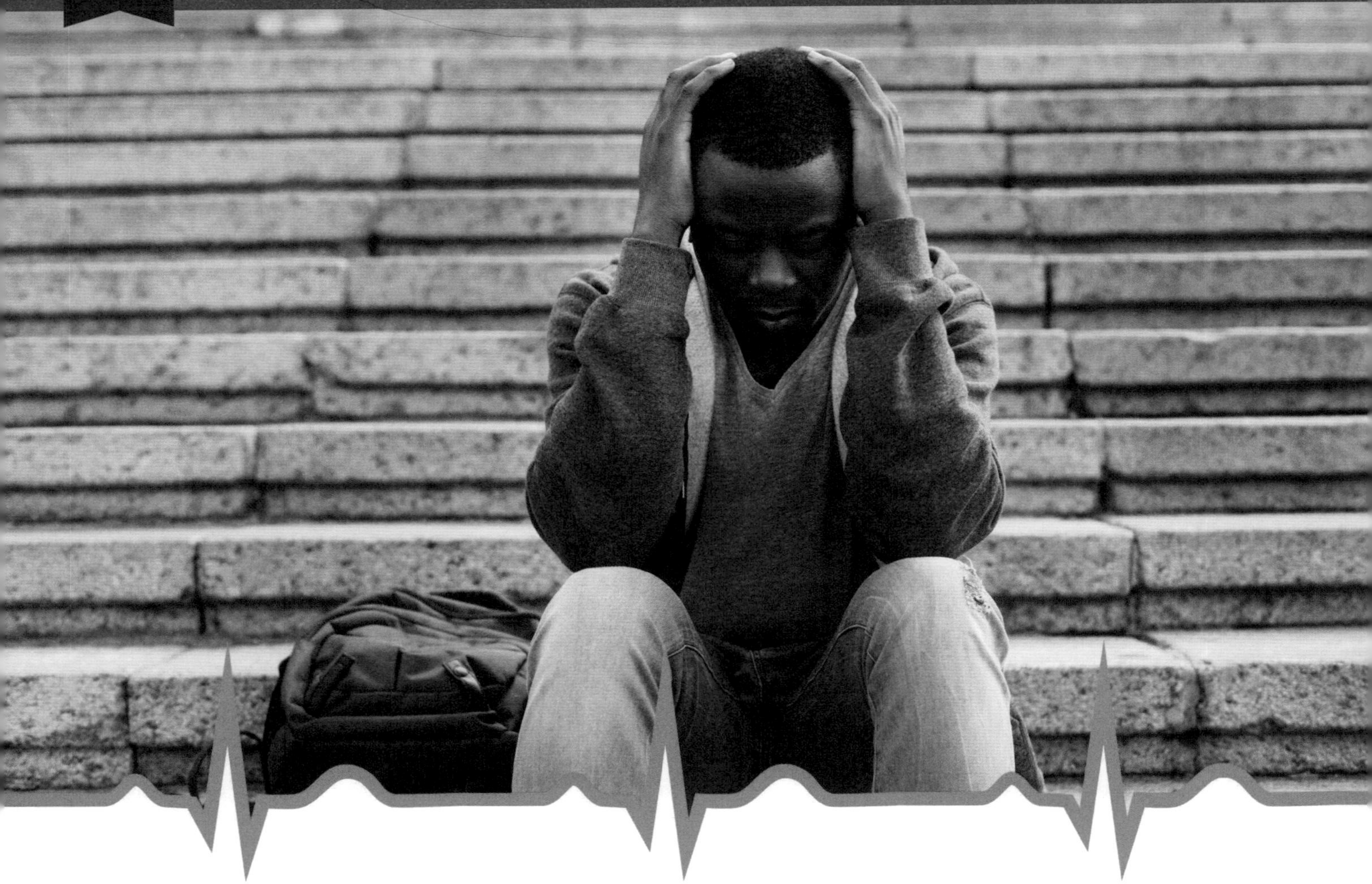

Go To Clinical Case 1

D.B. is a 20-year-old black male student at a university studying engineering. D.B. enters the university counseling center stating, "I am so down all the time. I just can't get out of bed some days. I am really behind on my work. My parents won't even talk to me, much less help me. They don't like that I am gay. They hate my boyfriend, Derek. I've had trouble with depression before, but this is bad. Derek is really worried about me. I'm drinking a lot, and sometimes I go days without a shower. I don't eat much. I've lost a bunch of weight."

D.B. appears disheveled and moves slowly. The nurse notes that his eyes are red and swollen and he seems to have a low level of energy. He appears to put a lot of effort into sharing his history with the nurse. The nurse takes the client's vital signs: 98.6°F (37°C), 88 beats/minutes, 16 breaths/minute, and blood pressure 124/66 mmHg.

NurseThink® Time

Using the NurseThink® system, complete the priorities. Check your answers designated by 💡 in the Depression Priority Exemplar.

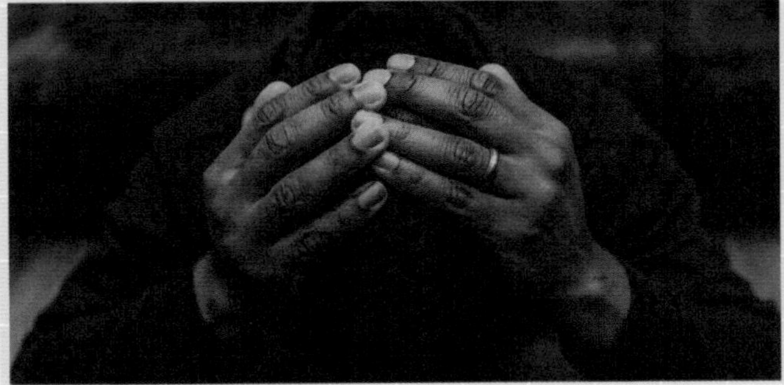

Image 16-2: As you complete NurseThink® Time, consider your own experiences related to stress, mental health issues, coping, and sadness. How do these feelings impact your nursing care of others who are experiencing similar issues?

NurseThink® Time

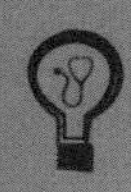

Priority Data Collection or Cues

1.

2.

3.

Priority Laboratory Tests/Diagnostics

1.

2.

3.

Priority Interventions or Actions

1.

2.

3.

Priority Potential & Actual Complications

1.

2.

3.

Priority Nursing Implications

1.

2.

3.

Priority Medications

1.

2.

3.

Reinforcement of Priority Teaching

1.

2.

3.

Depression

Pathophysiology/Description

- Depression is an alteration in mood manifested by sadness, despair, and pessimism
- Characterized as a chronic mood disorder
- Mood is defined as a significant and sustained emotion that impacts a person's perception of the world
- Lifetime prevalence of depression is 17%. Depression is a common psychiatric disorder
- Increasing incidence among adolescents and young adults, especially girls; twice as common in women than men
- May be linked to socioeconomic well-being
- May have seasonal links (research continues)
- Types
  - Major depressive disorder (MDD)
    - Symptomatic for at least two weeks
    - No mania associated
    - Not attributed to substances or medical condition
    - Single episode or recurrent
    - Transient, mild, moderate, or severe symptoms
    - May include anxiety and suicidality
    - May have psychotic or catatonic symptoms with lack of contact with reality
  - Persistent depressive disorder (dysthymia)
    - Less severe than MDD
    - No psychotic symptoms
    - Chronic mood depression and irritability
    - May be early onset (< 21 years) or late onset (> 21 years)
  - Premenstrual dysphoric disorder
    - Depressed mood, anxiety, mood swings and disinterest in activities one week prior to menstruation
    - Decreases/eliminated after menstrual cycle
  - Substance/medication-induced depressive disorder
    - Related to effects of a medication
    - Associated with intoxication/withdrawal
  - Depressive disorder due to another medical condition
  - Postpartum depression
    - Depressed mood after delivery-more significant than minor sadness
    - May have psychotic features
- Causality related to genetic, biochemical, and psychosocial influences

Priority Data Collection or Cues

- Monitor for depressed mood using standardized depression data collection tools, observe for anger, hopelessness, self-negating comments, pessimism, lack of control
- Determine potential risk of suicide including ideations, plan, energy level
- Collect data on client's self-esteem/feelings of hopelessness
- Observe for lack of interest in usual activities, changes in appetite (weight loss or gain), sleep patterns (insomnia or hypersomnia), and cognition (inability to concentrate, confusion, thoughts of death)
- Ask about client's ability or lack of ability to feel pleasure (anhedonia is the lack of ability to feel pleasure)
- Determine level of activity—client may be active or inactive
- Monitor fatigue level—may have decreased energy levels
- Observe hygiene and self-care, depression may decrease attention to self
- Monitoring depression in children
  - Infants/toddlers-feeding problems, lack of play, delays in speech/motor development
  - Preschool children-phobias, aggressiveness, auditory hallucinations
  - School age-vague physical complaints, poor social skills, aggressiveness, worry, poor self-esteem, lack of play
  - Adolescence-anger, aggressiveness, high-risk behaviors, apathy, social withdrawal, sexual acting out, restlessness, substance use
- Monitoring depression in older adults
  - Bereavement overload may compound sadness
  - Memory loss, confusion, or apathy may be manifested as pseudodementia

Priority Laboratory Tests/Diagnostics

- Serum toxicology to determine substance use
- Labs based on physiological needs (hydration/nutrition)

Priority Interventions or Actions

- Individualized psychotherapy, group therapy, family therapy
- Cognitive therapy
  - Designed to assist client to replace negative with positive automatic thoughts
  - Consider realistic potential complications
  - Focus on learning new methods to conceptualize and perceive life tasks
- Electroconvulsive therapy
- Transcranial magnetic stimulation-stimulates nerve cells in the brain
- Light therapy, exercise and activity (endorphin release)
- Medications
- Care for clients at risk for suicide
  - Create a safe environment—observe closely and stay with client as needed
  - Ensure room and surroundings are cleaned of any objects that may be used for self-harm. Constant observation is warranted
  - Determine for risk/lethality/ideations of suicide

- Demonstrate unconditional acceptance
- Allow for expression of feelings such as anger and guilt
- With depression
  - Develop a trusting relationship with an accepting attitude
  - Allow for ventilation of feelings such as anger
  - Provide education on mood and grief
  - Promote feelings of positive self-worth
  - Reassure that crying is healthy and acceptable
  - Provide distraction, physical activity, and outlets for anger and tension
  - Encourage group attendance
  - Promote assertiveness and positive communication
  - Promote realistic goal-setting and decision-making and means for goal attainment

Priority Potential & Actual Complications

- Catatonia, stupor
- Physiological impact of lack of meeting nutritional, sleep, and activity needs
- Suicide

Priority Nursing Implications

- Nurses should be aware of the "black box warning" wherein some antidepressants are associated with increased rates of suicide in young people when first starting medications
- Nurses need to ensure clients' safety when suicide is a concern. Nurses may need to ensure taking of medications (so they are not "stockpiled" for overdose) and by making frequent rounds at irregular times and observe clients closely
- Nurses may need to consider concurrent social and emotional issues in the client's life that may exacerbate depression (poverty, homelessness, gender and sexual identity, estrangement from family, lack of social supports)

Priority Medications

- Amitriptyline–oral administration
  - Tricyclic antidepressant
  - Takes 1-3 weeks to take effect
  - Avoid smoking—increases metabolism
- Fluoxetine–oral administration
  - Selective serotonin reuptake inhibitor (SSRI)-antidepressant
  - May take 2-3 weeks to work
  - Take in morning to avoid insomnia
- Phenelzine–oral administration
  - Monoamine oxidase inhibitor (MAOI), antidepressant
  - Large number of food interactions which could lead to hypertensive crisis
  - Later agent to be used-if depression refractory to other treatments
- Bupropion–oral administration
  - Atypical antidepressant
  - May decrease seizure threshold
  - Should not "double-up" doses if a dose is missed
  - Also used for smoking cessation
- Duloxetine–oral administration
  - Serotonin-norepinephrine reuptake inhibitor, antidepressant
  - May cause orthostatic hypotension
  - May cause sweating and constipation

Reinforcement of Priority Teaching

- Community resources including support groups, mental health clinics, crisis intervention
- Adherence to medication regimens
- Family education and support
- Awareness of client's risk for suicide, potential signs of suicidality, means to keep client safe, and emergency procedures

Next Gen Clinical Judgment

A nurse cares for a client in a group home who has major depression and is treated with an MAO inhibitor. The nurse implements a nutrition plan including the dietary restrictions associated with these medications.

1. What types of foods are restricted?
2. What types of foods are allowed?
3. What types of snacks could you suggest to have on hand to ensure adherence to these dietary restrictions?
4. What consequences may occur if the client does not comply with these restrictions?
5. How can this plan of care be communicated with the providers at the group home?

Go To Clinical Answers

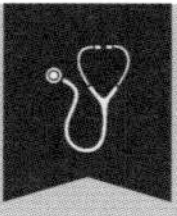

Text designated by [icon] are the top answers for the Go To Clinical related Depression.

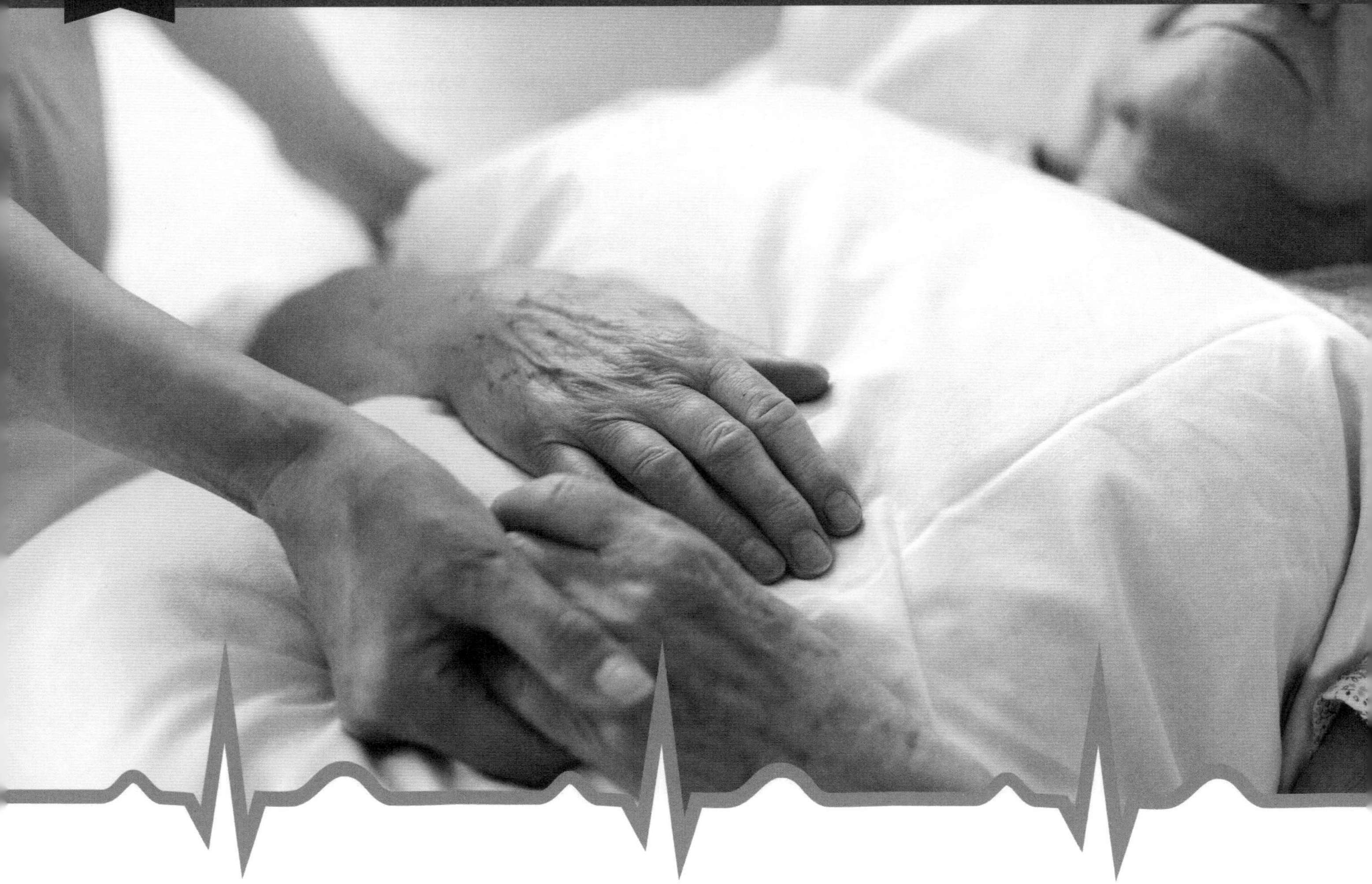

Go To Clinical

Go To Clinical Case 2

M.O. is a 98-year-old woman in a skilled nursing facility. M.O. was treated in an acute care setting three weeks ago for pneumonia, confusion, dehydration, and a urinary tract infection. Since returning to the skilled nursing facility, M.O. has been too weak to get out of bed or provide any self-care. She refuses to eat or drink, is incontinent, and slips in and out of consciousness. M.O.'s advanced directives indicate no heroic measures and her daughter is her durable power of attorney. The nurse notes these vital signs: 97°F (36.1°C), 124 beats/minute, 12 breaths/minute and irregular, and blood pressure 92/40 mmHg.

The client sometimes becomes agitated and restless. When she opens her eyes, she appears fearful and unable to focus. When she closes her eyes, the client groans with labored respirations.

M.O. is placed in hospice care; a hospice registered nurse visits to provide her morphine by mouth and to change the fentanyl patch. The client's daughter is at the bedside. The priest is called to provide Last Rights. The nurse notes that M.O.'s respiratory rate becomes slower, and the client's respirations sound "wet." M.O.'s skin becomes pale and cool. The nurse stays in the room as needed while other family members arrive. The nurse respects the client's and family's privacy and provides support as needed. The nurse notes that the client's respiratory rate has decreased to 2-4 breaths/minute and leaves the room to contact the nursing supervisor.

NurseThink® Time

Using the NurseThink® system, complete the priorities. Check your answers designated by in the Death and dying Priority Exemplar.

NurseThink® Time

Priority Data Collection or Cues

1.

2.

3.

Priority Laboratory Tests/Diagnostics

1.

2.

3.

Priority Interventions or Actions

1.

2.

3.

Priority Potential & Actual Complications

1.

2.

3.

Priority Nursing Implications

1.

2.

3.

Priority Medications

1.

2.

3.

Reinforcement of Priority Teaching

1.

2.

3.

Death and dying

Pathophysiology/Description

- There is specific care revolving around the dying process
- Also known as end-of-life care

Priority Data Collection or Cues

- Determine client's religious and spiritual preferences
- Ask about client's end-of-life wishes and advanced directive
- Consider other legal and ethical issues, including withdrawal of treatment, organ and tissue donation, legal documentation, cardiopulmonary resuscitation
- Monitor the physiological status of the client near death
  - Slowing of metabolism until organ function ceases
  - Decreases in sensory function such as changes in vision, taste, smell, pain, touch, loss of blinking/staring (hearing preserved until late in the process)
  - Respirations become shallow and irregular, with tachypnea or bradypnea, may develop audible crackles or wet sounds ("death rattle") or Cheyne-Stokes breathing (alternating deep and rapid breathing)
  - Skin may become cool and waxy, extremities become cool, pale, mottled, and cyanotic
  - Urine output decreases and client may be incontinent
  - Peristalsis slows leading to constipation and distension, client may be incontinent
  - Client moves less with depressed gag and swallow reflexes
  - Death occurs as organs fail, cardiac/respiratory arrest
  - Brain death occurs when the cerebral cortex ceases function/damage is irreparable
- Monitor clients frequently for status, need for comfort measures and need to notify or support family/others

Priority Interventions or Actions

- Encourage clients to have an advanced directive, including a living will and durable power of attorney
- Referral to hospice
  - Provides palliative and supportive care where focus is on comfort, rather than cure
  - Ensure the optimum pain management
  - The team of nurses, health care providers, social workers, and chaplains ensure comfort and symptom control
  - Encourage client and family to be involved in care as able
  - May be in the home, part of a hospital, or at a specific hospice center
  - Emotional support and respite care as needed
- Provide physical care
  - Provide pain management and hygiene measures, including oral care
  - Elevate the head of the bed, suction as needed, and provide oxygen
  - Provide rest as needed
  - Allow or restrict visitors to meet the needs of the client
  - Provide anti-emetics as needed
  - Offer small quantities of favorite foods or beverages
- Provide emotional care
  - Allow for privacy of client and family
  - Provide support and advocacy
  - Encourage family to communicate with client as able, using verbalizations and touch to relate with client
  - Encourage client and family to discuss fears at end-of-life, including pain, loneliness, and remorse
- Postmortem procedures
  - Close client's eyes, replace dentures (as needed), remove IV tubing, catheters, and dressings (check hospital policy and if autopsy is to be performed)
  - Wash client and redress (check policy and if autopsy is to be performed)
  - Place pads under client, place a pillow under head, and position client for family viewing
  - When transporting to the morgue, follow agency policy and ensure client identification, cover or use special bed for transport

Priority Nursing Implications

- Ensure that the client's dignity is preserved and family is respected
- Consider cultural practices, laws, and hospital policy when rendering postmortem care
- Provide privacy for family to spend time with the client after death
- Consider the nurse's own need for support when caring for dying clients

Priority Medications

- Morphine
  - Analgesic
  - End-of-life pain management
  - May slow respirations
  - May be given intravenously or orally
- Fentanyl
  - For severe, ongoing pain
  - Dose titrated to ensure safe pain relief
  - Patch provides sustained-release pain management
  - May also be given via buccal, nasal, and sublingual membranes
- Oral lubricant solution or spray
  - Available over-the-counter
  - Relieves dry mouth

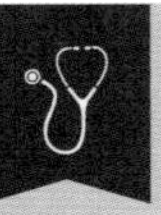

Go To Clinical Answers

Text designated by are the top answers for the Go To Clinical related Death and dying.

Pathophysiology/Description

- Bereavement is the human response characterized by grief and/or sadness in response to a loss
- Characterized by loss (when something of value is taken away) and grief (emotional grief subsequent to a loss)
- The real or perceived loss may be a person, pet, occupation, partner, health status or function, developmental milestone or crisis, or possession
- Anticipatory grief
  - Feeling grief before the loss
  - May lead to detachment prior to the loss
- Stages of grief
  - Kubler Ross
    - Denial
    - Anger
    - Bargaining
    - Depression
    - Acceptance
  - Worden
    - Accepting the reality of the loss
    - Processing the pain of grief
    - Adjusting to the world without the lost entity
    - Finding an enduring connection with the lost entity while resuming or finding a new life
  - Bowlby
    - Numbness/protest
    - Disequilibrium
    - Disorganization and despair
    - Reorganization
- Length of grief
  - Varies with the individual and the closeness of the individual that is lost
  - Acute grief period-6-8 weeks, may continue for a year or more
  - Nurses need to be sensitive to the individual response to loss and to the unique experiences of grieving

Priority Data Collection or Cues

- Determine client's developmental level. Grief responses vary based on developmental age, the client's understanding of death and permanence, and capacity of the client to cope with stressors and loss
- Monitor for financial or personal implications of the loss, coping skills, history of mental illness or substance abuse, history of trauma, number of previous losses, role of individual in the client's life
- Consider cultural and spiritual variables impacting the bereavement experience
- Observe client's stage of grief and risk factors associated with unresolved or maladaptive grieving

Priority Interventions or Actions

- Develop trust and show empathy
- Encourage discussion about the loss when appropriate—allow client to ventilate
- Help client identify emotions such as guilt, anger, anxiety, helplessness, bitterness
- Provide support and encouragement as appropriate
- Reassure the client and reinforce positive coping and periods of grief
- Examine previous coping or spiritual strategies used in the past to cope with loss
- Contact a spiritual leader as requested
- Provide referrals to local and other resources for counseling, support, and family assistance to address unresolved or maladaptive grief

Priority Potential & Actual Complications

- Delayed or inhibited grief
- Distorted or exaggerated grief
- Chronic or prolonged grief; unresolved grieving
- Maladaptive grieving/loss of self-esteem
- Clinical depression characterized by disturbed self-esteem, anhedonia, hopelessness, guilt, and dysphoria
- Suicidal ideations

Priority Nursing Implications

- Nurses may provide the role of listener and support person in the bereavement process
- Hospice services may provide support for the bereaved family or others in addition to the dying client. The interdisciplinary team focuses on client and family physical and emotional needs, especially pain and symptom management
- Stages of grief provide the nurse and client some structure and comfort as this process proceeds
- Nurses need to be aware of the individual, cultural, and spiritual dimensions of bereavement, along with the developmental factors impacting the grief response
- Nurses should examine their own belief system, reflect on their emotions, and be offered respite to ensure they can provide support to families

Reinforcement of Priority Teaching

- Have an advanced directive, including a living will and durable power of attorney
- Availability of resources to support the grief process

Anxiety disorders

Pathophysiology/Description

- Anxiety is the subjective response to stress
- Feelings of dread, impending doom, apprehension, fear, or discomfort which may or may not be associated with real stressors, may be out of proportion with stressor, and impairs functioning in social and work contexts
- Fear is the cognitive response to a threat, anxiety is the emotional response
- Most common of all psychiatric illnesses
- Twice as common in women than men; prevalence of 18% in adults; 25% in children
- Often exist with co-morbidities of depression, substance abuse, or other disorders
- Attributed to biological, genetic, cognitive, and psychological causative factors
- Types
  - Panic disorder
    - Sudden feelings of doom and physical symptoms
    - Are not triggered by a specific stressor or situation
    - Onset in early 20s
    - Variable frequency and severity
  - Generalized anxiety disorder
    - Unrealistic, persistent, and excessive worry and anxiety
    - Occur more days than not for duration of at least 6 months
    - Impaired social and occupational functioning
    - Onset may occur in childhood or adolescence, but also in the 20s
  - Phobias
    - Persistent, exaggerated, irrational, and intense fear of a situation, object, or activity
    - Agoraphobia is the fear of open spaces causing confinement to home environment
    - Social anxiety disorder is the fear that one might do something embarrassing or be negatively evaluated by others. May be specific to public speaking or performance or more vague and non-specific
    - Other phobias include fear of heights, snakes, dogs, strangers, homosexuals, spiders
    - Onset in the 20s and 30s
  - Obsessive-compulsive disorder (see Priority Exemplar)
  - Body dysmorphic disorder-exaggerated belief that the body is deformed
  - Trichotillomania is a hair pulling disorder
  - Hoarding disorder is the difficulty discarding or excessive acquisition of objects, regardless of value
- Client may hyperventilate and become lightheaded, short of breath, tachycardic, faint, or experience numbness/tingling of hands and feet

Priority Data Collection or Cues

- Consider use of standardized anxiety scales
- Observe for symptoms/signs of panic disorder including palpitations, tachycardia, diaphoresis, anxious expression, trembling, chest pain or pressure, nausea or vomiting, dizziness, chills, hot flashes, feelings of choking, shortness of breath, abdominal pain, feeling unsteady, paresthesias, depersonalization, feeling of losing control, or fear of dying
- Monitor for signs and symptoms of generalized anxiety disorder including muscle tension, restlessness, "feeling on edge," avoiding social events or activities, procrastination, or excessive worry. Manifestations may or may not have a trigger event or stressor
- Collect data on symptoms/signs of phobias including anxious response to a stressful object, activity, or situation including panic symptoms, sweating, tachycardia, and dyspnea
- Ask client about feelings of powerlessness such as feeling lack of control, expressions of doubt about personal capacity, withdrawal from decision-making or anxiety-producing situations, ritualistic behavior, preoccupation with the feared object

Priority Interventions or Actions

- Support client in therapies: Individual, cognitive, behavioral along with medications
- To address chronic anxiety
  - Explore client's perceptions of threat
  - Assist client to examine those factors that can and cannot be changed
  - Explore selected coping and stress-management strategies
  - Encourage independence and decision-making as able
  - Provide structured activity and distractions
  - Discuss replacing behaviors and thoughts with constructive thoughts and coping mechanisms
  - With phobias and specific anxieties--Consider use of controlled systematic desensitization (gradual exposure to stimuli) or implosion therapy (flooding with stimuli)
  - Allow for exploration, discussion, and reflection on thoughts and feelings
- During acute episode
  - Stay with client—do not leave alone when in a panic or highly anxious
  - Maintain a calm demeanor
  - Use brief messages—stay calm and describe agency routines
  - Manage hyperventilation, ask the client to take several breaths in a paper bag, then take slow deep abdominal breaths, repeat as needed
  - Decrease environmental stimuli
  - Use sedation as needed

- Once "attack" has subsided, explore sources of anxiety
- Assist client to identify triggers or early onset of anxiety and how to deal with these using deep breathing, imagery, prayer, meditation, or exercise

Priority Potential & Actual Complications

- Lack of social and occupational functioning
- Total social withdrawal
- Inability to meet personal daily needs

Priority Nursing Implications

- Anxiety is contagious. Nurses have a role to maintain calm when clients are escalating
- Deceleration techniques may be effective in addressing rising anxiety

Priority Medications

- Buspirone–oral administration
  - Anti-anxiety agent
  - Takes 10-14 days to be effective (not for PRN use)
  - Does not cause dependence or tolerance
  - Interacts with alcohol
- Lorazepam–oral administration, IV or IM
  - Benzodiazepine, calming agent
  - Client may become physically dependent and tolerant
  - Withdrawal if abruptly withdrawn
- Alprazolam–oral administration
  - Benzodiazepine, calming agent
  - Client may become physically dependent and tolerant
  - Withdrawal if abruptly withdrawn
- Imipramine–oral administration, IM injection
  - Tricyclic antidepressant
  - Higher doses needed to address panic with increased side effects

Reinforcement of Priority Teaching

- Healing is a long process and there may be times of regression
- Maintain therapy and medication regimen
- Most anti-anxiety agents cause sedation and orthostatic hypotension
- Community supports to deal with anxiety disorders
- Means to deal with signs and symptoms

Next Gen Clinical Judgment

A client who previously presented to the mental health clinic dirty and disheveled now appears neatly dressed and clean. What conclusions can you draw from these observations?

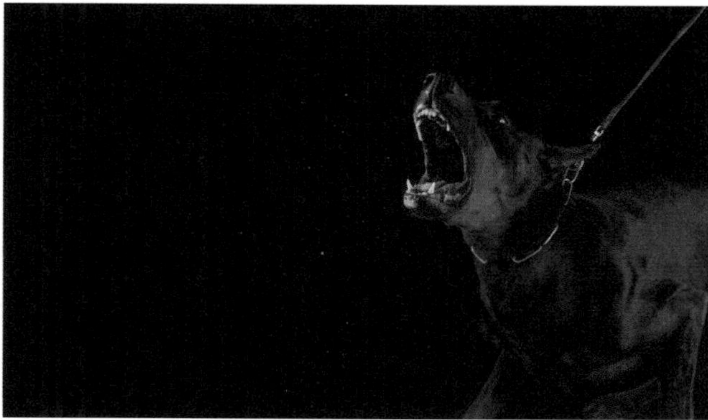

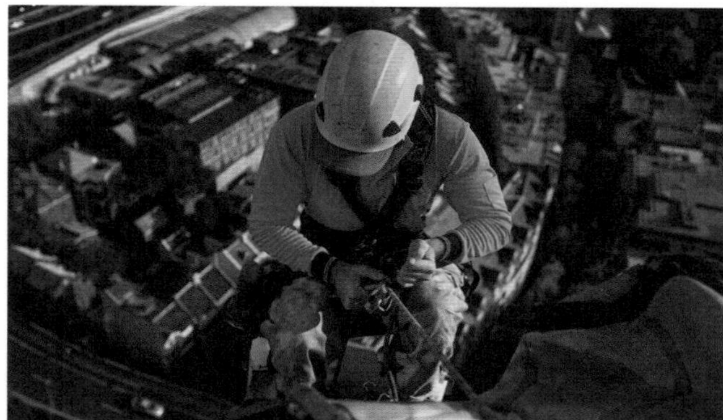

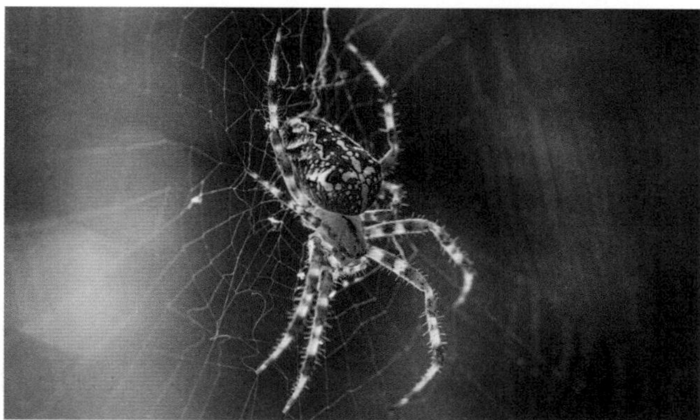

Image 16-3: Clients with phobias often fear the objects in these images. Compare and contrast the use of cognitive behavioral therapy, controlled systematic desensitization, and implosion therapy to treat these phobias. What advice would you provide to a client who suffers from phobias?

Pathophysiology/Description

- Characterized as a chronic mood disorder. Mood is defined as a significant and sustained emotion that impacts a person's perception of the world
- Affect is the external appearance of the emotional experience
- Bipolar disorders are manifested with cycles of depression and mania (elation in mood including exaggerated and risk-laden behaviors)
- Impacts about 2.6% of the US population. 83% are profoundly impacted. Impacts men and women equally, average onset is at 25 years
- Often misdiagnosed or undiagnosed
- Types
  - Bipolar I (major depression with mania)
  - Bipolar II (major depression with hypomania)
  - Cyclothymic disorder (mood cycling including less severe levels of depression and elevated mood not quite as significant as hypomania)
  - Substance/medication-induced bipolar disorder (directly caused by drugs during intoxication or withdrawal; or reaction to other medications such as steroids)
  - Bipolar disorder due to medical condition (electrolyte imbalance, brain tumor)
  - Disruptive mood dysregulation disorder is mainly a syndrome associated with childhood, manifested by irritability, temper tantrums, and mood swings
- Causation attributed to hereditary, genetic, and physiological (neurotransmitter/neuroanatomical) elements along with stress/trauma factors in the client's life or environment
- May occur in children and adults
- Comorbidity with attention-deficit/hyperactivity disorder(ADHD) in children (see ADHD Priority Exemplar)

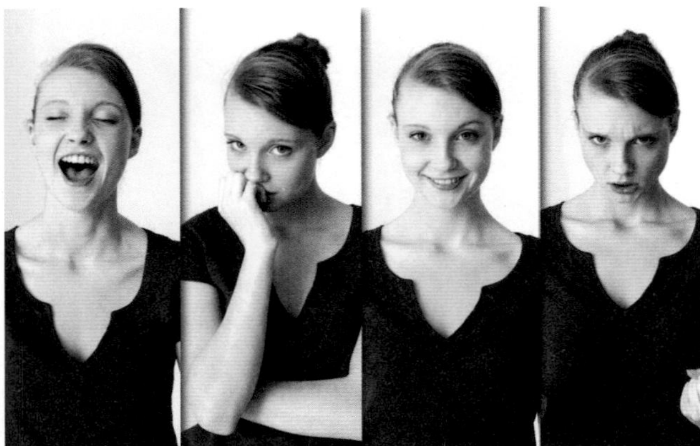

Image 16-4: Consider the strain bipolar disorder places on clients, their families, their partner/significant other, etc. How can nurses assist to reduce this stress?

Priority Data Collection or Cues

- Monitor for signs and symptoms of depression (see Depression Priority Exemplar)
- Observe for symptoms of mania including elation, inflated self-esteem, grandiosity, hyperactivity, agitation, racing thoughts/flight of ideas, distractibility, accelerated/forced speech, engagement in high-risk behaviors (substance use, promiscuity/exaggerated sexual behaviors, excessive shopping, gambling, investing), irritability, frenzied motor activity, decreased need for sleep, rapid mood swings, lack of hygiene/self-care
- Ask about impact on social and work life; to be considered mania it must have a significant impact on life functioning
- Observe for hypomania-behaviors similar to those above but not so severe as to cause significant social or work dysfunction, may begin as cheerful but devolve to irritability and volatility, may experience weight loss, engage in inappropriate and high-risk behaviors
- Collect data about delusions (false fixed beliefs) and hallucinations (distorted sensory experiences)
- Monitor for substance use

Priority Laboratory Tests/Diagnostics

- Electrolyte levels
- Drug and toxicology screens

Priority Interventions or Actions

- Medications including monotherapy with mood stabilizers
- Second-generation antipsychotics
- Psychoeducational focused family therapy concerning early warning signs and management
- Individual or group therapy (self-help or support groups) and cognitive therapy
- Electroconvulsive therapy
- Client management during acute episodes
  - Decrease external stimuli such as lights, noise
  - Remove dangerous objects
  - Check on client frequently/stay with client during increased agitation
  - Provide activities and distraction when feasible
  - Intervene as mood becomes anxious or agitated
  - Maintain calm attitude/set limits on manipulation and reinforce non-manipulative behaviors
  - Use a team approach to calm client including deceleration, medications, mechanical restraints
  - Implement gradual removal of client restraints as situation warrants

Priority Potential & Actual Complications

- Negative events related to poor decision-making/high-risk behaviors
- Physical exhaustion and life-threatening malnutrition
- Delirious mania may lead to intensified symptoms that threaten safety of self and others
- Confused thinking and stupor

Priority Nursing Implications

- Nurses need to work with dietician to ensure adequate calories such as use finger foods, high calorie shakes during acute episodes—maintain I & O, calorie counts
- During manic periods clients often feel powerful and capable. Clients may decide to not take medications, leading to exacerbations
- Nurses may need to assist in facilitating restful sleep

Priority Medications

- Lithium carbonate–oral administration, at times, IM
  - Mood stabilizer
  - Effective in about 1/3 of clients
  - Ensure adequate sodium and water intake
  - Cautious use of diuretics
  - Monitor serum levels (0.6-1.2 mEq/L)
- Valproic acid–oral administration, also IV
  - Anticonvulsant used to stabilize moods
  - May cause sedation
  - Cannot be discontinued abruptly
  - Avoid alcohol
  - May increase suicidal thoughts and behaviors
- Lamotrigine–oral administration, less commonly IV
  - Antiepileptic that is also a mood stabilizer-manages depression without inducing mania
  - Common side effects include dizziness, headache, and double vision

Reinforcement of Priority Teaching

- Avoid caffeine in diet to foster sleep
- Strict adherence with medication schedule
- Regular blood draws to monitor serum levels
- The need for therapy, in addition to medications, to manage chronic and acute elements of disorder

Next Gen Clinical Judgment

A client with bipolar disorder is prescribed lithium carbonate. List 5-7 elements that need to be included in the client's instructions to ensure safe medication administration, monitoring, minimizing side effects, and maximum therapeutic effect.

Bipolar Disorder Symptoms Includes

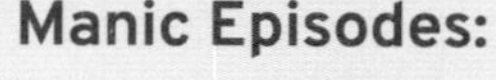
Manic Episodes:

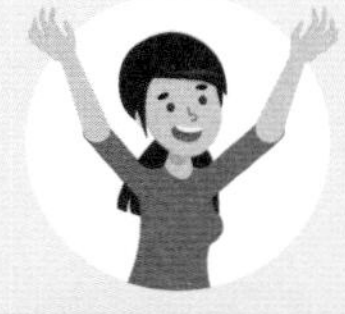
FEELING OVERLY HAPPY FOR LONG PERIODS OF TIME

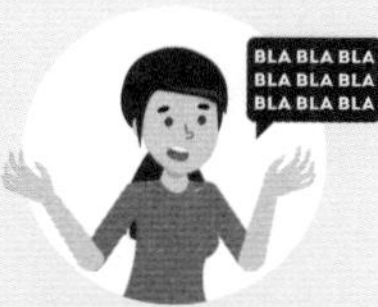

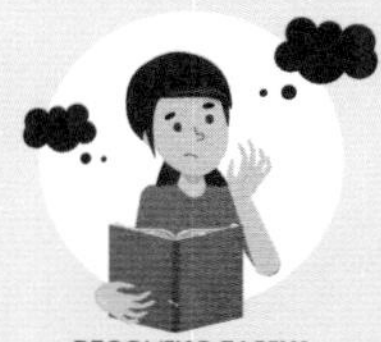
BECOMING EASILY DISTRACTED

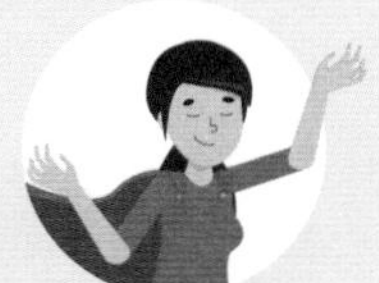
HAVING OVERCONFIDENCE IN ABILITIES

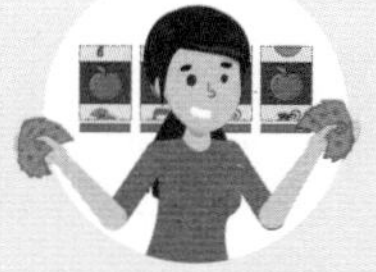
ENGAGING IN RISKY BEHAVIOR (E.G. GAMBLING)

Depression Episodes:

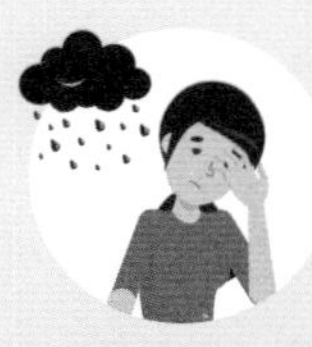
FEELING SAD OR HOPELESS FOR LONG PERIODS OF TIME

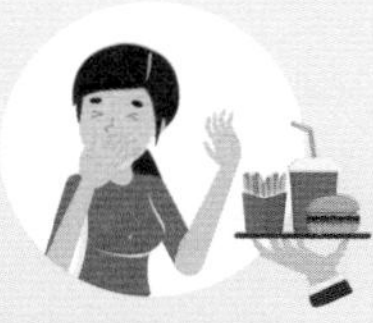
SIGNIFICANT CHANGE IN APPETITE

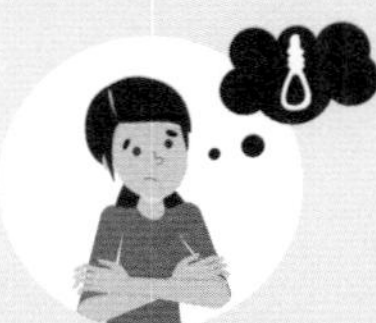
THINKING ABOUT OR ATTEMPTING SUICIDE

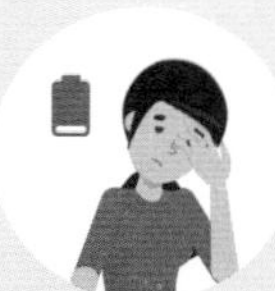
FEELING FATIGUE OR LACK OF ENERGY

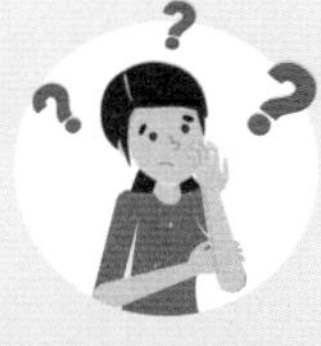
PROBLEMS WITH MEMORY AND CONCENTRATION

Image 16-5: Bipolar signs and symptoms. Name two nursing actions to address or alleviate each sign and/or symptom.

Schizophrenia

Pathophysiology/Description

- Known as a spectrum of disorders with a variety of etiological factors (biological, psychological, and environmental) and a wide variety of treatments that must be tailored to the individual and their symptoms
- Suicide is highly prevalent–1/3rd of clients have suicidal ideations, 10% die from suicide
- Affects about 1% of the Population
- Early onset begins in childhood, but generally begins during late adolescence and early adulthood
- Progressive disease with exacerbations and chronic course
- Phases of Schizophrenia
  - Premorbid
  - Prodromal
  - Active Psychotic/Acute schizophrenic episode
  - Residual
- Other psychotic disorders
  - Delusional disorders-clients have false, fixed beliefs without bizarre behaviors
    - Erotomaniac type-believes high status people are in love with them
    - Grandiose type–delusions of grand status, personal worth, and talents
    - Jealous type-perseverating that sexual partner is unfaithful
    - Persecutory-belief that one is being treated badly
    - Somatic type-false fixed beliefs about a medical condition
  - Brief psychotic disorder
    - Sudden onset of psychotic symptoms, including catatonia
  - Substance/medication-induced psychotic disorder
  - Psychotic disorders due to medical condition
  - Catatonic disorders due to a medical condition
  - Schizophreniform disorder-psychotic behaviors of short duration
  - Schizoaffective disorder-schizophrenic behaviors along with signs of depression and/or mania

Priority Data Collection or Cues

- Determine risk of suicide
- Monitor for symptoms of schizophrenia:
  - Positive symptoms
    - Delusions (false, fixed beliefs)
    - Hallucinations (distorted sensory perceptions)
    - Disorganized speech-echolalia (echoing previous word), incoherence, neologisms (new language), loose associations (speech or topics do not make sense)
    - Disorganized behavior-hyperactivity, hostility, agitation
  - Negative symptoms
    - Lack of speech/lack of intonation of speech/lack of gesturing
    - Withdrawal
    - Lack of ability to move or initiate activity
    - Blunted affect
    - Poor hygiene and lack of ADLs
- Obtain history from client, family, and others in the client's world to determine progression of symptoms
- Observe for: waxy flexibility (body stays in position and does not move after positioning), posturing, pacing and rocking, regression, eye movement abnormalities

Priority Interventions or Actions

- General
  - Pharmacotherapy with psychotherapy
  - Strategies that foster social skills, activities of daily living, and rehabilitation
  - Individual psychotherapy, group therapy, family therapy, assertive community therapy (team creates community experiences to regain skills), and behavioral therapy
- Suicide prevention strategies/Dealing with aggression
  - Observation of client at frequent, irregular intervals
  - Maintain a low-stimulus environment
  - Support client during agitated periods with additional staff and restraint as necessary
  - Initiate suicide precautions
    - Provide one-on-one supervision
    - No harmful objects/tell visitors no harmful objects
    - Observe for ideations of plan
    - Develop a no-suicide contract
- During hallucinations
  - Listen attentively and observe for hallucination behaviors
  - Avoid touch but convey an attitude of acceptance
  - Do not reinforce the client's perceptions-state you do not see, hear, and use words "the voices" to decrease credibility, etc.
  - Try to distract, listen to music/television, and engage in activities
  - Use "reasonable doubt" technique to relay lack of belief in hallucinations – "I don't believe this can be happening."
  - Assist client to see association between stress and hallucinations (I know you believe you see/hear them, but I do not. I know this is a very stressful time for you.)
  - Advise clients to use voice dismissal where they verbally tell the voice to go away

- Enhance relationships
  - Promote trust and avoid physical contact
  - Avoid talking or laughing around clients because they may suspect it is about them
  - Maintain an assertive, matter-of-fact means of dealing with the client
  - Encourage consistent caregivers
  - Orient client to surroundings
  - Use concrete communication techniques
- Physical priorities
  - Attempt to meet client needs if they are non-verbal and unable to do so on their own
  - Assist client with self-care needs and encourage hygiene
  - Develop a toileting schedule, as needed
  - Encourage independence and decision-making as able
  - Provide canned, packaged, or home foods if the client is suspicious of foods (client may also suspect foods from home)

Priority Potential & Actual Complications

- Total withdrawal from/lack of participation in society
- Suicide

Priority Nursing Implications

- Nurses need to be vigilant for clients who may be suicidal or at risk for self-harm
- Schizophrenia is associated with longer hospitalizations, higher costs, and greatest disruptions to family and personal life than any other mental health condition
- Evaluate and treat for extrapyramidal symptoms (EPS)
- Treatment for EPS may include changing the psychotropic medication, reducing the dose, or adding an anticholinergic agent (benztropine, diphenhydramine)

Priority Medications

- Chlorpromazine–oral, IV, IM
  - Phenothiazine antipsychotic
  - Leading antipsychotic medication
  - Watch for extrapyramidal symptoms
  - Monitor for gynecomastia and sedation
  - Watch for anticholinergic effects
- Risperidone–oral and IM administration
  - Atypical antipsychotic
  - Determine client's history—decreases seizure threshold
  - Encourage water or hard candy to alleviate dry mouth
  - May cause nausea and vomiting
- Clozapine–oral, IV, IM
  - Atypical antipsychotic
  - Need to have weekly blood levels monitored
  - Check for allergic reaction
  - May lead to weight gain
- Benztropine/diphenhydramine–generally oral, may be injected IM or IV in select circumstances
  - Anticholinergics
  - Decrease extrapyramidal symptoms (EPS)
  - Increased anticholinergic effects-sedation, dry mouth, orthostatic hypotension, constipation, urinary retention

Reinforcement of Priority Teaching

- Refrain from smoking due to increased metabolism of antipsychotic medications—or adjust dosage accordingly
- Be careful with activities and operating equipment due to orthostatic hypotension and sedation
- Potential for photosensitivity, need to use sunscreen

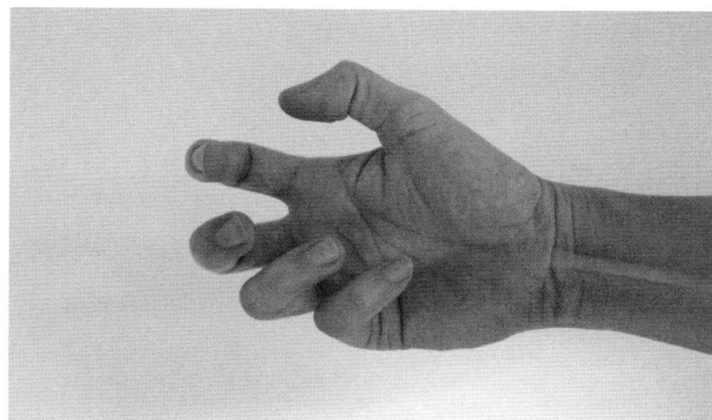

Image 16-6: A client taking antipsychotic medications contacts the telemedicine help desk and shares this photo of her hand. What might be happening? What management might the nurse anticipate? Why complications may occur if this situation goes untreated?

Next Gen Clinical Judgment

A client enters the ED expressing paranoid verbalizations and demonstrating agitation and restlessness.

1. What are the priorities of care for a client with schizophrenia in the emergency department?
2. How can a nurse ensure client safety and comfort during an emergency department visit?
3. What members of the interdisciplinary team are available to ensure safe and focused nursing care with this client?

Postpartum depression (PPD)

Pathophysiology/Description

- Postpartum depression affects up to 20% of women who give birth
- Changes in levels of hormones in the body after childbirth place some women at risk for postpartum depression
- There are many other factors that place women at risk for postpartum depression. Among them are marital discord, history of major depression, substance abuse, low self-esteem, severe psychological stressors, lack of social support and having a sick neonate, among others
- Treatment for postpartum depression includes psychotherapy, drugs or a combination of both

Priority Data Collection or Cues

- Monitor for:
    - Unprovoked irritability and rage
    - Intense feeling of dread and fear
    - Inability to sleep, or oversleeping
    - Sadness and crying without a cause
    - Feeling of guilt
    - Indifference to the newborn
    - Obsessions, including thoughts of injuring the newborn or self
    - Avoiding friends and family
    - Binging on food or eating too little
- Use validated screening scales:
    - Postpartum Depression Screening Scale
    - Edinburg Postnatal Depression Scale

Priority Interventions or Actions

- Probing questions to determine mother's state of mind and relationship with infant
- Empathetic discussion with mother and partner regarding feelings
- Initiate process for prescribed psychotherapy sessions
- Initiate antidepressant therapy

Priority Potential & Actual Complications

- Poor child/maternal bonding
- Developmental delays in baby
- Dysfunctional family relationship
- Major depression
- Suicide or homicide (of baby)

Priority Nursing Implications

- Nurses must be aware that even though postpartum depression impacts women primarily, a small percentage of men also experience the condition. When both parents are experiencing postpartum depression, measures to ensure proper care of the infant must become a priority

Priority Medications

- Fluoxetine–oral administration
    - May take 2-4 weeks to take effect
    - May be prescribed as immediate release (daily dosing) or delayed release (weekly dosing)
- Paroxetine–oral administration
    - May cause dizziness, diaphoresis, dry mouth, nausea
    - May take 1-3 weeks to take effect
- Escitalopram–oral administration
    - Common side effects are dizziness and irregular heartbeat, nausea, and diaphoresis
    - May take a few weeks to take effect
- Sertraline–oral administration
    - Side effects include diarrhea, constipation, nausea
    - May cause drowsiness so to take at bedtime

Reinforcement of Priority Teaching

- Maintain scheduled psychotherapy sessions and medication appointments
- Take antidepressants as prescribed
- Recognizing and reporting adverse effects of medications
- Who to contact if a crisis occurs at home that impacts safety of self or the baby
- Postpartum support groups
- Adequate sleep, nutrition, and relaxation
- Allowing friends and family to help with care of newborn
- Non-pharmacological treatment such as acupuncture, herbs and light therapy, among others
- Importance of partner offering ongoing affection and care

Clinical Hint

Every delivering family member (mother, father, parent, siblings, others) should be monitored for mood, safety, and capacity for caring. Postpartum depression is very real and is more significant than the "baby-blues." Nurses at the front line, in the ED, primary care, postpartum clinics, well-baby checks, and other resources should be vigilant and respond to cases of potential postpartum depression.

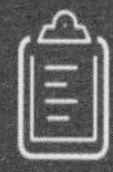

NurseThink® Quiz Questions

1. **Which finding on the pediatric client's data collection does the nurse recognize as a risk factor for their diagnosed general anxiety disorder?**
   a. Male gender.
   b. Low socioeconomic status.
   c. Under 2 years of age.
   d. Hispanic ethnicity.

2. **Which intervention does the nurse prioritize for an older adult newly diagnosed with anxiety disorder?**
   a. Check medications for interactions.
   b. Check for panic attacks.
   c. Review living arrangements.
   d. Determine ability to care for themselves.

3. **The nurse recognizes the client is experiencing severe anxiety when considering which finding?**
   a. Sleeplessness.
   b. Increased respirations.
   c. Nausea.
   d. Dilated pupils.

4. **What symptom unrelated to other childhood issues does the nurse classify as a symptom of early-onset schizophrenia in a child?**
   a. Hallucinations.
   b. Paranoia.
   c. Disordered speech.
   d. Social withdrawal.

5. **What symptoms cause the nurse to consider the client's screening positive for schizophrenia? *Select all that apply.***
   a. Paranoia.
   b. Abstract thinking.
   c. Female gender.
   d. Elaborate delusions.
   e. Hallucinations.

6. **A client was recently prescribed haloperidol for the treatment of schizophrenia. What side effects does the nurse emphasize need to be reported immediately to the health care provider?**
   a. Irritability and flaccid muscles.
   b. Headache and nausea.
   c. Weakness and fatigue.
   d. High fever and confusion.

7. **Which finding indicates the client suffers from major depression?**
   a. Symptoms lasting longer than 14 days.
   b. Symptoms develop three months after a trauma.
   c. Symptoms are present in the winter months only.
   d. Symptoms last beyond two years.

8. **Which statement by the client illustrates the need for further reinforcement of teaching regarding depression in the older adult?**
   a. "Depression is common in older adults."
   b. "Depression in older adults can cause social withdrawal and memory problems."
   c. "Depression is a normal part of aging, and I do not need treatment."
   d. "Life events and losses can compound depression in older adults."

9. **For which client does the nurse expect to implement light therapy to treat their diagnosis?**
   a. Client with major depressive disorder
   b. Client with adjustment disorder with depressed mood.
   c. Client with persistent depressive disorder.
   d. Client with seasonal affective disorder.

10. **When evaluating a client for postpartum depression, which findings indicate the client has the baby blues and not postpartum depression? *Select all that apply.***
    a. Resolves within 14 days.
    b. Lasts longer than 14 days.
    c. Tearfulness without cause.
    d. Loss of interest.
    e. Hopelessness.

11. **Which woman is most likely to develop postpartum depression after the birth of her child?**
    a. Multiparity and low income.
    b. Absence of child's father and lack of social support.
    c. Young age and supportive parents.
    d. Older age and primiparity.

12. **Which intervention does the nurse add to the care plan for a client with bipolar depression when they are in their manic state?**
    a. Enforce sleep time regardless of the client's desire to sleep.
    b. Change routine frequently to maintain pace with their mania.
    c. Reason with the client when they are experiencing delusions.
    d. Schedule a program of appropriate activities and exercise.

13. **Which documentation in the nurse's note indicates effective treatment for acute mania?**
    a. "Irritable, suggestible, distractible, napped for 10 minutes in the afternoon."
    b. "Converses without interrupting, clothing matches, participates in activities."
    c. "Attention span short, writing copious notes, intrudes in conversations."
    d. "Heavy makeup, seductive toward staff, pressured speech."

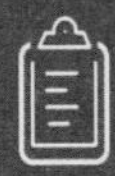

NurseThink® Quiz Questions

14. When collecting data findings, which type of bipolar disorder on the client's chart is the most difficult to treat?

a. Cyclothymic disorder.
b. Bipolar I.
c. Bipolar II.
d. Bipolar fluctuating.

15. Which client statement indicates the need for further reinforcement of teaching regarding perinatal loss?

a. "My grief can be just as strong as if I lost someone I have known for years."
b. "I don't have to worry about postpartum depression because I had a stillborn."
c. "My other children may grieve the loss of their sibling, too."
d. "Early miscarriage can still cause grief that I need to address."

16. When planning end-of-life care, which specific advance healthcare directive does the nurse discuss with the client to ensure their wishes are carried out?

a. Do not resuscitate order.
b. Living will.
c. Healthcare power of attorney.
d. Do not intubate order.

17. When monitoring a 6-year-old child for appropriate grief response related to the loss of their mother, which normal findings and responses does the nurse anticipate? *Select all that apply.*

a. "It is my fault mommy died because I didn't listen to her."
b. Changes in sleeping pattern.
c. "Mom will never come back."
d. Nightmares.
e. Discussing feelings with friends.

18. Which of the following symptoms of the classic grief response is the nurse most likely to observe in a client whose spouse died several weeks ago?

a. Excessive energy.
b. Weight gain.
c. Increased appetite.
d. Difficulty sleeping.

19. Which factor is most important in guiding the nurse's care of a pediatric client who lost their grandmother a few weeks ago?

a. The relationship they had with that grandparent.
b. Whether or not their parents are also sad.
c. Whether or not their siblings are also grieving.
d. Understanding that grief is the same no matter who they lose.

20. Which class of antidepressants does the nurse question the provider about when prescribed to an older adult client?

a. Selective serotonin reuptake inhibitors.
b. Serotonin and norepinephrine reuptake inhibitors.
c. Tricyclic antidepressants.
d. Atypical antidepressants.

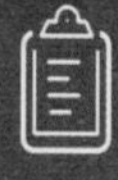

NurseThink® Quiz Answers

1. **Which finding on the pediatric client's data collection does the nurse recognize as a risk factor for their diagnosed general anxiety disorder?**
   a. Male gender.
   b. Low socioeconomic status.
   c. Under 2 years of age.
   d. Hispanic ethnicity.

   Topic/Concept: Emotion **Subtopic:** Anxiety disorder (peds) **Bloom's Taxonomy:** Applying **Clinical Problem-Solving Process:** Data Collection **NCLEX-PN®:** Psychosocial Integrity **QSEN:** Evidence-based Practice **CJMM:** Analyze Cues

   Rationale: Increased risks include being female and low socioeconomic background. Age plays more of a factor in separation anxiety disorder. There is not one identified race that is at higher risk of anxiety disorder.

   THIN Thinking: *Top Three* – Understanding risk factors alerts the nurse to focus screening in certain groups when symptoms are present. Early identification and treatment will lead to a better quality of life with emotional disorders.

2. **Which intervention does the nurse prioritize for an older adult newly diagnosed with anxiety disorder?**
   a. Check medications for interactions.
   b. Check for panic attacks.
   c. Review living arrangements.
   d. Determine ability to care for themselves.

   Topic/Concept: Emotion **Subtopic:** Anxiety disorder (adults) **Bloom's Taxonomy:** Applying **Clinical Problem-Solving Process:** Planning **NCLEX-PN®:** Safety and Infection Control **QSEN:** Safety **CJMM:** Prioritize Hypotheses

   Rationale: Anxiety disorder does not routinely cause the client to be unable to care for themselves. The biggest problem with older adults diagnosed with anxiety disorder is the potential for drug interactions between the antianxiety medication and those they are taking for other chronic illnesses.

   THIN Thinking: *Identify Risk to Safety* – Medication reconciliation for all clients, but older clients are more susceptible to medication side effects and interactions between their medications as they are often on multiple ones.

3. **The nurse recognizes the client is experiencing severe anxiety when considering which finding?**
   a. Sleeplessness.
   b. Increased respirations.
   c. Nausea.
   d. Dilated pupils.

   Topic/Concept: Emotion **Subtopic:** Anxiety disorder (adults) **Bloom's Taxonomy:** Applying **Clinical Problem-Solving Process:** Data Collection **NCLEX-PN®:** Physiological Adaptation **QSEN:** Evidence-based Practice **CJMM:** Recognize Cues

   Rationale: Sleeplessness is part of mild anxiety. Increased respirations are under moderate anxiety. Dilated pupils indicate panic. Nausea is a symptom classified under severe anxiety.

   THIN Thinking: *Top Three* – The level of anxiety can help the nurse understand what measures need to be taken to reduce the client's anxiety and how emergent the need to lessen their anxiety is.

4. **What symptom unrelated to other childhood issues does the nurse classify as a symptom of early-onset schizophrenia in a child?**
   a. Hallucinations.
   b. Paranoia.
   c. Disordered speech.
   d. Social withdrawal.

   Topic/Concept: Emotion **Subtopic:** Schizophrenia (peds) **Bloom's Taxonomy:** Analyzing **Clinical Problem-Solving Process:** Data Collection **NCLEX-PN®:** Psychosocial Integrity **QSEN:** Evidence-based Practice **CJMM:** Recognize Cues

   Rationale: Hallucinations could be fantasy play. Disordered speech and social withdrawal could be indicative of autism spectrum disorders. Paranoia is a symptom that does not fit into classic childhood behaviors or illnesses.

   THIN Thinking: *Clinical Problem-Solving Process* –A childhood diagnosis of schizophrenia is rare because it is difficult to diagnose definitively. Many providers will not officially assign the diagnosis to a child until they reach the age of 18.

5. **What symptoms cause the nurse to consider the client's screening positive for schizophrenia? *Select all that apply.***
   a. Paranoia.
   b. Abstract thinking.
   c. Female gender.
   d. Elaborate delusions.
   e. Hallucinations.

   Topic/Concept: Emotion **Subtopic:** Schizophrenia (adults) **Bloom's Taxonomy:** Analyzing **Clinical Problem-Solving Process:** Data Collection **NCLEX-PN®:** Pharmacological Therapies **QSEN:** Evidence-based Practice **CJMM:** Analyze Cues

   Rationale: Those with schizophrenia often have concrete thinking and have difficulty with abstract thought. Females are more at risk for late-onset schizophrenia, but this is not part of a screening. Paranoia, elaborate delusions, and hallucinations are all part of a positive screening.

   THIN Thinking: *Top Three* – Screening for mental illnesses should be done at every age as things may show up earlier or later in life. Mental illness needs to be identified and treated to ensure the client's safety and improve quality of life.

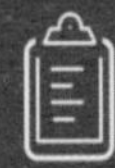

NurseThink® Quiz Answers

6. **A client was recently prescribed haloperidol for the treatment of schizophrenia. What side effects does the nurse emphasize need to be reported immediately to the health care provider?**
   a. Irritability and flaccid muscles.
   b. Headache and nausea.
   c. Weakness and fatigue.
   d. High fever and confusion.

   Topic/Concept: Emotion **Subtopic:** Schizophrenia (adults) **Bloom's Taxonomy:** Analyzing **Clinical Problem-Solving Process:** Evaluation **NCLEX-PN®:** Health promotion and maintenance **QSEN:** Patient-centered care **CJMM:** Evaluate Outcomes

   Rationale: High fever and confusion are symptoms of a serious side effect, neuroleptic malignant syndrome, that needs to be treated immediately, or it could be fatal. The other listed symptoms do not link to any other side effect of haloperidol: akathisia, dystonia, and tardive dyskinesia.

   THIN Thinking: *Identify Risk to Safety* – Many side effects of medications to treat schizophrenia are treatable or preventable if addressed as soon as possible. The nurse should encourage the client to report the first signs of any of these side effects to prevent injury.

7. **Which finding indicates the client suffers from major depression?**
   a. Symptoms lasting longer than 14 days.
   b. Symptoms develop three months after a trauma.
   c. Symptoms are present in the winter months only.
   d. Symptoms last beyond two years.

   Topic/Concept: Emotion **Subtopic:** Depression (adolescents/peds) **Bloom's Taxonomy:** Analyzing **Clinical Problem-Solving Process:** Data Collection **NCLEX-PN®:** Psychosocial Integrity **QSEN:** Patient-centered care **CJMM:** Recognize Cues

   Rationale: The timing and duration of symptoms help define the type of depression a client has. Seasonal affective disorder is a type of depression with symptoms during the winter months. Persistent depressive disorder lasts beyond two years. Adjustment disorder with depressed mood has symptoms that appear after a life trauma or event within about three months. Major depressive disorder requires the symptoms to be present for 14 days or longer.

   THIN Thinking: *Clinical Problem-Solving Process* – Determining the specific type of depression is imperative when determining the proper course of treatment.

8. **Which statement by the client illustrates the need for further reinforcement of teaching regarding depression in the older adult?**
   a. "Depression is common in older adults."
   b. "Depression in older adults can cause social withdrawal and memory problems."
   c. "Depression is a normal part of aging, and I do not need treatment."
   d. "Life events and losses can compound depression in older adults."

   Topic/Concept: Emotion **Subtopic:** Depression (adults) **Bloom's Taxonomy:** Analyzing **Clinical Problem-Solving Process:** Evaluation **NCLEX-PN®:** Coordinated Care **QSEN:** Teamwork and Collaboration **CJMM:** Evaluate Outcomes

   Rationale: While it is a common misconception because of the losses and illnesses that come with age, depression is not a normal part of aging. Depression is common in older adults and is compounded by losses in life and illnesses. Clients commonly withdraw socially and have impaired memory when they suffer from depression in their advanced age.

   THIN Thinking: *Clinical Problem-Solving Process* –Evaluating older clients for depression is extremely important as they are at increased risk for suicide because of the common issues they experience in their advanced age.

9. **For which client does the nurse expect to implement light therapy to treat their diagnosis?**
   a. Client with major depressive disorder
   b. Client with adjustment disorder with depressed mood.
   c. Client with persistent depressive disorder.
   d. Client with seasonal affective disorder.

   Topic/Concept: Emotion **Subtopic:** Depression (adults) **Bloom's Taxonomy:** Applying **Clinical Problem-Solving Process:** Planning **NCLEX-PN®:** Safety and Infection Control **QSEN:** Safety **CJMM:** Prioritize Hypotheses

   Rationale: Light therapy is effective in the treatment of seasonal affective disorder. It is not an effective therapy for the other forms of depression.

   THIN Thinking: *Top Three* – Seasonal affective disorder manifests during winter months when the days are shorter. The lack of light impacts mood and causes a depressed state; therefore, light therapy is an effective treatment.

10. **When evaluating a client for postpartum depression, which findings indicate the client has the baby blues and not postpartum depression? *Select all that apply.***
    a. Resolves within 14 days.
    b. Lasts longer than 14 days.
    c. Tearfulness without cause.
    d. Loss of interest.
    e. Hopelessness.

Topic/Concept: Emotion **Subtopic:** Postpartum depression **Bloom's Taxonomy:** Analyzing **Clinical Problem-Solving Process:** Data Collection **NCLEX-PN®:** Pharmacological Therapies **QSEN:** Patient-centered care **CJMM:** Analyze Cues

Rationale: The most significant differences between the blues and postpartum depression are that the clients with the blues usually have tearful outbursts that are not common in major depression, and it resolves on its own without treatment within 14 days. Lasting longer than 14 days classifies it as major depression. Both have symptoms of loss of interest, and major depression causes feelings of hopelessness.

THIN Thinking: *Clinical Problem-Solving Process* –The nurse must recognize the difference between postpartum depression and baby blues. The blues do not require treatment; the client needs emotional support to get through the acute period. Depression requires treatment and will not go away on its own.

11. **Which woman is most likely to develop postpartum depression after the birth of her child?**
    a. Multiparity and low income.
    b. Absence of child's father and lack of social support.
    c. Young age and supportive parents.
    d. Older age and primiparity.

Topic/Concept: Emotion **Subtopic:** Postpartum depression **Bloom's Taxonomy:** Analyzing **Clinical Problem-Solving Process:** Data Collection **NCLEX-PN®:** Psychosocial Integrity **QSEN:** Evidence-based Practice **CJMM:** Analyze Cues

Rationale: The woman that lacks social support and the child's father is absent is at the highest risk as she has two risk factors. Age does not impact risk. Primiparity does increase risk.

THIN Thinking: *Top Three* – Identifying those at higher risk before the baby's birth can help the nurse put preventative plans in place for the client and be more alert to identify the symptoms early if they do develop.

12. **Which intervention does the nurse add to the care plan for a client with bipolar depression when they are in their manic state?**
    a. Enforce sleep time regardless of the client's desire to sleep.
    b. Change routine frequently to maintain pace with their mania.
    c. Reason with the client when they are experiencing delusions.
    d. Schedule a program of appropriate activities and exercise.

Topic/Concept: Emotion **Subtopic:** Bipolar disorder **Bloom's Taxonomy:** Applying **Clinical Problem-Solving Process:** Planning **NCLEX-PN®:** Coordinated Care **QSEN:** Teamwork and Collaboration **CJMM:** Generate Solutions

Rationale: During manic phases, the clients may not be able to sleep; providing a quiet environment to allow rest is a better option as trying to force them to sleep may agitate the client. Consistency in routine is better for these clients, so the routine should not be changed frequently. It is not therapeutic to reason or argue with a client having delusions. A client in the manic phase can burn off excess energy when given assigned activities and exercise.

THIN Thinking: *Help Quick* – The nurse needs to guard the safety of the client and provide an outlet for their increased energy that will be safe in their manic phase.

13. **Which documentation in the nurse's note indicates effective treatment for acute mania?**
    a. "Irritable, suggestible, distractible, napped for 10 minutes in the afternoon."
    b. "Converses without interrupting, clothing matches, participates in activities."
    c. "Attention span short, writing copious notes, intrudes in conversations."
    d. "Heavy makeup, seductive toward staff, pressured speech."

Topic/Concept: Emotion **Subtopic:** Bipolar disorder **Bloom's Taxonomy:** Analyzing **Clinical Problem-Solving Process:** Evaluation **NCLEX-PN®:** Psychosocial Integrity **QSEN:** Informatics **CJMM:** Evaluate Outcomes

Rationale: Effective treatment for a patient with acute mania would produce the effects of being able to converse without interrupting, wearing appropriate matching clothing, and being able to participate in activities. The other options describe manic behavior.

THIN Thinking: *Clinical Problem-Solving Process* – Proper documentation is essential when evaluating the effectiveness of treatment. Documentation on behavior helps guide treatment in psychological disorders.

14. When collecting data findings, which type of bipolar disorder on the client's chart is the most difficult to treat?

a. Cyclothymic disorder.
b. Bipolar I.
c. Bipolar II.
d. Bipolar fluctuating.

Topic/Concept: Emotion **Subtopic:** Bipolar disorder **Bloom's Taxonomy:** Applying **Clinical Problem-Solving Process:** Data Collection **NCLEX-PN®:** Pharmacological Therapies **QSEN:** Evidence-based Practice **CJMM:** Recognize Cues

Rationale: Cyclothymic fluctuates between mood states extremely rapidly, making it the most unstable form and, therefore, the hardest to treat.

THIN Thinking: *Clinical Problem-Solving Process* –When planning care for a client, the nurse must understand the nature and expected disease progression to ensure proper care is being planned.

15. Which client statement indicates the need for further reinforcement of teaching regarding perinatal loss?

a. "My grief can be just as strong as if I lost someone I have known for years."
b. "I don't have to worry about postpartum depression because I had a stillborn."
c. "My other children may grieve the loss of their sibling, too."
d. "Early miscarriage can still cause grief that I need to address."

Topic/Concept: Emotion **Subtopic:** Death and dying **Bloom's Taxonomy:** Analyzing **Clinical Problem-Solving Process:** Evaluation **NCLEX-PN®:** Basic Care and Comfort **QSEN:** Patient-centered care **CJMM:** Evaluate Outcomes

Rationale: Even though the infant has died, the client can still have postpartum depression. In fact, they are more at risk due to the added grief from their loss. Early miscarriage needs to be addressed, siblings may mourn the loss and need to be emotionally cared for, and feelings of grief can be just as strong with an infant death as with someone the client knew for years.

THIN Thinking: *Clinical Problem-Solving Process* – Addressing all aspects and forms of grief the client may experience involves ensuring emotional support and addressing any signs of depression that may arise.

16. When planning end-of-life care, which specific advance healthcare directive does the nurse discuss with the client to ensure their wishes are carried out?

a. Do not resuscitate order.
b. Living will.
c. Healthcare power of attorney.
d. Do not intubate order.

Topic/Concept: Emotion **Subtopic:** Death and dying **Bloom's Taxonomy:** Applying **Clinical Problem-Solving Process:** Planning **NCLEX-PN®:** Psychosocial Integrity **QSEN:** Patient-centered care **CJMM:** Generate Solutions

Rationale: Legally, the best way to ensure the client's wishes are carried out is to have a healthcare power of attorney that understands and will follow your wishes. DNR and DNI orders can be overturned in the event the client is unable to make personal decisions. Living wills are just a statement outlining the client's wishes but do not hold legal weight. The healthcare power of attorney has legal rights to make all the medical decisions for the client if they cannot, and only they can do so, not other family members

THIN Thinking: *Clinical Problem-Solving Process* –A healthcare power of attorney is important. Without this, all other documents can be overturned by the legal next of kin to make decisions. The first next of kin for adults is the legal spouse, then children, then brothers, sisters, and parents. With a healthcare power of attorney, none of these people can make decisions any longer as the client designates that legal right to a specific individual.

17. When monitoring a 6-year-old child for appropriate grief response related to the loss of their mother, which normal findings and responses does the nurse anticipate? *Select all that apply.*

a. "It is my fault mommy died because I didn't listen to her."
b. Changes in sleeping pattern.
c. "Mom will never come back."
d. Nightmares.
e. Discussing feelings with friends.

Topic/Concept: Emotion **Subtopic:** Death and dying **Bloom's Taxonomy:** Analyzing **Clinical Problem-Solving Process:** Evaluation **NCLEX-PN®:** Coordinated Care **QSEN:** Teamwork and Collaboration **CJMM:** Evaluate Outcomes

Rationale: A child at this age still believes their actions can cause the death of their loved one and may blame themselves. They could have changes in sleeping or eating patterns. They may also experience nightmares. Older children from 8-11 understand that the parent is never coming back; at 6, the child still believes they are alive, but in a place they can't go. Adolescents tend to discuss their feelings with friends.

THIN Thinking: *Top Three* – Recognizing normal and abnormal grief responses allows the nurse to identify those clients that need interventions to prevent injury.

18. **Which of the following symptoms of the classic grief response is the nurse most likely to observe in a client whose spouse died several weeks ago?**
    a. Excessive energy.
    b. Weight gain.
    c. Increased appetite.
    d. Difficulty sleeping.

Topic/Concept: Emotion **Subtopic:** Bereavement **Bloom's Taxonomy:** Analyzing **Clinical Problem-Solving Process:** Data Collection **NCLEX-PN®:** Psychosocial Integrity **QSEN:** Patient-centered care **CJMM:** Recognize Cues

Rationale: Classic signs of grief include sleep disturbances, decreased appetite, weight loss, and somatic complaints such as abdominal pain or frequent headaches. In addition, clients experiencing grief often report intermittent periods of decreased motivation, energy, or activity.

THIN Thinking: *Top Three* – It is important to understand the stages and expectations of normal grief so that any dysfunctional grief can be identified and treated to prevent depression and other issues.

19. **Which factor is most important in guiding the nurse's care of a pediatric client who lost their grandmother a few weeks ago?**
    a. The relationship they had with that grandparent.
    b. Whether or not their parents are also sad.
    c. Whether or not their siblings are also grieving.
    d. Understanding that grief is the same no matter who they lose.

Topic/Concept: Emotion **Subtopic:** Bereavement **Bloom's Taxonomy:** Applying **Clinical Problem-Solving Process:** Planning **NCLEX-PN®:** Basic Care and Comfort **QSEN:** Patient-centered care **CJMM:** Prioritize Hypotheses

Rationale: When a child loses a grandparent, the biggest factor in how it impacts them is their relationship with that grandparent. How often they saw them and how well they knew them plays a role in how much they grieve over them. The grieving of others in the house does not impact them in their grief as much as their relationship with that person. Grief is different for each person and for each person lost based on the significance of that person in their life.

THIN Thinking: *Clinical Problem-Solving Process* –The loss of a grandparent is often the first experience with death a child has. Ineffective grieving with that loss can set a precedence for future losses.

20. **Which class of antidepressants does the nurse question the provider about when prescribed to an older adult client?**
    a. Selective serotonin reuptake inhibitors.
    b. Serotonin and norepinephrine reuptake inhibitors.
    c. Tricyclic antidepressants.
    d. Atypical antidepressants.

Topic/Concept: Emotion **Subtopic:** Depression **Bloom's Taxonomy:** Applying **Clinical Problem-Solving Process:** Implementation **NCLEX-PN®:** Pharmacological Therapies **QSEN:** Quality Improvement **CJMM:** Take Action

Rationale: Tricyclic antidepressants have an anticholinergic effect that can result in acute confusion, severe constipation, and urinary incontinence in older adult clients. They are better treated with other antidepressant medications like SSRIs, atypical antidepressants, and SNRIs.

THIN Thinking: *Identify Risk to Safety* – Proper medication prescription is important in all clients, but older adult clients are more susceptible to side effects and drug interactions. Evaluating their medications is essential to prevent injury.

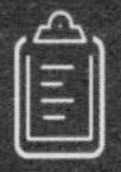

CHAPTER

17

Cognition

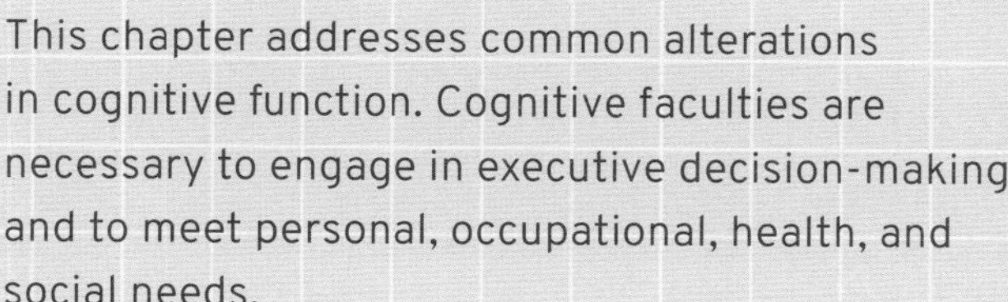

This chapter addresses common alterations in cognitive function. Cognitive faculties are necessary to engage in executive decision-making and to meet personal, occupational, health, and social needs.

Nurses provide care to clients that suffer cognitive issues which are reversible or irreversible, progressive or temporary, represent a wide range of cognitive abilities and disabilities, and may occur in clients across the lifespan.

Priority Exemplars:

- Dementia/Alzheimer's disease
- Autism
- Attention-deficit/hyperactivity disorder
- Delirium

Next Gen Clinical Judgment

Reflect on clients you have cared for in the past who suffered from cognitive impairments.

1. How did your communication strategies differ based on the client's cognitive abilities and disabilities?
2. Consider the QSEN competency of patient-centered care. How should the nurse ensure that patient-centered care is provided for clients with cognitive disabilities?
3. NCLEX® focuses on safety. Safety is also a QSEN competency. What safety priorities should be considered for clients with cognitive disabilities?
4. Demographic trends indicate that our population is aging. What implications does this hold for rates of cognitive disabilities, such as dementia and Alzheimer's disease?
5. Society often presumes that older adult clients have some degree of cognitive deterioration. How can nurses ensure that each client is addressed on an individual basis and without bias?

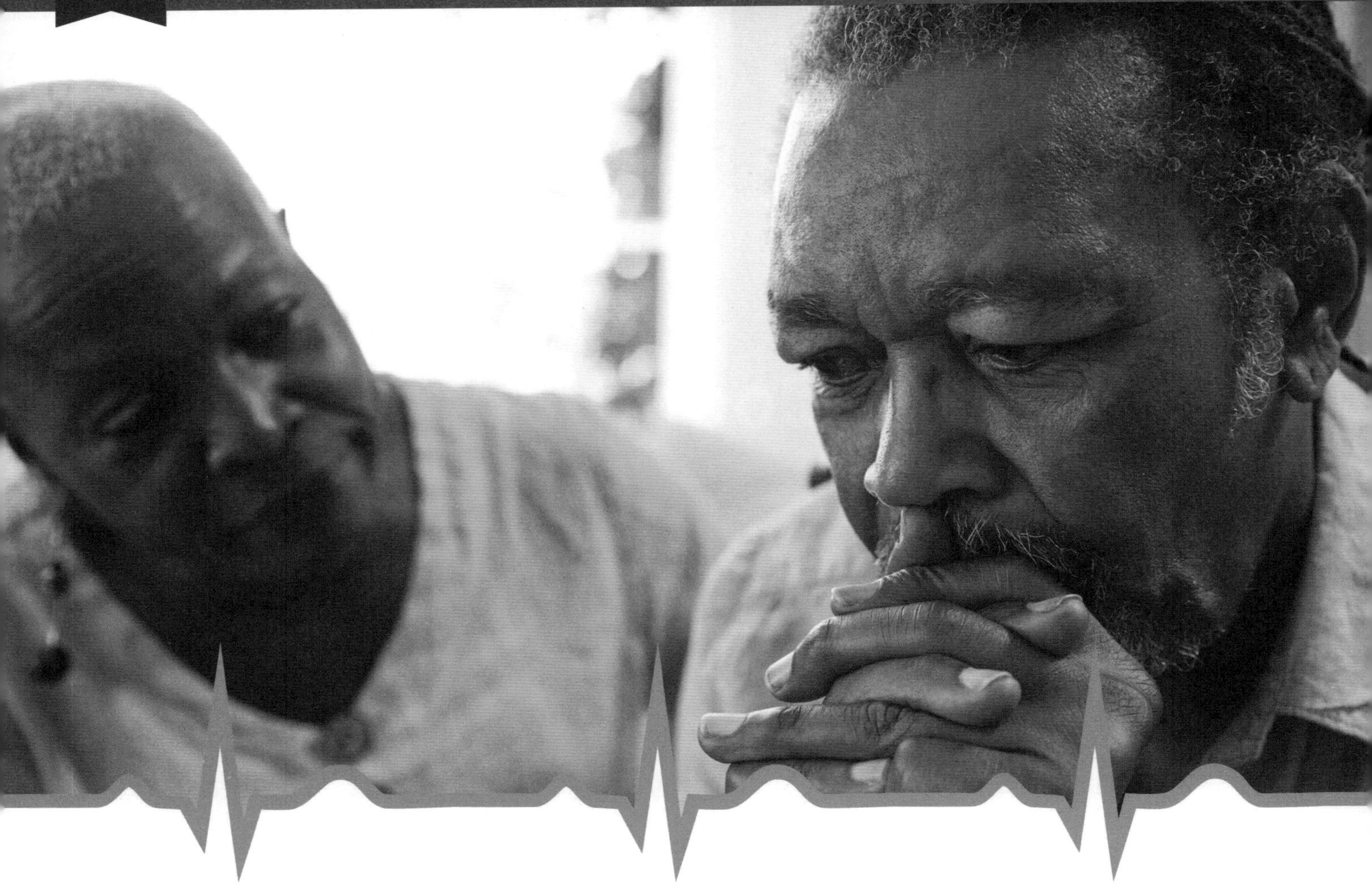

Go To Clinical Case 1

J.G. is a 74-year-old Black male born in the Caribbean. Until three years ago, J.G. was a practicing nephrologist. J.G. and his wife, Ella, visit the primary care provider with concerns about J.G.'s memory and changes in J.G.'s personality and behavior. Ella states, "My husband just isn't acting right. He called our son and just yelled at him over the weekend. He is cross all the time and doesn't seem like himself. Last night he put on the kettle to boil and let it boil dry." Upon further questioning, Ella and J.G. note that J.G. has been increasingly impulsive, very forgetful, socially isolated, irritable, and making poor choices. Ella found J.G. walking around the backyard in the middle of the night a few weeks ago and last night she caught him going out the back door at 3:00 AM. Ella said J.G. made up a story about going out to check on the dog. Ella stated their dog had died several years ago. They have not noted any changes in speech or physical abilities. Ella is worried that J.G. will hurt himself or others and neither of them are sleeping well. The nurse notes that all of J.G.'s vital signs are within normal limits. J.G. was diagnosed with pre-diabetes at his annual physical last year with a fasting serum blood glucose level of 120 mg/dL. J.G. has a history of hypothyroidism but he stopped taking the levothyroxine 10 years ago because "he didn't think he needed it." Ella and J.G. report that J.G. eats a healthy diet and takes walks daily. They both are trying to drink more water.

NurseThink® Time

Using the NurseThink® system, complete the priorities. Check your answers designated by 💡 in the Dementia/Alzheimer's disease Priority Exemplar.

NurseThink® Time

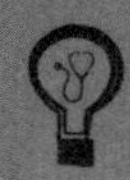

Priority Data Collection or Cues

1.

2.

3.

Priority Laboratory Tests/Diagnostics

1.

2.

3.

Priority Interventions or Actions

1.

2.

3.

Priority Potential & Actual Complications

1.

2.

3.

Priority Nursing Implications

1.

2.

3.

Priority Medications

1.

2.

3.

Reinforcement of Priority Teaching

1.

2.

3.

Pathophysiology/Description

- Dementia is the insidious and progressive decline in cognitive capacity and function while the client is conscious, these changes cause social and occupational dysfunction
- Categorized as neurocognitive disorders and classified based on severity of symptoms
  - Major Neurocognitive Disorder
    - Previously described as dementia
    - Significant decline in cognitive function
    - Conflict with ADLs and IADLs
  - Minor Neurocognitive Disorder
    - Mild cognitive impairment from previous level of functioning
    - May be responsive to early intervention
    - Still able to complete ADLs and IADLs but may employ compensatory mechanisms (writing lists, accommodations, or increased effort)
  - If disease is progressive, minor may precede major
- Causes/associated pathologies including Alzheimer's disease (AD), Huntington's disease, Parkinson's disease, HIV, substance/medication use, traumatic brain injury, vascular disease, Lewy body disease, frontotemporal lobar degeneration, or Prion disease
- May also be primary (such as AD) or secondary (to another disease or cause)
- Alzheimer's increase in incidence associated with increased life expectancy
- Stages of Alzheimer's Disease
  - Stage 1—no apparent symptoms-changes in brain function
  - Stage 2—forgetfulness-lose things or forget names
  - Stage 3—mild cognitive decline-interference with work, getting lost
  - Stage 4—mild to moderate cognitive decline-forgetfulness, depression, withdrawal, confabulation (making up stories to cover up memory loss)
  - Stage 5—moderate cognitive decline-lose ability to perform ADLs, disoriented
  - Stage 6—moderate to severe decline-disoriented, unable to do ADLs, sleeping problems, sundowners (agitation at nighttime), unable to communicate, institutionalization
  - Stage 7—severe cognitive decline-bedfast, aphasia, deteriorated cognitive function

Priority Data Collection or Cues

- Review findings from standardized cognitive assessment tests
- Monitor for changes in personal hygiene habits/ability to accomplish ADLs
- Observe for changes in judgment, abstract thinking, and impulse control
- Observe for speech and language-difficulty labeling objects, aphasia (inability to talk)
- Inquire of family members about personality changes, reports of wandering, changes in cognitive function, orientation, language difficulties, social issues
- Collect data about nutritional and hydration status
  - Ability to swallow
  - Ability to coordinate eating functions
  - Toleration of feedings
  - Measures of hydration including skin turgor, intake and output, mucous membranes, weight
- Determine history of drug or alcohol use
- Monitor for signs of potential abuse or neglect
- Determine ability to move, risk for wandering, or for apraxia (inability to initiate motor function). Determine pain level
- Monitor for incontinence/skin integrity
- Collect data about potential for injury, self-harm, and falls

Priority Laboratory Tests/Diagnostics

- Monitor serum electrolyte levels for abnormalities
- Serum albumin to monitor nutritional status
- Urine specific gravity for hydration status
- Monitor blood glucose level
- Collect data related to sexually transmitted infections and HIV as indicated
- Review diagnostic tests for thyroid dysfunction, nutritional/Vitamin B12 deficiencies, and liver and renal function studies
- Implement drug/alcohol screens for new admissions
- Lumbar puncture to rule out infection
- CT scanning and MRI to detect atrophy
- Positron emission tomography (PET)–measures metabolic activity of brain

Priority Interventions or Actions

- Determine and manage the underlying cause and check reversibility of potential causes
- Ensure that electrolytes, oxygenation, and blood glucose levels are within normal limits
- Provide nutritional interventions
  - Encourage favorite foods
  - Provide finger foods and easy-to-eat foods when agitated
  - Thicken liquids as tolerated
  - Ascertain client's wishes about tube feedings/potential for nasogastric or percutaneous endoscopic gastrostomy (PEG) tube feedings/hydration
- Gradually assume more physical care and feeding for client as condition deteriorates
  - Allow client to remain as independent as possible, allowing time as needed
  - Provide a structured schedule recognizing the individual's routine
  - Frequently monitor client's self-care abilities

- Prevent injury
  - Ensure the client's environment is arranged for convenience and safety
  - Keep highly used items and call light close to the client
  - Keep the bed in the lowest position or place a mattress on the floor and follow agency policy about side rails for safety. Pad head and foot boards as needed
  - Ensure client is supervised with ambulation, apply a bed alarm if appropriate
  - Move client to a room easily observed by nursing staff
  - Ensure nightlights are used
  - Consider use of soft restraints if indicated
- Re-orient client
  - Introduce yourself by name and use the client's name with each interaction
  - Use touch when appropriate
  - Approach client from the front and use simple words or single questions
  - Use clocks and calendars
  - Provide signs on rooms as indicated
  - Encourage personal items, a favorite chair, and pictures
  - Encourage visits from loved ones and friends, when appropriate
  - Encourage television, radio, and other diversions
  - Provide reminiscence therapy with movies, pictures, and photo albums
  - Keep staffing consistent
- Keep client safe when wandering
  - Maintain a structured time schedule for sleeping, meals, toileting, and hygiene
  - Provide a safe location to allow for pacing and wandering
  - When wanderer is a distance from the unit, walk with the client for a while and then redirect back to the unit
  - Ensure locking and alarm systems are in place
- If client has delusions and/or hallucinations
  - Do not reinforce or discuss false beliefs or experiences
  - Reinforce client safety
  - Change the subject or distract to another activity
  - Lavender oil may reduce anxiety and promote sleep

Priority Potential & Actual Complications

- Potential for hazards of immobility
- Malnutrition
- Dehydration
- May be fatal when confronted with potential co-morbidities
- Potential for injury to self and others
- Potential for injury with wandering

Go To Clinical Answers

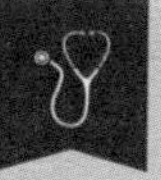

Text designated by [icon] are the top answers for the Go To Clinical related to Dementia/Alzheimer's disease.

Priority Nursing Implications

- Falls are prime risk as motor function deteriorates
- Ensure hearing aids and eyeglasses are at optimal functioning
- Some research indicates that use of ginkgo (an herbal supplement) may delay loss of memory
- Ensure that medications are reviewed for polypharmacy noting potential drug interactions and side effects
- Ensure monitoring of blood glucose, T3/T4/TSH levels which monitor thyroid function, and other physiological variables which may contribute to disorientation and personality or behavioral changes

Priority Medications

- Rivastigmine–oral administration, patch
  - Off-label use of antipsychotics to manage behavioral symptoms
  - Decrease memory loss
  - Slows disease progress, does not cure or stop the disease
- Memantine–oral administration
  - Improve cognitive function
  - Increases ability to conduct ADLs
- Risperidone–oral or IM administration
  - To treat psychotic symptoms
  - Black box warning-associated with cardiac deaths in elder adults
- Paroxetine–oral administration
  - SSRI
  - First line treatment for depression
  - Older adults should be monitored for hyponatremia
- Lorazepam–oral, IV, or IM administration
  - Anti-anxiety agent
  - Anxiety associated with loss of cognitive functioning
  - Shorter half-life anti-anxiety agents preferable with older adults
- Zolpidem–oral, rectal, sublingual, or oromucosal spray
  - Hypnotic
  - To enhance sleep
  - Watch for daytime sleeping, increased risk for falls, cognitive impairment, and paradoxical effects

Reinforcement of Priority Teaching

- Progress of illness, safety interventions, and other treatments
- Family support and means to share feelings and frustrations with the disease process
- Availability of community organizations for adult day care, respite services, disease-specific information, and hospice services (when appropriate)

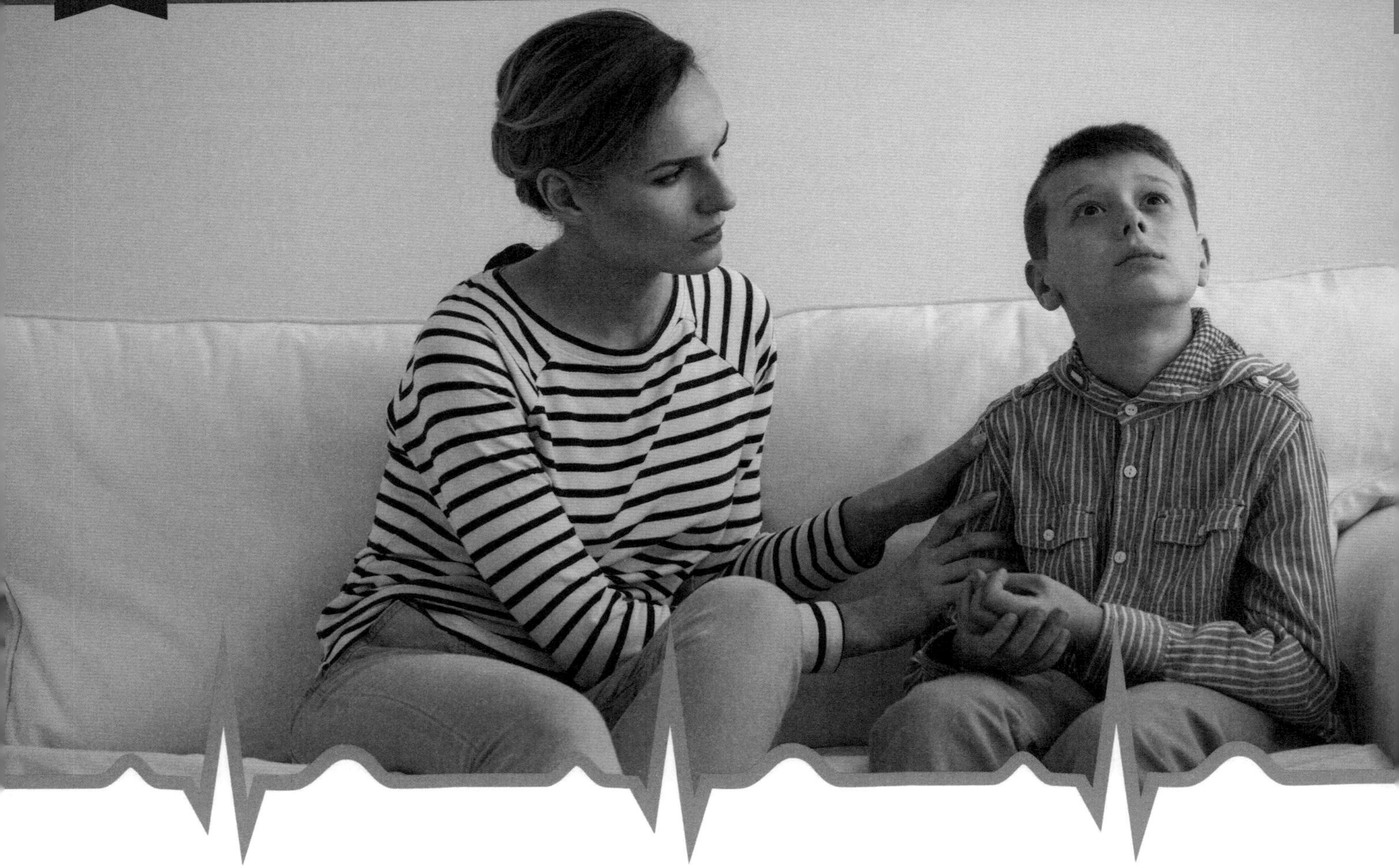

Go To Clinical Case 2

A.C. is a 10-year-old boy admitted to the pediatric unit for bilateral herniorrhaphies in the morning. A.C. was brought in the night before surgery to acclimate him to the unit and help him feel more comfortable with hospital routines. A.C. has autism and is in a mainstreamed fourth-grade class. A.C.'s math skills are above grade level; his reading is just below the 4th-grade level. A.C. is accompanied by his mother who is spending the night. According to A.C.'s mother, "When A.C. is stressed-out or hungry, he goes wild. He bangs his head on the wall, yells, and is difficult to console. I am really worried about tonight when he can not eat." A.C. is placed in a private isolation room with a parent bedroom attached. The pediatric nurses are skilled in working with children with autism and developmental disabilities. The nurse and the unlicensed assistive personnel (UAP) enter the room to take vital signs and reinforce pre-operative teaching. They allow the mother to place the blood pressure cuff on A.C.'s arm and allow A.C. to press the start button on the blood pressure machine. A.C. does not make eye contact but allows the nurse to take his temporal temperature and listen to his breath, cardiac, and bowel sounds. The nurse encourages A.C. to hold and touch the stethoscope. The nurse, UAP, and mother discuss ways to keep A.C. calm and feeling comfortable. The anesthesiologist completes a consult and allows a solid breakfast at 0700 and clear liquids until one hour before surgery (about 1030 AM). A.C. eats waffles with syrup and drinks apple juice every morning. The staff ensures those items are available tomorrow morning. The UAP moves A.C.'s mattress to the floor and provides padding around the bed.

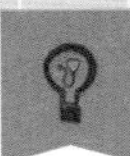

NurseThink® Time

Using the NurseThink® system, complete the priorities. Check your answers designated by the bulb icon in the Autism spectrum disorders (ASD) Priority Exemplar.

NurseThink® Time

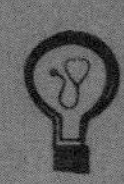

Priority Data Collection or Cues

1.

2.

3.

Priority Laboratory Tests/Diagnostics

1.

2.

3.

Priority Interventions or Actions

1.

2.

3.

Priority Potential & Actual Complications

1.

2.

3.

Priority Nursing Implications

1.

2.

3.

Priority Medications

1.

2.

3.

Reinforcement of Priority Teaching

1.

2.

3.

Autism spectrum disorders (ASD)

Pathophysiology/Description

- Characterized by a wide range of communication impairments, social withdrawal, lack of social interaction, and repetitive/unusual physical behaviors
- The spectrum includes autistic disorder, Rett syndrome, childhood disintegrative disorder, pervasive developmental disorder, and Asperger's disorder
- May be associated with other conditions including epilepsy, genetic disorders, and intellectual disabilities
- Incidence in the US is increasing. It is 5x's more common in males, 1/2 have average or above average intelligence
- Diagnosed early in childhood with chronic symptoms persisting into adulthood
- Cause unknown, may have genetic and perinatal etiologies

Priority Data Collection or Cues

- Collection of data depends upon where client is on the spectrum and level of functionality
- Observe eye contact, social interactions, interest in others, capacity to imitate others, demonstration and receipt of affection, attachment, and intro/extroversion
- Observe ability to empathize and process feelings of others, ability to hold a reciprocal conversation, verbal/non-verbal skills or echolalia, for idiosyncratic utterances or monotone speech, presence of facial expressions/gestures, lack of response to or overreaction to noise/sounds/stimuli
- Ask about imaginative activity and ability/capacity to play alone and with others and for friendships, observe for internal imaginative play
- Monitor intelligence and age-appropriate development (accelerated, delayed, or on par)
- Monitor for restricted/stereotyped physical activities/ interests: response to stimuli, irritability, compulsivity, fascination with objects, repetitive body movements (clapping, banging, rocking), self-injurious behaviors, restricted food choices/acceptance, repetitive verbalizations, and need for strict routine and sameness of surroundings

Priority Laboratory Tests/Diagnostics

- Diagnosed based on symptoms and history
- Early diagnosis increases effectiveness of interventions
- Diagnostic tests for potential co-morbidities (epilepsy)

Priority Interventions or Actions

- Ensure safety related to high levels of physical activity without cognitive controls. Create a safe, consistent environment for learning and play. Use safety devices to protect from self-injury. Provide familiar foods, objects, and routines
- Set realistic goals for success and provide clear, concrete instructions
- Form trusting relationships and ensure consistent caregivers/limit number of caregivers, convey acceptance, positive regard, and provide positive feedback/reinforce positive behaviors, eye contact, socially acceptable behavior, appropriate use of touch, and communication using the client's own methods of communicating
- Expose to group learning and play as tolerated, support client's interaction with others
- Follow client cues for hugging and touching
- Encourage self-care and capitalize on individual, personal strengths to meet future goals

Priority Potential & Actual Complications

- Potential exists for misdiagnosis and incorrect treatment
- Assumption of lower cognitive function related to communication impairment

Priority Nursing Implications

- Provide support with symptoms of self-injury, aggression, hyperactivity, impulsivity, and temper tantrums
- Be aware of savants who may excel in music, art, puzzles/ patterning, design, or memory
- Children with autism may seek healthcare related to other physical needs/diagnoses. Nurses need to be sensitive to and capable of working with clients across the lifespan

Priority Medications

- Risperidone–oral administration
  - Use for irritability controversial, ages 5-15 years
  - Monitor for neuroleptic malignant syndrome, tardive dyskinesia, and hyperglycemia/diabetes
- Aripiprazole–oral/IM administration
  - Use for irritability controversial, ages 6-17 years
  - May cause sedation, fatigue, weight gain, drooling, and tremoring

Reinforcement of Priority Teaching

- Ongoing healthcare and behavioral surveillance and collaboration with the school, family, caregivers, and health care providers
- Support family and client as the child grows and needs change
- Principles of safety
- Community resources, schools, and respite services. Consider legal rights afforded to clients with disabilities during planning of care

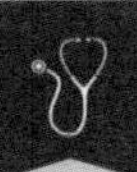

Go To Clinical Answers

Text designated by are the top answers for the Go To Clinical related to Autism spectrum disorders (ASD) disease.

Attention-deficit/hyperactivity disorder (ADHD)

Pathophysiology/Description

- Characterized by behaviors of inattention and/or hyperactivity with impulsivity (may be mild to severe)
- Hyperactivity is defined as increased psychomotor activity, may or may not be purposeful, may include rapid physical movements and verbal activity. May be inattentive or highly distractible
- Impulsivity is defined as acting without reflection or thought to consequences, unable to resist acting
- Difficult to diagnose in children less than 4 years of age, most often recognized when child enters school
- More common in boys, prevalence about 10% (among children in the US)
- May persist into adolescence and adulthood
- May have genetic, biochemical, anatomical, psychosocial, environmental, and perinatal origins of causality
- May occur with co-morbidities such as disruptive mood dysregulation, sleep disorders, oppositional defiance disorder, bipolar disorder, conduct disorder, learning disorders, and anxiety

Priority Data Collection or Cues

- Observe child and accessing history with family, teachers, and caregivers
- Extent of disorder measured using standardized psychiatric testing methods
- Determine ability to perform age-appropriate tasks, complete activities, and stay with activities until completed
- Observe ability to attend, length of attention span, ability to cooperate, ability to tolerate frustration, and level of distractibility
- Monitor ability to form relationships with peers, siblings, and classmates
- Observe level of activity, including fidgeting with hands/fingers, squirming in seat, or engagement in risky or dangerous behaviors
- Collect data on the client's ability to hear and listen to others, monitor for excessive talking or frequently using interruption to dominate conversation

Priority Laboratory Tests/Diagnostics

- Diagnosed based on symptoms and reports of child, family, teachers, and others
- Early diagnosis increases effectiveness of interventions
- Diagnostic tests for potential co-morbidities (sleep disorders)

Priority Interventions or Actions

- Ensure safety related to high levels of physical activity without cognitive controls
- Create a safe, consistent environment for learning and play. Consider distractibility and impulsivity
- Set realistic goals for success and provide clear, concrete instructions
- Encourage a highly nutritious diet, eat early in day to avoid impact of anorexia, and, although the role of sugar and caffeine in diet is unknown, these should be limited in diet
- Reinforce the need for family/individual therapy along with medication management
- Form trusting relationships and ensure consistent caregivers, convey acceptance, positive regard, and provide positive feedback
- Develop a behavior plan with logical consequences for engagement in high-risk behaviors
- Expose to group learning and play as tolerated

Priority Potential & Actual Complications

- Potential exists for misdiagnosis and incorrect treatment
- Exacerbation of behavioral issues due to mismanagement

Priority Nursing Implications

- Ensure that families understand the need for therapy along with medications such that children are managed as they grow and their needs change
- Children with ADHD may seek healthcare related to other physical needs/diagnoses. Nurses need to be sensitive to and capable of working with clients with ADHD

Priority Medications

- Dextroamphetamine/amphetamine–oral administration
  - Stimulant that calms hyperactivity and increases attentiveness
  - High-risk for dependence
  - Appetite depressant-give early in day and monitor for weight loss
  - May cause hypertension-monitor blood pressure and avoid over-the-counter medications
- Methylphenidate–oral administration
  - Stimulant that calms hyperactivity and increases attentiveness
  - May disturb sleep so given in morning or at least 6 hours before bedtime (14 hours for extended-release)
  - Appetite depressant-give early in day and monitor for weight loss
  - May cause growth retardation such that clients are encouraged to take a "drug holiday" to allow for growth during summer or breaks from school
- Bupropion–oral administration
  - To manage depression and mood swings
  - May cause headache, sedation, and dizziness

Reinforcement of Priority Teaching

- Ongoing healthcare and behavioral surveillance and collaboration with the school, family, caregivers, and health care providers

Pathophysiology/Description

- Changes in cognitive function, awareness, and ability to attend to stimuli. Occurs rapidly over a short period
- Cognitive impairment is manifested by changes in attention span, speech patterns, orientation, and decision-making
- Most often in older adults or those with serious illnesses
- May have hallucinations (false, sensory experiences) and illusions (misperceptions of environment)
- Symptoms may present immediately after the precursor (head injury, seizure) or more slowly (if related to electrolyte imbalance or medical condition)
- Causes and related factors include infections, seizures, electrolyte imbalances, hypercarbia, hypoxia, pain, hypoglycemia, and experiences of social isolation. Clients with a history of stroke, burns, migraine headaches, nutritional deficiencies (thiamine), hepatic or renal failure, a brain tumor, heat stroke, head trauma, or having surgery may also be at risk
- Other etiologies include:
  - Substance intoxication delirium
  - Substance withdrawal delirium
  - Medication-induced delirium
  - Delirium due to another medical condition

Priority Data Collection or Cues

- Observe vital signs for elevated heart rate and hypotension
- Monitor for distractibility, lack of ability to attend to conversations, restlessness
- Observe speech patterns. Verbalizations may be rambling, pressured, incoherent, or irrelevant. Client may change topics frequently
- Determine level of orientation. Clients may be disoriented to time and place and lacking in short-term memory
- Note sleep patterns, client may have distorted sleep, wakefulness, insomnia, day sleeping, hypersomnia, ask about dreams and nightmares
- Monitor for changes in state of awareness. Client may rapidly progress from hypervigilance to stupor to coma
- Observe physical behavior for restlessness, hyperactivity, hitting, tremoring, agitation, appearing to pick/pinch at air with fingers or punch objects that are not real; may also become stuporous
- Collect data on emotional stability. Client may be fearful, anxious, depressed, irritable, angry, euphoric, and lacking in response. Observe for crying, laughter, calling for help, muttering, moaning, violent acts against self or others, cursing, and trying to flee agency
- Observe physical signs including diaphoresis, facial flushing, dilated pupils
- Monitor for safety risks and potential for injury for self and others

Priority Laboratory Tests/Diagnostics

- Monitor serum electrolyte levels for abnormalities that may cause delirium
- Monitor blood glucose level
- Arterial blood gases for oxygenation and ventilation
- Test for sexually transmitted infections and HIV as indicated
- Include diagnostic tests for thyroid dysfunction, nutritional/Vitamin B12 deficiencies, and liver and renal function studies
- Implement drug/alcohol screens for new admissions
- Lumbar puncture to rule out infection

Priority Interventions or Actions

- Determine and manage the underlying cause
- Ensure that electrolytes, oxygenation, serum sodium levels, and blood glucose levels are within normal limits
- Maintain an environment of low stimulation
- Employ interventions to manage behaviors including distractibility
- Remain calm and assume an undemanding attitude
- Engage client in anxiety-reducing behaviors, such as dance or movement therapy
- Assume physical care and feeding for client
  - Allow client to be as independent as possible, allowing time as needed
  - Provide a structured schedule recognizing the individual's routine
  - Frequently observe client's self-care abilities. Ensure that clients have eyeglasses and hearing aids, as indicated
- For clients who are disoriented
  - Introduce yourself by name and use the client's name with each interaction
  - Use touch when appropriate
  - Approach client from the front and use simple words or single questions
  - Use clocks and calendars
  - Provide signs on doors for separate rooms
  - Encourage use of personal items, a favorite chair, and pictures
  - Encourage visits from loved ones and friends, when appropriate
  - Encourage television, radio, and other diversions
  - Provide reminiscence therapy with movies, pictures, and photo albums
  - Keep staffing consistent
- Ensure client is safe
  - Keep the bed in the lowest position and follow agency policy about side rails and bed alarm for safety
  - Consider putting the client in a bed closest to the nurses' station for safety and close observation
  - Consider one-on-one observation as needed
  - Pad head and foot boards as needed

Priority Potential & Actual Complications

- Potential for injury or safety threats to others
- Hazards of immobility associated with lack of movement/being bedridden
- Potential for malnutrition/dehydration/electrolyte imbalance

Priority Nursing Implications

- Monitor for side effects of new and previously taken medications
- Deal with complications of immobility including contractures, skin breakdown, constipation, depression, and pneumonia
- Instruct family on causes and management of delirium, may be very concerning due to rapid onset and troubling symptoms

Priority Medications

- Haloperidol–oral, IM, IV, or nasal spray
  - Antipsychotic
  - To manage psychotic symptoms
  - Monitor cardiac status-may prolong QT intervals
- Lorazepam–oral, IM, or IV administration
  - Anti-anxiety agent
  - For substance withdrawal and anxiety
  - Client may become physically dependent and tolerant
- Melatonin–generally oral administration, some research into IV and subcutaneous use
  - Homeopathic mood stabilizer
  - Available over-the-counter
  - May be combined with ramelteon (for insomnia)
  - Used to prevent and treat delirium
  - Additional studies are needed to confirm this as an evidence-based practice

Reinforcement of Priority Teaching

- Progress of illness, safety interventions, and other treatments
- Support for family including opportunities to share feelings and frustration about disease process
- Community organizations for adult day care, respite services, and hospice services (when appropriate)
- Family's ability to cope with delirium. This condition may be very frustrating due to the unpredictable nature and unknown outcome of delirium

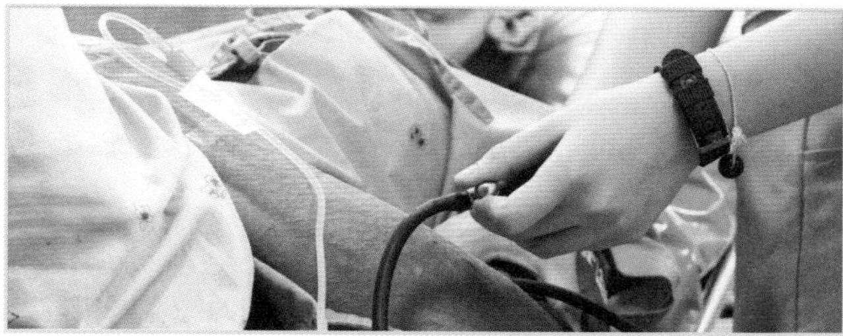

Image 14-1: Nurses frequently confront clients with altered cognitive function or delirium. What nursing measures are indicated to keep clients with delirium safe?

Briefly review various resources on the differences and similarities between delirium, dementia, and depression. Complete this table to help you Save Time Studying.

	DELIRIUM	DEMENTIA	DEPRESSION
Onset			
Duration			
Reversible			
Awareness			
Attention			
Hallucinations			
Memory			
Sleep			
Thoughts			

Table 17-1: Compare and Contrast: Delirium, dementia, depression

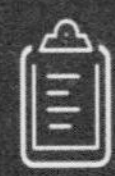

NurseThink® Quiz Questions

1. **Which data collection findings does the nurse expect to observe in a client with delirium?**
   a. Increased awareness, hypoxia, and anxiety.
   b. Increased awareness, arm drift, and slurred speech.
   c. Reduced awareness, impaired thinking, and behavioral changes.
   d. Reduced awareness, unilateral weakness, and slurred speech.

2. **The nurse determines that a client is at risk of developing delirium. Which factors caused the nurse to consider this possibility? *Select all that apply.***
   a. Infection.
   b. Excessive sleeping.
   c. Hypoxia.
   d. Trauma.
   e. Hyperglycemia.

3. **A pregnant client is hospitalized with delirium, and the nurse collects data to assist in determining the underlying cause. What conditions may have contributed to the client's delirium? (Select all that apply)**
   a. Preeclampsia
   b. Preterm labor
   c. HELLP syndrome
   d. Sepsis
   e. Hyperglycemia

4. **The nurse evaluates an older adult client who is very confused. What finding suggests they have delirium and not dementia?**
   a. Sudden onset confusion.
   b. Chronic cognitive decline.
   c. No apparent cause of the client's confused state.
   d. Confused state has lasted three months.

5. **The nurse gathers data on a client with dementia. What deficit areas does the nurse expect to find with this client? *Select all that apply.***
   a. Attention span.
   b. Communication.
   c. Learning.
   d. Judgment.
   e. Perception.

6. **The nurse cares for a client who has been diagnosed with vascular dementia. What probable cause does the nurse identify in the client's electronic health record?**
   a. History of stroke.
   b. Neuritic plaques on brain CT scan.
   c. Positive beta-amyloid precursor gene.
   d. History of traumatic brain injury (TBI).

7. **The health care provider considers a diagnosis of dementia for a client. The nurse reports deficits in the client's cognitive functions to assist with the diagnosis. Which cognitive functions does the nurse discuss with the provider? *Select all that apply.***
   a. IQ levels.
   b. Tactile perception.
   c. Communication.
   d. Reasoning.
   e. Attention span.

8. **The nurse cares for a client with Alzheimer's dementia who cannot find certain words when communicating. How does the nurse document this finding?**
   a. Apraxia.
   b. Aphasia.
   c. Anomia.
   d. Agnosia.

9. **Which finding indicates to the nurse that a client with Alzheimer's disease is in the middle stage or stage II of the disease?**
   a. Denies presence of symptoms.
   b. Wandering.
   c. Motor skills lost.
   d. Totally dependent care.

10. **The nurse evaluates the care plan for a client with delirium. Which nursing diagnosis listed on the care plan is appropriate for a client with Alzheimer's disease but not delirium?**
    a. Risk for compromised human dignity.
    b. Self-care deficit.
    c. Risk for injury.
    d. Caregiver role strain.

11. **Which lobe of the brain impaired by Alzheimer's disease is responsible for problems with judgment, an inability to make decisions, decreased attention span, and a decreased ability to concentrate?**

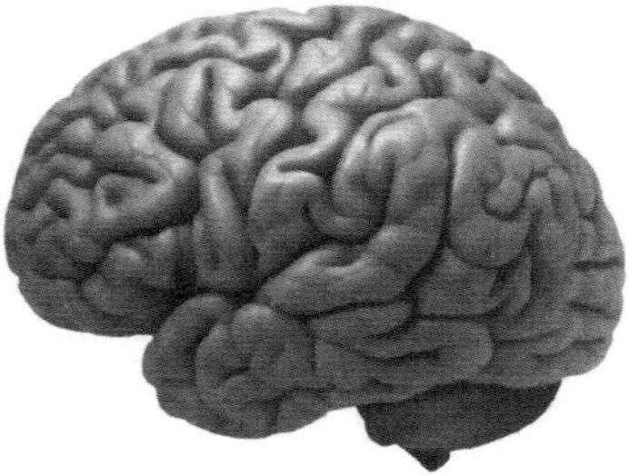

12. **Which part of the brain has been found to have congenital defects in many children diagnosed with autism?**

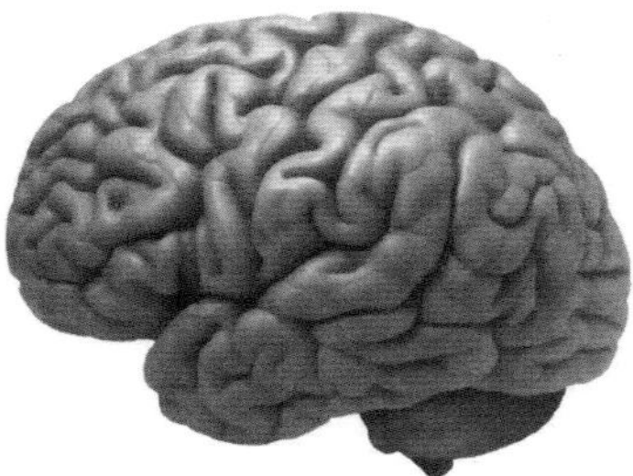

13. **The nurse observes a teenage client with autism spectrum disorder. What behavior is uncharacteristic of this disease process?**
    a. Does not hold eye contact.
    b. Unable to name common objects.
    c. Uses words repetitively.
    d. Tries to sit on their mother's lap.

14. **A 5-year-old client is brought into the provider's office by their mother, who states the child has autism. The client is new to this provider's office. Which observation causes the nurse to suspect emotional abuse or neglect instead of autism?**
    a. The child is wearing a diaper.
    b. They respond appropriately to questions.
    c. The client is banging their head against a padded chair.
    d. The child is sucking their thumb.

15. **The nurse evaluates a client for possible attention-deficit hyperactivity disorder (ADHD). What must be true about the client's symptoms to be diagnosed?**
    a. They must be present before the age of seven.
    b. They must be constant.
    c. They must be severe.
    d. They must be present at school.

16. **The nurse cares for an adolescent client with attention-deficit hyperactivity disorder (ADHD). What recommendation does the nurse provide to improve the client's ability to focus when studying?**
    a. Study in a quiet space.
    b. Study in a small group.
    c. Encourage long study periods.
    d. Review multiple subjects each session.

17. **The nurse supports the parents of a client with attention deficit hyperactivity disorder (ADHD). Which toy does the nurse recommend to help this child focus and remain calm?**

a. 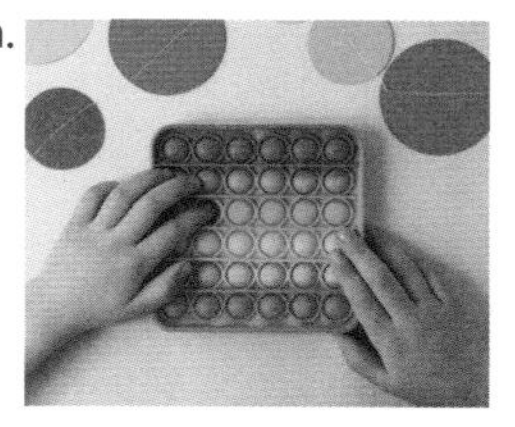

b. 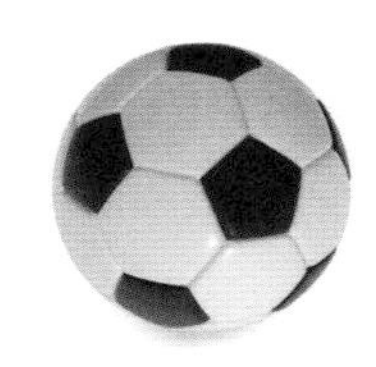

c. 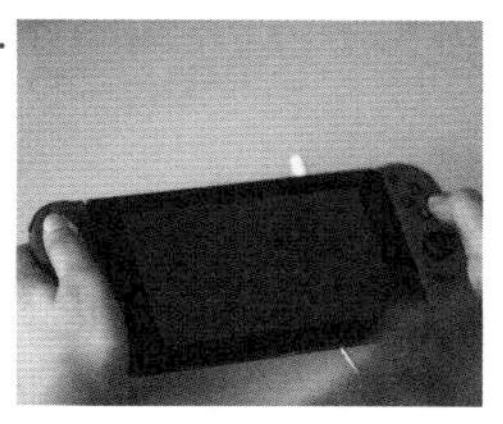

d. 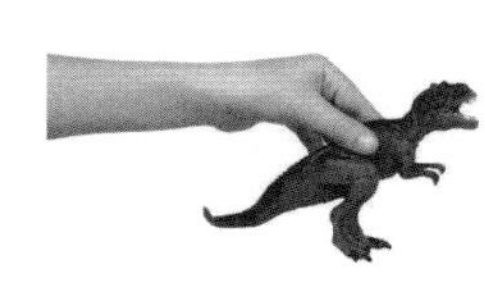

18. **The nurse reviews the plan of care for a client with hyperactivity disorder with their parents. Which trait of this disorder puts the client at most risk of injury?**
    a. Short attention span.
    b. Increased motor activity.
    c. Impulsiveness.
    d. Difficulty concentrating.

19. **The nurse considers the care plan for a client with hyperactivity disorder. Which treatment will be the most beneficial in building their ability to fit in socially with their peers?**
    a. Pharmacologic therapy.
    b. Behavioral therapy.
    c. Diet modifications.
    d. Neurofeedback therapy.

20. **The nurse cares for a client prescribed amphetamine-dextroamphetamine for the treatment of hyperactivity disorder. What does the nurse consider when a client is prescribed this medication? *Select all that apply.***
    a. The client's growth should be monitored.
    b. There can be "drug holidays."
    c. There is a high potential for abuse.
    d. Expect weight gain.
    e. It can cause insomnia.

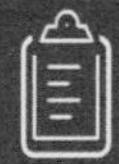

NurseThink® Quiz Answers

1. **Which data collection findings does the nurse expect to observe in a client with delirium?**
   a. Increased awareness, hypoxia, and anxiety.
   b. Increased awareness, arm drift, and slurred speech.
   c. ● Reduced awareness, impaired thinking, and behavioral changes.
   d. Reduced awareness, unilateral weakness, and slurred speech.

   Topic/Concept: Cognition **Subtopic:** Delirium **Bloom's Taxonomy:** Analyzing **Clinical Problem-Solving Process:** Data Collection **NCLEX-PN®:** Physiological Adaptation **QSEN:** Evidence-based Practice **CJMM:** Recognize Cues

   Rationale: Reduced awareness, impaired thinking, and behavioral changes are expected in delirium. Increased awareness is not expected, hypoxia and anxiety are related to an oxygenation issue, and arm drift, unilateral weakness, and slurred speech could all be indicative of a stroke.

   THIN Thinking: *Top Three* – It is important to differentiate between delirium and other similarly expressing medical emergencies that could be overlooked.

2. **The nurse determines that a client is at risk of developing delirium. Which factors caused the nurse to consider this possibility? *Select all that apply.***
   a. ● Infection.
   b. Excessive sleeping.
   c. ● Hypoxia.
   d. ● Trauma.
   e. Hyperglycemia.

   Topic/Concept: Cognition **Subtopic:** Delirium **Bloom's Taxonomy:** Applying **Clinical Problem-Solving Process:** Data Collection **NCLEX-PN®:** Safety and Infection Control **QSEN:** Safety **CJMM:** Recognize Cues

   Rationale: Hypoglycemia, sleep deprivation, trauma, infection, and hypoxia increase the risk of developing delirium.

   THIN Thinking: *Identify Risk to Safety* – The nurse should identify clients at high risk for specific conditions to prevent injury and provide early treatment.

3. **A pregnant client is hospitalized with delirium, and the nurse collects data to assist in determining the underlying cause. What conditions may have contributed to the client's delirium? (Select all that apply)**
   a. ● Preeclampsia
   b. Preterm labor
   c. ● HELLP syndrome
   d. ● Sepsis
   e. ● Hyperglycemia

   Topic/Concept: Cognition **Subtopic:** Delirium **Bloom's Taxonomy:** Analyzing **Clinical Problem-Solving Process:** Data Collection **NCLEX-PN®:** Physiological Adaptation **QSEN:** Evidence-based Practice **CJMM:** Analyze Cues

   Rationale: Preterm labor does not trigger delirium in pregnant women, but preeclampsia, HELLP syndrome, hyper and hypoglycemia, sepsis, and fluid and electrolyte imbalances can.

   THIN Thinking: *Clinical Problem-Solving Process* – It is very important to uncover the underlying cause of delirium as it is a syndrome related to another cause. Some causes can be life-threatening, and if not identified and corrected, the client could die.

4. **The nurse evaluates an older adult client who is very confused. What finding suggests they have delirium and not dementia?**
   a. ● Sudden onset confusion.
   b. Chronic cognitive decline.
   c. No apparent cause of the client's confused state.
   d. Confused state has lasted three months.

   Topic/Concept: Cognition **Subtopic:** Delirium **Bloom's Taxonomy:** Analyzing **Clinical Problem-Solving Process:** Data Collection **NCLEX-PN®:** Physiological Adaptation **QSEN:** Evidence-based Practice **CJMM:** Analyze Cues

   Rationale: Delirium is an acute confused state with a rapid onset and an identifiable underlying cause lasting no longer than one month.

   THIN Thinking: *Top Three* – The nurse needs to differentiate between delirium and dementia because delirium is reversible, and dementia is not. Delirium may also be caused by a life-threatening issue that needs to be addressed.

5. **The nurse gathers data on a client with dementia. What deficit areas does the nurse expect to find with this client? *Select all that apply.***
   a. ● Attention span.
   b. ● Communication.
   c. ● Learning.
   d. ● Judgment.
   e. ● Perception.

   Topic/Concept: Cognition **Subtopic:** Dementia **Bloom's Taxonomy:** Analyzing **Clinical Problem-Solving Process:** Data Collection **NCLEX-PN®:** Coordinated Care **QSEN:** Evidence-based Practice **CJMM:** Recognize Cues

   Rationale: With dementia, there is a global impact on the client's cognition, so there can be deficits expected in all areas of cognition like attention, concentration, judgment, perception, learning, memory, communication, language, and speed of information processing.

THIN Thinking: *Clinical Problem-Solving Process* – Thorough evaluation of clients with dementia is necessary to ensure they receive the proper care. Dementia is a degenerative disease that will eventually require total care, and the nurse needs to ensure they receive that care when appropriate.

6. **The nurse cares for a client who has been diagnosed with vascular dementia. What probable cause does the nurse identify in the client's electronic health record?**
   a. History of stroke.
   b. Neuritic plaques on brain CT scan.
   c. Positive beta-amyloid precursor gene.
   d. History of traumatic brain injury (TBI).

   Topic/Concept: Cognition **Subtopic:** Dementia **Bloom's Taxonomy:** Analyzing **Clinical Problem-Solving Process:** Data Collection **NCLEX-PN®:** Coordinated Care **QSEN:** Safety **CJMM:** Analyze Cues

   Rationale: Vascular dementia results from stroke. Neuritic plaques and beta-amyloid precursor genes are related to Alzheimer's dementia. TBI is structural dementia.

   THIN Thinking: *Clinical Problem-Solving Process* – Understanding the types of dementia can help the nurse predict the pattern and stage the client is in and will advance to.

7. **The health care provider considers a diagnosis of dementia for a client. The nurse reports deficits in the client's cognitive functions to assist with the diagnosis. Which cognitive functions does the nurse discuss with the provider? *Select all that apply.***
   a. IQ levels.
   b. Tactile perception.
   c. Communication.
   d. Reasoning.
   e. Attention span.

   Topic/Concept: Cognition **Subtopic:** Dementia **Bloom's Taxonomy:** Applying **Clinical Problem-Solving Process:** Data Collection **NCLEX-PN®:** Psychosocial Integrity **QSEN:** Patient-centered Care **CJMM:** Recognize Cues

   Rationale: IQ levels and tactile perception are not cognitive functions on the evaluation list. Communication, reasoning, and attention span are evaluation criteria for determining dementia.

   THIN Thinking: *Top Three* – The nurse needs to properly evaluate clients and their cognitive abilities even if dementia is not expected.

8. **The nurse cares for a client with Alzheimer's dementia who cannot find certain words when communicating. How does the nurse document this finding?**
   a. Apraxia.
   b. Aphasia.
   c. Anomia.
   d. Agnosia.

   Topic/Concept: Cognition **Subtopic:** Alzheimer's disease **Bloom's Taxonomy:** Applying **Clinical Problem-Solving Process:** Planning **NCLEX-PN®:** Basic Care and Comfort **QSEN:** Teamwork and Collaboration **CJMM:** Prioritize Hypotheses

   Rationale: Anomia is the inability to find words. Apraxia is the inability to use words or objects correctly. Aphasia is the inability to speak or understand words. Agnosia is the loss of sensory comprehension.

   THIN Thinking: *Clinical Problem-Solving Process* – It is important to identify the client's communication difficulties to ensure proper treatment planning to care for their individual needs effectively.

9. **Which finding indicates to the nurse that a client with Alzheimer's disease is in the middle stage or stage II of the disease?**
   a. Denies presence of symptoms.
   b. Wandering.
   c. Motor skills lost.
   d. Totally dependent care.

   Topic/Concept: Cognition **Subtopic:** Alzheimer's disease **Bloom's Taxonomy:** Analyzing **Clinical Problem-Solving Process:** Data Collection **NCLEX-PN®:** Basic Care and Comfort **QSEN:** Safety **CJMM:** Recognize Cues

   Rationale: Denying symptoms occurs in stage I; lost motor skills and total dependence fall into stage III. Wandering behavior is indicative of stage II.

   THIN Thinking: *Clinical Problem-Solving Process* – With progressive diseases that have no cure, the nurse must know how to stage it and what is needed and expected in each stage to get the appropriate treatment for the client.

10. **The nurse evaluates the care plan for a client with delirium. Which nursing diagnosis listed on the care plan is appropriate for a client with Alzheimer's disease but not delirium?**
    a. Risk for compromised human dignity.
    b. Self-care deficit.
    c. Risk for injury.
    d. Caregiver role strain.

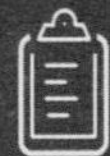

NurseThink® Quiz Answers

Topic/Concept: Cognition **Subtopic:** Alzheimer's disease **Bloom's Taxonomy:** Applying **Clinical Problem-Solving Process:** Planning **NCLEX-PN®:** Psychosocial Integrity **QSEN:** Patient-centered Care **CJMM:** Generate Solutions

Rationale: Delirium is acute, and long-term care isn't necessary with correction of the causative factor, so caregiver role strain is not applicable for delirium, but it would be for Alzheimer's. Both delirium and Alzheimer's could applicably use self-care deficit, risk for injury, and risk for compromised human dignity.

THIN Thinking: *Identify Risk to Safety* – The nurse should understand the disease process to ensure proper nursing care plan diagnoses as these drive the care p an goals and outcomes.

11. **Which lobe of the brain impaired by Alzheimer's disease is responsible for problems with judgment, an inability to make decisions, decreased attention span, and a decreased ability to concentrate?**

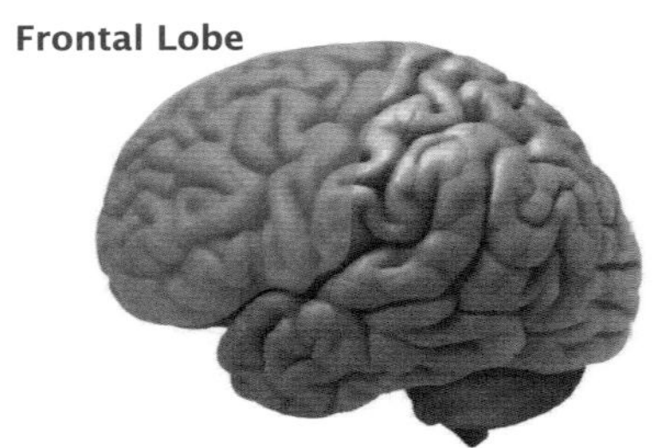

Topic/Concept: Cognition **Subtopic:** Alzheimer's disease **Bloom's Taxonomy:** Applying **Clinical Problem-Solving Process:** Data Collection **NCLEX-PN®:** Physiological Adaptation **QSEN:** Evidence-based Practice **CJMM:** Recognize Cues

Rationale: Impairment to the frontal lobe is responsible for problems with judgment, an inability to make decisions, decreased attention span, and a decreased ability to concentrate.

THIN Thinking: *Clinical Problem-Solving Process* – The nurse needs to be aware of what parts of the brain are affected by a disease to anticipate potential problems and symptoms the client will display and anticipate their needs.

12. **Which part of the brain has been found to have congenital defects in many children diagnosed with autism?**

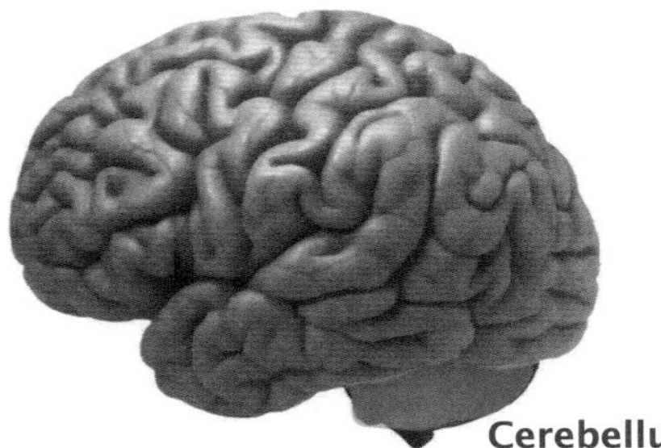

Topic/Concept: Cognition **Subtopic:** Autism spectrum disorder (child) **Bloom's Taxonomy:** Applying **Clinical Problem-Solving Process:** Data Collection **NCLEX-PN®:** Physiological Adaptation **QSEN:** Teamwork and Collaboration **CJMM:** Recognize Cues

Rationale: Three main congenital deformities in the cerebellum have been correlated to autism—cerebellar vermis hypoplasia, Dandy-Walker malformation, and Mega Cisterna Magna.

THIN Thinking: *Clinical Problem-Solving Process* – Any objective data and testing that can help identify a physical illness will help identify it earlier, assisting the nurse in ensuring earlier treatment and intervention.

13. **The nurse observes a teenage client with autism spectrum disorder. What behavior is uncharacteristic of this disease process?**
    a. Does not hold eye contact.
    b. Unable to name common objects.
    c. Uses words repetitively.
    d. Tries to sit on their mother's lap.

Topic/Concept: Cognition **Subtopic:** Autism spectrum disorder (adolescent) **Bloom's Taxonomy:** Applying **Clinical Problem-Solving Process:** Data Collection **NCLEX-PN®:** Psychosocial Integrity **QSEN:** Patient-centered Care **CJMM:** Analyze Cues

Rationale: Despite this being an overall odd behavior for a large adolescent, it is not common for an autistic child to seek human contact or physical contact so trying to sit on her mother's lap is not indicative of autism. It is common in autism to use words repetitively, not hold eye contact, and be unable to name common objects.

THIN Thinking: *Clinical Problem-Solving Process* – The nurse needs to know what to expect as a normal finding in a disease process to identify abnormal findings. What is abnormal for a person without a specific disease may be expected in a specific disease and vice versa.

14. **A 5-year-old client is brought into the provider's office by their mother, who states the child has autism. The client is new to this provider's office. Which observation causes the nurse to suspect emotional abuse or neglect instead of autism?**
    a. The child is wearing a diaper.
    b. They respond appropriately to questions.
    c. The client is banging their head against a padded chair.
    d. The child is sucking their thumb.

Topic/Concept: Cognition **Subtopic:** Autism spectrum disorder **Bloom's Taxonomy:** Analyzing **Clinical Problem-Solving Process:** Data Collection **NCLEX-PN®:** Coordinated Care **QSEN:** Evidence-based Practice **CJMM:** Recognize Cues

Rationale: The age-inappropriate behaviors combined with the capacity for appropriate verbal communication would indicate probable abuse or neglect. The mother stating the child is autistic could be a cover for her actions or a part of abuse through Munchausen syndrome.

THIN Thinking: *Help Quick* – It is important to recognize the symptoms of autism versus abuse as they can be similar. Emotional abuse and neglect do not have as obvious signs as physical abuse and can often be mistaken for other disease processes.

15. **The nurse evaluates a client for possible attention-deficit hyperactivity disorder (ADHD). What must be true about the client's symptoms to be diagnosed?**
    a. They must be present before the age of seven.
    b. They must be constant.
    c. They must be severe.
    d. They must be present at school.

Topic/Concept: Cognition **Subtopic:** Attention-deficit disorder (child) **Bloom's Taxonomy:** Applying **Clinical Problem-Solving Process:** Data Collection **NCLEX-PN®:** Coordinated Care **QSEN:** Patient-centered Care **CJMM:** Recognize Cues

Rationale: To be diagnosed with ADHD, the symptoms must be present in at least two settings and present before age seven. They can have varying degrees of severity and do not have to be constant.

THIN Thinking: *Clinical Problem-Solving Process* – ADHD can be inappropriately diagnosed when there are truly other issues present like abuse. The nurse needs to know how to differentiate between the symptoms to ensure proper interventions.

16. **The nurse cares for an adolescent client with attention-deficit hyperactivity disorder (ADHD). What recommendation does the nurse provide to improve the client's ability to focus when studying?**
    a. Study in a quiet space.
    b. Study in a small group.
    c. Encourage long study periods.
    d. Review multiple subjects each session.

Topic/Concept: Cognition **Subtopic:** Attention-deficit disorder (adolescent) **Bloom's Taxonomy:** Applying **Clinical Problem-Solving Process:** Planning **NCLEX-PN®:** Coordinated Care **QSEN:** Safety **CJMM:** Generate Solutions

Rationale: The client with ADHD would benefit from shorter study periods, focusing on a single topic each session, and studying alone in a quiet place away from distractions.

THIN Thinking: *Top Three* – Even on medications and even with the decrease many clients experience in symptoms in their later adolescence, many will still need environmental manipulation during learning periods as ADHD causes learning disabilities.

17. **The nurse supports the parents of a client with attention deficit hyperactivity disorder (ADHD). Which toy does the nurse recommend to help this child focus and remain calm?**

Answer: a.

Topic/Concept: Cognition **Subtopic:** Attention-deficit disorder **Bloom's Taxonomy:** Applying **Clinical Problem-Solving Process:** Planning **NCLEX-PN®:** Coordinated Care **QSEN:** Teamwork and Collaboration **CJMM:** Generate Solutions

Rationale: Fidget toys such as spinners or this popping toy have been shown to help with the hyperactivity of children with ADHD, especially during class and study. A figurine will not hold their attention as long and does not have as many moving parts to keep their interest. Gaming devices can exacerbate symptoms of ADHD. Playing with a ball may be a good motor activity for the child, but will not help with calm and focus.

THIN Thinking: *Clinical Problem-Solving Process* – The nurse needs to educate the client and their caregivers on nonpharmacological ways to care for their disorders and illnesses.

18. The nurse reviews the plan of care for a client with hyperactivity disorder with their parents. Which trait of this disorder puts the client at most risk of injury?

a. Short attention span.
b. Increased motor activity.
c. Impulsiveness.
d. Difficulty concentrating.

Topic/Concept: Cognition **Subtopic:** Hyperactivity disorder **Bloom's Taxonomy:** Applying **Clinical Problem-Solving Process:** Planning **NCLEX-PN®:** Safety and Infection Control **QSEN:** Safety **CJMM:** Prioritize Hypotheses

Rationale: Impulsiveness will put them at the highest risk of injury because they often do things without thinking, resulting in poor and dangerous decisions that may cause injury. Increased motor activity and short attention span can increase the risk when added to impulsivity but are not the highest risks by themselves. Poor concentration adds mostly to a level of frustration which will increase impulsivity in many cases.

THIN Thinking: *Identify Risk to Safety* – It is important to address the causes of potential complications so that they can be avoided as much as possible, reducing risks of injury from those complications.

19. The nurse considers the care plan for a client with hyperactivity disorder. Which treatment will be the most beneficial in building their ability to fit in socially with their peers?

a. Pharmacologic therapy.
b. Behavioral therapy.
c. Diet modifications.
d. Neurofeedback therapy.

Topic/Concept: Cognition **Subtopic:** Hyperactivity disorder **Bloom's Taxonomy:** Applying **Clinical Problem-Solving Process:** Planning **NCLEX-PN®:** Psychosocial Integrity **QSEN:** Patient-centered Care **CJMM:** Prioritize Hypotheses

Rationale: Behavioral therapy is the most beneficial psychosocially because it teaches them proper behavior in social settings and helps them learn impulse control to become more socially acceptable to their peers. Neurofeedback and diet modifications can be used, but their benefits are unproven. Pharmacological therapy will help with attention span, focus, and grades, but there is no magic pill; behavioral therapy is still needed.

THIN Thinking: *Clinical Problem-Solving Process* – The total care of each client is important. Every aspect that a disorder or disease impacts should be carefully considered and addressed.

20. The nurse cares for a client prescribed amphetamine-dextroamphetamine for the treatment of hyperactivity disorder. What does the nurse consider when a client is prescribed this medication? *Select all that apply.*

a. The client's growth should be monitored.
b. There can be "drug holidays."
c. There is a high potential for abuse.
d. Expect weight gain.
e. It can cause insomnia.

Topic/Concept: Cognition **Subtopic:** Hyperactivity disorder **Bloom's Taxonomy:** Analyzing **Clinical Problem-Solving Process:** Evaluation **NCLEX-PN®:** Pharmacological Therapies **QSEN:** Evidence-based Practice **CJMM:** Evaluate Outcomes

Rationale: Common side effects include insomnia, headache, and anorexia leading to weight loss. There is a high potential for abuse, and children may even sell it at school. They can be given drug holidays. Their growth can be affected and should be monitored.

THIN Thinking: *Top Three* – Understanding the expected side effects and risks of a medication is important when clients or their parents decide whether or not it is the right treatment for them. The nurse must ensure client understanding of pertinent information.

SECTION 3

Closing

CHAPTER

18

Health Promotion

Across the Lifespan

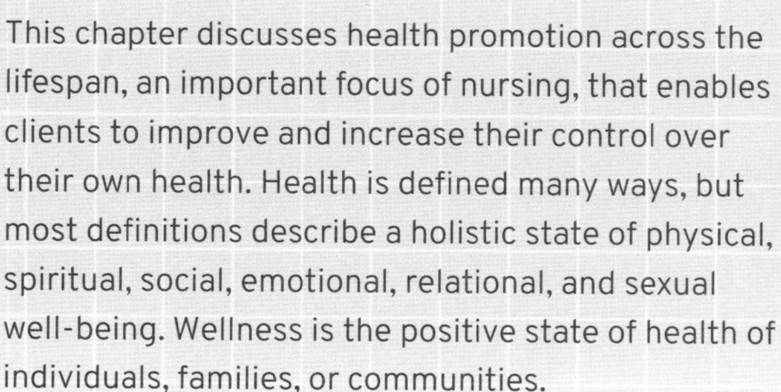

This chapter discusses health promotion across the lifespan, an important focus of nursing, that enables clients to improve and increase their control over their own health. Health is defined many ways, but most definitions describe a holistic state of physical, spiritual, social, emotional, relational, and sexual well-being. Wellness is the positive state of health of individuals, families, or communities.

This chapter also addresses development or the sequence of change over a person's lifetime in several domains (we address physical, motor, cognitive, psychoemotional, language, and play). Individuals across the lifespan may experience developmental delays in any of these domains, requiring nurses to adapt their plan of care. The ability to address clients on their developmental, not just chronological level, meet their health promotion needs, and reinforce client teaching and anticipatory guidance to promote health is integral of nursing practice.

As you read through this chapter, consider how principles of growth and development and health promotion may influence your answers to NCLEX® questions and your providing of holistic nursing care to clients in practice.

Priority Exemplars:

- Infants
- Toddlers
- Preschoolers
- School-age children
- Adolescents
- Adults
- Older adults

Pathophysiology/Description

- Includes ages from birth to 12 months (some sources indicate 18 months)
- Is a critical period for development in multiple domains, and infancy is the most rapid period of growth and development in the lifespan

Priority Data Collection or Cues

- Determine vital signs including newborn ranges (heart rate 120-160 bpm, respirations 30-60 bpm, blood pressures 80-90/40-50 mmHg) and infant ranges (heart rate 90-130 bpm, respirations 20-40 bpm, blood pressure 90/56 mmHg), temp. approximately 97-99°F axillary. For infants, cardiac output is heart rate dependent so bradycardia may markedly decrease perfusion
- Monitor clients for achieving developmental milestones in a variety of domains
  - Physical
    - Infants double birth weight by six months, triple birth weight by 12 months
    - Infant length increases by 50% at 1 year of age
    - Infants' heads are proportionally larger than the rest of the body
    - Determine the status of infant reflexes (see Newborn Care Priority Exemplar)
    - Collect data on the client's appearance to include muscle tone, behavior, level of consciousness, and mood. Observe client for developmentally appropriate smile
  - Motor
    - Fine motor skills demonstrated in infants as they learn reflexive movements, move from reflexive to simple repetitive movements, are able to bring toys to mouth, are able to use a pincer grasp, perform hand to hand transfer, and hold a pencil
    - Gross motor skills demonstrated in infants as they gain head control, learn to roll (front to back/back to front), sit, crawl, stand, and walk
  - Cognitive
    - Piaget's stage of sensorimotor phase in which learning begins by trial and error and learning through reflexive to purposeful movements
    - Infants learn object permanence as they develop a memory and understand disappearing/reappearing (peek-a-boo)
  - Psychoemotional
    - Erikson's phase of trust versus mistrust, as they form attachments, learn to trust caregivers, and negative feelings in response when needs are not met; infants learn to develop hope and faith. Lack of trust may contribute to attachment disorders and emotional strain
    - Learn boundaries of self with social games, responsive smiling, and understanding of self as separate from others
    - Monitor for eye contact, social smiling, and responsive hugging
    - Parents/caregivers are center of social circle
    - Separation anxiety is manifested and progresses from protest to despair to detachment to adjustment
  - Language
    - Progresses from crying to cooing to laughing to imitating sounds
    - Progresses to comprehending simple commands and repeating words
  - Play
    - Largely about manipulation of toys
    - Exploratory and solitary play
- Observe for potential child maltreatment including abuse and neglect

Priority Laboratory Tests/Diagnostics

- Newborn screening (see Newborn Care Priority Exemplar)
- Screening during infancy for congenital hip dysplasia
- Health screening and monitoring
- Length, weight, and head circumference and plot on a growth chart

Priority Interventions or Actions

- Reinforce health education
  - Reinforce infant care including bathing and bath safety, dressing, safe handling, and infant developmental milestones
  - Sleeping is a significant concern for many parents
    - Infants often establishing sleep patterns and many parents/caregivers may deal with sleep refusal, frequent waking, and mix up days and nights
    - Usually sleep about 9-11 hours a night with 1-2 naps/day
    - Reinforce safe sleep practices, including back-to-sleep, pacifiers, dressing lightly, no bumpers/pillows/blankets in bed, no co-bedding
  - Reinforce teaching about nutrition and feeding practices including bottle/breastfeeding, introducing solid foods at about 6 months
    - No whole cow's milk, egg whites, or honey until 12 months
    - Begin with well-cooked table foods, offer new foods one at a time
    - Encourage water between meals
    - Limit juice, use a cup to avoid bottle mouth caries
    - Use care with microwave, do not microwave bottles
  - Provide instruction about dental care, teeth begin to appear 6-10 months
    - Assist parents/caregivers to deal with irritability related to teething
    - Use of cold teething rings, over-the-counter topical pain relievers, and oral analgesics

- Prepare parents for infant's body self-exploration and infant's tendency to touch their genitals

Priority Potential & Actual Complications

- Poor attachment with lack of a secure caregiver
- Development delay
- Unintentional or intentional injury or illness

Priority Nursing Implications

- For hospitalized infants, nurses should:
  - Cuddle and hold infants
  - Encourage parent/caregivers to participate in care
  - Stimulate with toys
  - Allow for security objects
  - Encourage parent/caregiver involvement in care and rooming in
- Provide for non-nutritive sucking and oral stimulation if NPO or agitated
- Reinforce toy safety with hand to mouth infant behaviors, inquisitiveness, and lack of cognitive understanding of consequences
- Provide infant stimulation and counsel parents/caregivers on means to stimulate learning
- Nurses need to consider the cultural and spiritual aspects that may affect developmental care

Priority Medications

- Discuss the need for multivitamins with health care provider
- Determine the need for iron supplementation (after 6 months, may get iron from solids/cereals)
- Determine the need for Vitamin D
- Supplemental fluoride or access to fluoridated water
- Check recommendations for immunizations during the infant period (see www.aap.org)

Next Gen Clinical Judgment

A nurse assists with the insertion of an intravenous device in a 9-month old infant:

1. What challenges should the nurse anticipate in restraining the infant during this procedure?
2. What impact will the infant's developmental age have on their response to this procedure?
3. What impact will the infant's health status have on their response to this procedure?
4. How can the nurse assist parents or caregivers to console an infant after a painful procedure?

Reinforcement of Priority Teaching

- Anticipatory guidance for infant care with caregivers
  - Car seats and safe transporting of infants. Children less than two should be in a rear-facing car seat in the back seat. Provide access to information about state laws concerning passenger safety
  - Safety as infants become more mobile
  - Assist parents to choose and work with childcare arrangements
  - Monitor for achievement of developmentally appropriate milestones
- For infants with health issues and developmental delay, ensure early intervention into services and use of the multidisciplinary team to optimize development
- Encourage parents to post Poison Control Center Number

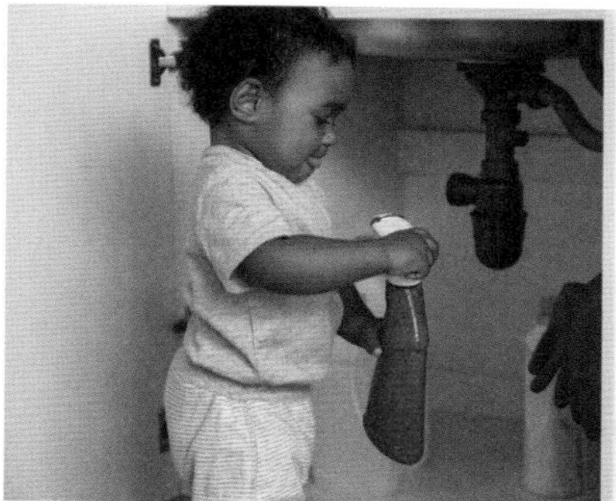

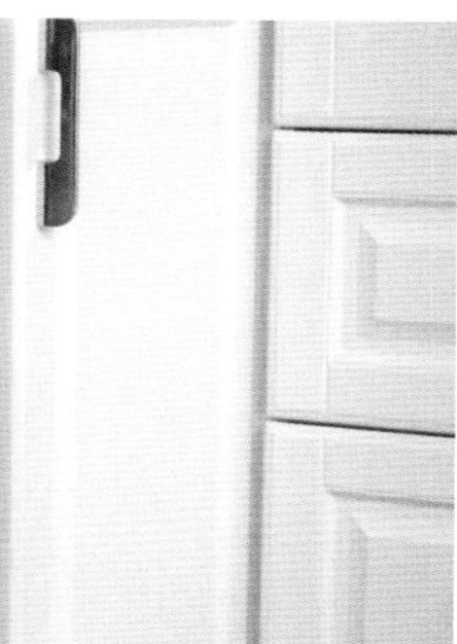

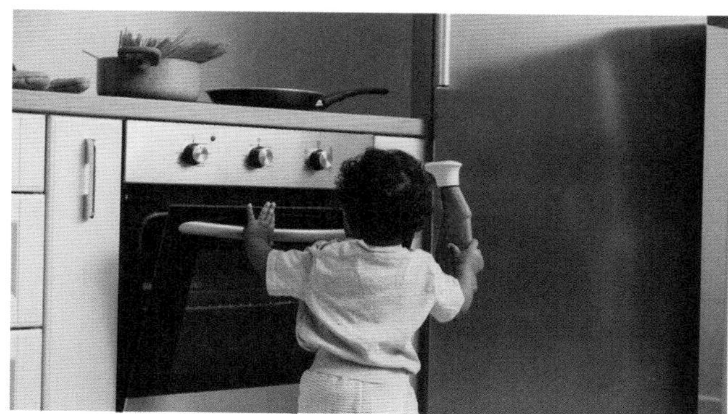

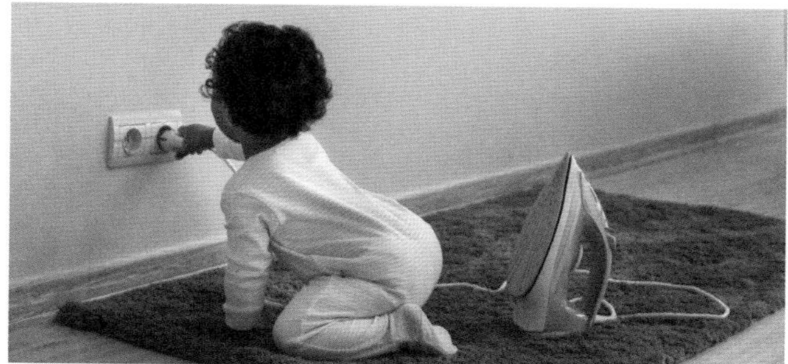

Image 18-1: What safety risks can you identify with the infants in these images? What prevention strategies can you identify? How can nurses assist parents and caregivers to keep their children safe and free from injury?

Pathophysiology/Description

- Includes ages 12 to 36 months
- Stage is characterized by growing mobility, independence, and learning

Priority Data Collection or Cues

- Determine vital signs including toddler ranges (heart rate 80-120 bpm, respirations 20-30 bpm, blood pressures 92/55 mmHg) temp. approximately 97.5-98.6°F axillary
- Monitor the client's achievement of developmental milestones in a variety of domains
    - Physical
        - Toddlers gain 4-6 kg/year
        - Body begins to thin-out as child becomes mobile
    - Motor
        - Gross motor development progresses such that toddlers learn to manage stairs, tricycles, running, and jumping
        - Fine motor skills typically progress to drawing circles and crosses, using blocks, using crayons, turning book pages, and turning doorknobs
    - Cognitive
        - Toddlers progress from sensorimotor period to pre-operational phase (Piaget)
        - Beginning reasoning skills based on own experiences
        - Begin to use symbols, imitate behaviors, and pretend
        - Enjoy completion of age-related tasks, beginning to learn chores and simple jobs
        - Beginning to master self-care, including feeding, dressing, and toileting
        - Begin to understand the past and the future
        - Are highly curious and "into everything." Need to provide safe supervision
    - Psychoemotional
        - Erikson's phase of autonomy versus shame and doubt. Lack of mastery of self-control/care may elicit feelings of shame and self-doubt
        - Learn self-control, willpower, and a sense of adequacy
        - Learn to increase independence in self-care including potty training
        - Often have negative behaviors (favorite word is "no") and may have temper tantrums
        - Can separate self from others, but can't empathize
        - Begin to assert self
        - Parents/caregivers are center of social circle
    - Language
        - Begin to use language to communicate
        - Usually have 10 words at 18 months to about 300 words at 24 months
        - Begin to use 2 words sentences
        - Understands language before able to use words to express needs
    - Play
        - Play moves from solitary to parallel where children play beside but not with others
        - Begin to have an imagination and participate in pretend play
        - Short attention span results in changing toys and activities often
    - Observe for potential child maltreatment including abuse and neglect

Priority Laboratory Tests/Diagnostics

- Lead screening is indicated for all children, especially those in old homes with lead-based paint or where the water supply may include unhealthy levels of lead
- The Denver II Developmental Screening test measures the gross motor, fine motor, adaptive/self-care, and social/language skills in children ages 1-6 years.Health screening and monitoring
- Length/height, weight, and head circumference all plotted on a growth chart

Priority Interventions or Actions

- Reinforce health education
    - Toddlers are at risk for injury due to their increased mobility and lack of judgment
    - Provide parents/caregivers with education about graded independence, dealing with negativism and temper tantrums, and addressing discipline
    - Guide parents through toilet training to include readiness for toilet training, the child recognizing they need to void or defecate, mobility skills, language skills to express personal needs, and consistency in process
    - Provide safety education about ingestions and poisoning, including household child-proofing, safe storage of harmful products, and child supervision. Discuss electrical, medication, stairway, toilet, pool, household cleaners, and other hazards
    - Address safe toys and age-appropriate play, including safe supervision
    - Nutrition
        - Toddlers may be "fussy" and go on "food jags"
        - Assist caregivers in providing a nutritious diet of grains, fruits, vegetables, dairy, and protein
        - Ensure table food is cut into small pieces to avoid choking and allow for self-feeding
        - Toddlers often go through physiological anorexia, if toddler refuses to eat, provide finger foods and nutritious snacks
        - Limit milk to 2-3 cups/day to ensure adequate appetite and prevent deficiencies of iron and other nutrients
        - Low-fat or skim milk not to be used until after 2 years of age
        - Dilute juices to prevent diarrhea and excessive intake of sugar

- Prepare parents for toddler's body self-exploration and toddler's tendency to touch their genitals, begin to discuss body parts using appropriate names and about body privacy

Priority Potential & Actual Complications

- Unintentional or intentional injury or illness
- Toddlers may be prone to poisoning, ingestions, lead poisoning, water accidents, and motor vehicle accidents (risk for unrestrained toddlers who may react violently to confinement)

Priority Nursing Implications

- For hospitalized toddlers, provide choices and convey a positive attitude toward child
  - Allow child to express protest and accept regressive behaviors
  - Provide favorite objects and activities that allow for mobility
  - Choose words carefully because toddlers take words very literally
  - Monitor for pain carefully, toddlers may react to pain, restraint, and frustration with aggressive responses
  - Toddlers are at risk for falls and require injury prevention care while hospitalized
  - Hospitalized toddlers fear loss of control, injury, and pain
  - Encourage parent/caregiver involvement in care and rooming in
- Encourage parents to see positive sides of toddler learning, including curiosity and exploration while providing safe supervision
- Nurses need to consider the cultural and spiritual aspects that may affect developmental care

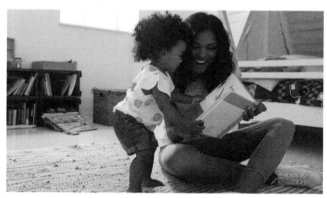

Image 18-2: Reading to toddlers assists with language, emotional, and cognitive development. Consider the answer to a parent who states: "I don't have to read to my child yet, she is only 18 months old. I'll start reading to her when she goes to school."

Priority Medications

- Determine the need for multivitamins and iron
- Check recommendations for immunizations during the toddler period (see www.aap.org)

Reinforcement of Priority Teaching

- Anticipatory guidance for toddler care with caregivers
  - Car seats and safe transporting of toddlers. Children less than two should be in a rear-facing car seat in the back seat. Children over two should be in a front facing car seat in the back seat. Provide access to state laws and encourage caregivers to consult car seat manufacturer recommendations regarding placement of children in car seats
  - Assist parents to deal with the issues associated with toddlerhood, including negativism, temper tantrums and use of "no" and "me do it"
  - Safety as toddlers become more mobile. This may include risks for poisoning/ingestions, falls, drowning (bath/pool), choking, and car safety
  - Assist parents to choose and work with childcare arrangements
  - Monitor for achievement of developmentally appropriate milestones
  - Encourage strategies that foster language skills
  - Reinforce the importance of reading to children on a daily basis
  - Ensure that family has ready access to Poison Control center number

Next Gen Clinical Judgment

A toddler undergoes surgery and will be in a hip spica cast for 4-6 months. The child is active and the parents are concerned about how to keep their child occupied and content while in the cast. List 4 suggestions for play, activities, and distraction that may assist the parents during this time of immobility.

1. ______________________________

2. ______________________________

3. ______________________________

4. ______________________________

 Pathophysiology/Description

- Ages 3-5 years

Priority Data Collection or Cues

- Determine vital signs preschool ranges (heart rate 70-110 bpm, respirations 16-22 bpm, blood pressures 95/57 mmHg), temp. approximately 97.5-98.6°F axillary
- Monitor clients for achieving developmental milestones in a variety of domains
    - Physical
        - Few physical changes in the preschool years
        - Preschoolers gain about 5 pounds/year and double birth length at four years
    - Motor
        - Develop mastery of body
        - Gross motor skills include jumping rope, skating, swimming, going up and down steps, skipping, and running; children able to build coordination skills
        - Increase in fine motor skills; skills include copying squares and crosses, scribbling, drawing letters or numbers, and ability to work with fine/small toys
    - Cognitive
        - Preoperational stage of development including prelogical thinking and understanding of the past/present/future. Thinking is concrete and egocentric
        - Preschool children learn to plan, categorize and classify
        - Children begin to learn to empathize and socialize with peers
        - Increase in understanding of cause and effect and reasoning. Preschool children are curious and frequently ask "Why?"
        - Increase in magical thinking and belief of personal role in illness, negative effects, and impacts on siblings/peers
        - Increase in fears of things they do not understand
        - High levels of energy may be manifested as episodes of anger or tantrums
    - Psychoemotional
        - Period of initiative versus guilt wherein children develop a sense of purpose and initiate activities. Children may over-anticipate their ability, do new activities, but may fail, leading to guilt
        - Develop new skills in making and keeping friends; child's world moves from the family to the neighborhood/community
        - Less negative in demeanor
        - Preschoolers often want to please adults and authority figures
        - Stressors may begin related to school, siblings, illness, moving, or other life changes. Mutilation anxiety (fear of pain and injury) begins
        - Regression is normal
    - Language
        - Shares thoughts, interacts, and communicates
        - Take words at their literal meaning, may misinterpret messages
        - Vocabulary contains 8000-14000 words
        - Preschool children ask lots of questions
    - Play
        - Social/associative play
        - Begin to demonstrate cooperative play behaviors
        - Develop imaginative play, pretending, and imaginary playmates
        - Pretend play very critical for dealing with stress and learning new skills
        - Like to build and create things
- Observe for potential child maltreatment including abuse and neglect

Priority Laboratory Tests/Diagnostics

- The Denver II Developmental Screening test measures the gross motor, fine motor, adaptive/self-care, and social/language skills in children ages 1-6 years
- Health screening and monitoring
- Height and weight plotted on a growth chart

Priority Interventions or Actions

- Reinforce health education
    - Potty training is completed, ensure the child is clean and reinforce hygienic toileting in preschool children
    - Dental health and hygiene habits begin, encourage children to brush and floss. Ensure routine dental examinations and care
    - Reinforce safe car seat use and need for continued car seat use. Children should be in the back seat. State laws differ about the use of booster seats. Provide access to information about state laws concerning passenger safety
    - As their world expands, encourage the child to try diversified foods. Preschoolers are known for food jags and frequent changing favorite and detested foods. Often focus on social aspects of eating and mealtime
    - Encourage water consumption
    - Prepare parents for child's body self-exploration and children's tendency to touch their genitals, begin to instruct on body parts using appropriate names and encourage preschooler to use those names, address about body privacy, introduce concepts of other gender, and safe and appropriate touching by others. Introduce concepts of safe touch and stranger safety
    - Preschool children may experience sleep problems, encourage the use of pre-sleep routines, nightlights, and security blankets or objects

Priority Potential & Actual Complications

- Unintentional or intentional injury or illness
- Preschoolers may be prone to water accidents, pedestrian/ bicycle, and motor vehicle accidents if not properly restrained

Priority Nursing Implications

- For hospitalized preschoolers
  - Magical thinking and fears make illness and injury particularly stressful during this time frame
  - Regression is a normal manifestation. May be unable to separate from parents
  - Fear bodily harm and pain
  - Fear invasive procedures and loss of control
  - Try to continue normal routines as much as possible and allow for self-care activities
  - Provide simple medical play using dolls, puppets, pictures, and harmless medical equipment. Adapt information to the child's level of understanding using simple words and concepts
  - Allow for play and diversional activities
  - Avoid invasive procedures as much as possible
  - Allow child to wear underwear and own clothes if possible, allow favorites toys and books to be part of child's life during hospitalization
  - Encourage parent/caregiver involvement in care and rooming in
- Reinforce instruction about strangers and personal body safety. Inform the child about the need to seek out assistance from a trusted adult
- Encourage swimming lessons and water safety
- Nurses need to consider the cultural and spiritual aspects that may affect developmental care

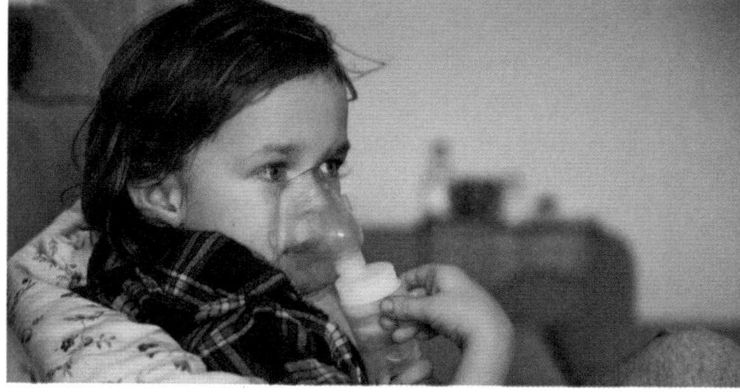

Image 18-3: This preschool child receives a bronchodilator via nebulizer when in respiratory distress.

What signs and symptoms would indicate the need for this medication?

How is a medication given via a nebulizer?

How should the nurse prepare a child of this age for this treatment?

How would the nurse know that the treatment was effective?

Priority Medications

- Consult health care provider about use of multivitamins
- Check recommendations for immunizations during the preschool period (see www.aap.org)

Reinforcement of Priority Teaching

- Recommend judicious use of television, computers, and video games
- Reinforce teaching with parents/caregivers about how to prepare child for the rigors and schedule of school
- Encourage creative arts, drawing, reading, and quiet play, in addition to time outdoors building skills in gross motor activities
- Encourage parents/caregivers to foster safe and independent self-care in their preschool child
- Ensure that parents/caregivers teach their child their full name, parents'/caregivers' names, phone number, address, and how to dial 911

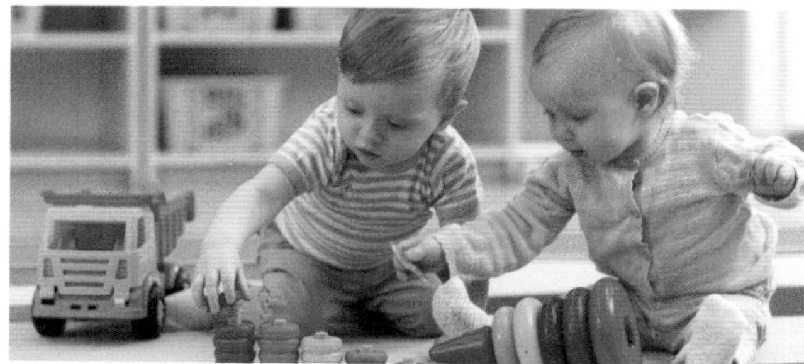

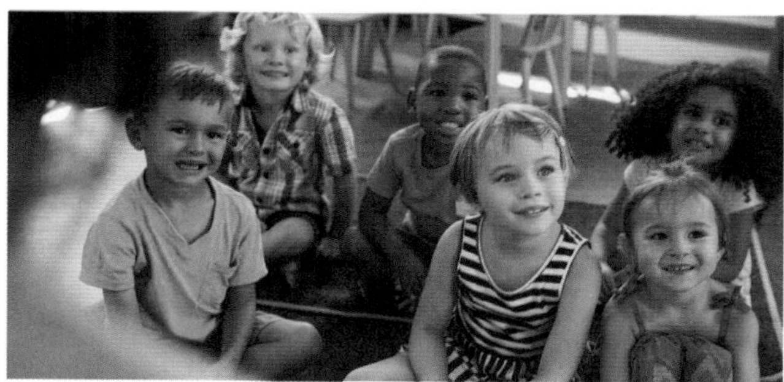

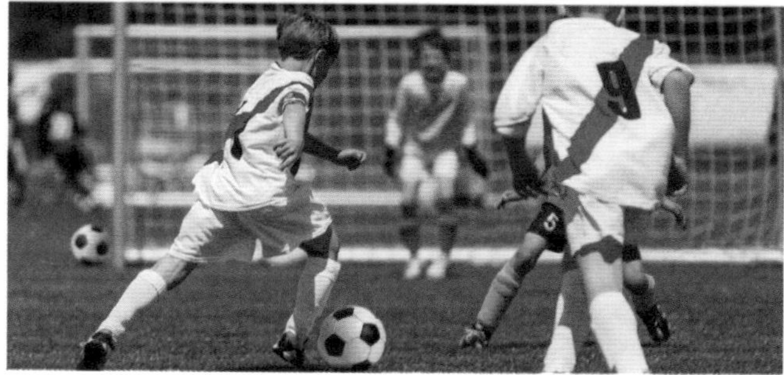

Image 18-4: Consider the children in each of these pictures. What age group do they portray? How should the describe the play for children of each age? How can nurses foster development in each age group through play?

Pathophysiology/Description

- Ages 6-12 years
- This is a period of rapid changes in skills, thoughts, and behaviors with expanded physical, psycho-emotional, social, and cognitive skills

Priority Data Collection or Cues

- Determine vital signs including school-age children ranges (heart rate 60-100 bpm, respirations 18-20 bpm, blood pressures 107/64 mmHg) temp. approximately 97.5-98.6°F axillary
- Monitor clients for achieving developmental milestones in a variety of domains
  - Physical
    - Period of slowed physical growth until the pre-puberty growth spurt
    - Gains about 4-7 pounds/year and grows about 2 inches/year. Girls tend to be taller and heavier than boys until puberty
  - Motor
    - Gross motor skills become increasingly graceful with running, jumping, balancing, throwing, and catching. Enjoy games and activities
    - Fine motor skills develop as children have more control over their wrists and fingers. Able to draw, paint, write, and manipulate computer games
    - Develop increased strength and endurance
  - Cognitive
    - In Piaget's stage of concrete operational thought. Children use logical thought and problem solving
    - May progress to formal operational thought with abstract reasoning at the end of the school-age period
    - Beginning to make decisions and accept responsibility
    - Learn to function within the rules and expectations of school and other settings. Able to attend to content, adjust to school routine, control activity, and control impulsivity. Increased concentration
    - Learn conservation of size, shape, and volume
    - Can categorize and put objects in series. Begin to collect and sort objects. Collections are valued possessions of school-age children
    - Observe for learning disabilities and differences and the potential for accommodations to aid in learning
  - Psychoemotional
    - The child's world becomes broadened to include friends and the community, church/places of worship, school, and neighborhood
    - Erikson's task of industry versus inferiority includes achieving competency, learning to learn and work, taking on tasks and mastering activities, ongoing development of self-esteem and sense of worth
    - Increasingly empathic, less egocentric, and able to see the perspectives of others
    - Desire to please adults and authority figures
    - Developing personal preferences to meet needs and independence in activities and routine. Still need guidance in making good choices
    - Peers become more important. Emphasis is on same-gender peers. Develop "best friends" and small groups. Increase in group identity as they near adolescence
  - Language
    - Rapid language acquisition
    - Learning to use the rules of grammar
    - Learning to understand jokes and meaning of content when out of context
  - Play
    - Play in small or large groups
    - Play is cooperative with rules. Breaking rules is reacted to with anger and frustration
    - Interest in competition and sports
- Observe for potential child maltreatment including abuse and neglect

Priority Laboratory Tests/Diagnostics

- Scoliosis screening in children 11-12 years (preteen screening)
- Health screening and monitoring
- Vision and hearing screening usually completed at school
- Height and weight measurement and calculation of body mass index (BMI)

Priority Interventions or Actions

- Reinforce health education
  - Provide instruction about safe car restraints including children 8-16 in a properly fitted seatbelt. Children less than 12 years of age should be in the back seat. Provide access to information about state laws concerning passenger safety
  - Reinforce bike, car, fire, and water safety
  - Reinforce sexuality education at an age appropriate level to include forms of sexual identity, sexual self-esteem, and about impending puberty with physical, psychoemotional, and social impacts. Prepare parents and caregivers for school-age children's sexual curiosity, using appropriate names, about body privacy, concepts of other gender, and safe and appropriate touching by others. Reinforce concepts of safe touch and stranger safety
  - Reinforce teaching about dental care and routine dental examinations
  - Begin focusing health education at the child as they assume greater levels of self- care

- Reinforce nutritious diet habits and drinking adequate water. Ensure that eating and exercise habits lay the foundation to avoid obesity later in life. Encourage new and different food
  - Begin to discuss peer pressure with child and parents/caregivers and explore family values and means to deal with pressure from friends, the media, and other sources
  - Encourage judicious use of television, computer, and video games; encourage active exercise, time outdoors, and sports

Priority Potential & Actual Complications

- Unintentional or intentional injury or illness
- School-age children are capable of self-care but still require the monitoring and supervision of a caring adult
- Beginning of risk behaviors that may result in accidents (pedestrian, car, bicycle, fires)
- Increased exposure to infections as world broadens

Priority Nursing Implications

- For hospitalized school-age children
  - May fear separation from parents/caregivers, stress may cause regressed behavior
  - May miss school, peers, and routine
  - Fear bodily injury, illness, and disability
  - Fear immobilization and restrictions
  - Respond well when provided choices whenever possible, provide limits on behaviors
  - Prepare for procedures using medical play, body diagrams, pictures, and movies
  - Provide privacy when warranted
  - Encourage visitation of peers, siblings, and pets
  - Encourage parent/caregiver involvement in care and rooming in
- School-age children are stressed about peers, parental expectations, school expectations, and self-care after school if they spend time alone (latch-key issues). Inform children how to use stress management techniques such as exercise, hobbies, music, care of pets, and other diversional activities
- Bullying and dealing with bullies are two areas prompting an increased focus by nurses and others working with school-age children
- Nurses need to consider the cultural and spiritual aspects that may affect developmental care

Priority Medications

- Consult health care provider about use of multivitamins
- Human papilloma vaccine recommended in girls ages 11-12, boys ages 9-26 (may be earlier in cases of sexual abuse)
- Check recommendations for immunizations during the school-age period (see www.aap.org)

Reinforcement of Priority Teaching

- School-age children are highly responsive to environmental stimuli and enrichment. Reinforce teaching with parents/caregivers to provide diversified experiences during this period
- School age children should know how to call 911 if needed

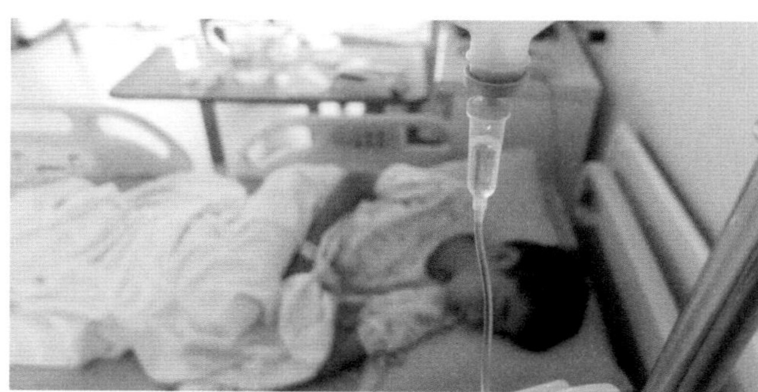

Image 18-5: Boredom is one of the leading stressors of school-age children when hospitalized. List several diversional activities that the nurse may recommend for a school-age child who is in the hospital.

1. ______________________________
2. ______________________________
3. ______________________________
4. ______________________________

Next Gen Clinical Judgment

A nurse cares for a client who is in the 6th grade and uses a wheelchair for movement. The child has a history of myelomeningocele with paraplegia.

- What skin integrity issues should the nurse address?
- How would the nurse know if the child has grown out of the current wheelchair?
- What body mechanics principles should the nurse consider to avoid personal injury when transferring the client from the bed to the wheelchair? The wheelchair to the car?
- How can the nurse ensure that the client gets enough exercise and range of motion when using a wheelchair?
- What safety issues should the nurse address?
- How can the nurse foster vicarious play with a child who is wheelchair-bound?
- How should the nurse foster optimal growth and development in children with physical disabilities?

Pathophysiology/Description

- Ages 13-20 years
- Begins around puberty, when reproduction is possible
- Often a healthy period, with teens needing encouragement to obtain physical examinations and routine care

Priority Data Collection or Cues

- Determine vital signs including adolescent ranges (heart rate 55-90 bpm, respirations 12-20 bpm, blood pressure 121/70 mmHg) temp. approximately 97.5-98.6°F axillary
- Monitor clients for achieving developmental milestones in a variety of domains
  - Physical
    - During pre-pubertal growth spurt, teens may grow 4-12 inches and gain 15-65 pounds
    - Period of increased growth, gender specific changes, secondary sexual organ development and changes, and changes in the distribution of fat and muscle
    - Adolescents begin to have acne and body odor
    - Onset of secondary sexual characteristics and menstruation begins
  - Motor
    - Continue to develop fine and gross motor skills
    - Puberty may be a period of awkwardness
    - Determine personal talents in motor areas
    - Increasing strength and endurance
  - Cognitive
    - Able to engage in future-oriented, deductive reasoning
    - Can base new knowledge on past experiences
    - Engages in abstract, formal operations according to Piaget characterized by logical thinking and maturing problem solving skills. Able to determine and rank options
    - The developing prefrontal cortex provides cognitive controls when faced with risk, temptation, impulsiveness, and new sensations or stimuli
    - Standardized screening tools measure intelligence and cognitive functioning
    - Need opportunities for independent decision-making to build skills
    - Observe for learning disabilities and differences and the potential for accommodations to aid in learning
  - Psychoemotional
    - Erikson identified as identity versus role confusion where teens develop a sense of personal identity. Inability to master this task may lead to decreased self-esteem/decreased self-awareness, and frustration or depression related to role confusion
    - Become independent from parents/family and depend more on peers
    - Preoccupied with body and body image, imagine everyone is looking at them with a critical eye
    - Developing a sexual and gender identity, and family, health, and group identity
    - Usually skilled in empathy though may regress when stressed
    - May no longer be focused on pleasing adults or adhering to the rules of authority
  - Language
    - Vocabulary continues to develop and expand
    - Language is often regionalized or based on local word choice or syntax, peer, and media influences
    - Beginning to articulate thoughts and feelings to family, teachers, peers, and others
    - Building personal communication skills and style
  - Play
    - Building talents and interests into hobbies
    - Games and athletics are common forms of play, friends are key in age-appropriate play and activities
    - May begin to work outside the home for money
    - Importance of chores, value of money, and budgeting should be explored with adolescents
    - May need assistance to schedule time for diversional activities along with routine or scheduled ones
- Observe for potential child maltreatment including abuse and neglect, intimate partner violence, and other threats to home safety

Priority Laboratory Tests/Diagnostics

- Standardized nutrition screening, including body mass index
- Testing for sexually transmitted diseases in sexually active teens
- Screen for depression, anxiety, or other mental health issues, including risk for suicide (see Priority Exemplars)
- Screen for eating disorders (see Priority Exemplar)
- Reinforce instruction about self-breast and self-testicular exams

Priority Interventions or Actions

- Reinforce health education
  - Inform parents and teens about the changes and characteristics inherent of adolescence
  - Address mental health during the teen years and importance of early detection and intervention. Determine risk for suicide and make immediate referrals. Be attuned to such signs of suicide as absenteeism, social withdrawal, verbalization of suicidal ideations, and changes in sleep or eating patterns. Directly ask about ideas, methods, or intent of self-harm
  - Reinforce and support education related to car safety/seatbelts, avoiding risk behaviors, and the hazards of tobacco, alcohol, and illicit drugs

- Reinforce sexual education including the pleasures and responsibilities associated with sexual activity, understanding consent, prevention of sexually transmitted diseases, and contraception
  - Reinforce instruction on risk reduction and harm reduction related to substances, smoking, driving, activities, swimming, firearms, biking, and other threats to safety
  - Discuss with teens and parents about privacy and confidentiality
  - Address the stressors associated with adolescence (peers, school, etc.) and coping mechanisms. Identify less constructive coping methods (cutting, substances) and refer or address as needed while exploring healthy coping mechanisms
  - Encourage teens to sleep about eight hours per night. Most teens do not get enough sleep
  - Reinforce instructions on the importance of an adequate diet. Most teens lack calcium, zinc, iron, folic acid, and protein in their usual diet. Advise teens to avoid empty calories and the need for high protein/moderate carbohydrate food choices
- Determine teen's receptivity to teaching and learning

Priority Potential & Actual Complications

- Adolescents who are not provided with opportunities to make and learn from mistakes may remain dependent on adults in their world
- High-risk behaviors, related to dopamine surges and desire for risk, may lead to accidents or injury
- Unintentional or intentional illness or injuries
- Injuries related to substance use, motor vehicles, and other high-risk behaviors
- Homicide and suicide are two common causes of mortality in teens

Priority Nursing Implications

- The hospitalized adolescent
  - May vacillate between dependence on and independence from parents
  - May miss peers and be concerned about missing school
  - Fear being different from peers
  - May not admit to being fearful of procedures or healthcare
  - May respond with anger, withdrawal, or uncooperativeness
  - May seek help and then reject it
  - Nurses should provide complete explanations and support positive coping
  - Allow clients to wear their own clothes, make some choices in care, provide an appropriate warning prior to treatments, and allow favorite foods
  - Ensure privacy and confidentiality are respected. This may cause difficulty with parents or caregivers. Ensure conditional confidentiality, wherein one must divulge any information that reflects harm of self or others. Explore state laws related to minors, emancipated minors, and mature minors and their implications for consent, confidentiality, and care
  - Provide books, apps, websites, and videos as appropriate to provide health education
  - Encourage parent/caregiver involvement in care and determine teens' need for parent/caregiver rooming in
- Nurses may encounter teens who are pregnant or parenting. Teens who have prenatal care, receive adequate nutrition, and avoid risk behaviors have the capacity to have healthy pregnancies. Teen parents may require health supervision, psychosocial support, and assistance with the logistics of parenting, such as childcare and managing school and children
- Bullying and dealing with bullies are two areas prompting an increased focus by nurses and others working with teens
- Peers are often a positive force in teens' lives. Consider using peer or group focused interventions when working with teens
- There is growing concern that teens may be homeless, living in poverty, lack access to healthcare, or are subjected to intimate partner violence or human trafficking
- School Based Health Centers provide access to teen-friendly, convenient, low/no cost, and comprehensive healthcare
- Nurses need to consider the cultural and spiritual aspects that may affect developmental care

Priority Medications

- Human papilloma vaccine if not previously vaccinated; may be given to girls 13-26 and boys 9-26 (see school age Priority Exemplar)
- Consult health care provider about use of multivitamins
- Check recommendations for immunizations during the adolescent period (see www.aap.org)

Reinforcement of Priority Teaching

- Adolescents may begin to self-advocate and manage their healthcare needs, with the support of parents, caregivers, and health care providers
- Previously considered only a period of stress and conflict, adolescence is a time to gain knowledge and skills, learn about self, and learn to manage in the world

Clinical Hint

Nurses should carefully observe each teen for developmental age and abilities. Although they may be the physical size of adults, teens' cognitive and emotional capacities are not yet fully developed.

Pathophysiology/Description

- 18-25-year-old individuals comprise a new category of emerging adults. This is a newly defined category, wherein individuals are increasingly independent of parental control but may be dependent on them for support and financial assistance
- Young adult defined as 18-35 years
- Middle adult defined as 36-64 years
- This cohort of individuals is more racially/ethnically diverse than ever before
- This is a growing cohort as the life expectancy increases

Priority Data Collection or Cues

- Determine vital signs including adult ranges (heart rate 55-90 bpm, respirations 12-18 bpm, blood pressures 128/80 mmHg) temp. approximately 97.5-98.6°F axillary. Need to know client baseline vital signs
- Monitor clients for achieving developmental milestones in a variety of domains
    - Physical
        - Obtain height, weight, and body mass index
        - Completes physical growth around 20 years of age (except for childbearing and breastfeeding women)
        - Changes in weight associated with nutrition and lifestyle issues
        - Physical strength peaks in the young adult years
        - Body function may begin to decline in the middle adult years
        - Tend to be active during the adult years with few illnesses; chronic and other illnesses increase in incidence as adults age
        - Changes in appearance to include wrinkling of skin, graying of hair, decreased hearing and visual acuity, and body composition
        - Posture may change
    - Motor
        - Fine and gross motor skills are mature and may change with decreased muscle mass, decreased bone strength, and increase in fat deposits
        - Adulthood is a time to cultivate hobbies and talents and use fine and gross motor skills (sports, golf, hobbies, gardening, crafts, and walking, among others)
    - Cognitive
        - Ability to reason using formal operations, decision-making is stable, although adults may still make poor choices
        - Critical thinking improves throughout the adult years with experience and increased contextual thinking
        - Flexibility with life changes, responses to aging, and cognitive function associated with temperament and personality characteristics
        - Education, life experiences, and occupation impact thinking skills
    - Psychoemotional
        - Young adults in Erikson's stage of intimacy versus isolation, individuals develop the ability to love and commit one's self; establish intimate bonds of love and friendship. Lack of achievement may lead to anger, bitterness, and isolation
        - Middle adults are in Erikson's stage of generativity versus stagnation wherein efforts are devoted to life goals for family, career, and community; giving care to others is a priority. Focus is on passing on qualities and assets to the next generation and providing support to the previous generation. Failure to meet the goals of this stage may lead to lack of personal growth and egocentricity
        - Roles have changed as male and female roles in intimate relationships, parenting, and gender responsibilities/expectations, have changed
        - Adult years are ones of personal and career achievement, as adults deal with biological changes of the body
        - Described as the "sandwich generation" in the caring of and balancing of the needs of aging parents and children and/or grandchildren
        - Changes in social norms related to marriage, parenting, and aging may impact adult development; influenced also by social media, technology, and current social issues
        - In these years adults address and resolve social and personal tasks, from ages 23-28, adults may focus on self-perception and intimacy, ages 29-34 years may focus on achievement and mastery, and ages 35-43 may consider the quality of their life and their relationships
        - Mid-life crises may occur in career, marriage, parenting, and lifestyles
        - Adults deal with changes in career, mobility, sexual performance, family and marital transitions, and depression and anxiety
    - Language
        - Adults are generally articulate
        - May require support with local/regional language
        - May speak better than able to read and illiteracy continues to persist in modern society
    - Play
        - Usually a financially stable period, but current economic conditions may jeopardize this stability
        - Time for building hobbies and diversional activities
    - Ask about family history of disease as it may impact personal disease trajectory
    - Determine functional ability as one grows older and determine ability to care for self and others
    - Monitor for exposure to occupational and environmental hazards
    - Discuss life satisfaction, hobbies, interests, habits (sleep, diet, exercise, sexual activity, alcohol, cigarettes, caffeine, substances, home, and pets)
    - Ask about personal safety, violence in the home, and intimate partner violence

Priority Laboratory Tests/Diagnostics

- Screen using self-breast and self-testicular exams
- Screen for hypertension, hypercholesterolemia, blood glucose levels, and conduct genetic screening
- Screen for drug, alcohol, and nicotine use
- Screen for sexually transmitted infections
- Screen for exposure to occupational or environmental factors
- Screen for eating disorders
- Conduct mammograms (annually after age 40 years), colonoscopies (every 10 years after age 45), and other screenings as recommended

Priority Interventions or Actions

- Reinforce health education
    - Consider lifestyle enhancements including diet, exercise, healthy sleep, balancing stress, smoking, risky and under-the-influence driving, binge drinking, use of seatbelts, sun safety, age related changes, and healthy stress management
    - Reinforce sexual health education to promote healthy sexual behaviors, contraception, protection, consent, sexual pleasure and responsibilities, and the psychodynamic aspects of sexual activity. Also address pregnancy, birth, and childbearing (see Chapter 5)
    - Provide support during the perimenopausal period in women (decreased menses, sleep disturbances, weight changes, hot flashes, and mood changes) and the climacteric period in men (less rigid erections, fatigue, mood changes, longer refractory periods between erections)
    - Identify modifiable risk factors and reinforce information to assist with lifestyle change
- Provide assistance with minor or chronic health issues (see appropriate Priority Exemplars)
- Assist clients to deal with unplanned pregnancy or infertility
- Encourage adequate sleep and encourage use of sleep hygiene interventions
- Ensure that adults are able to deal with life stresses, including family and job stressors

Priority Potential & Actual Complications

- Unintentional or intentional injury or illness
- Accidental injury including motor vehicle accidents, suicide, and homicide
- Potential for intimate partner violence, including physical, verbal and emotional aspects

Priority Nursing Implications

- Many young adults are healthy and active, they tend to postpone health seeking and ignore symptoms. As adults age, they may be more inclined to seek care
- Nurses may be involved in encouraging preconception health (those behaviors that enhance the positive outcomes of pregnancies)
- Nurses need to consider the cultural and spiritual aspects that may affect developmental care

Priority Medications

- Folic acid during the preconception years to prevent neural tube defects in offspring
- Travel immunizations to selected areas
- Multivitamins to enhance nutrition
- Calcium and Vitamin D supplements to prevent osteoporosis

Reinforcement of Priority Teaching

- Establish internal and external support systems to assist them into the older adult years
- Determine client's ability to learn and grow and desire to adhere to recommendations of a healthy lifestyle
- Observe for health literacy and ability to understand health instruction and recommendations

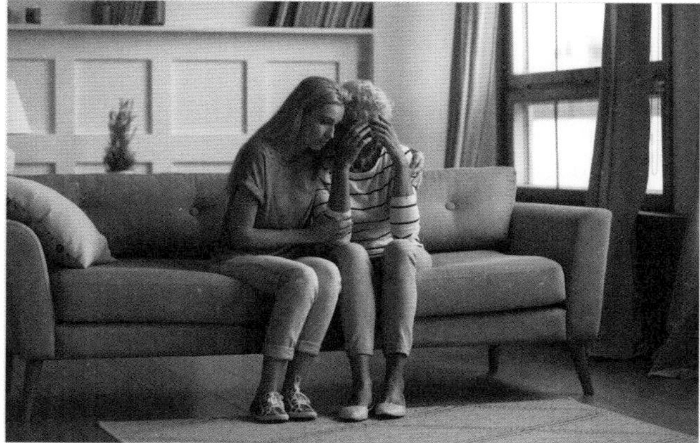

Image 18-6: A nurse provides home-based care for a woman and her 96-year-old mother. The woman and mother wish to keep the mother in the home despite her progressive dementia, wandering, and poor judgment.

1. *What community resources will assist the clients to attain their wish?*
2. *What safety hazards confront the mother and how can the house be adapted to prevent injury?*
3. *What respite services may also provide support for this family?*
4. *What developmental tasks confront the woman and the mother?*

Pathophysiology/Description

- Young-old adult ages 65-75 years
- Middle-old adult 76-85 years
- Old-old adult over 85 years
- High degree of variability in how each individual ages
- Increasing percentages of the population are older adults, increasing diversity of this cohort
- Most older adults live in non-institutional settings, or at home, despite common misperceptions

Priority Data Collection or Cues

- Recognize that a comprehensive collection of data of an older adult may take a long time and require more detail as a person ages
- Determine vital signs including older adult ranges (heart rate 55-90 bpm, respirations 12-18 bpm, blood pressures 130/80 mmHg) temp. approximately 97.5-98.6°F axillary. Need to know client baseline vital signs
- Monitor clients for achieving developmental milestones in a variety of domains
    - Physical
        - Obtain weight and height, with the knowledge that height will decrease, and body mass index will decrease
        - Changes include loss of pigment and wrinkling of skin, slowed reflexes, decreased balance, decreased short-term memory, decreased muscle mass, brittle bones, changes in gait, decreased cardiac output, decreased exercise tolerance, decreased pulmonary function, suppressed cough, decreased immune function, decreased need for calories, decreased thirst, constipation, dehydration, decreased glucose tolerance, decreased metabolic rate, decreased continence and bladder capacity, and decreased visual/hearing acuity, among other changes
        - Observe for impact of changes in hearing and vision. Changes in taste cause older adults to want salt and sweets. Changes in smell and taste hamper appetite
    - Motor
        - May deteriorate with changes in muscle tone, strength, bone structure, and balance
        - Tremors, arthritis, stiffness, or pain may change fine motor abilities
        - Changes in visual acuity may alter fine motor abilities
    - Cognitive
        - Monitor level of consciousness and orientation
        - Confusion is often related to physical illness, including urinary tract infections
        - Observe for depression, delirium, and dementia (See Priority Exemplars)
        - Observe for sudden changes in neurological status or functional/cognitive status; notify a registered nurse of changes in status
    - Psychoemotional
        - Erikson's period of integrity versus despair, when one looks back over one's life, accepts meaning out of life, and finds integrity and fulfillment or becomes sad and full of despair
        - Psychological adjustment to deterioration and threats to independent living
        - Dealing with loss of income and loss of skills
        - Changes in role function
        - Coping with loss (spouse, friends, job, body image, functioning), depression, grief, potential for suicide, and isolation/loneliness
        - Changes in memory
            - Fluid knowledge is acquired recently and may be forgotten
            - Crystallized knowledge is learned long ago and often remembered by older adults
    - Language
        - Remain articulate
        - Language may be hampered by hearing impairment
    - Play/work/functional abilities
        - ADLs (Activities of daily living) including hygiene, self-feeding, moving, and meeting personal needs
        - IADLs (Instrumental activities of daily living) including procuring and preparing food, shopping, paying bills, and talking via the phone
- Ask about health history, genetic history, and for co-morbidities
- Monitor for pain and impact of pain on functional abilities
- Discuss lifestyle and habits, including alcohol, cigarettes, diet, exercise, drugs, sleep, and stress management

Priority Laboratory Tests/Diagnostics

- Monitor renal, hepatic, and cardiac function
- Monitor serum calcium levels
- Monitor serum albumin levels to determine nutritional status
- Screen for hypertension, depression, changes in vision or hearing acuity, skin changes, and other health alterations
- Conduct mammograms (annually after age 40 years), colonoscopies (every 10 years after age 45), and other screenings as recommended

Priority Interventions or Actions

- Goals are to stabilize chronic conditions, promote health, and promote independence
- Reinforce health education as individuals adjust to changes of aging
    - Reinforce teaching about dental health and means to maintain teeth or substitutes

- Counsel about proper weight, exercise, low-fat diet, moderate alcohol use, smoking cessation, stress management, and handwashing
  - Provide nutrition counseling to include small, frequent feedings. Older adults often eat most for breakfast and appetite decreases throughout the day
  - Reinforce sleep hygiene interventions because older adults tend to experience sleep disturbances; older adults frequently sleep during day, making nighttime sleep difficult; older adults require moderate levels of sleep and rest
  - For clients with incontinence, reinforce instruction on hygiene, protection, and Kegel exercises
  - Assist clients to deal with constipation including fluids, fiber, exercise, and laxatives. Some clients experience diarrhea, encourage fluids and analyze diet
  - Assist client to deal with changes in housing, social situation, sexuality, grieving, and life transitions
- With decreased thirst, encourage adequate fluid intake except at night when trips to the bathroom may precipitate falls
- Provide opportunities for reality orientation, validation, and reminiscence
- Reinforce instructions as clients are able to manage and comprehend information

Priority Potential & Actual Complications

- Unintentional or intentional injury or illness
- Elder abuse (monitor and refer/manage related to domestic, institutional or self) emotional financial, physical, verbal, financial, or sexual abuse or neglect or abandonment
- Older adults are highly prone to infections related to suppressed immune systems
- At risk for dehydration and clients may become malnourished. Dehydration is a greater concern
- Social isolation, despair, unresolved pain, and other sorrows may drive older adults to suicide
- Multiple co-morbidities may tax the client's ability to live a quality life

Priority Nursing Implications

- Hospitalized older adults
  - Protect from hospital-acquired infections and falls, determine level of continence, skin for breakdown, mobility issues, and for poor nutrition/hydration
  - Provide favorite foods and fluids and use restraints sparingly
  - Round hourly for observations, toileting, and meeting client needs
  - Encourage aseptic technique and handwashing, use invasive procedures only when needed
- Increased incidence of falls related to physical and other factors
- Nurses need to consider the cultural and spiritual aspects that may affect developmental care
- Consider ageism and personal bias toward older adults as it impacts care

Priority Medications

- Monitor older adult medications and for polypharmacy, medication errors, interactions, side effects, non-compliance, use of over-the-counter medications, and use of complementary or alternative medications
- Observe effects and use lower dosages, understanding the potential for accumulation and toxicity
- Monitor for changes in neurological status as it may relate to medications
- Immunizations to include influenza, shingles, tetanus, diphtheria, pertussis (if around young children), and pneumococcal disease. Older adults may need boosters of selected immunizations if titers are not adequate
- Consider the use of probiotics to regulate bowel function

Reinforcement of Priority Teaching

- Safety aspects for clients with decreased cognitive function
- Home safety including lighting, limiting of physical obstacles, moving of throw rugs, limit use of heat therapies such as heating pads, easy access to phone, home set up for current living needs and desires, and ability to adapt home to physical limitations
- Case management to ensure safe and adequate home environment, access to resources, and healthcare surveillance

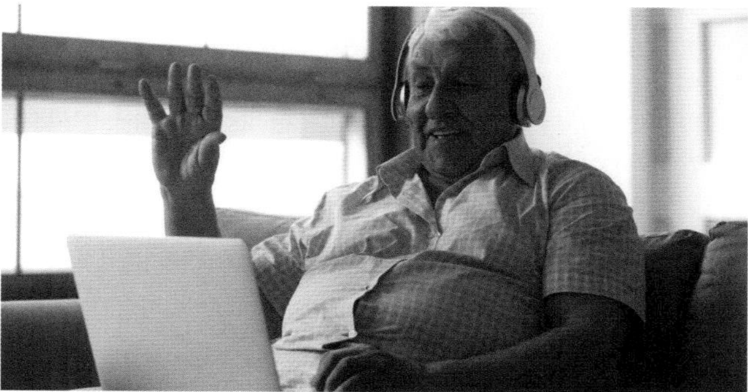

Image 18-7: How might technology address social isolation, mobility issues, learning, and connectedness with older adults?

What barriers might older adults confront when learning to use technology to communicate with others?

How might a nurse address these barriers?

How could telehealth assist older adults in accessing healthcare services?

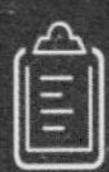

NurseThink® Quiz Questions

1. **The nurse reviews the proper introduction of solid foods with a client's parents. Which food does the nurse encourage as the most appropriate first food for the infant?**
   a. Rice infant cereal.
   b. Citrus fruits.
   c. Eggs.
   d. Meats.

2. **The nurse addresses ways the client can protect their 3-month-old infant from injury. What does the nurse include in this conversation?**
   a. Prop the bottle if not holding during feeding.
   b. Do not use the microwave to warm bottles.
   c. Shake powder onto perineum only.
   d. Allow the infant to sleep in the bed with you.

3. **The parent of a toddler asks the nurse about proper nutrition for their child. The nurse explains each food group and indicates the number of daily servings the toddler should be eating. Place the food types in order from most to least number of daily servings that a toddler should be eating.**
   a. Meat.
   b. Fruit.
   c. Milk.
   d. Bread.
   e. Vegetables.

4. **The nurse reinforces education with the parent of a toddler on choking prevention. Which food does the nurse emphasize needs to be avoided for their child?**
   a. Popcorn.
   b. Macaroni and cheese.
   c. Bananas.
   d. Hot dogs cut lengthwise.

5. **The nurse participates in a community education fair, focusing on the proper use of vehicle restraints to prevent injury in children. Which example does the nurse give of a child who requires a safety seat?**
   a. 9-year-old.
   b. Child is 5 feet tall.
   c. Child weighs 65 pounds.
   d. 3-year-old.

6. **The nurse speaks with the parents of a preschooler about ways to prevent injury. What recommendation does the nurse include in this discussion?**
   a. Teach their child about hazards.
   b. Use safety devices to prevent injury in the house.
   c. Pad furniture in case of falls.
   d. Keep cleaning supplies in lower cabinets.

7. **Which child is more likely to have awakened from a night terror versus a nightmare?**
   a. 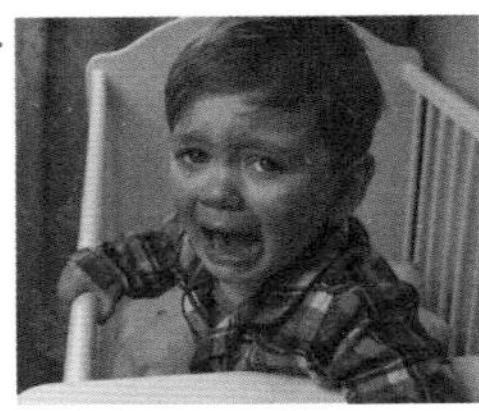
   b. 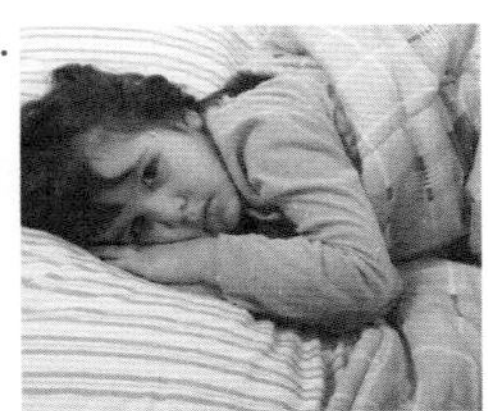

8. **The school nurse provides information to parents on the proper care of their preschooler's dental hygiene. What does the nurse include in this education? *Select all that apply.***
   a. Dental check-ups every 6-12 months.
   b. Avoid flossing until older.
   c. Discontinue fluoride supplements in this age group.
   d. Brush teeth twice daily.
   e. Increase sugars in the diet.

9. **The school nurse evaluates a client brought into the office from their third-grade class. Which reported symptom indicates the possible need for specialized treatment of continued stress?**
   a. Fatigue.
   b. Weight gain.
   c. Bed-wetting.
   d. Dizziness.

10. **The nurse collects information from the parent of a 9-year-old client. Which reported behavior is cause for concern in this client?**
    a. The client sucks their thumb.
    b. The client prefers to sit on the floor while doing homework.
    c. The client tends to procrastinate on school work.
    d. The client is well-behaved most of the time.

11. **A child playing on the school playground falls and has their tooth avulsed. The off-duty nurse is picking their child up from school and is requested to assist. Place in order the emergency treatment for an avulsed tooth.**
    a. Rinse gently with water if dirty.
    b. Recover tooth.
    c. Insert tooth in socket or place in cup of cold milk or under child's tongue.
    d. Hold tooth by the crown; do not touch the root.
    e. Transport the child to a dentist immediately.

12. **The nurse cares for an adolescent client and reviews education regarding injury prevention. Which education does the nurse include for the client and their parents? *Select all that apply.***
    a. Avoid the use of medications not prescribed to them.
    b. Wear restraints when driving.
    c. Wear a helmet in contact sports.
    d. Avoid or minimize the use of kitchen cooking appliances.
    e. Drive no more than five miles per hour over the speed limit.

13. **Which activity places the adolescent at the highest risk for serious or fatal injury?**

a. 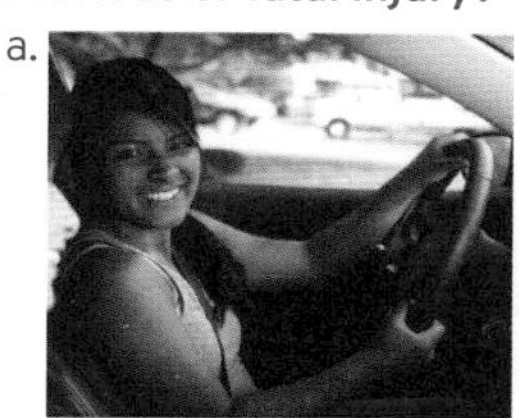

b. 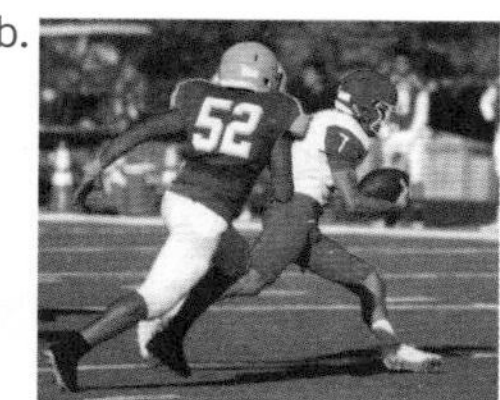

c. 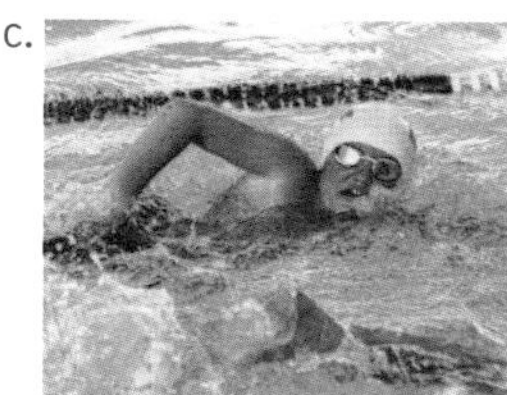

d. 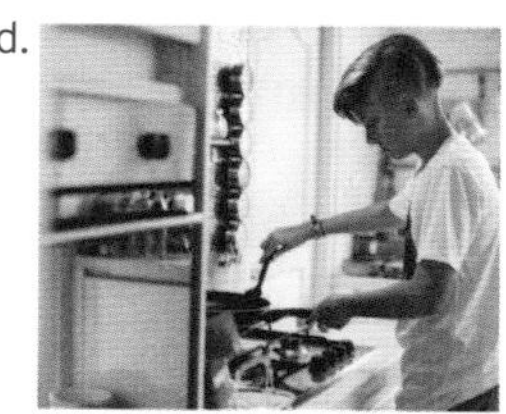

14. **The nurse utilizes screening protocols for an adolescent client. What screening does the nurse not include for this client?**
    a. Sexual transmitted infection screening.
    b. Scoliosis screening.
    c. Hearing and vision screening.
    d. Autism screening.

15. **The nurse discusses infection prevention with an adolescent client. Which priority information does the nurse include for a client in this age range?**
    a. Dental hygiene practices.
    b. Proper bathing practices.
    c. Using a qualified professional for piercings.
    d. Avoiding condom use.

16. **The nurse provides information about injury prevention to a young adult client. What does the nurse include as a priority instruction?**
    a. Avoidance of mixing alcohol with other drugs.
    b. Swimming safety.
    c. Locking cleaning supplies in an upper cabinet.
    d. Removal of fall risks around the house.

17. **The nurse screens an adult client for depression. Which symptoms does the nurse include as indicative of a positive screening? *Select all that apply.***
    a. Loss of interest in things.
    b. Irritability.
    c. Change in eating habits.
    d. Change in sleeping habits.
    e. Lack of concentration.

18. **The nurse cares for an older adult client who has had several falls the previous night. After being quiet most of the shift, the client is now screaming and attempting to get out of bed. What is the nurse's first action?**
    a. Identify potential causes of the client's behavior.
    b. Get a prescription for restraints to prevent another fall.
    c. Medicate with prescribed lorazepam IV to sedate the client.
    d. This is expected older adult behavior and should just be monitored.

19. **The home health nurse collects data in the home of an older adult client. Which of the findings is a fall hazard?**

a. 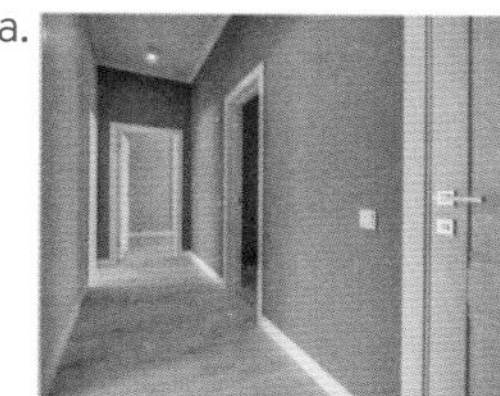

b. 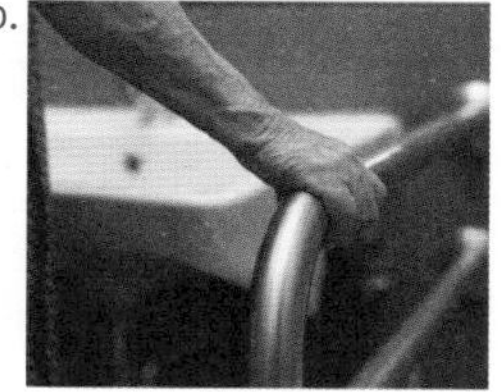

c. 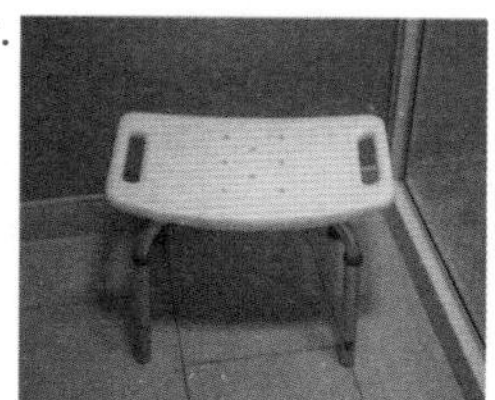

d. 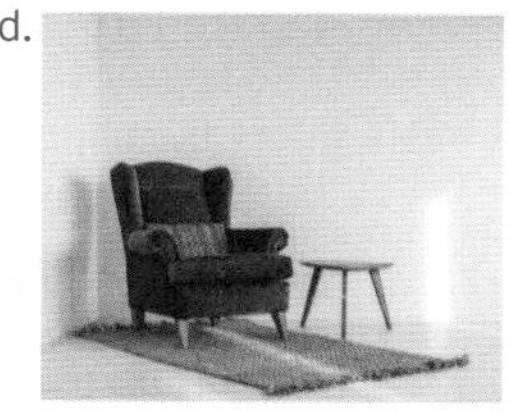

20. **The nurse prepares a client for discharge and reviews their medication prescriptions. Which prescription does the nurse clarify with the provider?**

HEALTH CARE PROVIDER PRESCRIPTIONS	
June 7	1. Lisinopril 10 mg PO daily 2. Amitriptyline 100 mg PO daily 3. Metoprolol 50 mg PO daily 4. Sertraline 200 mg PO daily

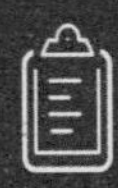

NurseThink® Quiz Answers

1. **The nurse reviews the proper introduction of solid foods with a client's parents. Which food does the nurse encourage as the most appropriate first food for the infant?**
   a. Rice infant cereal.
   b. Citrus fruits.
   c. Eggs.
   d. Meats.

   Topic/Concept: Health Promotion **Subtopic:** Infants **Bloom's Taxonomy:** Applying **Clinical Problem-Solving Process:** Planning **NCLEX-PN®:** Coordinated Care **QSEN:** Teamwork and Collaboration **CJMM:** Generate Solutions

   Rationale: Due to the higher chance of allergy formation, eggs, meats, and citrus fruits are generally reserved for introduction later in the process, with milder things like vegetables and grains introduced earlier on. Solid foods should not be introduced until after six months of age when their GI tract is more mature and less likely to develop an allergy.

   THIN Thinking: *Clinical Problem-Solving Process* – Proper diet in infancy has been tied to many long-term health effects for children, so proper dietary practices for infants can have far-reaching consequences. The nurse must inform new parents the importance of a proper diet and what that consists of for their infant.

2. **The nurse addresses ways the client can protect their 3-month-old infant from injury. What does the nurse include in this conversation?**
   a. Prop the bottle if not holding during feeding.
   b. Do not use the microwave to warm bottles.
   c. Shake powder onto perineum only.
   d. Allow the infant to sleep in the bed with you.

   Topic/Concept: Health Promotion **Subtopic:** Infants **Bloom's Taxonomy:** Applying **Clinical Problem-Solving Process:** Planning **NCLEX-PN®:** Reduction of Risk Potential **QSEN:** Safety **CJMM:** Generate Solutions

   Rationale: The bottle should not be propped, and powder should be placed in the hand before applied, not shaken, as both of these increase risks for aspiration in this age group. The infant should not sleep in the bed with anyone as this increases the risks of smothering and suffocation. Bottles should be warmed under lukewarm running water and not in the microwave as this can cause hot spots in the bottle that can burn the baby.

   THIN Thinking: *Identify Risk to Safety* – Prevention is the top priority for nursing interventions surrounding any form of injury. If the injury can be prevented altogether, then there is no morbidity or mortality increase to address.

3. **The parent of a toddler asks the nurse about proper nutrition for their child. The nurse explains each food group and indicates the number of daily servings the toddler should be eating. Place the food types in order from most to least number of daily servings that a toddler should be eating.**
   a. Meat.
   b. Fruit.
   c. Milk.
   d. Bread.
   e. Vegetables.

   Answer: D, B, E, C, A

   Topic/Concept: Health Promotion **Subtopic:** Toddlers **Bloom's Taxonomy:** Applying **Clinical Problem-Solving Process:** Planning **NCLEX-PN®:** Coordinated Care **QSEN:** Evidence-based Practice **CJMM:** Prioritize Hypotheses

   Rationale: A toddler should have 6-7 servings of bread, 3-4 servings of fruit, 3 servings of vegetables, 2-3 servings of milk, and 2 servings of meat daily for a healthy diet.

   THIN Thinking: *Top Three* – A healthy diet is good preventative practice for many lifelong and chronic illnesses that a child can develop. Starting them on the right path early helps form proper dietary habits to continue as they grow.

4. **The nurse reinforces education with the parent of a toddler on choking prevention. Which food does the nurse emphasize needs to be avoided for their child?**
   a. Popcorn.
   b. Macaroni and cheese.
   c. Bananas.
   d. Hot dogs cut lengthwise.

   Topic/Concept: Health Promotion **Subtopic:** Toddlers **Bloom's Taxonomy:** Applying **Clinical Problem-Solving Process:** Planning **NCLEX-PN®:** Reduction of Risk Potential **QSEN:** Patient-centered Care **CJMM:** Generate Solutions

   Rationale: Parents should avoid things large enough to be swallowed that will block the airway like nuts, popcorn, marshmallows, whole hot dogs, big chunks of meat, fruits with pits, fish bones, dried beans, chewing gum, and hard candies.

   THIN Thinking: *Identify Risk to Safety* – Parents often give toddlers snacks that are choking hazards without realizing it. Education should be provided to prevent injury as choking is a high risk in this age group.

5. **The nurse participates in a community education fair, focusing on the proper use of vehicle restraints to prevent injury in children. Which example does the nurse give of a child who requires a safety seat?**
   a. 9-year-old.
   b. Child is 5 feet tall.
   c. Child weighs 65 pounds.
   d. 3-year-old.

   Topic/Concept: Health Promotion **Subtopic:** Toddlers **Bloom's Taxonomy:** Applying **Clinical Problem-Solving Process:** Planning **NCLEX-PN®:** Safety and Infection Control **QSEN:** Safety **CJMM:** Prioritize Hypotheses

   Rationale: To be considered safe to ride without a safety seat, the child should be greater than 40 pounds, taller than 4 feet 9 inches, and between four and eight years old, or greater than eight years old.

   THIN Thinking: *Clinical Problem-Solving Process* – Motor vehicle trauma is the leading cause of trauma and death across age groups. Parents must understand how to properly restrain their children to prevent injury.

6. **The nurse speaks with the parents of a preschooler about ways to prevent injury. What recommendation does the nurse include in this discussion?**
   a. Teach their child about hazards.
   b. Use safety devices to prevent injury in the house.
   c. Pad furniture in case of falls.
   d. Keep cleaning supplies in lower cabinets.

   Topic/Concept: Health Promotion **Subtopic:** Preschoolers **Bloom's Taxonomy:** Applying **Clinical Problem-Solving Process:** Planning **NCLEX-PN®:** Health Promotion and Maintenance **QSEN:** Patient-centered Care **CJMM:** Generate Solutions

   Rationale: In this age group, it is best to educate the child on hazards and avoiding injury as they can comprehend this information and are more able to listen to instructions. A toddler would have a greater risk for falls and need safety devices around the house. Cleaning supplies should still be kept in either a locked cabinet or a high cabinet out of reach as poisoning is still a risk.

   THIN Thinking: *Identify Risk to Safety* – To prevent injury, the nurse must provide age-appropriate education. Prevention is the priority nursing intervention for injury.

7. **Which child is more likely to have awakened from a night terror versus a nightmare?**

   Answer: b.

   Topic/Concept: Health Promotion **Subtopic:** Preschoolers **Bloom's Taxonomy:** Analyzing **Clinical Problem-Solving Process:** Data Collection **NCLEX-PN®:** Coordinated Care **QSEN:** Teamwork and Collaboration **CJMM:** Analyze Cues

   Rationale: Children with night terrors are usually only in distress during them and forget them when they wake. Children with nightmares are usually distressed after the dream is over and awaken crying as they remember the dream.

   THIN Thinking: *Clinical Problem-Solving Process* – Identifying the differences in sleep issues will help the nurse address the issues the client is experiencing and identify potential causes.

8. **The school nurse provides information to parents on the proper care of their preschooler's dental hygiene. What does the nurse include in this education? *Select all that apply.***
   a. Dental check-ups every 6-12 months.
   b. Avoid flossing until older.
   c. Discontinue fluoride supplements in this age group.
   d. Brush teeth twice daily.
   e. Increase sugars in the diet.

   Topic/Concept: Health Promotion **Subtopic:** Preschoolers **Bloom's Taxonomy:** Applying **Clinical Problem-Solving Process:** Planning **NCLEX-PN®:** Coordinated Care **QSEN:** Evidence-based Practice **CJMM:** Prioritize Hypotheses

   Rationale: Children in the age group should continue to have fluoride supplementation, brush twice daily, floss daily, decrease sugary and other cariogenic foods in their diet, and get dental check-ups regularly every 6-12 months depending on the condition of their teeth and family history.

   THIN Thinking: *Top Three* – Healthy teeth are important for maintaining a healthy diet and preventing other lifelong illnesses like heart issues.

9. **The school nurse evaluates a client brought into the office from their third-grade class. Which reported symptom indicates the possible need for specialized treatment of continued stress?**
   a. Fatigue.
   b. Weight gain.
   c. Bed-wetting.
   d. Dizziness.

   Topic/Concept: Health Promotion **Subtopic:** School-aged children **Bloom's Taxonomy:** Analyzing **Clinical Problem-Solving Process:** Data Collection **NCLEX-PN®:** Coordinated Care **QSEN:** Safety **CJMM:** Analyze Cues

   Rationale: Symptoms that could indicate chronic stress that may require specialized treatment include things like bed-wetting, stomach pains, headache, sleep problems, change in eating habits, aggressive or stubborn behavior, reluctance to participate, and regressive behaviors—especially if chronically a problem.

THIN Thinking: *Clinical Problem-Solving Process* – Bed-wetting and other regressive behaviors is a serious symptom in a school-aged child that could indicate chronic stress and the need for advanced treatment. The stress can come from many factors as minor as friend conflict to as serious as abuse in the home.

10. The nurse collects information from the parent of a 9-year-old client. Which reported behavior is cause for concern in this client?

a. The client sucks their thumb.
b. The client prefers to sit on the floor while doing homework.
c. The client tends to procrastinate on school work.
d. The client is well-behaved most of the time.

Topic/Concept: Health Promotion **Subtopic:** School-aged children **Bloom's Taxonomy:** Analyzing **Clinical Problem-Solving Process:** Data Collection **NCLEX-PN®:** Health Promotion and Maintenance **QSEN:** Patient-centered Care **CJMM:** Recognize Cues

Rationale: A child at this age should not be sucking their thumb; this is a regressive behavior that needs to be investigated. The other behaviors are all normal variations of school-age children.

THIN Thinking: *Clinical Problem-Solving Process* – Regressive behaviors can be related to stress or the addition of a new sibling, but because these can be caused by a wide range of problems, some of which are severe, they should always be investigated and addressed.

11. A child playing on the school playground falls and has their tooth avulsed. The off-duty nurse is picking their child up from school and is requested to assist. Place in order the emergency treatment for an avulsed tooth.

a. Rinse gently with water if dirty.
b. Recover tooth.
c. Insert tooth in socket or place in cup of cold milk or under child's tongue.
d. Hold tooth by the crown; do not touch the root.
e. Transport the child to a dentist immediately.

Answer: B, D, A, C, E

Topic/Concept: Health Promotion **Subtopic:** School-aged children **Bloom's Taxonomy:** Applying **Clinical Problem-Solving Process:** Implementation **NCLEX-PN®:** Safety and Infection Control **QSEN:** Evidence-based Practice **CJMM:** Take Action

Rationale: If transported correctly and immediately, the tooth may be saved and replaced by the dentist.

THIN Thinking: *Help Quick* – An appropriate and timely response can save the avulsed tooth. Dental health is linked to nutrition and overall health. Therefore, maintaining all aspects of dental health is important for overall health.

12. The nurse cares for an adolescent client and reviews education regarding injury prevention. Which education does the nurse include for the client and their parents? *Select all that apply.*

a. Avoid the use of medications not prescribed to them.
b. Wear restraints when driving.
c. Wear a helmet in contact sports.
d. Avoid or minimize the use of kitchen cooking appliances.
e. Drive no more than five miles per hour over the speed limit.

Topic/Concept: Health Promotion **Subtopic:** Adolescents **Bloom's Taxonomy:** Applying **Clinical Problem-Solving Process:** Planning **NCLEX-PN®:** Reduction of Risk Potential **QSEN:** Patient-centered Care **CJMM:** Generate Solutions

Rationale: Accidental poisoning with unprescribed medications/narcotics and alcohol is prevalent in this age group. Safe driving practices like using restraints and driving under the speed limit will reduce the risk of motor vehicle trauma. Sporting injuries are also common, so proper protective equipment use should be encouraged in contact sports. Adolescents should be able to use cooking appliances without burning themselves at this age; bigger burn risks at this age are surrounding smoking, sun exposure, and electrical hazards.

THIN Thinking: *Identify Risk to Safety* – Age-appropriate prevention is the most important nursing intervention for injury of any type. Proper education is the first step to prevention.

13. Which activity places the adolescent at the highest risk for serious or fatal injury?

Answer: a.

Topic/Concept: Health Promotion **Subtopic:** Adolescents **Bloom's Taxonomy:** Analyzing **Clinical Problem-Solving Process:** Data Collection **NCLEX-PN®:** Reduction of Risk Potential **QSEN:** Evidence-based Practice **CJMM:** Analyze Cues

Rationale: Driving is the highest risk activity as 40% of all teen deaths in the United States are related to motor vehicle accidents. Contact sports are safer as long as protection is worn. Swimming is safer as long as they know how to swim. Cooking is something they are well able to do at this age with minimal risk.

THIN Thinking: *Identify Risk to Safety* – Education on proper vehicle safety is extremely important for adolescents. They have just learned to drive and do not always follow the safety rules and therefore are more vulnerable to accidents and injury or death surrounding the use of a vehicle.

14. The nurse utilizes screening protocols for an adolescent client. What screening does the nurse not include for this client?

a. Sexual transmitted infection screening.
b. Scoliosis screening.
c. Hearing and vision screening.
d. Autism screening.

Topic/Concept: Health Promotion **Subtopic:** Adolescents **Bloom's Taxonomy:** Applying **Clinical Problem-Solving Process:** Planning **NCLEX-PN®:** Health Promotion and Maintenance **QSEN:** Patient-centered Care **CJMM:** Generate Solutions

Rationale: By adolescence, autism should be well-identified, and screening should not be necessary. Scoliosis, STIs, and vision and hearing deficits are all potential problems that should be screened in this age group.

THIN Thinking: *Top Three* – Screenings are imperative when it comes to early interventions to address health concerns. The nurse must understand what age groups are at risk for which problems to screen effectively.

15. The nurse discusses infection prevention with an adolescent client. Which priority information does the nurse include for a client in this age range?

a. Dental hygiene practices.
b. Proper bathing practices.
c. Using a qualified professional for piercings.
d. Avoiding condom use.

Topic/Concept: Health Promotion **Subtopic:** Adolescents **Bloom's Taxonomy:** Applying **Clinical Problem-Solving Process:** Planning **NCLEX-PN®:** Safety and Infection Control **QSEN:** Safety **CJMM:** Priority Hypotheses

Rationale: Sexually transmitted infection prevention, including condoms, should be included, and piercings/tattoos should be done by professionals rather than at home with unsterilized items causing infection. They already understand proper dental hygiene and bathing practices at this age and usually follow them.

THIN Thinking: *Identify Risk to Safety* – Infection prevention can be accomplished in this age group through education of preventative practices. These clients can comprehend and follow instructions in their best interests.

16. The nurse provides information about injury prevention to a young adult client. What does the nurse include as a priority reinforcement of teaching?

a. Avoidance of mixing alcohol with other drugs.
b. Swimming safety.
c. Locking cleaning supplies in an upper cabinet.
d. Removal of fall risks around the house.

Topic/Concept: Health Promotion **Subtopic:** Adults **Bloom's Taxonomy:** Applying **Clinical Problem-Solving Process:** Planning **NCLEX-PN®:** Health Promotion and Maintenance **QSEN:** Patient-centered Care **CJMM:** Prioritize Hypotheses

Rationale: Older adults are at higher risk of falls. Children are at risk of poisoning from cleaning supplies. Swimming safety is important but not the highest risk in this age group. The highest risks of injury and death in young adults include accidental poisoning by mixing alcohol and medications, gun injury, and motor vehicle accidents.

THIN Thinking: *Identify Risk to Safety* – Adults still need education on injury prevention as they are still at risk for specific types of trauma and injury.

17. The nurse screens an adult client for depression. Which symptoms does the nurse include as indicative of a positive screening? *Select all that apply.*

a. Loss of interest in things.
b. Irritability.
c. Change in eating habits.
d. Change in sleeping habits.
e. Lack of concentration.

Topic/Concept: Health Promotion **Subtopic:** Adults **Bloom's Taxonomy:** Applying **Clinical Problem-Solving Process:** Data Collection **NCLEX-PN®:** Psychosocial Integrity **QSEN:** Patient-centered Care **CJMM:** Recognize Cues

Rationale: Depression puts an adult at higher risk of suicide. Signs for depression include a change in eating or sleeping habits, irritability, lack of concentration, and loss of interest in things.

THIN Thinking: *Clinical Problem-Solving Process* – Potential depression needs to be identified and treated to prevent risks of suicide.

18. **The nurse cares for an older adult client who has had several falls the previous night. After being quiet most of the shift, the client is now screaming and attempting to get out of bed. What is the nurse's first action?**
    a. Identify potential causes of the client's behavior.
    b. Get a prescription for restraints to prevent another fall.
    c. Medicate with prescribed lorazepam IV to sedate the client.
    d. This is expected older adult behavior and should just be monitored.

    Topic/Concept: Health Promotion **Subtopic:** Older adults **Bloom's Taxonomy:** Applying **Clinical Problem-Solving Process:** Implementation **NCLEX-PN®:** Coordinated Care **QSEN:** Safety **CJMM:** Take Action

    Rationale: This is not expected behavior, and the nurse should evaluate the client to try and determine the cause of the behavior change. Restraints should not be the first recourse, and using prescribed lorazepam in this manner is a restraint.

    THIN Thinking: *Clinical Problem-Solving Process* – Restraints of all types should always be the last resource. A change in client behavior such as this may be directly related to a problem that can be addressed.

19. **The home health nurse collects data in the home of an older adult client. Which of the findings is a fall hazard?**

    Answer: d.

    Topic/Concept: Health Promotion **Subtopic:** Older adults **Bloom's Taxonomy:** Analyzing **Clinical Problem-Solving Process:** Data Collection **NCLEX-PN®:** Safety and Infection Control **QSEN:** Evidence-based Practice **CJMM:** Analyze Cues

    Rationale: Throw rugs increase the risk of falls in the older adult and should be removed. Shower chairs, well-lit hallways, and hand railings all help to decrease the risks of falls.

    THIN Thinking: *Identify Risk to Safety* – When checking an older adult client's home environment, the nurse should pay close attention to fall risks and address them to prevent falls. Falls are the highest risk for older adult clients, increasing morbidity and mortality in this age group.

20. **The nurse prepares a client for discharge and reviews their medication prescriptions. Which prescription does the nurse clarify with the provider?**

    Answer: 2. admitriptyline 100 mg PO daily

    Topic/Concept: Health Promotion **Subtopic:** Older adults **Bloom's Taxonomy:** Applying **Clinical Problem-Solving Process:** Implementation **NCLEX-PN®:** Pharmacological Therapies **QSEN:** Patient-centered Care **CJMM:** Take Action

    Rationale: The client is 79 years old; tricyclic antidepressants like amitriptyline should not be used in the older adult because they have anticholinergic properties that can cause acute confusion and urinary incontinence. SSRIs like sertraline are preferred for older adult clients with depression. Metoprolol and Lisinopril are both safe for older adult clients as well.

    THIN Thinking: *Help Quick* – The nurse must address the possible provider error before the client is discharged. An alternative will need to be prescribed; depression needs to be addressed in the older adult as untreated depression can lead to suicide and poor management of chronic illness.

CHAPTER

19

Role of the Nurse in Quality and Safety

Clinical Judgment Connections

It goes without saying that clinical judgment is a key concept of NCLEX-PN®. In other words, as you answer each question, consider the role of the nurse in attending to client needs. As discussed in Chapter 2, the Client Needs make up the blueprint of the NCLEX-PN®. As you answer questions about these needs, think about the nurse's responses—How would a nurse think in the case? What cues or data are important for this client with this illness? How the nurse thinks, processes the cues, and makes decisions based on that information is clinical judgment.

Next Gen Clinical Judgment

Consider the scope of practice of LPNs/LVNs in your state. How should the nurse respond if an assignment appears to be outside the practical nurse's scope of practice?

So what elements are critical components that we should address? The nurse's first priority is the CLIENT. Next, remember NCLEX-PN® is an examination of safety. Keeping clients safe is always a priority—both in real life and on the exam.

The QSEN competencies (Quality and Safety Education for Nurses—www.qsen.org) are designed to guide students and nurses in the safe delivery of quality care. We will discuss each competency and types of NCLEX-PN® questions that may be related to each concept. As we unpack the NCLEX-PN®, think about how this information will enhance your success!

Next Gen Clinical Judgment

Search the Internet for schools and agencies in your area that use the QSEN competencies to guide their practices.

Patient-centered care

As you answer questions, think about the most client-centered or family-centered options. Clients and families are actively involved in decisions that impact them and are partners in care. When answering questions, consider the option that demonstrates the highest level of respect for the client and ensures that the client's and family's needs are a priority over nursing, institutional, and agency priorities. For example, review the following question and see how patient-centered care is the priority:

Q: A nurse assists to prepare a client for placement of a dialysis shunt. The client states "I am not sure I am ready to have this surgery." How would the nurse respond?

1. "Why don't you want to have surgery today?"
2. "You signed the consent and the operating room is ready."
3. "You are just nervous, the medicine will calm you down."
4. "Would you like to speak to the surgeon about your surgery?"

The answer is 4 and is the most client-centered response. Ensuring that care is focused on the client and the client's concerns is an important role of the nurse as client advocate. Advocacy is a fundamental role for nursing. Advocacy is speaking up for and providing support for another person or group who may not be able to speak or act for themselves. The nursing profession offers a voice for clients, ensuring that clients have their questions answered, concerns expressed, and priorities attended to while receiving care. Client-centered care also emphasizes cultural data collection and culturally aware nursing care. The client may represent the individual, family, group, or community.

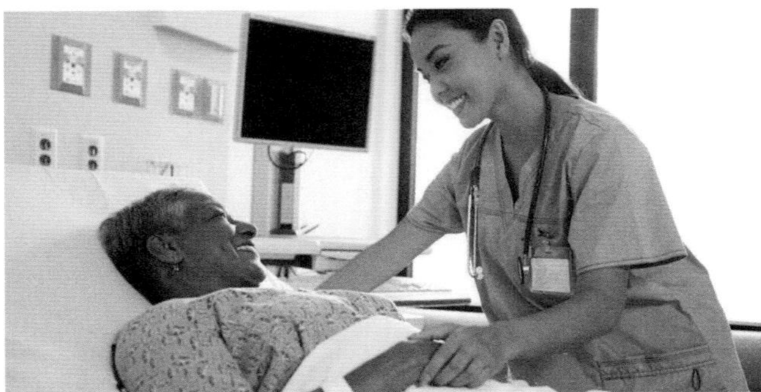

Image 19-1: How should the nurse ensure that clients are well-informed about their care?

Teamwork and collaboration

Nursing does not practice alone, nor does a nurse practice nursing in solitude. Even in home care or when you are the only nurse present, nurses are members of the healthcare team and nurses collaborate to attain better client outcomes. To be successful on NCLEX-PN®, you need to know the roles of members of the healthcare team, ensure that team members are informed of changes in client's needs and status, advocate for clients within the team, and coordinate the team's cohesive, well-communicated, and client-centered plan of care! Consider teamwork and collaboration as you answer this question:

Q: A nurse cares for a client who has disclosed that she is homeless and does not know where she will go after discharge. Which referral is of highest priority at this time?

1. Social work for housing assistance and follow-up.
2. Dietitian for assisting with meal planning.
3. Chaplain for assisting with spiritual needs.
4. Discharge nurse to prepare for discharge immediately.

The correct answer is 1. The social worker is the best person to assist the client who has disclosed that they are homeless. The nurse may need the other members of the healthcare team for various reasons, but for this situation, the highest priority is to ensure the client has a plan after discharge.

Inherent with teamwork and collaboration are the concepts of leadership. As a leader, nurses guide the healthcare team, coordinate the team to enhance communication, ensure quality care, and assign to other practical/vocational nurses and unlicensed assistive personnel to get the job done! As discussed in Chapter 4, NCLEX-PN® questions may pertain to assigning appropriate tasks to UAPs or other LVN/LPNs. Always consider the rights of safe assignments: the right task, to the right person, with the right instructions, with the right supervision, and with the right communication.

Clinical Hint

In a test question about assigning UAPs responsibilities, usually assign the simplest task to the UAP.

When assigning others, consider the skill level required of the task and the skill level of the potential completer of the task. For example, if a test question mentions years of experience, years of working with a specific client population, special training/certification, and education level, it is asking you to consider these elements as you assign that task. Think about client factors—what is the question asking you to think about prior to answering the question? Does it specify a client's age, diagnosis, or treatment that requires appropriate knowledge and skills? See how this is operationalized in this question:

Q: An LPN/LVN assists in caring for several clients on a medical-surgical unit. Which client should the nurse assign to the unlicensed assistive personnel to receive morning hygiene care?

1. A 48-year-old client who had a posterior spinal fusion one day ago.
2. A 83-year-old who sustained a head injury and is on strict activity restrictions.
3. A 61-year-old client who developed COVID and requires specific positioning.
4. A 28-year-old client who had shoulder surgery and has some limited range of motion.

The correct answer is option 4. The UAP should provide morning care to the client with the least complex needs. The UAP may need additional training or assistance to log-roll a client after a spinal fusion, adhere to strict activity restrictions, or prone clients with COVID. The client with shoulder surgery requires the least complexity in decision-making when providing care and would be most appropriate for the UAP.

One exercise you may want to do is to visit the board of nursing's website in the state where you would like to be licensed. Look for the statements about assigning. They usually focus on the clinical problem solving (nursing process) and the need for nurses to gather data, reinforce education and evaluate nursing care. Although the nurse practice acts of each state are unique, they all include some statements about the role of the practical nurse.

Another part of teamwork and collaboration is communication! Consider the chaos of the healthcare environment if people were not communicating effectively. A current evidence-based practice being launched is bedside reporting. The practice of nurses providing shift-change, handoff reports at the client's bedside is one that is sweeping the nation. This change in practice is thought to increase client satisfaction and involvement in care, the efficacy of report, and comprehensive environmental rounds during report. You may hear some downsides, too! Confidentiality, the need to have a positive working relationship with the clients, and other issues may impede the effectiveness of bedside reporting. In an evidence-based project, researchers analyzed bedside reporting practices in their institution and validated its usefulness in enhancing client safety and promoting professionalism among the nurses. Let's do this test question about bedside reporting:

Q: An LPN/LVN receives bedside report at the change of shift. About which part of the report should the nurse ask for clarification?

1. The client has a history of hypertension managed with lisinopril.
2. The client is allergic to cephalosporins and penicillin medications.
3. The client reports abdominal pain unrelieved by pain medication.
4. The client's family is unable to visit because they live far away.

The correct answer is option 3. The options about the client having hypertension managed by medications, the client's allergies, and family visiting issues are not essential information. The client having pain that is not addressed by pain medication should be clarified. The nurse should consider if an analgesic was administered, if non-pharmacological strategies were attempted, and if the health care provider was notified. Just from this example, one can see the power of bedside reporting in allowing the nurse to be there and discuss findings with fellow colleagues and the client! A great evidence-based practice to enhance client outcomes and may serve as potential subjects of questions on your exam!

Evidence-based practice

Remember NCLEX-PN® World in Chapter 4? In NLCEX-PN® World, the nurse has nearly endless resources in terms of time, supplies, money, and friends (or help/assistance to carry out a task). When answering a question, the nurse is charged with conducting nursing practice without "cutting corners" or breaching policy standards and best practices. As such, the nurse is responsible to sustain a "spirit of inquiry" for using best practices to provide client care, to ensure that current research informs care, and continue to seek out evidence to support nursing practice. Let's review this question to see EBP concepts in action:

Q: A nurse provides care for a client receiving nasogastric feedings. The nurse confirms placement of the tube and begins the feeding. Which action should the nurse implement to ensure safe feeding administration?

1. Place the client in the high-Fowler's position.
2. Take the client's abdominal girth before and after each feeding.
3. Ensure that the feeding is instilled as quickly as it will infuse.
4. Listen for bowel sounds during the feeding to ensure toleration.

The correct option is 1. There is strong evidence that elevating the head of the bed allows gravity to ensure the feeding is safely administered. There is no need to measure the abdominal girth or to auscultate bowel sounds. The feeding should be administered slowly to avoid diarrhea or abdominal discomfort. A comprehensive review of the literature affirms this answer and demonstrates the power of and need for evidence-based practices!

These EBP are interpreted in terms of changing practices. Models exist to examine and assimilate research findings into policies and procedures. On a bigger scale, changes in practice may influence health policy and make positive health status changes for people around the world! (And, specifically will be reflected in NCLEX-PN® items!)

Quality Improvement

In line with EBP, nurses are concerned with advancing the quality of care through ongoing quality improvement practices. Nurses at the bedside are able to identify client care issues and participate in projects to determine best practices. Not every nurse can be a nurse researcher but all should be involved in quality improvement projects regardless of setting. One of the best ways to ensure safety is to carefully monitor concerns, near misses, and errors that may arise in the nurses' practice setting.

After data and trends are analyzed, an initiative is developed to address concerns. Here is an important example of quality improvement in action since SBAR is becoming more important on the NCLEX-PN®.

Many of us learned about SBAR in our nursing education. Those initials denote:

- S-situation
- B-background
- A-assessment
- R-recommendations

The SBAR model provides a framework for nurses to call health care providers with changes in status. The nurse is charged to provide information on each of the SBAR criteria to ensure comprehensive communication among the healthcare team and to inform health care providers of in-time information upon which to make decisions. You may be asked questions about SBAR, as in the following question:

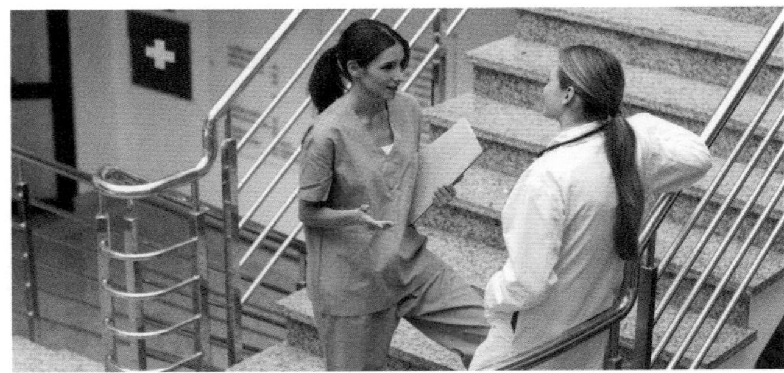

Image 19-2: If these nurses were discussing a client, what HIPAA violations should the nurse anticipate?

Q: A nurse cares for a client who was admitted three days ago for diabetes mellitus. The client has been improving, but is now experiencing a headache and has no order for pain medication. Which statement would be appropriate to include in the recommendation section of the SBAR when speaking to the health care provider?

1. "The client has a headache. He rates his pain a 4/10."
2. "The client was admitted three days ago for a high blood glucose level."
3. "For his headache, what would you like to prescribe?"
4. "His current vital signs are stable."

The correct answer is 3 because it is a nursing recommendation. The other answers are correct for the other letters of the acronym.

One example of a quality improvement project at work is the use of SBAR within computer communication systems. Their organization placed the SBAR report within a computer platform and was found to positively impact communication practices and client safety—a nurse-led initiative effecting positive change in nursing practice. This is an example of a quality improvement project designed to increase client safety and positive client outcomes!

Safety

Nurses use their thinking, clinical judgment, and decision-making skills to enhance client safety. Medication errors, falls, and other safety issues are threats to our healthcare system and to clients. We've said several times that NCLEX-PN® is an examination of safety.

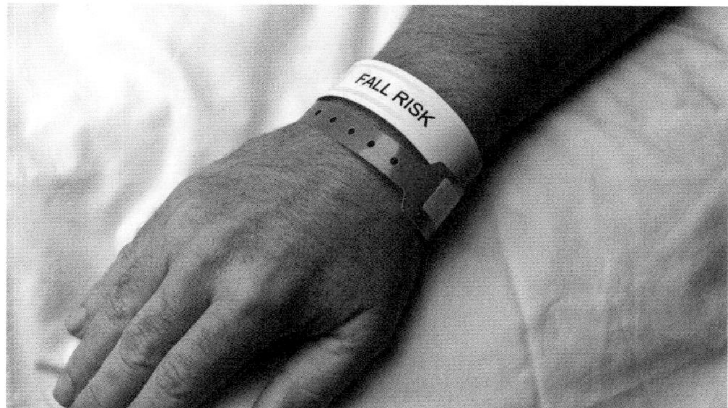

Image 19-3: How does a client identification band contribute to client safety? How does a fall risk identification band contribute to client safety?

When employed as a nurse you will hear more about safety in client care and organizations' goals to promote a culture of safety. For many questions, keeping the client safe is of highest priority. Let's view this question to validate the importance of safety.

Q: A client received an opioid pain medication and is experiencing dizziness. He is a fall risk due to a history of falls. What instruction is of highest priority?

1. Use the call bell when needing to use the restroom.
2. Do not eat or drink if you experience any nausea.
3. How to use the bedside controls to raise the head of the bed.
4. Let the nurse know if you are still in pain in two hours.

The correct answer is option 1. The client is already considered a fall risk due to a history of falls. The client has now received medication that increased this risk. The highest priority for this client to ensure he does not attempt to get out of bed without assistance. This is an example of a question in which you need to focus on safety and think about what makes the client more at risk than other clients. Remember the client need Reduction of Risk Potential? Again, using good decision-making and clinical judgment skills while setting sound priorities will ensure that you select the correct response on questions in this domain, and others!

Informatics

Informatics is a QSEN competency that uses information and technology to enhance safe, quality care. So what is informatics? It is the use of the internet, internal intranet platforms, computers/digital methods and new mechanisms to improve client care, safety, and outcomes. How does informatics increase communication and safety? We know that many states and agencies have adopted electronic health records (EHR) or electronic medical records (EMR). These mechanisms allow for health records to be communicated between healthcare professionals and facilities to ensure comprehensive care. Functionality such as medication reconciliation, home medication review, and holistic case management promotes safety in medication management and administration. Telehealth, or using telephones, computers, and technologies to provide healthcare at a distance or between separate settings, brings healthcare and expertise to remote locations, homes or across miles. This is another informatics role for nursing!

Nurses are involved with the use of informatics at many levels. Let's use a test question to demonstrate nursing informatics:

Q: A nurse cares for a client and documents in the electronic health record following morning care. What would be included in the documentation? Select all that apply.

1. The client yelled at the staff last night according to the morning report.
2. The nurse provided oral care for the client.
3. The UAP will be in later to change the client's linens.
4. The client ate a good breakfast.
5. The client's vital signs as checked by the nurse.
6. The nurse shaved the client as his request.

The answers to this question are 2, 5, and 6. The nurse should document only the tasks they perform. The nurse should not include hearsay from previous shifts, vague terms, or futuristic charting. This documentation question demonstrates how informatics can appear in NCLEX-PN® items. Finally, using technology to seek out information and search the literature reflects a significant use of informatics in nursing practice. Consider the breadth of information available on the World Wide Web to use to enhance client care and outcomes.

In this chapter, we reinforced concepts of client safety, the role of the nurse, and the QSEN framework. These topics may infuse any client need of the NCLEX-PN®, especially Coordination of Care, Safety and Infection Control, and Reduction of Risk Potential. Now, take the NurseThink® Quiz on these concepts.

Next Gen Clinical Judgment

Consider your last or previous clinical assignment. What QSEN principles did you use to ensure client safety?

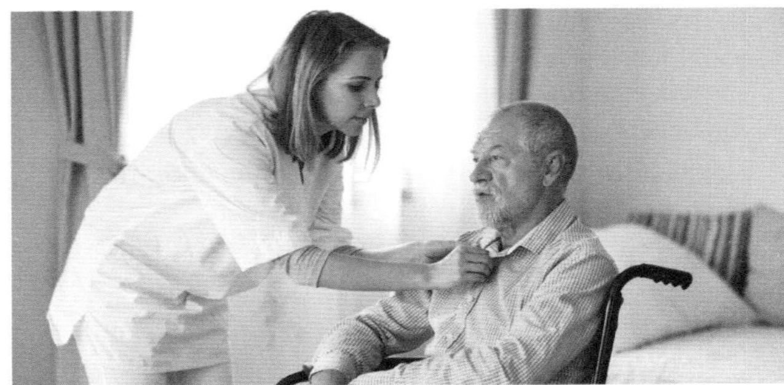

Image 19-4

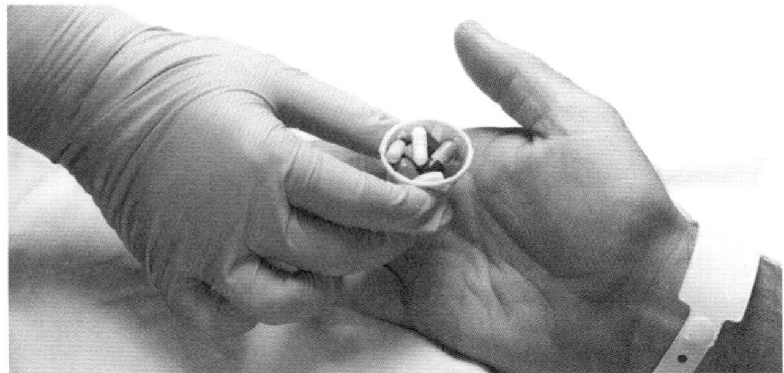

Image 19-5

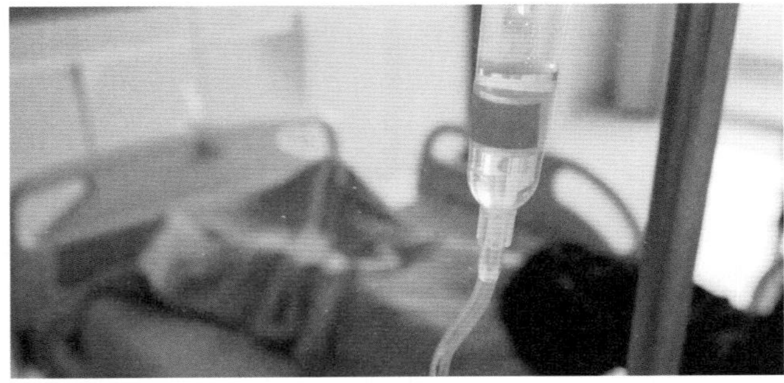

Image 19-6

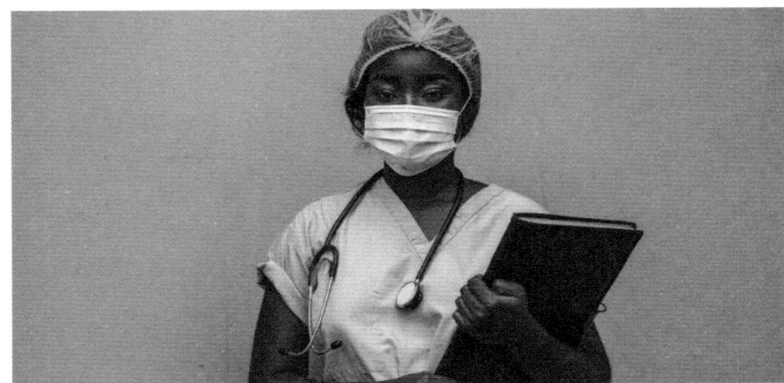

Image 19-7

How do each of these images depict QSEN principles:

- *Patient-centered care*
- *Teamwork and collaboration*
- *Evidence-based practices*
- *Quality improvement*
- *Safety*
- *Informatics*

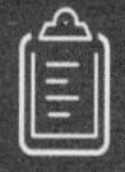

NurseThink® Quiz Questions

1. **The nurse plans reinforcement of discharge teaching for a client with newly diagnosed Type II Diabetes Mellitus (DM). Which priority consultation does the nurse incorporate into the client's plan of care?**
   a. Counseling consultation.
   b. Dietary consultation.
   c. Social work referral.
   d. Finance counselor.

2. **When collecting data, the nurse collects as much evidence as possible to support subsequent care and treatment of the client, including subjective and objective data. Which findings are considered objective data? *Select all that apply.***
   a. Blood pressure.
   b. Fever.
   c. Pulse.
   d. Stiff neck.
   e. Photophobia.
   f. Slurred speech.

3. **The nurse delegates vital signs to the unlicensed assistive personnel (UAP) but is unsure of the UAP's level of experience. Which statement by the UAP requires additional instruction by the nurse?**
   a. "I will document vital signs in the client's electronic medical record."
   b. "I will report abnormal vital signs immediately to the nurse."
   c. "I will only report vital signs to the nurse if the client appears ill."
   d. "I will document the type of temperature obtained."

4. **The nurse arrives to work and checks the assignment board. Due to staffing shortages, the nurse is instructed to report to the labor and delivery unit as a float nurse. The nurse has never worked in the labor and delivery unit before. What is the nurse's best action?**
   a. Report the assignment to the supervisor.
   b. Clarify the assignment with the nurse manager.
   c. Refuse to float to labor and delivery.
   d. Ask a senior nurse what action to take.

5. **The nurse delegates tasks to the client care team. Which task does the nurse assign to the unlicensed assistive personnel (UAP)?**
   a. Sterile dressing change.
   b. Discharge education.
   c. Check a post-op incision.
   d. Obtaining vital signs.

6. **The nurse evaluates a client who presents to urgent care with a severe diabetic foot wound. The client speaks Spanish and appears to have a limited understanding of English. The nurse does not speak Spanish. What is the nurse's best response?**
   a. The nurse should speak slowly and articulate words.
   b. The nurse should request a family member to interpret.
   c. The nurse should obtain a medical interpreter for the client.
   d. The nurse should continue the questions in English.

7. **The nurse is aware of Quality and Safety Education for Nursing (QSEN) competencies to guide safe and quality care for all clients. Which competency guides interprofessional teams for improved quality of care?**
   a. Quality Improvement.
   b. Patient-Centered Care.
   c. Teamwork and Collaboration.
   d. Informatics.

8. **The nurse manager asks the nursing practice council to plan a quality improvement project. Which proposal is accepted by the nurse manager?**
   a. Using client satisfaction scores to change the emergency room registration process.
   b. Changing the brand of a product based on a wealth of research evidence.
   c. Conducting a state-wide survey of nurses to determine hourly pay rates.
   d. Interviewing family members about their experiences with ICU visitation.

9. **The nurse finds a client lying on the floor next to the bed with a laceration to the right arm. The client reports getting up to go to the sink, getting caught in the bedsheet, and falling to the floor from the bed. Which documentation by the nurse is most appropriate for an incident report?**
   a. "Client found lying on right side after tripping on sheet and falling to the floor."
   b. "Client found lying on right side on floor. Client states, 'I got caught in the sheet.'"
   c. "Client tripped over bedsheet. 2 cm superficial laceration to right forearm."
   d. "Client leg caught on bedsheet, causing client to fall in the floor and lacerate right forearm."

10. **The nurse preceptor discusses documentation with the new nurse. Which statements by the new nurse demonstrate understanding? *Select all that apply.***
    a. "When documenting my opinions, I'll be sure to keep my comments respectful."
    b. "I will remember that all of my documentation is actually a legal document."
    c. "Any written documentation should be legible to avoid errors."
    d. "Prioritizing the information I include will make my documentation more useful for other team members."
    e. "It doesn't matter what time I document things, as long as they are accurately documented."

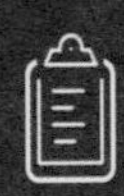

NurseThink® Quiz Questions

11. **The nurse cares for a client with middle-stage Alzheimer's Disease. Which finding does the nurse determine to be consistent with this stage of the disease?**
    a. Lack of awareness of the environment.
    b. Occasional memory lapses.
    c. Slower movements when dressing.
    d. Forgetting personal events.

12. **The nurse prioritizes a client's care using Maslow's Hierarchy of Basic Needs. Because the client's physiological needs are met, which safety need does the nurse address?**
    a. Clean drinking water.
    b. Protective housing.
    c. Belongingness.
    d. Self-fulfillment.

13. **The nurse cares for a client in diabetic ketoacidosis (DKA) and evaluates the client's response to intravenous fluids and intravenous insulin. Which data indicates the client is responding positively to treatment?**
    a. Rate and depth of respirations increase.
    b. Pulse and respiratory rate increase.
    c. Client becomes more alert; respirations slow.
    d. Blood pressure decreases; pulse increases.

14. **The nurse begins a daily report to the unlicensed assistive personnel (UAP) on the nursing team. The nurse notes that the UAP has a flushed face, nasal congestion, moist cough, and appears pale. The nurse asks the UAP how she feels, and the UAP states, "I have a bit of a fever, and I'm tired, but I need to work." What is the nurse's best action?**
    a. Delegate tasks to the UAP as previously planned.
    b. Assist the UAP to an empty client room to lie down.
    c. Provide the UAP with a surgical mask before seeing clients.
    d. Insist the UAP see the charge nurse about going home.

15. **The nurse plans to discuss electronic health records (EHRs) with older adults at a local senior center. Which information regarding EHRs is incorrect and not included in the nurse's presentation?**
    a. The Health Insurance Portability and Accountability Act applies to EHRs.
    b. EHRs are generally facility-specific and not shared across institutions.
    c. EHRs are relatively safe from hacking and releases of information.
    d. Only physicians have access to the information in EHRs.

16. **The oncoming nurse receives report from the previous nurse. What additional information is a priority for the nurse to obtain from the client's electronic health record (EHR)? *Select all that apply.***
    a. Recent and trending laboratory results.
    b. Recent and trending vital signs.
    c. Client's insurance information.
    d. Specific cultural or spiritual requests.
    e. Client's marital status and living situation.

17. **The nurse prepares to administer an analgesic to a client for post-operative pain. Which information is the priority for the nurse to obtain from the electronic health record?**
    a. Medication allergies.
    b. Medication route and dosage.
    c. Last time of administration.
    d. Pain relief from last administration.

18. **The emergency room nurse cares for an older adolescent client brought to the facility for substance use. The nurse implements which patient-centered approach to communicating with the adolescent?**
    a. Communicate only with the parents, not the adolescent.
    b. Give the adolescent choices in the delivery of care.
    c. Take a direct, authoritative approach to communicating.
    d. Allow the adolescent sole decision-making rights.

19. **The registered nurse (RN) delegates tasks to the licensed practical nurse (LPN) and unlicensed assistive personnel (UAP). Which action by the nurse indicates an understanding of the role of the care team?**
    a. The RN requests the LPN complete a new admission assessment.
    b. The RN asks the LPN to change bed linens and refill water pitchers.
    c. The RN asks the UAP to refill water pitchers and assigns the LPN oral medications.
    d. The RN asks the LPN to administer packed red blood cells.

20. **The nurse assists the health care provider in a procedure requiring informed consent. What is the nurse's role in the informed consent process?**
    a. Explain the purpose of the procedure.
    b. Explain the risks and benefits of the procedure.
    c. Witness the client's signature on the consent form.
    d. Answer any of the client's remaining questions.

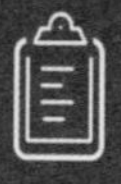

NurseThink® Quiz Answers

1. **The nurse plans discharge reinforcement of teaching for a client with newly diagnosed Type II Diabetes Mellitus (DM). Which priority consultation does the nurse incorporate into the client's plan of care?**
   a. Counseling consultation.
   b. Dietary consultation.
   c. Social work referral.
   d. Finance counselor.

   Topic/Concept: Role of the Nurse **Subtopic:** Patient-centered Care **Bloom's Taxonomy:** Applying **Clinical Problem-Solving Process:** Planning **NCLEX-PN®:** Coordinated Care **QSEN:** Patient-centered care **CJMM:** Prioritize Hypotheses

   Rationale: Diet plays a major role in the management of DM. It is the nurse's role to recognize client risks in improving client outcomes. Counseling and social work referrals are not necessarily indicated with a new diagnosis of DM. Nurses do not typically make referrals to finance counselors.

   THIN Thinking: *Top Three* – The nurse should consider the needs of the client upon discharge. For the new diabetic, dietary education, as well as a consultation with a diabetic educator, are priority areas of education in improving client outcomes.

2. **When collecting data, the nurse collects as much evidence as possible to support subsequent care and treatment of the client, including subjective and objective data. Which findings are considered objective data? *Select all that apply.***
   a. Blood pressure.
   b. Fever.
   c. Pulse.
   d. Stiff neck.
   e. Photophobia.
   f. Slurred speech.

   Topic/Concept: Role of the Nurse **Subtopic:** Patient-centered Care **Bloom's Taxonomy:** Applying **Clinical Problem-Solving Process:** Data Collection **NCLEX-PN®:** Psychosocial Integrity **QSEN:** Patient-centered care **CJMM:** Recognize Cues

   Rationale: Objective data, which can be observed and measured, includes blood pressure, temperature, heart rate, and slurred speech. Subjective data is based on the client's perception, such as stiffness or sensitivity to light.

   THIN Thinking: *Clinical Problem-Solving Process* – The nurse should be aware of the type of data they are collecting and whether or not that data is observable and measurable or based on the client's report. Both types of data are important and must be considered in the client's data collection and plan of care.

3. **The nurse delegates vital signs to the unlicensed assistive personnel (UAP) but is unsure of the UAP's level of experience. Which statement by the UAP requires additional reinforcement of teaching by the nurse?**
   a. "I will document vital signs in the client's electronic medical record."
   b. "I will report abnormal vital signs immediately to the nurse."
   c. "I will only report vital signs to the nurse if the client appears ill."
   d. "I will document the type of temperature obtained."

   Topic/Concept: Role of the Nurse **Subtopic:** Patient-centered Care **Bloom's Taxonomy:** Analyzing **Clinical Problem-Solving Process:** Evaluation **NCLEX-PN®:** Coordinated Care **QSEN:** Patient-centered care **CJMM:** Evaluate Outcomes

   Rationale: The UAP should document all vital signs, including the route of temperature measurement, and report any abnormal vital signs to the nurse.

   THIN Thinking: *Clinical Problem-Solving Process* –The nurse must determine the knowledge and skill level of the UAP before delegating tasks.

4. **The nurse arrives to work and checks the assignment board. Due to staffing shortages, the nurse is instructed to report to the labor and delivery unit as a float nurse. The nurse has never worked in the labor and delivery unit before. What is the nurse's best action?**
   a. Report the assignment to the supervisor.
   b. Clarify the assignment with the nurse manager.
   c. Refuse to float to labor and delivery.
   d. Ask a senior nurse what action to take.

   Topic/Concept: Role of the Nurse **Subtopic:** Evidence-based Practice **Bloom's Taxonomy:** Applying **Clinical Problem-Solving Process:** Implementation **NCLEX-PN®:** Coordinated Care **QSEN:** Evidence-based Practice **CJMM:** Take Action

   Rationale: Refusal of an assignment could be considered insubordination and the supervisor would likely refer the nurse back to the nurse manager. A senior nurse may not give sound advice. The nurse's best action is to clarify the assignment with the nurse manager, discussing whether the 5 rights of delegation are being met.

   THIN Thinking: *Help Quick* – The nurse manager delegates assignments to the nurses who are responsible for the delegated duties. In this case, the nurse's first action is to clarify the assignment.

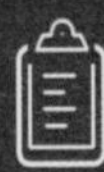

NurseThink® Quiz Answers

5. **The nurse delegates tasks to the client care team. Which task does the nurse assign to the unlicensed assistive personnel (UAP)?**
   a. Sterile dressing change.
   b. Discharge education.
   c. Check a post-op incision.
   d. ● Obtaining vital signs.

   Topic/Concept: Role of the Nurse **Subtopic:** Evidence-based Practice **Bloom's Taxonomy:** Applying **Clinical Problem-Solving Process:** Planning **NCLEX-PN®:** Basic Care and Comfort **QSEN:** Evidence-based Practice **CJMM:** Generate Solutions

   Rationale: Obtaining vital signs can be delegated to the UAP if the Five Rights of Delegation are met. Sterile procedures, discharge education, and assessments are not within the scope of practice of a UAP.

   THIN Thinking: *Clinical Problem-Solving Process* – Delegation is important for safe, timely, and efficient care. The nurse must be aware of the knowledge, skill, and experience of care team members when delegating tasks to ensure safe and accessible care. The nurse must also know which interventions require the knowledge and skill of a licensed nurse.

6. **The nurse evaluates a client who presents to urgent care with a severe diabetic foot wound. The client speaks Spanish and appears to have a limited understanding of English. The nurse does not speak Spanish. What is the nurse's best response?**
   a. The nurse should speak slowly and articulate words.
   b. The nurse should request a family member to interpret.
   c. ● The nurse should obtain a medical interpreter for the client.
   d. The nurse should continue the questions in English.

   Topic/Concept: Role of the Nurse **Subtopic:** Evidence-based Practice **Bloom's Taxonomy:** Applying **Clinical Problem-Solving Process:** Implementation **NCLEX-PN®:** Psychosocial Integrity **QSEN:** Evidence-based Practice **CJMM:** Take Action

   Rationale: An interpreter is advised when the nurse and client do not speak the same language and important information needs to be communicated. Family members should only be used as a last resort as information may be misconstrued or miscommunicated. Continuing in English, even if speaking slowly, will lead to frustration and confusion.

   THIN Thinking: *Help Quick* – Data Collection requires good communication between the client/family/caregiver and the nurse. A medical interpreter may be necessary and is advised when sharing and receiving important health information.

7. **The nurse is aware of Quality and Safety Education for Nursing (QSEN) competencies to guide safe and quality care for all clients. Which competency guides interprofessional teams for improved quality of care?**
   a. Quality Improvement.
   b. Patient-Centered Care.
   c. ● Teamwork and Collaboration.
   d. Informatics.

   Topic/Concept: Role of the Nurse **Subtopic:** QSEN Competencies **Bloom's Taxonomy:** Applying **Clinical Problem-Solving Process:** Planning **NCLEX-PN®:** Coordinated Care **QSEN:** Teamwork and Collaboration **CJMM:** Prioritize Hypotheses

   Rationale: Teamwork and Collaboration is the delivery of care among an interprofessional team to achieve continuity of care and improved client outcomes. Quality improvement includes organization and care-related processes that develop and implement plans to improve healthcare services and client outcomes. Patient-centered care is safe, compassionate, and culturally competent care; decision-making includes the client. Informatics is the use of technology for communication and management of information that supports decision-making and evidence-based practice.

   THIN Thinking: *Help Quick* – In many client scenarios, the nurse can quickly implement a nursing intervention that will improve the client's condition. Sometimes, the best immediate action the nurse can take for a client is to collaborate with another member of the healthcare team that can address a specific client concern.

8. **The nurse manager asks the nursing practice council to plan a quality improvement project. Which proposal is accepted by the nurse manager?**
   a. ● Using client satisfaction scores to change the emergency room registration process.
   b. Changing the brand of a product based on a wealth of research evidence.
   c. Conducting a state-wide survey of nurses to determine hourly pay rates.
   d. Interviewing family members about their experiences with ICU visitation.

   Topic/Concept: Role of the Nurse **Subtopic:** Quality Improvement **Bloom's Taxonomy:** Applying **Clinical Problem-Solving Process:** Planning **NCLEX-PN®:** Reduction of Risk Potential **QSEN:** Quality Improvement **CJMM:** Prioritize Hypotheses

   Rationale: Using internal data to develop a plan or implement improvements in healthcare services is quality improvement. Using research evidence to make changes is an example of evidence-based practice. A survey of nursing salaries is an example of survey research, and family interviews are an example of qualitative research.

THIN Thinking: *Top Three* – The nurse must understand approaches to change practice or implement new processes for improving healthcare and client outcomes. Quality improvement, evidence-based practice, and research are all different approaches to identifying the need for change and making practice changes.

9. **The nurse finds a client lying on the floor next to the bed with a laceration to the right arm. The client reports getting up to go to the sink, getting caught in the bedsheet, and falling to the floor from the bed. Which documentation by the nurse is most appropriate for an incident report?**
   a. "Client found lying on right side after tripping on sheet and falling to the floor."
   b. "Client found lying on right side on floor. Client states, 'I got caught in the sheet.'"
   c. "Client tripped over bedsheet. 2 cm superficial laceration to right forearm."
   d. "Client leg caught on bedsheet, causing client to fall in the floor and lacerate right forearm."

Topic/Concept: Role of the Nurse **Subtopic:** Quality Improvement **Bloom's Taxonomy:** Applying **Clinical Problem-Solving Process:** Data Collection **NCLEX-PN®:** Health promotion and maintenance **QSEN:** Quality Improvement **CJMM:** Analyze Cues

Rationale: Incident reports are an important part of a quality improvement plan. Accurate, factual documentation is vital. The correct documentation states what the nurse noted and what the client stated; this does not imply that the nurse witnessed the incident. Additional details would be helpful here, but this is an accurate response.

THIN Thinking: *Top Three* – When completing an incident report, the nurse should prioritize factual and accurate information. Conjecture should be avoided.

10. **The nurse preceptor discusses documentation with the new nurse. Which statements by the new nurse demonstrate understanding? *Select all that apply.***
    a. "When documenting my opinions, I'll be sure to keep my comments respectful."
    b. "I will remember that all of my documentation is actually a legal document."
    c. "Any written documentation should be legible to avoid errors."
    d. "Prioritizing the information I include will make my documentation more useful for other team members."
    e. "It doesn't matter what time I document things, as long as they are accurately documented."

Topic/Concept: Role of the Nurse **Subtopic:** Quality Improvement **Bloom's Taxonomy:** Analyzing **Clinical Problem-Solving Process:** Evaluation **NCLEX-PN®:** Coordinated Care **QSEN:** Informatics **CJMM:** Evaluate Outcomes

Rationale: All paper and electronic documentation is part of a client's health record and is a legal document. Written documentation should be legible, and all documentation should be timely as other team members rely on current documentation for providing client care. Prioritizing data will keep documentation succinct, and therefore, more helpful. Opinions are not appropriate and should not be included.

THIN Thinking: *Top Three* – While a client data collection is documented thoroughly, documentation such as a nursing note highlights priority information that is relevant to client care and helpful for other members of the care team.

11. **The nurse cares for a client with middle-stage Alzheimer's Disease. Which finding does the nurse determine to be consistent with this stage of the disease?**
    a. Lack of awareness of the environment.
    b. Occasional memory lapses.
    c. Slower movements when dressing.
    d. Forgetting personal events.

Topic/Concept: Role of the Nurse **Subtopic:** Safety **Bloom's Taxonomy:** Analyzing **Clinical Problem-Solving Process:** Data Collection **NCLEX-PN®:** Physiological Adaptation **QSEN:** Safety **CJMM:** Analyze Cues

Rationale: Occasional memory lapses and slowed movements are consistent with early-stage progression of Alzheimer's Disease. Forgetting one's personal history and experiences is consistent with middle-stage progression. Losing awareness of one's environment is consistent with late-stage progression.

THIN Thinking: *Top Three* – The nurse can evaluate the stage of the disease by being aware of the symptoms indicating progression from one stage to the next.

12. **The nurse prioritizes a client's care using Maslow's Hierarchy of Basic Needs. Because the client's physiological needs are met, which safety need does the nurse address?**
    a. Clean drinking water.
    b. Protective housing.
    c. Belongingness.
    d. Self-fulfillment.

Topic/Concept: Role of the Nurse **Subtopic:** Safety **Bloom's Taxonomy:** Applying **Clinical Problem-Solving Process:** Planning **NCLEX-PN®:** Basic Care and Comfort **QSEN:** Safety **CJMM:** Prioritize Hypotheses

Rationale: Clean drinking water is a physiologic need; shelter and security are safety needs; belongingness is a love and belonging need; self-fulfillment is an element of self-actualization.

THIN Thinking: *Top Three* – The nurse should implement care based on level of priority, using Maslow's hierarchy of needs and addressing physiological and life-threatening issues first.

13. The nurse cares for a client in diabetic ketoacidosis (DKA) and evaluates the client's response to intravenous fluids and intravenous insulin. Which data indicates the client is responding positively to treatment?

a. Rate and depth of respirations increase.
b. Pulse and respiratory rate increase.
c. Client becomes more alert; respirations slow.
d. Blood pressure decreases; pulse increases.

Topic/Concept: Role of the Nurse **Subtopic:** Safety **Bloom's Taxonomy:** Analyzing **Clinical Problem-Solving Process:** Evaluation **NCLEX-PN®:** Physiological Adaptation **QSEN:** Safety **CJMM:** Evaluate Outcomes

Rationale: The client in DKA is typically lethargic or sleepy and may be confused or disoriented. A slowing of respirations towards baseline and an increase in alertness indicate improvement in DKA. Rapid pulse and deep, rapid respirations (Kussmaul respirations) are often seen in DKA and do not indicate improvement. Hypotension may be present with DKA, and pulse may increase to compensate; this does not indicate improvement.

THIN Thinking: *Clinical Problem-Solving Process* –When providing nursing care, the nurse should continuously evaluate the client's status and response to treatment. It is important for the nurse to monitor the client in DKA to determine the need for a change in treatment.

14. The nurse begins a daily report to the unlicensed assistive personnel (UAP) on the nursing team. The nurse notes that the UAP has a flushed face, nasal congestion, moist cough, and appears pale. The nurse asks the UAP how she feels, and the UAP states, "I have a bit of a fever, and I'm tired, but I need to work." What is the nurse's best action?

a. Delegate tasks to the UAP as previously planned.
b. Assist the UAP to an empty client room to lie down.
c. Provide the UAP with a surgical mask before seeing clients.
d. Insist the UAP see the charge nurse about going home.

Topic/Concept: Role of the Nurse **Subtopic:** Teamwork and Collaboration **Bloom's Taxonomy:** Applying **Clinical Problem-Solving Process:** Implementation **NCLEX-PN®:** Safety and Infection Control **QSEN:** Teamwork and Collaboration **CJMM:** Take Action

Rationale: The nurse must consider the team member's wellbeing while also protecting the clients and other team members. To reduce the risk of spreading infection, the UAP needs to see the charge nurse about going home.

THIN Thinking: *Help Quick* – The nurse not only collects data on the client but should be observant of issues that may arise in team members and co-workers.

15. The nurse plans to discuss electronic health records (EHRs) with older adults at a local senior center. Which information regarding EHRs is incorrect and not included in the nurse's presentation?

a. The Health Insurance Portability and Accountability Act applies to EHRs.
b. EHRs are generally facility-specific and not shared across institutions.
c. EHRs are relatively safe from hacking and releases of information.
d. Only physicians have access to the information in EHRs.

Topic/Concept: Role of the Nurse **Subtopic:** Informatics **Bloom's Taxonomy:** Applying **Clinical Problem-Solving Process:** Planning **NCLEX-PN®:** Health Promotion and Maintenance **QSEN:** Informatics **CJMM:** Generate Solutions

Rationale: EHR access is provided on a need-to-know basis; thus, all medical providers, registration staff, etc. may have access to some elements of electronic records. The other statements are all accurate.

THIN Thinking: *Clinical Problem-Solving Process* –When planning care or education for the client, the nurse must share the most important information with the client and address concerns correctly.

16. The oncoming nurse receives report from the previous nurse. What additional information is a priority for the nurse to obtain from the client's electronic health record (EHR)? *Select all that apply.*

a. Recent and trending laboratory results.
b. Recent and trending vital signs.
c. Client's insurance information.
d. Specific cultural or spiritual requests.
e. Client's marital status and living situation.

Topic/Concept: Role of the Nurse **Subtopic:** Informatics **Bloom's Taxonomy:** Applying **Clinical Problem-Solving Process:** Planning **NCLEX-PN®:** Coordinated Care **QSEN:** Teamwork and Collaboration **CJMM:** Prioritize Hypotheses

Rationale: Trending lab values and vital signs are critical in planning client care. Cultural or spiritual requests are helpful but not the priority. Insurance information and marital status are unnecessary to provide nursing care.

THIN Thinking: *Top Three* – The nurse should use the EHR to collect data that was not received in the nursing report or to confirm information received that is important in providing nursing care.

17. **The nurse prepares to administer an analgesic to a client for post-operative pain. Which information is the priority for the nurse to obtain from the electronic health record?**
    a. Medication allergies.
    b. Medication route and dosage.
    c. Last time of administration.
    d. Pain relief from last administration.

Topic/Concept: Role of the Nurse **Subtopic:** Informatics **Bloom's Taxonomy:** Applying **Clinical Problem-Solving Process:** Planning **NCLEX-PN®:** Basic Care and Comfort **QSEN:** Evidence-based Practice **CJMM:** Prioritize Hypotheses

Rationale: Checking medication allergies is the priority response to ensure the client's safety. The other information is important but not the priority.

THIN Thinking: *Identify Risk to Safety* – The nurse should follow the six rights of medication administration when preparing medications. If the client has an allergy to a drug, it is not appropriate for administration and continued implementation of the rights would not be relevant.

18. **The emergency room nurse cares for an older adolescent client brought to the facility for substance use. The nurse implements which patient-centered approach to communicating with the adolescent?**
    a. Communicate only with the parents, not the adolescent.
    b. Give the adolescent choices in the delivery of care.
    c. Take a direct, authoritative approach to communicating.
    d. Allow the adolescent sole decision-making rights.

Topic/Concept: Role of the Nurse **Subtopic:** QSEN Competencies **Bloom's Taxonomy:** Applying **Clinical Problem-Solving Process:** Planning **NCLEX-PN®:** Psychosocial Integrity **QSEN:** Patient-centered Care **CJMM:** Prioritize Hypotheses

Rationale: Adolescents may be resistant to authoritative approaches and decisions made by adults. They should be given choices and included in their own plan of care whenever possible, but they are still minors and do not have sole decision-making rights.

THIN Thinking: *Top Three* – The nurse should approach clients at their level of development, which is not always correlated with their age. For adolescents, it is important to remember their need for autonomy and provide them with choices when possible.

19. **The registered nurse (RN) delegates tasks to the licensed practical nurse (LPN) and unlicensed assistive personnel (UAP). Which action by the nurse indicates an understanding of the role of the care team?**
    a. The RN requests the LPN complete a new admission assessment.
    b. The RN asks the LPN to change bed linens and refill water pitchers.
    c. The RN asks the UAP to refill water pitchers and assigns the LPN oral medications.
    d. The RN asks the LPN to administer packed red blood cells.

Topic/Concept: Role of the Nurse **Subtopic:** Teamwork and Collaboration **Bloom's Taxonomy:** Analyzing **Clinical Problem-Solving Process:** Evaluation **NCLEX-PN®:** Coordinated Care **QSEN:** Teamwork and Collaboration **CJMM:** Evaluate Outcomes

Rationale: Admission assessments and administering blood products are not within the LPN scope of practice, and the LPN should decline these assignments. Changing linens and filling water pitchers is not a good use of the LPN's knowledge and skills and should be assigned to the UAP. Asking the UAP to fill waters and the LPN to administer oral medications is appropriate delegation.

THIN Thinking: *Clinical Problem-Solving Process* –The nurse should determine if nursing care is within the scope of practice for their degree and licensing. If care is outside that scope of practice or not in the knowledge or skill level of the nurse, they should decline to perform or ask for assistance in completing the task.

20. **The nurse assists the health care provider in a procedure requiring informed consent. What is the nurse's role in the informed consent process?**
    a. Explain the purpose of the procedure.
    b. Explain the risks and benefits of the procedure.
    c. Witness the client's signature on the consent form.
    d. Answer any of the client's remaining questions.

Topic/Concept: Role of the Nurse **Subtopic:** Teamwork and Collaboration **Bloom's Taxonomy:** Applying **Clinical Problem-Solving Process:** Planning **NCLEX-PN®:** Basic Care and Comfort **QSEN:** Teamwork and Collaboration **CJMM:** Generate Solutions

Rationale: Witnessing the client's signature is the responsibility of the nurse. The other components of obtaining informed consent are the provider's responsibility.

THIN Thinking: *Clinical Problem-Solving Process* –The nurse should act within their scope of practice regarding informed consent. The nurse's role is not to inform or obtain the consent but to serve as a client advocate, ensure the client is competent to provide informed consent, and witness the signing of the consent form.

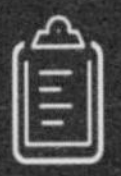

NurseThink® Quiz Answers

CHAPTER

20

Where do I go from here?

Next steps: Set your study goals—Plan your study time and stick with it

You have been successful thus far. You've completed nursing school...you're dedicated to a career in nursing. Let's just get you through the next hurdle...NCLEX-PN®! We know you have a career goal...let's set up some study goals!

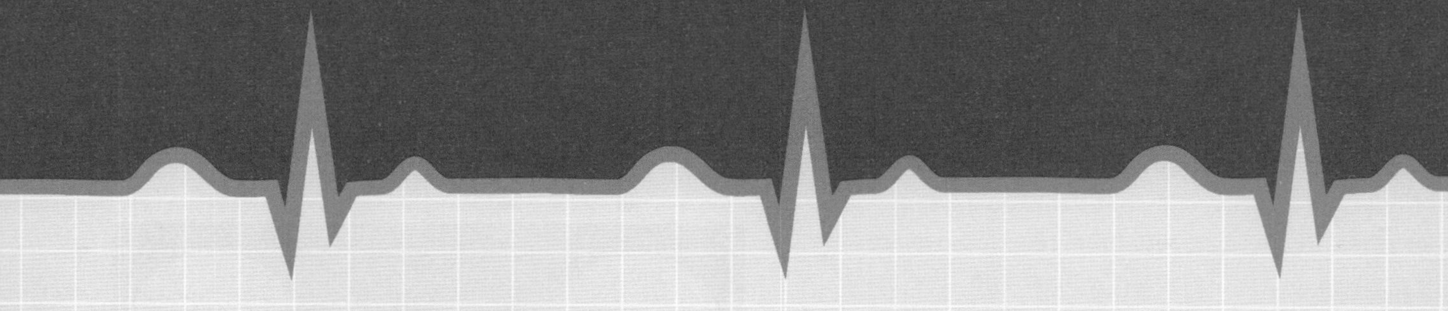

In case you are one of those people who skip to the last chapter or routinely just start at the end, let's talk about using this book. Using a calendar or your phone calendar to establish a study schedule is a good way to get started. Split this text up in sections and assign sections to days or weeks. End the week or time period with a test, from here, online, another text, or from test banks. Make sure the tests you take represent areas of study (as at the end of chapters in this text) or are based upon the NCLEX-PN® blueprint (like the quizzes available with this text).

Then, when you've read through the **Priority Exemplars**, completed the **Go To Clinical Cases**, and **NurseThink® Quizzes** you may set some additional goals for your study or prep time. First, look at your time – if you've scheduled the exam, look at the days you have until the exam. If you haven't scheduled yet—remember what we discussed in Chapter 3. Schedule the exam with enough time to study-but soon enough to avoid memory lag! What commitments do you have in between now and then? Work? Family? Personal? Then, plot out your time. Make a commitment to study EVERY day! Some find it helpful to use a calendar, planner, or computer calendar to make a visual representation of their study plan. Remember the 50/100 study rule. Every day complete a 50-item quiz—as you check your answers, write down or take note of the topics you get wrong. Read the rationales carefully. If you still have questions, use this book or other resources to dig deeper into the topic. Remember to study the topics you don't know or you don't feel as comfortable answering questions about—don't study the material you have mastered! Look up information about the questions you don't understand—remember to study to learn, not memorize.

Once a week, complete a 100-item or more test. Longer tests allow you to maintain your "test-taking stamina" that will be needed for NCLEX-PN®. Again, focus on the questions and topics you get wrong! These larger tests are also a good time to determine why you are getting items wrong. Is it a lack of knowledge? Are you missing keywords when you are reading? Did you look at the question and you believed that you knew the material—but missed the intent of the question? As discussed previously, so much of success on the NCLEX-PN® is quiet, calm reading! Taking your time is critical as you progress toward NCLEX-PN®.

Other strategies have demonstrated effectiveness in enhancing the quality of your studying. Many set apart a designated room or area for studying. Make sure it is a comfortable spot, but not too comfortable! You don't want to sleep through your study time! Surround yourself with water, plenty of pencils/pens, a computer and textbooks to look up information, and some "creature comforts." These may include your favorite slippers, soft music, heartwarming pictures of friends and family, or inspirational posters or messages. Remember, your brain responds well to the messages of affirmations, wherein positive self-talk bolsters your confidence and your test-taking abilities! Then, when you are taking a test or quiz—make sure you simulate the testing environment. Consider the testing session as a real testing event—no interruptions, no snacks, no phones, no talking, no music, no fun—just testing.

Some find that *group* studying helps reinforce concepts and information. The benefits of group studying include the ability to garner many perspectives while studying. For example, other people may identify topics, approaches, or potential issues that you haven't thought about yet! These groups also offer the opportunity for discussion about testing and processes. Other opinions or questions, answers, and interpretations of the test plan may broaden your knowledge and the ability to prepare for NCLEX-PN®.

Your healthy NCLEX® lifestyle

We want to reiterate the importance of healthy lifestyle choices during this stressful time. Researchers tell us that the average adult needs 7-8 hours of sleep per night. Our society rewards those who don't appear to need as much sleep, posing accolades for those who sleep 3-4 hours per day. In fact, many people in our society live in chronic sleep deprivation and most people would benefit from more sleep. If you have trouble falling asleep or are wakeful during the night, investigate sleep hygiene practices. Habits such as limiting screen time a few hours before bed, a warm bath or shower, reading before bed, placing a notepad and pen near the bed to make lists of things (rather than worrying about them), listening to soft music, not studying in bed but reserving the bed for sleep, and practicing calming meditation or imagery while preparing for sleep may all assist in getting that good night's rest. Exercise is great... but make sure you complete your work-out a few hours prior to bedtime to ensure a "winding down" time before bed.

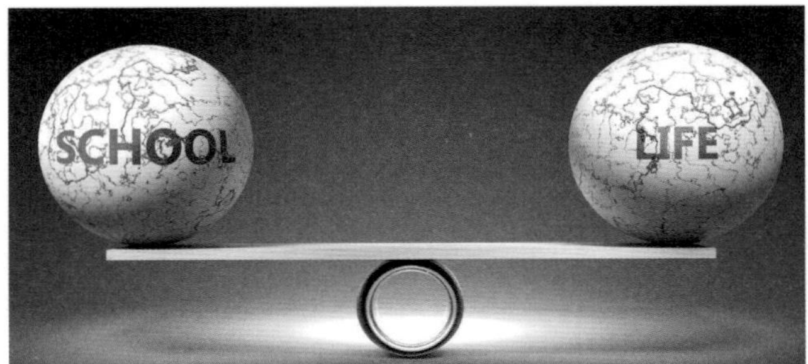

Image 20-1: Think about the various elements of your life you needed to balance while in school. Many find this balance just as challenging as you carve out study time to prepare for NCLEX®.

What will assist you in making your study plan successful?

How will you balance work, study, life, and personal demands?

Next Gen Clinical Judgment

A healthy lifestyle includes components of nutrition, exercise, sleep, stress management, play, relationships, intellectual stimulation, sense of worth, spiritual faith, and reduction of risk behaviors. Which element most requires your attention to make the greatest improvement in your health?

Neuroscience studies demonstrate that adequate sleep enhances learning by increasing our ability to attend in learning situations, in processing information to memories, and in organizing memories for later retrieval. In fact, it is during sleep that our brain transfers short-term memories into long-term storage such that we can make connections to previously learned information when exposed to new ideas and retrieve information. The implications for a sound night's rest are evident here—so sleep well!

Just as critical as sleep is the need to fuel your body for optimum functioning. Research into high protein/low carbohydrate diets and others that espouse balanced nutrition all point to the need for your body to be at its best physically when studying for and taking the exam. Many sources support the use of B-complex vitamin supplementation to enable the body to best deal with stress. Others support adequate fiber in your diet to ensure gastrointestinal regularity. Most sources affirm the universal "goodness" of adequate water intake. Think for a moment of your last busy day—during classes or on the job—if you were on day shift, somewhere around 3:00 PM you may have become drowsy. You went in search of a "pick-me-up." That may have led you to a caffeinated soda or coffee, a sweet snack, or something salty. Instead, many authorities contend that your "slump" was more related to dehydration than hypoglycemia (unless you have a medical diagnosis). So, try drinking 12-16 ounces of water the next time you feel lethargic and see if it really is more about hydration. Remember that caffeine and alcohol are dehydrating so imbibe within reason—this study period is not the time for excesses. That being said, also strictly avoid stimulants. Not only do they make you jittery but they may hamper your ability to make connections and think critically—essential skills in NCLEX-PN® preparation.

Next Gen Clinical Judgment

Although the Next Gen revisions will not start until 2023, make sure you practice with Next Gen style items as part of your NCLEX® preparation!

Other aspects of the healthy lifestyle—to put you at your best—include balancing your life. Make sure you exercise—find something you enjoy doing—running, walking, dancing, yoga, sports, swimming—and try to find time five days per week to work your muscles and enhance your oxygenation. A lot of time writing, reading, or on a computer may lead to neck and back pain—muscle stretches, twists, progressive relaxation, or even a massage, may enhance your endurance and ability to really attend as you adhere to your study goals.

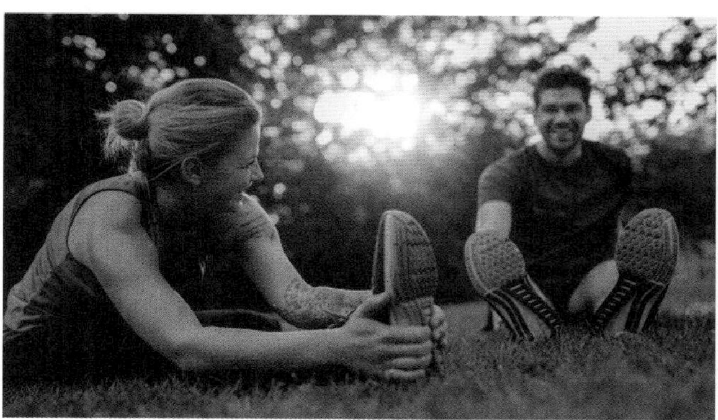

Image 20-2: Make a commitment to adhere to a healthy lifestyle. What sleep, nutrition, stress management, exercise, hydration, and play improvements will you make in your life?

Now is also the time to make sure you play! Spend an afternoon with friends and family! Engage in retail therapy (within reason)! Enjoy the sunshine when you can (buildup your Vitamin D stores) and hunker down to study on rainy days. Consider your hobbies—what do you love to do? What activities help you get away from it all? Let's think about that calendar you made to study—many individuals find it helpful to identify times in the calendar for play and time with family and friends. Sometimes, it is easier to engage in hard-core studying when you know something fun is on the horizon! Still not sure of how to fill up your time? See the article on NCLEX-PN® Boot Camp listed on the reference list in the back of this book to develop your own boot camp of work, play and lifestyle activities around your studying and preparation.

Clinical Hint

See the Online Quizzing resources for Next Gen and other test items.

That also brings up your support systems. Consider the people in your world that are also invested in your success. Think about those who have supported you throughout nursing school and, perhaps, other life crossroads. Ask them to stick with you just a few more months. Seek their assistance in managing home, family, and other obligations. Sometimes support systems need a reminder that, although you are done with school, your study time hasn't ended. Remind them that this exam is **important** and implore that they stand by you for just a little longer.

This also may be a time that your "BFFs" from nursing school (or other arenas) provide a significant amount of support. Not only do they know what you are going through, but they may be in the same situation! We all know that "misery loves company" and, although we don't want you to think of this as total misery—those in the same situation may best empathize with your current concerns. If you are working in a clinical area, engage in conversations with the staff. Talk to the other nurses about their role, daily lives, and memories of NCLEX-PN®. This may offer some encouraging support.

Focus on your goals and the nearness of these goals! That may energize and inspire you for continued success!

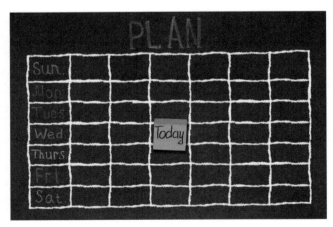

Image 20-3: How will you plan your time when studying for NCLEX®? What resources , in addition to this text, will you use to create a comprehensive study plan?

Be Successful!

So now it is up to you! We have shared information on testing, studying, and nursing content. We have made suggestions on how to best prepare yourself for NCLEX-PN®. Now the hard work is up to you! We can say, unequivocally, that your time and effort, your sweat and tears, are worth it! Nursing is a privilege! No other profession can boast the assets of our life's work! We reach people in so many ways, we make a difference, and we enjoy so many personal moments of success and humility every day! We wish you well and offer sincere wishes of success on the NCLEX-PN® exam! In a short period of time, we hope to welcome you to the rewarding and vital profession of nursing! Good luck on this next step in your professional life!

Next Gen Clinical Judgment

Consider how you will study for NCLEX® to focus on clinical judgment. When answering questions, visualize a client experiencing the issue, problem, or disorder.

- What signs or cues would the client be manifesting?
- What additional data would you need to collect to care for this client?
- How should a nurse respond to this problem or issue?
- What should the nurse consider when planning the care of this client?
- What interventions or actions might be indicated?
- How would a nurse know that their interventions are effective?
- How would the client look if the client was deteriorating?
- How would the client look if the client was improving?
- How does this client's care compare with those for whom you have cared in the past?
- How does this client's care contrast (appear different from) those for whom you have cared in the past?
- How will you use this information to care for future clients or answer questions in the future?

References

Altmiller, G. (2017). Content validation of quality and safety education for nurses-based clinical evaluation instrument. Nurse Educator, 42(1), 23-27.

American Automobile Association. (2018). Car seat safety laws. Retrieved from https://drivinglaws.aaa.com/tag/child-passenger-safety/

American Cancer Society. (Revised 2016). Cancer A-Z. Retrieved from https://www.cancer.org/cancer.html

American Cancer Society. (2018). Guidelines for the early detection of cancer. Retrieved from https://connection.cancer.org/Consumer/PDF/Product/P2070.00.pdf

American Cancer Society. (2018). How are Wilms tumors diagnosed? Retrieved from https://www.cancer.org/cancer/wilms-tumor/detection-diagnosis-staging/how-diagnosed.html

American Stroke Association. (2015). Complications after stroke. Retrieved from www.strokeassociation.org/letstalkaboutstroke

Bello, J., Quinn, P., & Horrell, L. (2011). Maintaining patient safety through innovation: An electronic SBAR communication tool. CIN: Computers, Informatics, Nursing, 29 (9), 481-483.

Black, B. P. (2017). Professional nursing: Concepts and challenges (8th ed.). St. Louis, MO: Elsevier.

Cancer Treatment Centers of America. (2018). About your cancer. Retrieved from https://www.cancercenter.com/cancer/

Centers for Disease Control and Prevention. (2018). Lung cancer. Retrieved from https://www.cdc.gov/cancer/lung/

Children's Hospital of Wisconsin. (2018). Hydrocephalus. Retrieved from https://www.chw.org/medical-care/fetal-concerns-center/conditions/infant-complication/hydrocephalus

Comprehensive Cancer Center, University of Michigan Health System. (2013). A Patient and family guide to blood and marrow transplant. Retrieved from http://www.med.umich.edu/cancer/files/bmt-patient-family-handbook.pdf

Cronenwett, L. & Sherwood, G. (2011). Lecture: Innovations for integrating quality and safety in education and practice: The QSEN project [Power Point slides]. Retrieved from http://www.qsen.org/docs/qsen_cronenwett_sherwood_STTI_2011_special_session.pdf

Cronenwett, L., Sherwood, G., Barnsteiner, J., Disch, J., Johnson, J., Mitchell, P., Sullivan, D., & Warren, J. (2007). Quality and safety education for nurses. Nursing Outlook, 55 (3), 122-131.

Cuellar, E.T. (2017). HESI comprehensive review for the NCLEX-RN® examination. St. Louis, MO: Elsevier.

Dickinson, P., Luo, X., Kim, D., Wood, A., Muntean, W., & Bergstrom, B. (2016). Assessing higher-order cognitive constructs by using an information-processing framework. Journal of Applied Testing Technology, 17 (1), 1-19.

Giddens, J. F. (2017). Concepts of nursing practice (2nd ed.). St. Louis, MO: Elsevier.

Giordano, S.H. (2018). Breast cancer in men. New England Journal of Medicine, 378, 2311-2320.

Halter, M.J. (2018). Varcarolis' foundations of psychiatric-mental health nursing (8th ed.). St. Louis, MO: Elsevier.

Hinkle, J.L. & Cheever, K.H. (2018). Brunner & Suddarth's textbook of medical-surgical nursing (14th ed.). Philadelphia, PA: Wolters Kluwer.

Herrman, J.W. & Johnson, A. (2009). From beta-blockers to boot camp: A nursing course approach to NCLEX® success. Nursing Education Perspectives, 30 (6), 384-388.

Hockenberry, M.J., & Wilson, D. (2015). Wong's nursing care of infants and children. St. Louis, MO: Elsevier.

Hogan, M. (2018). Comprehensive review for NCLEX-RN® (3rd ed.). New York, NY: Pearson.

Institute of Medicine. (2003). Health professions education: A bridge to quality. A. C. Greiner, & E. Knebel (Eds.). Washington, DC: Author.

Institute of Medicine of the National Academies. (2010). The future of nursing: Leading health, advancing change. Retrieved from http://nationalacademies.org/hmd/reports/2010/the-future-of-nursing-leading-change-advancing-health.aspx

Irving, S.Y., Lynam, B., Northington, L., Bartlett, J.A., & Kemper, C. (2014). Nasogastric tube placement and verification in children: A review of the current literature. Critical Care Nurse, 34 (3), 67-76.

Isaacs, D. (2017). Antibiotic prophylaxis for infective endocarditis: A systematic review and meta-analysis. Journal of Paediatrics and Child Health, 53 (9), 921-922.

Johns Hopkins Medicine, Sydney Kimmel Cancer Center, Blood and Bone Marrow Cancers Program. (n.d.). Blood and bone marrow cancer basics. Retrieved from https://www.hopkinsmedicine.org/kimmel_cancer_center/centers/blood_bone_marrow_cancers

Kaufman, J.S. (2017). Acute exacerbation of COPD: Diagnosis and management. The Nurse Practitioner, 42 (6), 1-7.

Koning, C., Young, L., & Bruce, A. (2016). Mind the gap: Women and acute myocardial infarctions: An integrated review of literature. Canadian Journal of Cardiovascular Nursing, 26 (3), 8-14.

Lewis, S.L., Dirksen, S.R., Heitkemper, M.M., & Bucher, L. (2017). Medical-surgical nursing: Assessment and management of clinical problems (10th ed.). St. Louis, MO: Elsevier.

Lilley, L.L., Collins, S.R., & Snyder, J.S. (2017). Pharmacology and the nursing process (8th ed.). St. Louis, MO: Mosby.

Lim, C.L., Byrne, C., & Lee, J.K. (2008). Human thermoregulation and measurement of body temperature in exercise and clinical settings. Annals Academy of Medicine Singapore, 37(4), 347-353.

Lowdermilk, D.L., Perry, S.E., Cashion, M.C., & Alden, K.R. (2015). Maternity and women's healthcare. St. Louis, MO: Elsevier.

Mangin, D. et al. (2012). Chlamydia trachomatis testing sensitivity in midstream compared with first void specimens. Annals of Family Medicine, 10 (1), 50-53.

Mayo Clinic. (2018). Amyotrophic lateral sclerosis. Retrieved from https://www.mayoclinic.org/diseases-conditions/amyotropic-lateral-sclerosis/diagnosis-treatment/drc-20354027

Mayo Clinic. (2018). Cleft lip and cleft palate. Retrieved from https://www.mayoclinic.org/diseases-conditions/cleft-palate/symptoms-causes/syc-20370985

Mayo Clinic. (2018). Diseases and conditions. Retrieved from https://www.mayoclinic.org/diseases-conditions

Mayo Clinic. (2018). Guillain-Barré syndrome. Retrieved from https://www.mayoclinic.org/diseases-conditions/guillain-barre-syndrome/symptoms-causes/syc-20362793

Mayo Clinic. (2018). Pyloric stenosis. Retrieved from https://www.mayoclinic.org/diseases-conditions/pyloric-stenosis/symptoms-causes/syc-20351416

Mayo Clinic. (2018). Spina bifida. Retrieved from https://www.mayoclinic.org/diseases-conditions/spina-bifida/symptoms-causes/syc-20377860

McAllister, T.W. (2011). Neurobiological consequences of traumatic brain injury. Dialogues in Clinical Neuroscience, 13(3), 287-300.

McCuistion, L., Vuljoin-DiMaggio, K., Winton, M.B., & Yeager, J.J. (2018). Pharmacology: A patient-centered nursing process approach (9th ed.). St. Louis, MO: Elsevier.

McKinney, E., James, S., & Murray, S. (2018). Maternal-child nursing (5th ed.). Philadelphia, PA: W.B. Saunders.

Metheny, N.A., Pawluszka, A., Lulic, M., Hinyard, L.J., & Meert, K.L. (2017). Testing placement of gastric feeding tubes in infants. American Journal of Critical Care, 26(6), 466-473.

Nagel, D.A. & Penner, J.L. (2016). Conceptualizing telehealth in nursing practice. Journal of Holistic Nursing, 34 (1), 91-104.

National Council of State Boards of Nursing. (2017). Next generation NCLEX® news. Retrieved from www.ncsbn.org/NCLEX_Next_Fall17_Eng.pdf

National Council of State Boards of Nursing. (2017). Exam to licensure: Your career gateway. Retrieved from www.ncsbn.org

National Council of State Boards of Nursing. (2018). Next generation NCLEX® news. Retrieved from https://www.ncsbn.org/11435.htm

National Institute of Neurological Disorders and Stroke. (2018). All disorders. Retrieved from https://www.ninds.nih.gov/Disorders/All-Disorders?title=&page=6

National Institute of Diabetes and Digestive and Kidney Diseases. (2018). Cushing's syndrome. Retrieved from https://www.niddk.nih.gov/health-information/endocrine-diseases/cushings-syndrome

National Institute of Health and Care Excellence, NICE guideline [NG14]. (2015). Melanoma: Assessment and management. Retrieved from https://www.nice.org.uk/guidance/ng14

O'Grady, N.P., Alexander, M., & Burns, L.A. (2011). Guidelines for the prevention of intravascular catheter-related infections. Atlanta, GA: Centers for Disease Control and Prevention. Retrieved from www.cdc.gov/hicpac/pdf/guidelines/bsi-guidelines-2011.pdf

Pearson Education. (2019). Nursing: A concept-based approach to learning (Vol. 1-3). Minneapolis, MN: Author.

Perry, S.E., Lowdermilk, D.L., Cashion, K., Alden, K.R., Olshansky, E.F., Hockenberry, M.J., Wilson, D., & Rodgers, C.C. (2018). Maternal child nursing care (6th ed.). St. Louis, MO: Elsevier.

Pop, V., & Badaut, J. (2011). A neurovascular perspective for long-term changes after brain trauma. Translational Stroke Research, 2(4), 533-545.

Potter, P.P., Perry, A.G., Stockert, P.A., Hall, A.M., & Ostendorf, W. (2017). Fundamentals of nursing. St. Louis, MO: Elsevier.

QSEN Institute. (2018). Quality and safety education for nurses. Retrieved from www.qsen.org

Ricci, S. (2017). Essentials of maternity, newborn, and women's health nursing (4th ed.). Philadelphia, PA: Wolters Kluwer.

Schirm, V., Banz, G., Swartz, C., & Richmond, M. (2018). Evaluation of bedside shift report: A research and evidence-based practice. Applied Nursing Research, 40, 20-25.

Sherwood, G. & Zomorodi, M. (2014). Anew mindset for quality and safety: The QSEN competencies redefine nurses' roles in practice. Nephrology Nursing Journal, 41, 15-23.

Silvestri, L.A. & Silvestri, A. (2017). Saunders comprehensive review for the NCLEX-RN® examination (7th ed.). St. Louis, MO: Elsevier.

Stalter, A. & Mota, A. (2018). Using systems thinking to envision quality and safety in healthcare (QSEN). Nursing Management, 49(2), 32-39.

Stanhope, M. & Lancaster, J. (2016). Public health nursing: Population-centered health care in the community (9th ed.). St. Louis, MO: Elsevier.

St Jude's Children's Research Hospital. (2018). Wilms tumor. Retrieved from https://www.stjude.org/disease/wilms-tumor.html

Taylor, C., Lillis, C., Lynn, P., & LeMone, P. (2015). Fundamentals of nursing (8th ed.). Philadelphia, PA: Wolters Kluwer.

Townsend, M. (2015). Psychiatric mental health nursing: Concepts of care in evidence-based practice. Philadelphia, PA: FA Davis.

University of California San Francisco (2018). Acute lymphoblastic leukemia treatment. Retrieved from https://www.ucsfhealth.org/conditions/acute_lymphoblastic_leukemia/treatment.html

U.S. Department of Health and Human Services, Centers for Disease Control and Prevention. (2018). Bacterial meningitis. Retrieved from https://www.cdc.gov/meningitis/bacterial.html

U.S. Department of Health and Human Services, Centers for Disease Control and Prevention. (2018). Information on avian influenza. Retrieved from https://www.cdc.gov/flu/avianflu/index.htm

U.S. Department of Health and Human Services, Centers for Disease Control and Prevention. (2018). Information on swine influenza/variant influenza virus. Retrieved from https://www.cdc.gov/flu/swineflu/index.htm

U.S. Department of Health and Human Services, Centers for Disease Control and Prevention. (2018). Pink eye: Usually mild and easy to treat. Retrieved from https://www.cdc.gov/Features/Conjunctivitis/

U.S. Department of Health and Human Services, Centers for Disease Control and Prevention. (2018). Prevention strategies for seasonal influenza in healthcare settings. Retrieved from https://www.cdc.gov/flu/professionals/infectioncontrol/healthcaresettings.htm

U.S. Department of Health and Human Services, Centers for Disease Prevention and Control. (2016). The ABCs of hepatitis. Retrieved from https://www.cdc.gov/hepatitis/resources/professionals/pdfs/abctable.pdf

U.S. Department of Health and Human Services, National Institute of Diabetes and Digestive and Kidney Disease. (2018). Adrenal insufficiency and Addison's disease. Retrieved from https://www.niddk.nih.gov/health-information/endocrine-diseases/adrenal- insufficiency- addisons- disease

U.S. Department of Health and Human Services, National Institute of Diabetes and Digestive and Kidney Disease. (2018). Cushing's syndrome. Retrieved from https://www.niddk.nih.gov/health-information/endocrine-diseases/cushings-syndrome

U.S. Department of Health and Human Services, National Institutes of Health, National Cancer Institute. (2018). Cancer types. Retrieved from https://www.cancer.gov/types

U.S. Department of Health and Human Services, National Institutes of Health, National Heart, Lung, and Blood Institute. (2018). Polycythemia Vera. Retrieved from https://www.nhlbi.nih.gov/health-topics/polycythemia-vera

U.S. Department of Health and Human Services National Institutes of Health, National Institute of Neurological Disorders and Stroke. (2018). Myasthenia gravis fact sheet. Retrieved from https://www.ninds.nih.gov/disorders/patient-caregiver-education/fact-sheets/myasthenia-gravis-fact-sheet

U.S. Department of Health and Human Services National Institutes of Health, National Institute of Neurological Disorders and Stroke. (2018). Peripheral neuropathy fact sheet. Retrieved from https://www.ninds.nih.gov/Disorders/Patient-Caregiver-Education/Fact-Sheets/Peripheral-Neuropathy-Fact-Sheet#3208_1

Vallerand, A.H., Sanoski, C.A., & Deglin, J.H. (2017). Davis's drug guide for nurses (15th ed.). Philadelphia, PA: FA Davis.

Varcarolis, E.M. (2017). Essentials of psychiatric mental health nursing (3rd ed.). St. Louis, MO: Elsevier.

Venes, D. (Ed). (2017). Taber's cyclopedic medical dictionary (23rd ed.). Philadelphia, PA: FA Davis.

Whelton, P.K, & Carey, R.M. (2017). The 2017 guideline for high blood pressure. JAMA: Journal of the American Medical Association, 318(21). 2073-2074.

Wilmot Cancer Institute. (2018). Blood and marrow transplantation. Retrieved from https://www.urmc.rochester.edu/cancer-institute/services/bmt/patient-discharge.aspx

World Health Organization. (2017). Fact sheets: Hepatitis E. Retrieved from http://www.who.int/en/news-room/fact-sheets/detail/hepatitis-e

Yan, S., Wang, X., Lv, C., Wang, Y., Wang, J., Yang, Y., & Wu, N. (2017). Intermittent chest tube clamping may shorten chest tube duration and postoperative hospital stay. Journal of Thoracic Oncology, 12 (1), S1402-S1403.

Yoder-Wise, P. (2014). Leading and managing in nursing (5th ed.). St. Louis, MO: Elsevier.

Index

T

U

V

W

Z

NurseThink® Quick Laboratory and Diagnostics

LAB TEST	NORMAL RANGE	CRITICAL CONCERNS	INCREASED
HEMATOLOGY			
CBC			
*Red Blood Cells / Erythrocytes (RBC)	4.2 - 5.9 × 10^6/µL		(Polycythemia), Hemoconcentration
Reticulocytes	0.5 - 1.5%		Acute Hemorrhage
*Hemoglobin (Hgb)	12 - 17 g/dL	< 5.0 g/dL or > 20 g/dL	
*Hematocrit (Hct)	36 - 51%	< 15% or > 60%	
*White Blood Cells / Leukocytes (WBC)	4,000-10,000 µL or mm^3	< 2,500 or > 30,000 µL or mm^3	Infections, Inflammation, Stress
*Neutrophils (polys/segs)	> 75%		Bacterial Infections
Bands	< 10%	> 10%	Acute Bacterial Infection
*Absolute Neutrophil Count (ANC)	> 1000 µL or mm^3	< 1000 µL or mm^3	
*Platelets	150,000-350,000 µL or mm^3	< 50,000 or > 1 million µL or mm^3	Malignancies
COAGULATION			
Bleeding time	Less than 10 minutes	> 10 minutes	Low Platelets, DIC, ASA
Prothrombin Time (PT)	11 - 12.5 seconds	> 20 seconds	Liver dysfunction, Coumadin, Vit K Deficiency
*International Normalized Ratio (INR)	0.8 - 1.1	> 5.5	Liver dysfunction, Coumadin, Vit K Deficiency
Activated Partial Thromboplastin Time (aPTT)	25 - 35 seconds	> 70 seconds	Coagulation Deficiencies, Heparin
Partial Thromboplastin Time (PTT)	60 - 70 seconds	> 100 seconds	Coagulation Deficiencies, Heparin
D-dimer	< 0.5 mcg/mL		Thrombus
IMMUNE & INFLAMMATORY			
C-Reactive Protein (CRP)	< 1.0 mg/dL		Bacterial Infection, Inflammation
Erythrocyte Sedimentation Rate (ESR)	0 - 20 mm/h		Inflammation, Renal Failure, Malignancy
FLUID, ELECTROLYES & RENAL			
URINE			
*Urine Specific Gravity	1.005 - 1.030		Dehydration, SIADH
METABOLIC PANEL			
*Blood Urea Nitrogen (BUN)	8 - 20 mg/dL	> 100 mg/dL	Renal Failure, Dehydration, ↑Protein Intake
*Creatinine	0.7 - 1.3 mg/dL	> 4 mg/dL	Renal Disease
Electrolytes			
*Potassium (K)	3.5 - 5.0 mEq/L	< 2.5 mEq/L or > 6.5 mEq/L	Acidosis, Renal Failure
*Sodium (Na)	136 - 145 mEq/L	< 120 mEq/L or > 160 mEq/L	Diabetes Insipidus, Cushing's, HHNK
*Calcium (Ca)	9 - 10.5 mg/dL	< 6 mg/dL or > 13 mg/dL	Hyperparathyroidism, Renal Failure
Chloride (Cl)	98 - 106 mEq/L	< 80 mEq/L or > 115 mEq/L	Dehydration, Metabolic Acidosis
*Magnesium (Mg)	1.5 - 2.4 mEq/L	< 0.5 mEq/L or > 3 mEq/L	Renal Failure
Phosphorus (Ph)	3.0 - 4.5 mg/dL	< 1 mg/dL	Hypoparathyroidism, Renal Failure
*Glucose	70 - 100 mg/dL	< 50 mg/dL or > 400 mg/dL	Diabetic Ketoacidosis, HHNK
*Protein - Total	6 - 7.8 g/dL		Hemoconcentration
*Protein - Albumin	3.5 - 5.0 g/dL		Dehydration
FLUID STATUS			
* Serum Osmolality	275 - 295 mOsm/kg	< 265 or > 320 mOsm/kg	Diabetes Insipidus, HHNK, Hyperglycemia
CARDIOPULMONARY			
ABG's			
*pH	7.35 - 7.45	< 7.25 or > 7.55	Alkalosis (resp/metabolic)
*pO_2	80 - 100 mmHg	< 40 mmHg	Hyperoxygenation
*pCO_2	35 - 45 mmHg	< 20 mmHg or > 60 mmHg	Hypoventilation
*HCO_3	22- 26 mEq/L	< 15 mEq/L or > 40 mEq/L	Metabolic alkalosis
*O_2 saturation	> 94%	< 75%	
Brain natriuretic peptide (BNP)	< 100 pg/mL		Heart failure
METABOLISM & WASTE			
Ammonia	40 - 80 mcg/dL		Liver dysfunction
Bilirubin - Total	0.3 - 1.2 mg/dL	Adult: > 12 mg/dL	Liver failure, RBC hemolysis, GB obstruction
Thyroid Stimulating Hormone (TSH)	0.5 - 5 mU/L		Thyroid dysfunction
ENZYMES			
Alkaline Phosphatase (ALP.)	36 - 92 U/L	Enzymes will be released and rise with cell damage. Once the damage stops, the enzymes will return to normal.	Liver, Biliary Tract, Bone
Aminotransferase, Alanine (ALT)	0 - 35 U/L		Liver, (Less in Kidneys, Heart, Muscles)
Aminotransferase, Aspartate (AST)	0 - 35 U/L		Liver
Amylase	0 - 130 U/L		Pancreas
Creatine Kinase (CPK)	30 - 170 U/L		Heart, Brain, Muscle
Lactic Dehydrogenase (LDH)	60 - 100 U/L		Heart, Liver, Kidneys, Muscles, Brain, Lungs
Lipase	< 95 U/L		Pancreas
Troponin I & T	< 0.5ng/mL & < 0.10 ng/mL		Cardiac
THERAPUETIC DRUG LEVELS			
Peak and Trough			
Digoxin	0.8-2.0 ng/mL	> 2.4 ng/mL = toxic level	
Lithium	0.6- 1.2 mEq/L	> 1.5 mEq/L = toxic level	Renal Failure, ↓consciousness, ECG changes

* Know APPROXIMATE Normal for NCLEX® Exam

References: American College of Physicians & Mosby's Diagnostic and Laboratory Test Reference, 10th ed.

Do not memorize specific lab numbers – they vary greatly.
It is more important to know **approximate** normal and recognize **critical concerns** – this is when a nursing action is required.

DECREASED	SPECIAL NOTES
(Anemia), Blood Loss, Hemodilution	↑ with Epoetin; Too High = Clot formation; Too Low = O_2 Transport
Bone Marrow Failure	Immature RBCs
	Oxygen Carrying Capacity; PRBC < 7 g/dL
	Hydration Dependent
Chemo, Bone Marrow Failure	↑ with Filgrastim
Chemo, Bone Marrow Failure	Poly/Segs are Mature WBCs
Bone Marrow Failure	Increase = Left Shift
(Neutropenia)	ANC = WBC x (% Neutrophils + % Bands); < 1000 = Isolation
ITP, Leukemia, Chemo	< 20,000: = Spontaneous Bleed; ↑ with Oprelvekin
	Therapeutic is > 1.5 - 2 times control with warfarin therapy
	Therapeutic is 1.5 to 4 with warfarin therapy
	Therapeutic is 1.5-2.5 times the control with heparin therapy
	Cardiac marker but not specific to myocardium
Sickle Cell Anemia, Polycythemia Vera	
Excessive Diuresis, Diabetes Insipidus	Fluctuates Fluid Status
Hepatic Failure, Overhydration	End By-Product of Protein Breakdown
Decreased Muscle Mass	Doubling of level indicates 50% reduction in the GFR
Diuretics, Gastrointestinal Loss	Abnormal level leads to arrhythmias, muscle cramps
SIADH, Addison's	↓ = Lethargy, Stupor, Coma, Seizures; ↑ = Agitation, Seizures
Hypoparathyroidism, Pancreatitis, Low Protein	↓ = Tetany; ↑ = Osteomalacia, Dehydration
Gastrointestinal Loss, Low Na Diet	↓ = Hyperexcitability; ↑ = Weakness, Lethargy
Alcoholism; Renal Disease	Abnormal level leads to arrhythmias, muscle irritability
Hyperparathyroidism, Vit D Deficiency	↓ = Osteomalacia; ↑ Hypocalcemia (tetany)
↓ Glucose intake or absorption, Exercise	
Malnutrition, Burns, Blood Loss	Needed for wound healing
Liver Dysfunction, Nephrotic Syndrome	Impacts fluid shift in and out of the vascular space
SIADH, Overhydration	Measures concentration of dissolved particles in blood
Acidosis(resp/metabolic)	pH is inversely proportional to H+ concentration
Hypoxemia (pneumonia, etc.)	Indirect measure of O_2 concentration in arterial blood
Hyperventilation	Measurement of ventilation
Metabolic acidosis	Measures metabolic component of acid-base balance
Hypoxemia/Anemia	Indication of the % of Hgb saturated with oxygen
	The higher the number the weaker the left ventricular contractions
	Product of protein breakdown; Neurotoxic; Treated with Lactulose
	Neurotoxic to newborns
Pituitary dysfunction, Hyperthyroidism	T3, T4, T7 often needed to rule out thyroid dysfunction
	Biochemical Markers for Cardiac Disease
	Monitors therapeutic drug levels of nephrotoxic medications
Subtherapeutic	Cardiac Glycoside
Subtherapeutic: symptoms poorly controlled	Lithium clearance from the body is increased during pregnancy

PRIORITY LABS

Infection, Inflammation & Immunity
WBCs, Segs, Bands, ANC, CRP, ESR

Liver Disorders
Liver Enzymes; PT/PTT/INR; Albumin; Ammonia, Bilirubin Na, K, Glucose

Renal Disorders
BUN; Creatinine; Osmolality, K, Na, Ca, Ph, RBCs, Urine SG

Cardiac Disorders
Cardiac Enzymes, BNP, ABGs, Digoxin Level

Pancreas Disorders
Amylase, Lipase, Ca, Glucose

Hemorrhage - DIC
RBCs, Reticulocytes, Hgb, Hct, Platelets, Coagulation Studies

Fluid Imbalance
Protein, Albumin, Na, Urine SG, Osmolality, RBCs, Hgb, Hct, BUN

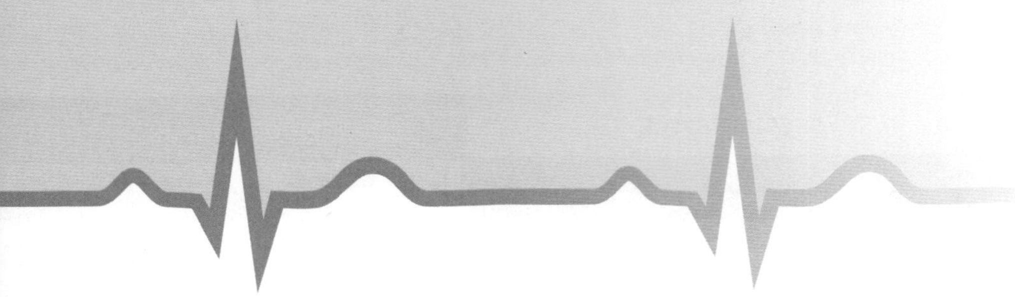

Go To Clinical Cases – Patient Assignments

Chapter 5: Sexuality

Case 1: Pregnancy

Case 2: Postpartum hemorrhage

Chapter 6: Circulation

Case 1: Hypertension

Case 2: Stroke – cerebrovascular accident (CVA)

Chapter 7: Protection

Case 1: Urinary tract infection

Case 2: Influenza

Chapter 8: Homeostasis

Case 1: Overhydration/Fluid Overload

Case 2: Dehydration/Fluid Deficit

Chapter 9: Respiration

Case 1: Asthma

Case 2: Tuberculosis

Chapter 10: Regulation

Case 1: Skin cancers

Case 2: Hyperthermia

Chapter 11: Nutrition

Case 1: Gastroesophageal reflux

Case 2: Constipation

Chapter 12: Hormonal

Case 1: Gestational diabetes

Case 2: Hypothyroidism

Chapter 13: Movement

Case 1: Multiple sclerosis

Case 2: Fractures

Chapter 14: Comfort

Case 1: Pressure ulcers

Case 2: Sleep disorders

Chapter 15: Adaptation

Case 1: Eating Disorders

Case 2: Substance abuse

Chapter 16: Emotions

Case 1: Depression

Case 2: Death and dying

Chapter 17: Cognition

Case 1: Dementia/Alzheimer's disease

Case 2: Autism spectrum disorders (ASD)